Introduction to Communication Disorders

A Lifespan Evidence-Based Perspective

ROBERT E. OWENS, JR.

College of St. Rose

KIMBERLY A. FARINELLA

Northern Arizona University

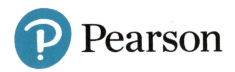

Pearson

Content Development: Brenda Hadenfeldt
Content Management: Bridget Daly
Content Production: Shruti Joshi
Product Management: Drew Bennett
Product Marketing: Krista Clark
Rights and Permissions: Jerrell Forschler

Please contact https://support.pearson.com/getsupport/s/ with any queries on this content

Cover Image by Jasmin Merdan/Getty Images

Library of Congress Cataloging-in-Publication Data

Names: Owens, Robert E., Jr., 1944- author. | Farinella, Kimberly A.,
   author.
Title: Introduction to communication disorders : a lifespan evidence-based
   perspective / Robert E. Owens, Jr., Kimberly A. Farinella.
Description: Seventh edition. | Hoboken, NJ : Pearson, [2024] | Includes
   bibliographical references.
Identifiers: LCCN 2023000060 | ISBN 9780137878925 (paperback) | ISBN
   9780137871902 (paperback)
Subjects: LCSH: Communicative disorders--Textbooks. | Speech
   disorders--Textbooks.
Classification: LCC RC423 .O95 2024 | DDC 616.85/5--dc23/eng/20230214
LC record available at https://lccn.loc.gov/2023000060

3 2023

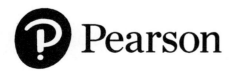

ISBN-10:   0-13-787892-3
ISBN-13: 978-0-13-787892-5

To Our Many Friends with Communication Disorders

Pearson's Commitment to Diversity, Equity, and Inclusion

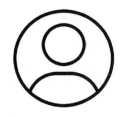

Pearson is dedicated to creating bias-free content that reflects the diversity, depth, and breadth of all learners' lived experiences.

We embrace the many dimensions of diversity, including but not limited to race, ethnicity, gender, sex, sexual orientation, socioeconomic status, ability, age, and religious or political beliefs.

Education is a powerful force for equity and change in our world. It has the potential to deliver opportunities that improve lives and enable economic mobility. As we work with authors to create content for every product and service, we acknowledge our responsibility to demonstrate inclusivity and incorporate diverse scholarship so that everyone can achieve their potential through learning. As the world's leading learning company, we have a duty to help drive change and live up to our purpose to help more people create a better life for themselves and to create a better world.

Our ambition is to purposefully contribute to a world where:

- Everyone has an equitable and lifelong opportunity to succeed through learning.
- Our educational content accurately reflects the histories and lived experiences of the learners we serve.

- Our educational products and services are inclusive and represent the rich diversity of learners.
- Our educational content prompts deeper discussions with students and motivates them to expand their own learning (and worldview).

Accessibility

We are also committed to providing products that are fully accessible to all learners. As per Pearson's guidelines for accessible educational Web media, we test and retest the capabilities of our products against the highest standards for every release, following the WCAG guidelines in developing new products for copyright year 2022 and beyond.

 You can learn more about Pearson's commitment to accessibility at
https://www.pearson.com/us/accessibility.html

Contact Us

While we work hard to present unbiased, fully accessible content, we want to hear from you about any concerns or needs with this Pearson product so that we can investigate and address them.

 Please contact us with concerns about any potential bias at
https://www.pearson.com/report-bias.html

 For accessibility-related issues, such as using assistive technology with Pearson products, alternative text requests, or accessibility documentation, email the Pearson Disability Support team at **disability.support@pearson.com**

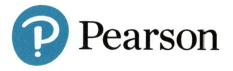

The seventh edition of *Introduction to Communication Disorders: A Lifespan Evidence-Based Perspective* has been a yearlong project of dedication and work. We hope you're pleased with the result. As with previous editions, this one is an exhaustive compilation of hundreds of professional studies conducted by our colleagues in the field.

As the title says, this text is an introduction to the fields of speech-language pathology and audiology. For some of you this will be an eye-opener. You may be surprised by everything these fields encompass and all the various roles and work venues.

Our goal is to educate and inform and also to entice you to want to know more. If you choose to become a speech-language pathologist (SLP) or audiologist, we can promise that there will be many things to learn and skills to master. Coursework will be followed by clinical experiences. Your reward in the end will be a fulfilling and respected career working with other dedicated and knowledgeable professionals.

We stand at a point in history when many aspects of life are changing quickly. Assessment and intervention of communication and swallowing disorders are also changing. By the time you are a licensed SLP or audiologist, new technologies and techniques will have changed the scope of our practice and the ways we interact with clients. Embrace this field and embrace the change. That is where life becomes rewarding.

With each new encounter, we all have the opportunity to change and to grow. Whether you do or not is up to you. Be open to the new experiences at the same time that you hold your beliefs in place.

New to This Edition

A new edition of a text confronts authors with new challenges. One is which content to include and how much. Another is finding a better way to do so than in the previous edition. We hope we've accomplished all those tasks well and that you'll be pleased with this edition.

Professors who have used the text before will notice some new additions and changes in emphasis. These are based on professional feedback, reviewers' comments, student input, and the changing nature of communication disorder services. Here is a partial list of updates and modifications.

- **NEW Case Study Approach.** Each chapter features a case study that is introduced at the beginning of the chapter, carried through the chapter, and revisited at the end of each chapter. In this way, the chapter's academic discussion refers the reader back to an actual client, enlivening the content.

- **NEW Notes from Professionals.** Chapter-opening stories, end-of-chapter Reflections sections, and other quotations from SLPs and audiologists working in the area described in each chapter give the reader a taste of the field from a practitioner's point of view. These additions further humanize the discussion.

- **NEW Sources Throughout.** The text is thoroughly updated with the addition of several hundred new sources. This is the result of nearly as many hours of reading or perusing journal articles.
- **NEW Focus in Chapter 1 on Professional Opportunities and Perspectives.** The emphasis in Chapter 1 has moved from a list of professional requirements to a sampling of all the areas addressed in this field and the opinions and feelings of those working with communication disorders.
- **NEW Topics.** New areas are explored, such as the expanding use of telepractice (Chapter 1) and developmental language disorders (Chapter 4).

As a student, approach this text seriously, acknowledging the range of areas discussed and the diversity found within the individuals being served by SLPs and audiologists and the variation found in those providing those services.

There's a place for you in this field that is attainable with study, hard work, and application. It begins here with this book and your college course. Again, we encourage you to embrace it.

Key Content Updates by Chapter

- **Chapter 1:** Introduces students to the field of speech-language pathology and audiology with expanded examples and testimonials and a totally revamped chapter; explores education and work environments in a more personal manner without overwhelming a reader with details; as is done throughout the text, addresses comments directly to the reader.
- **Chapter 2:** Answers the question "What is a communication disorder?" by comparing typical behavior with not-so-typical behavior; introduces topics such as how we measure communication and how a speech-language pathologist or audiologist decides if a child has a disorder; in broad brushstrokes and with increased emphasis on culture, introduces the areas of communication and swallowing, which are explored in depth in subsequent chapters.
- **Chapter 3:** Incorporates the anatomy and physiology of swallowing; provides greater detail for anatomy and physiology of speech production subsystems with additional figures, photos, and other information; provides a comprehensive case study on the complications that may be encountered with COVID-19 and the short- and long-term effects on swallowing and speech production; provides greater detail on breathing for life plus a brief introduction to mechanical ventilation and the role of the speech-language pathologist in evaluating and treating individuals who may require mechanical ventilation.
- **Chapter 4:** Through new videos and examples, introduces language, typical language development, and language disorders; incorporates the newest terminology such as *developmental language disorder* and *intellectual developmental disorder*; increases emphasis on the bilingual and bidialectal child occurs throughout and with an expanded section on assessment of the language of these children.
- **Chapter 5:** Reduces reliance on knowing/understanding IPA symbols and deleted IPA chart; includes a detailed case study of a bilingual child to

highlight evidence-based practices/procedures in evaluating and treating speech sound disorders in culturally and linguistically diverse populations; provides brief discussion of the importance of highly trained interpreters when assessing/treating multilingual populations; updates research on speech sound acquisition in children across the world; updated information on cerebral palsy; uses more bulleted information to increase readability and highlight key concepts; gives general information about treatment of speech sound disorders in the text, with specific treatment approaches described in the Evidence-Based Practice (EBP) box, reducing redundant information.

- **Chapter 6:** Incorporating the newest research, relates reading and writing disorders to other disorders of speech and language explored in previous chapters; addresses potential causes of reading and writing disorders in the assessment and intervention sections on both.

- **Chapter 7:** After describing the ways in which our brains process language, builds on that base to discuss the various disorders associated with brain injury or disfunction; adds a new differential diagnosis diagram to aid the reader in understanding the different types of aphasia based on a client's behavior, making the discussion less theoretical; bases discussion of assessment and intervention on practical considerations and less on a list of tests or materials; includes new topics such as *primary progressive aphasia*.

- **Chapter 8:** Updates information to reflect current theories and models associated with onset and persistence of stuttering; uses its case study to provide comprehensive information related to assessment of stuttering; provides more general treatment information in the text, with specific evidence-based treatment approaches detailed in the EBP box to reduce redundancy; adds discussion of the importance of counseling, with greater overall focus on the feelings/attitudes of individuals who stutter.

- **Chapter 9:** Uses its case study to provide detailed information on 22q11.2 deletion syndrome and its potential impact on voice and resonance; includes detailed description of the compounding effects of a complex medical history and its impact on all aspects of communication, including a brief review of Chapter 5's assessment and treatment of speech sound disorders; includes the intersection of medical and school-based speech-language pathology practices; provides a greater focus on feelings/attitudes toward communication impairments and the impact on social/educational participation; highlights key concepts more simply in tables, reducing information in text; updates instrumental voice and resonance assessment techniques; explains voice disorder versus voice difference; reorganizes treatment sections; includes a more holistic and sensitive description of gender-affirming care.

- **Chapter 10:** Updates introductory-level discussion of neural structures important for speech motor control with accompanying figures; deletes cerebral palsy (CP) sections with focus on adults with neuromotor impairments in this chapter, with neuromotor impairments in children (e.g., CP) confined to Chapter 5; reduces and simplifies content related to etiologies, with key information highlighted in tables; briefly introduces the construct of communicative participation; adds photos and figures to highlight several management strategies for individuals with dysarthria; briefly introduces interprofessional practice (i.e., combined speech and physical therapy treatment for adult client with neuromotor speech impairment); adds a treatment video highlighting integral stimulation and backward-chaining management techniques for individuals with apraxia of speech.

- **Chapter 11:** Updates and simplifies content pertaining to etiologies, provided in tables instead of text; updates evidence-based content for evaluation and treatment of swallowing disorders across the lifespan; adds photos and videos to highlight several evaluation and treatment techniques for swallowing disorders; defines new terminology pertaining to nonoral feeding options; revisits expiratory muscle training from Chapter 3, demonstrating the interconnection between respiration and swallowing; adds new description of principles related to exercise physiology and their importance in treatment of swallowing disorders.

- **Chapter 12:** Updates information from the literature regarding the associated physical, cognitive, and emotional challenges that accompany hearing loss in adults, including overall impact on general health, mental health, and risk for cognitive decline; expands discussion of the role of the audiologist and related professionals who also serve people who have hearing loss; introduces students to the role of the listening and spoken language therapist; features greater detail and updated literature regarding bone conduction hearing aids, as well as an introduction to over-the-counter aids; updates literature on cochlear implants, including FDA guidelines and benefits for children with cochlear hearing loss as well as for those with auditory neuropathy spectrum disorder (ANSD).

- **Chapter 13:** Updates content to include new research on assessment, intervention, and best practices; dispels myths concerning augmentative and alternative communication (AAC); highlights the importance of collaboration and communication partner training; updates information on new technology; includes information on the process to fund and implement an AAC device; stresses the importance of the individual's ability to interact with others using a multimodal approach that includes the home language and culturally competent service.

Pearson eTextbook, Learning Management System (LMS)–Compatible Assessment Bank, and Other Instructor Resources

Pearson eTextbook

The Pearson eTextbook is a simple-to-use, mobile-optimized, personalized reading experience. It allows you to easily highlight, take notes, and review key vocabulary all in one place—even when offline. Seamlessly integrated videos and other rich media will engage you and give you access to the help you need, when you need it. To gain access or to sign in to your Pearson eTextbook, visit https://www.pearson.com/pearson-etext. Features include:

- **Video Examples** Each chapter includes *Video Examples* that illustrate principles or concepts aligned pedagogically with the chapter. These video clips demonstrate key concepts to further your understanding of chapter material and provide opportunities for you to see expert practitioners working with clients with communication impairments. They are meant to be practical and are for you to enjoy—and, more importantly, for you to take into account and reflect on as part of your education.

- **Interactive Glossary** All key terms in the eTextbook are bolded and provide instant access to the full glossary.

LMS-Compatible Assessment Bank

With this new edition, all assessment types—quizzes, application exercises, and chapter tests—are included in LMS-compatible banks for the following learning management systems: Blackboard, Canvas, D2L, and Moodle. These packaged files allow maximum flexibility to instructors when it comes to importing, assigning, and grading. Assessment types include:

- **Learning Objective Quizzes** Each chapter learning objective is the focus of a Learning Objective Quiz that is available for instructors to assign through their Learning Management System. Learning objectives identify chapter content that is most important for learners and serve as the organizational framework for each chapter. The higher-order, multiple-choice questions in each quiz will measure your understanding of chapter content, guide the expectations for your learning, and inform the accountability and the applications of your new knowledge. Each multiple-choice question includes feedback for the correct answer and for each distractor to help guide students' learning.

- **Application Exercises** Each chapter provides opportunities to apply what you have learned through Application Exercises. These exercises are usually short-answer format and are typically based on a video example in the Pearson eTextbook, or on a written scenario. A model response written by experts is provided to help guide learning.

- **Chapter Tests** Suggested test items are provided for each chapter and include questions in multiple-choice and short-answer/essay formats.

Instructor's Manual

The Instructor's Manual is provided as a Word document and includes resources to assist professors in planning their course.

PowerPoint® Slides

PowerPoint slides are provided for each chapter and highlight key concepts and summarize the content of the text to make it more meaningful for students. Oftentimes, these slides also include questions and problems designed to stimulate discussion and to encourage students to elaborate and deepen their understanding of chapter topics.

Note: All instructor resources—LMS-compatible assessment bank, instructor's manual, and PowerPoint slides—are available for instructor download at www.pearson.com. After searching for your title, be sure you have selected "I'm an educator," then select the "Instructor resources" tab.

About the Authors

Robert E. Owens, Jr., PhD ("Dr. Bob"), is a retired professor at the College of St. Rose in Albany, New York, and a New York State Distinguished Teaching Professor. He holds Honors from the American Speech-Language-Hearing Association and the New York Speech-Language-Hearing Association. Dr. Owens is the author of:

- *Language Development: An Introduction* (10 editions)
- *Language Disorders: A Functional Approach* (7 editions)
- *Early Communication Intervention*
- *Program for the Acquisition of Language with the Severely Impaired (PALS)*
- *Help Your Baby Talk: Introducing the New Shared Communication Method*
- *Queer Kids: The Challenge & Promise for Lesbian, Gay & Bisexual Youth*

Dr. Owens's *Language Development* text is the most widely used in the world and has been translated into Spanish, Korean, Mandarin, and Arabic. His latest project is SUGAR (Sampling Utterance and Grammatical Analysis Revised), a free, valid, easy, quick language sample analysis method that he has coauthored with Stacey Pavelko, PhD. Dr. Owens has presented over 230 professional papers and workshops around the globe. His professional interests are language disorders in infants, toddlers, and preschoolers who are also some of his best friends. And he's a gran'pa!

Kimberly A. Farinella, PhD, CCC-SLP, is a clinical professor in the Department of Communication Sciences and Disorders at Northern Arizona University, where she teaches Motor Speech Disorders at the graduate level and Speech Science at the undergraduate level. She also serves as Clinic Director of the Northern Arizona University Speech-Language-Hearing Clinic and supervises graduate student clinicians with pediatric and adult clients with various speech sound disorders of neurological origin.

Dr. Farinella has presented nationally on the differential diagnosis and treatment of children with severe speech sound disorders. She completed her doctoral training at the University of Arizona and her postdoctoral fellowship in the Division of Speech Pathology in the Department of Neurology at the Mayo Clinic in Rochester, Minnesota. Dr. Farinella's research interests include treatment efficacy for childhood apraxia of speech, interprofessional practice, and the systematic study of the principles of motor learning.

Acknowledgments

No text is written without much-needed help of other people. It seems appropriate at this point to acknowledge that we, the authors, are indebted to many others. We can begin with the pioneers who went before us and for our contemporaries who have brought the field of communication disorders to its present state. Next, we thank the reviewers of this edition; we've tried to heed their sound advice.

In addition, we are indebted to our colleagues David DeBonis and Kelly Fagan for their contributions in authoring the chapters on audiology and on augmentative and alternative communication, respectively. Without their expertise we would have been hard pressed to address these essential areas well.

Robert E. Owens, Jr.

I'm fortunate to have the support of some wonderful people. First, I must acknowledge my colleagues at The College of Saint Rose. My Department of Communication Sciences and Disorders co-chairs, Drs. Dave DeBonis and Jack Pickering, are two perfect examples of leading by example. I'm blessed to co-teach Counseling in Communication Disorders with Jack.

Other incredible colleagues include in alphabetical order Katelynn Carroll, Sarah Coons, Lottie Dunbar, Jessica Evans, Kelly Fagan, Julie Hart, Nathan Holt, Wendy Kolakowski, Zhaleh Lavasani, Dr. Deirdre Muldoon, Grace Paster, Melissa Spring, Lynn Stephens, Dr. Julia Unger, and Victoria Vestal. Somehow through the pandemic, by working together, we managed to fulfill our teaching and supervising mission. What a truly marvelous group of dedicated professionals and all-around warm and wonderful individuals! Our program at The College of St. Rose is exciting, innovative, and dynamic.

My family also deserve special thanks for their understanding and support. This includes my three children, Jason, Todd and his wife Jami, and Jessica, and my grandchildren, The Divine Ms. Cassidy, Dakota, and Zavier.

Over the last several years, I've had the great joy to work closely with Dr. Stacey Pavelko, SUNY Binghamton, in the development of SUGAR (Sampling Utterances and Grammatical Analysis Revised). She's an innovative colleague and tireless worker.

I would also be remiss if I didn't acknowledge the inspiration of my dearest friend, Addie Haas, PhD, a former department chair in Communication Disorders at SUNY New Paltz and previous coauthor of this text. Though we've both aged and our adventures have matured some, she remains my kind, generous, loving friend of over 40 years.

In addition, special thanks and much love to my partner at O and M Education, Moon Byungchoon, for his patience, support, and perseverance. He was of great help with this text, doing work I did not have time to accomplish.

Other dear and supportive friends and colleagues in alphabetic order include Wendy Bower, Katie Guevara, Regina Grantham, Gloria Lopez, Clara Ines Merchan, Cleste Roseberry-McKibbin, Anne Rowley, and Cata, Sergio, Natalia, and Nico Quevedo. If I have forgotten someone, chalk it up to my age, not to my lack of love and caring.

Kimberly A. Farinella

I want to thank the contributors to this newest edition of the textbook. First, I thank Carolyn Abraham, MS, CCC-SLP, a board-certified expert in dysphagia, for her contributions to Chapter 11. I also thank my good friend Margo Zelenski, MS, CCC-SLP, a dysphagia expert from the Mayo Clinic in Scottsdale, Arizona, for her contributions to this chapter as well.

Many thanks to Karina Kadhi, BS, SLPA, for appearing in a photograph in Chapter 8; Steven R. Knight, CRNA APRN, for the medical photographs used in Chapter 9; Nikkol Anderson, MA, OTR/L, ATP, for photographs contributed to Chapter 11; and former Northern Arizona University (NAU) graduate students Sarah Cullimore, Jocilyn Benninger, and Myra Crimmel for their willingness to contribute photos of themselves. I especially want to thank Dr. Ehud Yairi, Dr. Fe' Murray, Sherril Howard, Emily Flores, Myra Crimmel, and Carolyn Abraham for their heartfelt and thoughtful written reflections provided for students throughout the text.

Thank you to my husband who supports me in everything I do. Thank you to Brenda Hadenfeldt, our development editor, who has worked diligently to ensure our vision for this version of the textbook was realized. Finally, I want to thank our patients who were willing to contribute photographs and videos to benefit the educational training of current and future students in the fields of speech-language pathology and audiology.

BRIEF CONTENTS

CONTENTS

1 The Field, the Professionals, and the Clients

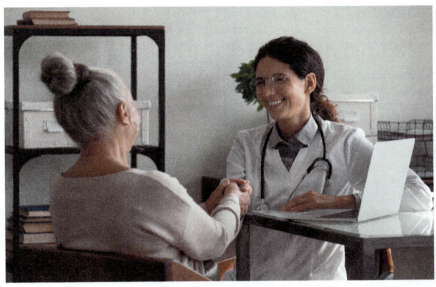

© Fizkes/Shutterstock

Learning Objectives

When you have finished this chapter, you should be able to:

1.1 Describe communication disorders.

1.2 Discuss the roles of audiologists, speech-language pathologists, and speech, language, and hearing scientists.

1.3 Explain how intervention services change through the lifespan.

1.4 Describe how evidence-based practice influences clinical decisions.

1.5 Outline the history of changing attitudes toward individuals with communication disabilities over the centuries and legislation over the past several decades.

> ❝ Being an SLP affords me the opportunity to work with incredible people across the lifespan, to be a valued member of a healthcare team, and to give a voice through other means to those who can't speak. I've been lucky to collaborate with other professionals to make real and meaningful changes for my patients/clients. It's a real privilege to be a speech-language pathologist.
>
> —*A rehabilitation hospital-based speech-language pathologist (SLP)*

Can you imagine life without communication? No talking, no listening, no interacting with others? Communication is part of what makes us human. Even minor or temporary problems with communication, such as temporary laryngitis, are often frustrating. Imagine problems with eating and swallowing. We've all experienced the temporary inconvenience of trying to eat with a sore throat. What would life be like if these problems were more lasting?

CASE STUDY   Mike

Mike was a 16-year-old. We first met in his hospital room. He had Wilson's syndrome a rare genetic disorder in which copper accumulates in the liver, brain, and other organs. Mike's condition had deteriorated to the point where he needed almost continuous care and he was in the hospital awaiting a donor for a liver transplant. Without the surgery he would continue to worsen.

Mike's most visible characteristic was tremors in his body that seemed to be continual. His speech was slurred and difficult to understand. Swallowing was difficult. His short-term memory was also affected.

Through some experimentation and with Mike's patient help, we found that if I held his hand as if we were arm wrestling, his tremors could be somewhat controlled, his speech improved, and swallowing difficulties reduced. I helped Mike eat and we worked

on his speech. At that time speech-language pathologists did little with swallowing but I was encouraged by both his occupational and physical therapists. They offered a few pointers relevant to his condition.

I had to school myself quickly on Wilson's syndrome and we worked diligently, but Mike's doctors weren't hopeful about the ultimate outcome without a transplant. I continued to sit sat on his bed and gripped his hand as we worked. Mike was deteriorating but we worked to hold the speech and swallowing abilities that he had. He was an easy patient who smiled often and laughed easily.

We developed a ritual whenever I had to leave. I'd begin, "Okay, Mike, gotta go; see you when I see you." To which he replied, "Not if I see you first."

Mike is just one of millions of people who face daily communication challenges. We hope through this text to explore these challenges to communication, as well as to feeding and swallowing. In the process, we hope we'll convince you that being a speech-language pathologist (SLP) is a career path for you.

> *This field is phenomenal. . . . I wholeheartedly love the work I do. . . . Going into speech-language pathology comes with great responsibility. As clinicians, we can be generalists, clinical counselors, advocates, and, for our peers, a community. I am humbled to learn that other SLPs in this community are also researchers, software developers, lobbyists, children's book authors, and so much more. It gives me hope to know that I can make a difference in other avenues. It is our responsibility as a field to create safe and equitable environments for our clients, colleagues, and peers. Everyone deserves access to communication.*
>
> —A school-based SLP

In this first chapter, we introduce communication and swallowing disorders and the professionals who work with individuals who have challenges in these areas. These highly trained professionals are called audiologists, speech-language pathologists, or speech/language scientists. We explore their roles and explain the need for evidence-based practice (EBP) and why it's important to intervention. EBP is one of the bases of this text. In addition, this first chapter provides a historical perspective and outlines the laws that mandate appropriate care for those in need. Finally, along the way, we'll explore why people choose these careers.

In the remainder of the text, we begin with some background material so we have a similar understanding of what comes next. We take a **holistic** approach to diagnosis and treatment of people with communicative disorders and examine the sometimes-perplexing contrast between "typical" and "disordered." There are separate chapters that discuss speech characteristics such as voice, fluency, and phonology. We also provide chapters that are organized on the basis of etiology or cause, such as neurogenic and craniofacial disorders. Within each chapter, we examine the interconnectedness of age, time of a disorder's onset, social and cultural factors, and causes of the presenting disorder, and we describe evidence-based assessment and treatment practices. Although our chapter topics may be somewhat arbitrary and we recognize that it's common for an individual to demonstrate difficulties with more than one aspect of communication, we hope that the organization of this text offers you an overall view of this exciting field.

> *Valery has loved baseball for as long as she can remember. She got it from her dad, a devoted Yankees fan. She loves to watch it and talk about it, but most of all she loves playing it. Unfortunately, she now believes because of her head injury in an auto accident that she'll never be able to even express how much she misses it. Even so, today may be momentous. Her SLP, Pam, plans to introduce Valery to an assistive technology device that has a speech generator. Who knows what we'll hear from Valery next?*

Before we go too far, we should make a distinction between four terms, *impairment*, *disability*, *handicap*, and *disorder*. Although simplistic, think of a progression. We begin with **impairment**, a biological or physiological condition that involves the loss of physical, social, or cognitive functioning. This can lead to **disability** or a restriction in ability to perform a function as a result of the impairment. According to the Americans with Disabilities Act of 1990 (ADA), a **disability** is "a physical or mental impairment that substantially limits one or more major life activity." This may or may not lead to a **handicap**, which is a social disadvantage that accrues to the individual with an impairment or disability, often in the form of barriers that can prevent an individual from reaching a goal or a person's potential.

Throughout this text, we use the term *disorder*. For example, we discuss language and voice disorders. The terms *disorder* and *impairment* are often used interchangeably, although there is a subtle difference. While an impairment may involve loss of a function, a **disorder** disrupts that function. I have a visual impairment; I'm farsighted, but with glasses I can read well. If I were blind, reading via the typical means may be disrupted completely. Thus, blindness is considered a disorder. Disorders are a matter of degree. In the next chapter, we discuss to what degree: When is a difference in ability considered a disorder?

Why does someone decide to become a speech-language pathologist or audiologist? It is mostly because of the satisfaction this person receives from helping others to live a fuller life. Many—maybe even you—first became interested through a personal or family encounter with a communication disorder or through work or volunteer experience with individuals having communication difficulties. SLPs and audiologists may also have chosen their careers because they want to be useful to society, to contribute to the general good.

> *I love the variation in this field. I can work in a variety of settings with a variety of clients with different ages and disorders. And the field keeps changing as new disorders are included and new research put forward. I've often surprised myself with the satisfying challenge of exploring other areas of being an SLP.*
>
> —A university-based SLP

Pearson eTextbook
Video Example 1.1

Before you begin, you might want to check out this video on what it means to be a speech-language pathologist.

https://youtu.be/SPgR5DK5PFI

Communication Disorders

Learning Objective 1.1 Describe communication disorders.

We've mentioned communication disorders, but we haven't been very specific. It's always good to agree on our topic in any type of communication, so let's begin here.

A **communication disorder** impairs the ability to both receive and send and also process and comprehend concepts or verbal, nonverbal, and graphic information. A communication disorder may affect hearing, language, and/or speech processes; may range from mild to profound severity; and may be developmental or acquired. One or a combination of communication disorders may be presented by an individual and may result in a primary disability or may be secondary to other disabilities.

That's a lot. In short, a communication disorder may affect any and all aspects of communication, even gesturing. All aspects of communication may be involved: hearing, language (the code we use to communicate), and/or speech (our primary mode or manner of communication). This is reflected in the American Speech-

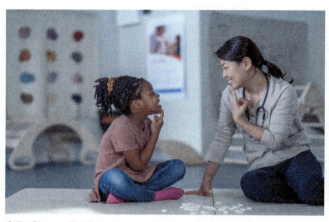

© FatCamera/E+/Getty Images

Language-Hearing Association's (ASHA) name. (The Appendix describes ASHA's professional role in more detail.) Currently, ASHA has 223,000 members and affiliates who are audiologists; speech-language pathologists; speech, language, and hearing scientists; audiology and speech-language pathology support personnel; and students. (ASHA, n.d.).

Although we work primarily with people having communication disorders, SLPs are not limited to just speech and language. As mentioned, SLPs are involved in feeding and swallowing disorders and nonspeech (called *nonverbal*) forms of communication. Similarly, audiologists are involved in more than testing hearing.

Ken was in his early 50s when he first became aware of a slight muscle twitch in his hands. He was driving a long distance and attributed the muscle spasm to fatigue. It reoccurred periodically. When it became more consistent, he sought medical advice and was informed after several tests that he had Parkinson disease. In the later stages of Parkinson, Ken decided to retire and his home care became a family responsibility. In addition to speech difficulties, he developed the dementia that sometimes accompanies Parkinson. This, in turn, affected his language and finally reduced him to single-word responses. Eating and swallowing became challenging. A proud man, Ken refused certain therapeutic interventions. As he deteriorated, he never lost his sense of humor, even as walking, balance and speech, language, and swallowing became more difficult. Luckily, he had a team of specialists, including his SLP.

A **speech disorder** may be evident in the atypical production of speech sounds, interruption in the flow of speaking, or abnormal production and/or absences of voice quality, including pitch, loudness, resonance, and/or duration. For example, if you've had laryngitis your voice was temporarily affected. A **language disorder**, in contrast, is an impairment in comprehension and/or use of spoken, written, and/or other symbol systems, such as English. Finally, a **hearing disorder** is a result of impaired sensitivity of the auditory or hearing system. No doubt you've heard individuals referred to as having deafness or difficulty hearing. In addition, auditory disorders may include **central auditory processing disorders**, or deficits in the processing of information from audible signals. It's important to note here that SLPs may also be part of a team working with cognitive or brain functioning.

> *I love knowing that despite all the challenges we are helping clients have more fulfilling lives.*
>
> —An audiologist in a rehabilitation facility

It's appropriate to note that communication disorders do not include communication differences, such as dialectal differences or speaking another language. In the United States, we all speak a dialect of American English that sometimes makes it difficult to communicate with one another. If you've been to a country where you don't speak the language well, you know that this definitely can impede communication. While these differences may lead to communication difficulties, they are simply differences, not disorders, and cannot be treated by SLPs as if they are.

Another communication variation is the use of **augmentative/alternative communication** systems. Far from being a communication disorder, these systems, whether signing or the use of digital methods, are attempts often taught by SLPs to compensate and facilitate, on a temporary or permanent basis, for impaired or disabled communication disorders.

We would be remiss if we didn't at least note that an SLP's responsibility also extends to feeding and swallowing disorders. These vary from the preterm infant with a weak sucking response to the adult patient recovering from a stroke and slowly regaining the motor control needed to chew and swallow easily.

Some SLPs work with those who do not have disorders but seek services to modify and/or protect their voice or to help them strengthen their English. These clients would include professional singers and acters, transgender voice clients, and those who speak other languages.

> *Dominique, a professional singer, began to notice "a scratchiness in my throat." It became more persistent. She cancelled a few performances to give her voice a rest. Finally, she scheduled an appointment with an ear, noise, and throat doctor or ENT, who diagnosed early-stage polyps or growths on her vocal folds. Located in your larynx, your vocal folds are tissue that vibrate to help you make sounds. The ENT recommended therapy with an SLP. Dominique is now enjoying her vocation again and performing in regional theater. She's using her voice in an efficient way that does not abuse it and lead to polyps. Potential disorder was averted.*

Prevention of communication disorders is also a portion of what some SLPs and audiologists do. For example, audiologists help government agencies, the military, and industry with sound abatement to protect hearing. Children and adults may also be counseled on voice abuse to forestall disorders later.

As you can see, communication and feeding and swallowing disorders cover a wide range of challenges with varying severities that can be related to several other disorders. Assessment and intervention may involve a team of professionals. Our purpose in preparing this text is to help you understand and appreciate the many varied disorders that fall within the scope of practice of the SLP and audiologist.

Pearson eTextbook
Video Example 1.2

In this video from the American Speech-Language-Hearing Association, you learn about becoming an audiologist or speech-language pathologist.
www.youtube.com/
watch?v=_OIcPbndZMo

Maybe a few pages ago you had some vague recollection of an SLP in your elementary school who worked with children correcting their production of difficult speech sounds. That's part of disordered communication, but it's only a small part, as you are about to find out.

The Professionals and Their Roles

Learning Objective 1.2 Discuss the roles of audiologists, speech-language pathologists, and speech, language, and hearing scientists.

Today, professionals who serve individuals with communication disorders come from several disciplines. They often refer clients to one another or work together in teams to provide optimal care. Depending on the disorder and the cause, a team may consist of physicians, neurologists, psychologists, physical and occupational therapists, teachers, audiologists, and speech-language pathologists.

> *Marie is in her 90s. An independent woman, she lived alone and socialized with friends until she fell, broke her hip, and struck her head, resulting in a traumatic brain injury. Eight months later she walks about a mile a day with the help of a walker and receives speech and language services for motor-speech and language difficulties. Marie enjoys going to therapy in a group program based on a projects approach in which she decides on a goal, such as teaching a Bible lesson in her church and works on it diligently. She also enjoys the interest groups and discussions run by her SLP. She is free to go to whichever groups she wishes and is currently in the political and gardening discussions.*

Opportunities for SLPs and audiologists include serving individuals of all ages, from infants to older adults, with varied disorders, from mild to profound, in a wide assortment of settings.

Audiologists and SLPs are employed in early intervention programs with infants and toddlers, in preschools, schools, colleges and universities, hospitals, independent clinics, nursing care facilities, rehabilitation programs, nursing homes, research laboratories, and home-based programs. Many are in private practice. Although it is still evolving, **telepractice**—provision of speech and language assessment and intervention via the Internet—is slowly expanding, especially in underserved geographical areas (Waite et al., 2010). The COVID pandemic caused a shift to telepractice in many areas of service. Let's discuss audiologists, speech-language pathologists, and speech, language, and hearing scientists.

Audiologists

Audiologists are specialists who measure hearing ability and identify, assess, manage, and prevent disorders of hearing and balance. They use a variety of technologies to measure and appraise hearing in people from infancy through old age.

Although they work in educational settings to improve communication and programming for people with hearing disabilities, audiologists also contribute to the prevention of hearing loss by recommending and fitting protective devices and by consulting with government and industry on the detrimental effects and management of environmental noise. In addition, audiologists evaluate and assist individuals with **auditory processing disorders (APD)**, sometimes called central auditory processing disorders. They also select, fit, and dispense hearing aids and other amplification devices and provide guidance in their care and use (DeBonis & Moncrieff, 2008).

Licensed audiologists are independent professionals who practice without a prescription from another health care provider (ASHA, 2001b). Box 1.1 contains an audiologist's comments on some of the challenges and rewards of the profession. As you will note, being a good detective, or problem solver, is one of the skills that is needed. Websites of interest are found at the end of the chapter.

Credentials for Audiologists

At the present time, the educational requirement for an audiologist is 3 to 5 years of professional education beyond the bachelor's degree. An audiologist's studies will culminate in a doctoral degree that may be an audiology doctorate (AuD) or a doctor of philosophy (PhD) or doctor of education (EdD) degree in audiology.

After a person has earned a doctorate, obtained the required preprofessional as well as paid clinical experience, and passed a national examination, they are eligible for the Certificate of Clinical Competence in Audiology (CCC-A) awarded by ASHA. The ASHA CCC-A (sometimes referred to as ASHA "Cs") is the generally accepted standard for most employment opportunities for audiologists in the United States. In addition, states require audiologists to obtain a state license. The requirements for state licensure tend to be the same as or similar to the ASHA standards (ASHA, 2020a).

Jermain was born 1-month preterm and failed his neonatal or newborn hearing screening. He also failed to pass a second hearing screening 6 weeks later. His mother was especially concerned and desperate to know what to do. The audiologist introduced her to a colleague who was an SLP working in early intervention. After evaluation by a team that included a pediatrician, an audiologist, an early childhood specialist, and an SLP, Jermain was enrolled in an early intervention program. The SLP comes to his home twice weekly and collaborates with his mother and sisters to further his communication. Jermain signed "Eat," his first word, when he was 8 months old. Currently, at 13 months of age, he is developing typically, signs eight words, and is awaiting funding for a cochlear implant. He is tested regularly by the audiologist to confirm his eligibility and to advise the team on further developmental considerations.

Pearson eTextbook
Video Example 1.3
Before you read any further about rewarding careers in audiology and in working with children with hearing disorders, you might want to check out this video from the Oregon Speech-Language & Hearing Association.
www.youtube.com/ watch?v=3qq9CaMsJe4

BOX 1.1   **An Audiologist Reflects**

I chose to become an audiologist because I enjoyed the challenge. Most clients come in and are frightened or apprehensive. I try to set them at ease while I explain each test I will perform. At each step, I try to bring the client along and make sure that they understand what I will be doing and why. Children are often the biggest challenge and sometimes refuse to cooperate. This is when I have to be at my best.

If I confirm the presence of a hearing loss, then my task becomes one of counseling and referral. It takes time to walk a client through the results and the possibilities. Older clients are often not willing initially to accept a diagnosis of hearing loss.

Counseling is very important, especially for family members. It is all too easy for family members to adopt an "I told you so" attitude, but we must be sensitive to the needs of the client with the loss who will need time to adjust to their now-diagnosed disorder. It is this detective work and the counseling that give me satisfaction and motivate me to come to work every day.

Pearson eTextbook
Video Example 1.4

Before you read about SLPs, we suggest watching these testimonials from the Oregon Speech-Language & Hearing Association.

www.youtube.com/
watch?v=3BlfadNmUF0

You can further explore a career in audiology at three websites. The Acoustical Society of America (www.acousticalsociety.org) has materials of special interest to hearing scientists and audiologists. The American Academy of Audiology (www.audiology.org) provides consumer and professional information regarding hearing and balance disorders as well as audiological services. Finally, ASHA (www.asha.org) provides information for professionals, students, and others who are interested in careers in audiology or hearing science. Simply select "Careers" in the upper-left corner of the website.

Speech-Language Pathologists

Speech-language pathologists (SLPs) are professionals who provide an assortment of services related to communication disorders. The distinguishing role of an SLP is to identify, assess, treat, and prevent communication disorders in all modalities (including spoken, written, pictorial, and manual), both receptively and expressively. This includes attention to physiological, cognitive, and social aspects of communication. SLPs also provide services for disorders of swallowing and may work with individuals who elect to receive services as mentioned previously.

> *The thing I love most about being a speech-language pathologist is empowering families through caregiver coaching. . . . I love when we get to the point in therapy when caregivers realize they don't have to have the latest and greatest toys in order to inspire change and progres. . . . [T]hey look at their recycling bins in a whole new light and that brings me great joy.*
>
> —An early-intervention SLP

Like audiologists, licensed SLPs are independent professionals who practice without a prescription from another health care provider (ASHA, 2020b). Box 1.2 contains reflections by an SLP who believes in setting his imagination free and not giving up in the challenge to help others.

Some states employ **speech-language pathology assistants** (SLPAs) in the schools. These professionals can administer tests and therapy under an SLP's direction but cannot diagnose a disorder or provide intervention independently. SLPAs usually have a bachelor's degree in communication sciences and disorders from an ASHA-certified SLP program.

BOX 1.2   A Speech-Language Pathologist Reflects

For me, the exciting part of my job is the problem solving and the satisfaction of helping others. Similar to a fictional detective who collects all the clues, synthesizes the information, and deduces the guilty party, I evaluate each client and determine the best course of intervention. The more severe the impairment, the greater the challenge, and I love a challenge. How can I help a young man who attempted suicide and is now brain injured to access the language within him? How can a young child with autism begin the road through communication to language? How can I help parents communicate with their infant who has deafness, blindness, and cerebral palsy? When is the best time to introduce signing with a nonspeaking client? These are all challenges for me and the children and adults I serve. We work together as I try to solve each communication puzzle and propose and implement possible intervention strategies. Sometimes I'm very successful and sometimes I have to reevaluate my methods, but as I said, I love a challenge.

Credentials for Speech-Language Pathologists

Even with technology, the task of an SLP can be changing. Technologies for digital speech recording and analysis are now readily available, as are new and exciting assistive technologies for those with great difficulty communicating via speech (Ingram et al., 2004). Computers and computer programs alone are not enough. Accurate assessment and successful intervention rest on the knowledge, experience, and expertise of the SLP.

> *Ron has struggled to speak from about age 3. At that time, he began to repeat words and to halt before saying some words, as if they were stuck in his throat. His parents became concerned and sought professional help. Now in fifth grade, Ron sees an SLP at school who is working with him to ease the onset of words. His speech is characterized by some fear in specific situations, although he socializes easily with peers who seem to ignore his dysfluencies, which are primarily characterized by repetition of initial sounds in some words. The SLP has helped Ron identify situations and sounds that are especially challenging and they are working diligently to modify his speech as much as possible prior to middle school.*

SLPs have a master's or doctoral degree and have studied typical communication and swallowing development; anatomy and physiology of the speech, swallowing, and hearing mechanisms; phonetics; speech and hearing science; and disorders of speech, language, and swallowing.

ASHA issues a Certificate of Clinical Competence in Speech-Language Pathology (CCC-SLP) to an individual who has obtained a master's degree or doctorate in the field, completed a monitored clinical fellowship year, and successfully passed a national qualifying examination. Ongoing professional development must be demonstrated through a variety of continuing education options. Since 2004, the United States, the United Kingdom, Australia, and Canada have allowed mutual recognition of certification in speech-language pathology (Boswell, 2004). The ASHA website lists the credentials that are needed in the professions of both audiology and speech-language pathology.

Individual states have licensure laws for SLPs. A license may be needed if you plan to engage in private practice or work in a hospital, clinic, public school, or other setting. Most states accept a person with an ASHA CCC-SLP as having met licensure requirements, although you will need to check with your state licensing board on the specifics.

> *I love the moment when I get to sit back and just watch my clients doing the thing that was once so hard for them. There's that pause followed by a glimmer in their eye when they realize, "I'm doing it!"*
>
> —A former school-based SLP, now teaching at a university

REFLECTION QUESTION 1.1

Were you surprised by the scope of possible intervention for SLPs and audiologists? Did you begin reading thinking only of speech and hearing? What surprised you the most, and why?

If you want to further explore a career in speech-language pathology, check out the ASHA website (www.asha.org). You'll find a wealth of information, as well

Pearson eTextbook

Video Example 1.5

Why choose a career in speech-language pathology or audiology?

www.hearingandspeechcareers .org/?_ga=2.174918695 .426052360.1656512710- 1066178008.1594126986

as discussion of various disorders that affect children and adults who may benefit from the help of a SLP. Type in the disorder you wish to explore in the search box in the upper right of the website. If you wish to read about a career as a SLP, select "Careers" at the top left of the website.

Speech, Language, and Hearing Scientists

Individuals who are employed as speech, language, or hearing scientists typically have earned a doctorate degree, either a PhD or an EdD. They are employed by universities, government agencies, industry, and research centers to extend our knowledge of human communication processes and disorders. Some may also serve as clinical SLPs or audiologists.

What Speech, Language, and Hearing Scientists Do

The professions of speech-language pathology and audiology require lifelong learning. Clinicians need to be able to intelligently use relevant research findings in their practice.

Speech scientists may be involved in basic research exploring the anatomy, physiology, and physics of speech-sound production. Using various technologies, these researchers strive to learn more about typical and pathological communication. Their findings help clinicians improve service to clients with speech disorders. Recent advances in knowledge of human genetics provide fertile soil for continuing investigation into the causes, prevention, and treatment of various speech impairments. Some speech scientists are involved in the development of computer-generated speech that may be used as a substitute or compliment for individuals who are unable to speak or speak only with great difficulty. Box 1.3 contains some observations by a speech-language scientist who enjoys the interdisciplinary nature of his work.

Language scientists may investigate the ways in which children learn their native tongue. They may study the differences and similarities of different languages. Over the past half-century or so, the United States has become increasingly linguistically and culturally diverse; this provides an excellent opportunity for cross-cultural study of language and communication. Some language scientists explore the variations of modern-day English (dialects) and how the language is changing. Others are concerned with language disabilities and study the nature of language disorders in children and adults. An in-depth knowledge of typical language is critical to understanding language problems.

Tami was diagnosed with severe cerebral palsy (CP) shortly after birth. Although she had many of the reflexive behaviors of a typically developing child, these behaviors continued for a longer period. Otherwise, she appeared to be floppy and to have poor muscle tone. As she matured during the first year, her CP became apparent. Tami was a bright child and her learning and interaction seemed only limited by her poor motor control.

BOX 1.3   A Speech-Language Scientist Reflects

I work as a speech scientist and college professor specializing in voice science. In this profession I'm able to combine my love of communication with my interest in biology. As a student I hadn't realized the possibilities that would be open to me in this profession. I instruct students in the structure and functioning of the speech mechanism and in voice disorders. In the clinic, I use instrumentation to measure different parameters of voice. This enables me to objectify my diagnosis and provide accurate measurement of speech changes that may result from any number of disorders as varied as laryngeal cancer and neuromuscular dysfunction. I also work with transgender clients, helping them adopt a new voice. I love my work because it combines science and technology with speech-language pathology.

She learned to recognize spoken words early but was extremely limited in the sounds she could produce. Within the first year, Tami's SLP suggested to her parents that they continue with motor speech intervention but also introduce an assistive communication device. Initially, the device consisted of a simple switch that activated a single prerecorded message.

Hearing scientists investigate the nature of sound, noise, and hearing. They may work with other scientists in the development of equipment to be used in the assessment of hearing. They are also involved in the development of techniques for testing the hard-to-test, such as infants and those with severe physical or psychological impairments. Hearing scientists develop and improve assistive listening devices such as hearing aids and telephone amplifiers to help people who have limited hearing. In addition, they are concerned with conservation of hearing and are engaged in research to measure and limit the impact of environmental noise.

Related Professions: A Team Approach

Specialists in communication disorders do not operate in a vacuum. They work closely with family members, regular and special educators, psychologists, social workers, doctors and other medical personnel, and occupational, physical, and music therapists. They may collaborate with physicists and engineers. Box 1.4 shows an SLP's typical schedule, showing a tremendous amount of teamwork.

BOX 1.4   A Team Approach

Alicia is the senior speech-language pathologist in a community-based rehabilitation center in New York State. During the mornings, Alicia works with infants, preschoolers, and school-age children at the center. In the afternoons, she directs the Augmentative/Alternative Communication Program and assists severely impaired individuals of all ages to improve their communication abilities. The schedule outlined below has a bit more collaboration than is normally found in any one day, but it suggests the kinds of activities that are typical within a workweek.

8:30 a.m. — Education staff meeting for preschool children: classroom teacher, psychologist, social worker, occupational therapist, physical therapist

9:00 — Preschool class activity: eight children age 3–4, one classroom teacher, two aides

10:00 — Individual half-hour therapy sessions with children in the preschool and school programs

11:30 — Combined physical and speech therapy for Jeramy, age 4, diagnosed with spastic cerebral palsy; work with physical therapist

noon — Lunch

12:30 p.m. — Prepare for the afternoon

1:00 — Consult with engineer on wheelchair switch for Lucretia, age 7, who has multiple disabilities

1:30 — Outpatient, David, age 24, had been in a motorcycle accident and experiences some speech and language difficulties

3:00 — Conference with Bettina, Bettina's foster mother, and Barbara Sloane, the social worker for the family

3:30 — Communication Disorders Department meeting; Malcolm, an audiologist, reports on a 3-hour course he took on Saturday on cochlear implants. Group will discuss who will give a brief summary of the articles of interest in the latest issue of the professional journal *Language, Speech, and Hearing Services in the Schools* at the next meeting.

Service Through the Lifespan

Learning Objective 1.3 Explain how intervention services change through the lifespan.

This text is organized on the basis of two aspects of communication disorders that are important for your understanding, service throughout the lifespan and evidence-based practice. Before we move on, let's discuss each one briefly and why it's important.

Individuals with communication and swallowing disorders may be of any age, and SLPs and audiologists address their needs from birth through old age. According to U.S. government data, 1 in 7 people has a disability. This percentage translates into over 44 million people in the United States (Institute on Disability, 2021). These figures do not include the many millions of individuals with chronic health issues who may also be in need of communications disorder services (Boersma et al., 2020). In general, the likelihood of having a disability or chronic health issue increases as we age.

CASE STUDY   **Mike** *(continued)*

Mike, mentioned at the beginning of the chapter, is one of many individuals you will meet throughout this text. Each chapter features a case study like Mike's, demonstrating the many ways that SLPs and other professionals make a difference for people across the lifespan.

Although the exact number of individuals in the United States who have communication disorders is difficult to determine (ASHA, 2008), they are in the millions. For example, each year nearly 1 in 12 or 7.7% of American children age 3–17 has a disorder related to voice, speech, language, or swallowing (Black et al., 2016). That percentage translates into nearly 6 million children who may be in need of communication intervention services. Additionally, 1 in 25 people will experience some form of dysphagia or swallowing disorder during their lifetime, including 22% of those over age 50 (ASHA, 2008; Bhattacharyya, 2014).

The U.S. Census Bureau reports that about 2% of all children born in the United States have some existing disabling condition and that hearing loss occurs more often than any other physical problem (Brault, 2005). All infants in the United States must be screened for hearing loss. Babies and toddlers may also exhibit developmental delay and have physical problems, including those involving movement, hearing, and vision, that may impact their communication and feeding abilities.

Pearson eTextbook
Video Example 1.6

Our clients. It's all about them. In this video is an honest discussion about how it feels to work in the field of speech-language pathology.

https://youtu.be/ma7yFjNv5OU

An interdisciplinary approach is necessary in the assessment and treatment of very young children and an individualized family service plan (IFSP) is developed for each child treated. Such plans address the needs of the entire family, with sensitivity to that family's language and culture. Early identification and intervention has been demonstrated to be highly valuable in facilitating optimum results and potentially preventing later difficulties. Some children will be diagnosed later as having developmental difficulties not evident at birth.

Preschoolers with communication difficulties must also be identified and helped. For some, services begun earlier may now be handled by different agencies. The youngster may be placed in a special preschool, and professionals may continue to assist the family in addressing the child's needs.

John had worked in construction nearly his entire adult life. Although his wife worked in a local market after her children were grown, John had always been considered to be the head of the household and the family breadwinner. Needless to say, it was a shock when he experienced a massive stroke at age 47. He experienced difficulty with the motor aspects of speech, with language production and comprehension, and with swallowing. As soon as his condition stabilized, the hospital SLP made a bedside evaluation. The SLP shared his findings with both John and the family. John was facing a lengthy rehabilitation. Naturally, the family had concerns and John's SLP tried to answer their questions, counsel them, and refer them to other agencies and professionals. After approximately a week in intensive care, he was released to a rehabilitation hospital and into the care of another SLP.

Almost half of all SLPs are employed by school systems. They work with youngsters in all grades, addressing a full range of communication and swallowing problems. These are described in the chapters that follow. School-age children with communication difficulties often experience academic and social difficulties, which add additional urgency to the work of communication experts. Some young adults, such as those who were identified earlier as being developmentally delayed or with physical disabilities, may continue to receive services until they are 21 years old.

> **REFLECTION QUESTION 1.2**
>
> *As you think about intervention across the lifespan and working as a member of a team, think about variations in this arrangement. Are there ages of clients or severities of disorders in which you as an SLP might work alone with a client, times when you might consult with other specialists, and still other times when you might serve as a member of a team?*

Other individuals may find themselves in need of communication services for the first time later in life. For example, between 1.5 and 2 million Americans sustain traumatic brain injury each year in the United States (see Chapters 4 and 7) stemming from bicycle, motorcycle, or motor vehicle accidents; falls; or firearms. As a result, they may have cognitive and/or motor problems that interfere with their ability to communicate and/or eat. The SLP plays an important role in rehabilitative efforts.

Although almost anyone can experience aphasia, or the inability to produce and comprehend language, usually as the result of a stroke or other neurological condition that may impair motor and cognitive abilities, most individuals with aphasia are middle age or older. Almost 180,000 Americans acquire this disorder annually; approximately 2 million individuals currently live with the disorder (National Aphasia Association, n.d.)

Among those over age 65, stroke, neurological disorders, and cognitive impairments may interfere with effective communication and swallowing. Hearing loss may affect at least one-quarter of people in this age group, creating a need for assessment and treatment. For example, 8.5% of those over age 55 have disabling hearing loss in both ears. This percentage increases to 25% of those between 65 and 74 years of age and 50% of those above age 75 (National Institute on Deafness and Other Communication Disorders, 2021).

SLPs and audiologists work directly with individuals with communication disorders. They often also work with parents and teachers and with spouses and children of adult clients. In addition, SLPs and audiologists collaborate with other health care professionals as well as staff members of nursing homes and other adult facilities. Along with direct service for communication disorders, SLPs and audiologists provide counseling and guidance directed toward improving quality of life, especially in the later years (Lubinski & Masters, 2001).

> After contracting meningitis as a camp counselor, Natalia experienced motor difficulties that affected her speech and swallowing. Although, thanks to her age, she seemed to recover relatively quickly, she benefited greatly from the intervention of her SLP. Within 6 months, Natalia was back in college with only minor problems in the higher cognitive functions required for abstract thought and language. She continued to see her SLP on an outpatient basis for the rest of the year.

SLPs and audiologists work in the neonatal intensive care unit and in nursing homes for seniors and anywhere in between where individuals with communication disorders live or attend school. Clinical intervention may be short term or long term, continuous or intermittent, in-home or outpatient, in-person or via telehealth—almost any configuration you can imagine. In addition, assessment and intervention of a broad variety of communication and swallowing disorders are usually accomplished in collaboration with other health care and/or educational professionals. That said, SLPs and audiologists are independent professionals, free to exercise their professional judgment and expertise.

Evidence-Based Practice

Learning Objective 1.4 Describe how evidence-based practice influences clinical decisions.

As in other professions, SLPs and audiologists use evidence-based practice to provide the best services possible.

Throughout this text, we try to report the best information we can, based on the research evidence available. As an SLP or audiologist (if either is your career choice), it will be your responsibility to provide the best and most well-grounded research-based intervention that is humanly possible. In other words, you should do what has been proven to work best and to be most effective.

Deciding on the most efficacious intervention is a portion of something called **evidence-based practice (EBP)**. EBP is an essential part of effective and ethical intervention. The primary benefit is the delivery of optimally effective care to each client (Brackenbury et al., 2008).

In EBP, decision making is informed by a combination of scientific evidence, clinical experience, and client needs. EBP is based on two assumptions (Bernstein Ratner, 2006):

- Clinical skills grow not just from experience but from the currently available data.
- An expert SLP or audiologist continually seeks new therapeutic information to improve efficacy.

Professional journals, called peer-reviewed journals, in which each manuscript is critiqued by other experts in the field and accepted or rejected on the basis of the quality of the research, are the best sources of clinical research-based evidence. Simply put, research, specifically the portion of research directly relevant to decisions about clinical practice, is combined with reason when making decisions about treatment approaches (Dollaghan, 2004).

Ideally, for each of us, EBP is a work in progress with updates as we learn more. New information may come to light through research that changes previous assumptions about that evidence. None of this relieves SLPs and audiologists of the responsibility to provide the best, most efficacious assessment and intervention possible. See the ASHA online resource at the end of the chapter.

In this discussion, we've used two terms: *efficacy* and *effectiveness*. These are sometimes difficult to discern, so it's important that you understand the generally accepted meanings of these terms from a clinical and research perspective. Technically, **efficacy** as it relates to clinical outcomes is the probability of benefit from an intervention method under ideal conditions (Office of Technology Assessment, 1978). There are three key elements to this definition:

- It refers to an identified population, such as adults with global aphasia, not to individuals.
- The treatment protocol should be focused, and the population should be clearly identified.
- The research should be conducted under optimal intervention conditions (Robey & Schultz, 1998). Of course, results in real-life clinical situations may differ somewhat.

Of interest is the therapeutic effect or the positive benefits resulting from treatment. The ideal treatment, then, would seem to be the one that results in the largest changes to meaningful client outcomes, with only limited variability across clients (Johnson, 2006).

SLPs are tasked with determining which treatment approach is best for each client. It is also important for SLPs to recognize that efficacy is never an all-or-nothing proposition (Law et al., 2004; Rescorla, 2005).

Lingyun was identified as having a language disorder in preschool. His family was initially reluctant to accept this diagnosis and blamed it on his bilingual upbringing and on cultural misunderstanding by his preschool SLP. Luckily, the SLP was knowledgeable about multilingual development and reassured his parents and grandparents. By working with the family and being sensitive to their concerns, the SLP gained the family's trust. She convinced them that many children have difficulty with language initially and that there was no stigma attached to being in speech and language therapy. After approximately a year and a half receiving speech and language services, Lingyun is now a happy, precocious, well-adjusted second-grader with no language disorder.

Effectiveness is the probability of benefit from an intervention method under average conditions (Office of Technology Assessment, 1978). The effectiveness of treatment is the outcome of the real-world application of the treatment for individual clients or subgroups. In short, effectiveness is a measure of "what works." Valid clinical studies must be realistically evaluated for the feasibility of applying them to intervention with specific populations and individuals (Guyatt & Rennie, 2002).

One way of determining potential effectiveness, but not the only one, may be a clinical approach's reported **efficiency** (Kamhi, 2006a). Efficiency results from application of the quickest method involving the least effort and the greatest positive benefit, including unintended effects. For example, an unintended benefit of working to correct difficult speech sounds is that it improves the production of untreated easier sounds, although the reverse is not true (Miccio & Ingrisano, 2000). Targeting more difficult sounds would seem to be more efficient.

As mentioned, other factors in decision making include the clinician's expertise and experience, client values, and service delivery variables. In addition to clinical experience and expertise, individual SLP factors such as attitude and motivation are important. Clients vary widely and respond differently to intervention based on each client's unique characteristics, such as family history and support, age, hearing ability, speech and language reception and production, cognitive abilities, and psychosocial traits, such as motivation. Finally, service delivery factors include the targets and methods selected, the treatment setting, participants, and the schedule of intervention.

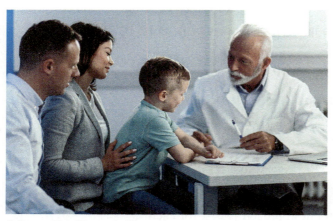

© Drazen Zigic/Shutterstock

An SLP or audiologist must carefully discuss possible intervention options with a client and/or family, including an explanation of the research evidence. The goal is to provide sufficient information to enable the client and/or family to make an informed choice or to collaboratively plan and refine the options to suit the client and/or family preferences.

Making good clinical decisions is not always easy. High-quality evidence-based research must be evaluated critically by each SLP and applied to specific clients with specific communication disorders. EBP requires the judicious integration of scientific evidence into clinical decision making (Johnson, 2006). Although EBP can improve and validate clinical services, we must acknowledge that some research can be difficult to incorporate into everyday clinical settings because of the time required for SLPs to comb through relevant research. In addition, evidence may be limited, contradictory, or nonexistent (Brackenbury et al., 2008). In the last analysis, however, the necessity of providing the best intervention services possible must be the foremost professional concern.

Some help comes in the form of **meta-analysis**. In studies employing meta-analysis, research on a topic is ranked according to the strength of the data and then examined to see the statistical trends. If strong studies show that an assessment or intervention method is effective, then other studies are examined to see if they support this finding. In this way, SLPs and audiologists are provided with information on the most effective and efficient findings from a variety of sources.

Michele is a college student and a transgender female. She knew early in her life that she was a girl but was punished by her parents for dressing as a girl and playing with "girl" toys. When she came to college, she presented as male and had close-cut hair. Michele "punked" her hair and dressed gender-neutral for her first year. Her appearance attracted other individuals who were transitioning. Luckily, in her second year, she was able to rent an apartment with these friends. Michele attends the university's

*transgender voice program, a group run by the Communication Science and Disorders
department. There she works on efficient use of her voice and socializes with other
transgender clients of all ages. Every session has a confidence-building component along
with voice therapy. Although not confident enough to tell her parents, Michele is more
secure in herself and feels supported by the staff and by other clients.*

You can explore EBP further at two websites. The ASHA site (www.asha.org)
describes EBP and offers guidance for clinical practice. Select "Practice Management" to find the "Practice Portal" which will take you to a choice of disorders you
may wish to explore. The National Institute on Deafness and Other Communication Disorders (NIDCD) site (www.nidcd.nih.gov) contains relevant health and
research information. Just type the disorder in the search box in the upper right
of the website.

*These students want us to be creative, and want us to be resourceful, and want us to be
able to change really quickly and come up with something fun. They really, at the end
of the day, just want to be loved.*

—A school-based SLP

Communication Disorders in Historical Perspective

Learning Objective 1.5 Outline the history of changing attitudes toward individuals
with communication disabilities over the centuries and legislation over the past several
decades.

For students, it's easy to think that services for those with disorders of all types were
always readily available. This is not the case. Even in the United States, rights for
those with disabilities or chronic health issues are a relatively recent phenomenon
that has not reached full fruition. As an SLP, you'll find that advocating for your
clients and for others with disorders is a constant challenge. Sadly, many admin-
istrative bodies still see services for those with disabilities as an area of the budget
ripe for budget cuts.

It is believed that many early human groups shunned less able individuals.
They sometimes abandoned children who were malformed or who had obvious
physical disabilities. Some but not all groups also abandoned, deprived of food, or
even killed aged people who could no longer contribute. There is also archaeologi-
cal data to suggest that in some early cultures those with physical disabilities were
sometimes considered to have special powers and were treated accordingly.

Over the centuries, attitudes have changed. By the late 1700s to early 1800s
in some parts of the world, societal efforts were being made to help those who
were unable to care for themselves. Individuals began to be classified and grouped
according to their disorder. Special residences for individuals with deafness, blindness, mental illness, and intellectual limitations were established, although most
were little more than warehouses providing no services other than what was necessary to keep the residents alive (Karagiannis et al., 1996). The institutions were
often sponsored by religious organizations and were local in nature.

The first U.S. "speech correctionists" were educators and others in the helping
or medical professions who took an interest in speech problems (Duchan, 2002).
These were accompanied by a few "quacks" who promised curing therapies or
drugs. The more legitimate therapists came from already established professions.

Among them were Alexander Melville Bell and his father, Alexander Graham Bell, of telephone fame. Other Americans trained with famous "speech doctors" in Germany and Austria or became interested in what was called "speech correction" because of their own difficulties, often with stuttering. The first professional journal, *The Voice*, which appeared in 1879, focused primarily on stuttering research and interventions that were available.

Early interest groups were formed primarily among teachers within the National Education Association and among physicians and academics belonging to the National Association of Teachers of Speech. The latter group formed the American Academy of Speech Correction in 1925, a precursor to ASHA, and attempted to promote scientific inquiry and to set standards for training and practice. ASHA has had varying names over the years; it finally settled on American Speech-Language-Hearing Association in 1978.

The profession of audiology originated in the 1920s, when audiometers were first designed for measuring hearing. Interest surged in the 1940s when returning World War II veterans exhibited noise-induced hearing loss due to gunfire or prolonged and unprotected exposure to noise. Others had psychogenic hearing loss as a result of trauma. The Veterans Administration provided hearing testing and rehabilitation.

Gradually, ASHA was able to establish professional and educational standards and to advocate for the rights of individuals with disabilities. During the 1960s in the United States and elsewhere, intense energy was directed toward the advancement of civil rights for all people. Just as the rights of women, ethnic minorities, and the LGBTQ community have been and are being recast, the status of individuals with disabilities has been reevaluated, and bold reforms have been initiated.

> *I've learned that you can pass every test and receive every degree, but you won't be successful in a field like this if you don't love what you do and have a passion for helping every person you work with.*
>
> —A graduate student in communication sciences and disorders

A series of laws passed by the U.S. Congress over the past 50 years mandates appropriate treatment for individuals with disabilities.

The American Coalition of Citizens with Disabilities was created in 1974; legislative action on behalf of all Americans with disabling conditions began in earnest around the same time. In many cases, people with disabilities occupied leadership roles in the push for change. As a result of this work, providing opportunities for individuals with disabilities to develop to their full potential was no longer simply an ethical position. It became federally mandated through a series of laws.

Finally, in 1974, Congress enacted the Education for All Handicapped Children Act (EAHCA) as Public Law 94–142. It mandated that a free and appropriate public education must be provided for all children with disabilities between the ages of 5 and 21. Several years later, Public Law 99–457 extended the age of those served to cover youngsters between the ages of birth and 5 years. In 1990, Congress reauthorized the original law and renamed it the Individuals with Disabilities Education Act (IDEA). IDEA addressed the multicultural nature of U.S. society. The needs of English language learners (ELLs) and those from racial-ethnic minorities were targeted for special consideration. Reauthorized in 2004, IDEA established birth-to-6 programs as well as new early intervention services. ASHA has been a vital advocacy agency throughout this long legislative process.

Pearson eTextbook
Video Example 1.7

Here's an example of self-advocacy and education of the larger community.

www.youtube.com/watch?v=WQsA_ItnGeg

In recent years, there has been a positive movement among those with disabilities to organize and to express pride in their identity and self-advocacy. This has been called the Disability Rights Movement and mirrors other civil rights actions. This movement and burgeoning organizations it spawns are often modeled on the community of those with deafness, often called the Deaf Community.

Although self-advocacy is not always possible for those with severe disorders, many groups have coalesced within different disorders, such as individuals with high-functioning autism spectrum disorder. These groups, in turn, can offer a voice to their community. Some communities see the person-first designation, as in "a person with autism," to be demeaning and an attempt to hide their disorder, claiming instead older terms, such as identifying as an "autistic person." There is still much discussion and debate and these developments will continue for some time.

Pearson eTextbook
Video Example 1.8
Here's a second, very enjoyable video on self-advocacy. Let your true colors shine! www.youtube.com/watch?v=_q XxrUyTCcE&t=265s

Summary

Speech-language pathologists, audiologists, and other specialists work together to assist those with communicative disorders. They work in a variety of settings and with people of all ages. They are rewarded by contributing to the well-being of others.

The American Speech-Language-Hearing Association is the largest organization of professionals working with communication disorders. ASHA's missions include the scientific study of human communication, provision of clinical service in speech-language pathology and audiology, maintenance of ethical standards, and advocacy for individuals with communication disabilities. As a result, federal legislation currently mandates services for all people with disabilities.

Are you ready to begin your journey? Communication is a fascinating process. Helping people communicate is a rewarding career.

Pearson eTextbook
Video Example 1.9
Hopefully, by now you have a spark that will ignite your passion for the fields of audiology and speech-language pathology. In this video an inspired undergraduate student, possibly like you, discusses his hopes for working with individuals with communication disorders. www.hearingandspeech careers.org/?_ga=2 .111077504.426052360 .1656512710-1066178008 .1594126986

Epilogue   Case Study: Mike

Mike and I had worked together for about a month. Although his health deteriorated, we somehow managed to keep his speech skills. We also worked on his language and short-term memory by recalling recent events. I met with his parents, who seemed pleased with what we had done together and were happy, when possible, to help him with memory tasks.

On one routine visit, I was surprised to find Mike's bed empty. After inquiring of the nursing staff, I learned that he had passed away. As you can imagine, I was overcome with a sense of loss. Sitting next to him and holding his hand meant that Mike had gotten inside my personal space, which at some level had bound us together.

As time passed, I dealt with my emotions of anger, helplessness, and grief. I came to peace with what had happened. I took comfort from what we had accomplished, helping Mike hold the communication skills he had. Given his deteriorating health, we did not see nor expect to see improvement. My work had added to his quality of life.

I realize that this is not the uplifting therapy story you might desire in a first chapter, but it's real life and it doesn't detract from the good things we can do for our clients. Mike kept what skills he could and he and I could be proud of that. As SLPs, we work with those in both the beginning and ending stages of life and of course, with all of life that is in the intervening years. Mike's story is just one more in a long line. We affect our clients and they, in turn, affect us as well.

At times shortly after Mike's passing, I would smile over something I recalled from our therapy sessions. I remember thinking that Mike had fulfilled his tease. I never didn't see him again because as he had threatened, "Not if I see you first."

Reflections from a Retired Speech-Language Pathologist and University Professor

Speech-language pathology became my dream career in undergraduate school. The desire to develop and support communication skills for individuals of all ages has been most rewarding. It does not end with retirement as many opportunities still make my career choice phenomenal.

Suggested Readings/Sources

American Speech-Language-Hearing Association (ASHA). (n.d.-a). *Careers that grow with you: The future of audiology and speech-language pathology*. www.asha.org/Careers/Careers-That-Grow-With-You/.

American Speech-Language-Hearing Association (ASHA). (n.d.-b). *Learn about the CSD professions: Make a difference, make a change*. www.asha.org/Students/Learn-About-the-CSD-Professions/.

2 Typical and Disordered Communication

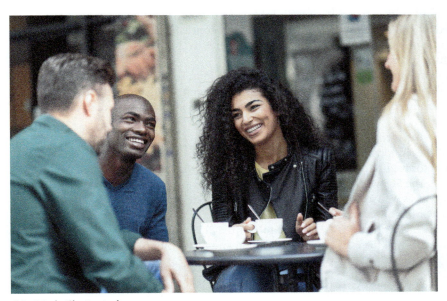

© javi_indy/Shutterstock

Learning Objectives

When you have finished this chapter, you should be able to:

2.1 Explain the role of culture and environment in human communication.

2.2 Describe the different aspects of human communication.

2.3 Demonstrate how communication disorders may be classified, including the names and frequency of occurrence of different types of communication disorders.

2.4 Describe in general the assessment and intervention process.

> " One afternoon, I received a phone call from a mom—a friend of an acquaintance—who explained that she hoped to enroll her son in a special summer remedial education program and wanted me to evaluate him and find that he had a learning disability. After I informed her that I didn't make that type of decision, she backed up and asked me just to find a communication disorder. I then informed her that I was bound by the ASHA Code of Ethics and could not do that either. I could evaluate her son and the results would tell the story. She hung up somewhat disappointed.
>
> The line between typical and disordered communication is not something we can move to fit our needs. To do so would not only be unethical but it would do a disservice to everyone we serve.
>
> –Robert Owens

What is **communication**? It's important for us to answer that question before we can explore communication disorders. In general, we can say that communication is an exchange of ideas between sender(s) and receiver(s). It involves message transmission and response or feedback. Communication requires two parties.

> **CASE STUDY**   Billy John
>
> Billy John had been born with a cleft palate, a condition that occurs when the roof of the mouth or the palate doesn't close during gestation. Because he was born at home in a rural area, few early services were available. A community visiting nurse tried to advise his parents on feeding and swallowing but had little helpful advice because of lack of experience, although she thankfully recommended a special feeding bottle. The delivering physician warned the parents to expect multiple challenges with feeding, dentation, middle ear infections, and speech issues.
>
> Within just a few days an early-intervention speech-language pathologist (SLP) began to visit the home and provide intervention for feeding and swallowing and sound making. The SLP was concerned about speech development as well as feeding, and felt that Billy John's hearing might also be affected. Unlike other infants she had worked with, Billy John seemed uninterested in making eye contact or being held and cuddled. She attributed this avoidance to his difficulties feeding and worked to make these times as positive as possible.
>
> Billy John had a series of middle ear infections as an infant. He had his first surgery for his cleft palate at age 10 months. There was very little tissue to use for the repair and his cleft remained partially open.
>
> Now 5, Billy John has had two subsequent surgical procedures and his SLP in preschool is working on his speech and language, both of which were delayed.
>
> As you read the chapter, think about:
>
> - Cultural and social factors influencing communication
> - Possible causes of delayed speech and language development
> - The role of the SLP in disorder prevention, assessment, and intervention

The Role of Culture and the Environment

Learning Objective 2.1 Explain the role of culture and environment in human communication.

Possibly the worst punishment for a prisoner is to be sentenced to isolation or solitary confinement. Milder discipline for a teenager might include limitations on texting or social media use. These restrictions are punitive because we humans are social beings. We have powerful drives to be with and to communicate with others.

As humans, not communicating is nearly impossible. Even a lack of response to someone sends a message to "leave me alone."

We communicate to make contact or to reach out to others and to satisfy our needs, reveal feelings, share information, and accomplish a host of purposes. Communication is interactive; it is a give-and-take. The importance of effective communication is highlighted when it fails or is hindered in some way. Think about how frustrated you get by a temporary lapse in Internet or cell phone service. Now imagine if that was a permanent, semi-permanent, or recurring condition.

Several variables affect communication and its success or failure. These include cultural identity, setting, and participants, to name a few. The study of these influences on communication is called **sociolinguistics**.

Cultural Identity

Each of us is a member of a language community. The more you understand about your own culture and that of the people with whom you communicate, the more effective your interaction will be. Perhaps you have traveled to a country in which a language that you did not know was spoken. You might have been able to communicate by gesture and pantomime or through *Google Translate* or another app; however, you would have to agree that while you could exchange some meaning, it fell far short of optimal communication. If this text were written in perfectly good Mandarin Chinese and you could not read that language, it would communicate nothing meaningful to you. Speakers and listeners must share competence in a common language if they are to communicate fully.

Even when two people come from the same language background, "perfect" communication is rare. This is because successful communication depends not just on language and speech, writing, or other means but on related factors, such as age, socioeconomic status, geographical background, ethnicity, gender, and ability.

The location and the participants also influence the nature of communication. Where you interact affects how and what you'll say. You communicate differently at home, in school, in a noisy restaurant, and at a ballgame. Similarly, you might speak quite differently to your best friend, your mother, your father, your boss, your grandmother, and to large audiences.

As a practical issue for an SLP, you'll be expected to work with individuals and families from the mainstream U.S. population and with many others. For example, according to the National Center for Educational Statistics (NCES; 2022b), the percentage of White non-Hispanic students in the public schools is below 50%. Over 10% of children will be English language learners (ELLs) (NCES, 2022a) and others will be speakers of nonmainstream American English dialects.

Your challenge will be to provide services in a culturally competent and culturally humble manner. **Cultural competence** is understanding, appreciating, and responding appropriately to a full range of diversity dimensions that you and clients and families bring to an interaction (American Speech-Language-Hearing Association [ASHA], n.d.-a). **Cultural humility** is recognition that to be truly effective we must recognize that learning and self-reflection are lifelong, that power imbalances exist and must be addressed, and that institutions must be accountable. For the SLP, this client-first approach can be stated as "I don't and can't know it all but let's explore culture together and craft a collaborative response."

REFLECTION QUESTION 2.1

As the U.S. population continues to diversify, it's important to consider the impact of culture on communication and on communication assessment and intervention. Can you think of any communication differences that might be culturally based but might seem to the unaware person to be a disorder? Most of these, but not all, will affect pragmatics or language use.

The Environment

Not only does communication reflect the cultures of the speakers but it also occurs within an environment or context. In fact, the act of communication often only makes sense within a context. "Can you take out the garbage on the way?" would seem odd if uttered during a haircut. Likewise, "You're hilarious!" would seem out of place at a funeral. There are places to ask questions and places where it would seem inappropriate.

The communication environment includes not only the location in which communication occurs but also the people involved and the event in which they are involved. Often, the communication itself is the context. "Sure, honey" would only work as a response to the request about garbage but wouldn't make sense as a reply to being called hilarious at a funeral, especially if you had just met the individuals involved. Even when we write, we must consider the reader and must build the context on paper from the language available to us.

As an SLP, you'll be expected to provide culturally appropriate services and to consider the environment in which language occurs. It's only when we consider the environment in which communication occurs that we can ensure generalization or carryover to that environment. For example, if a client's speech is most dysfluent in classroom presentations, it would be a disservice to not address that environmental situation in intervention.

Aspects of Communication

Learning Objective 2.2 Describe the different aspects of human communication.

As noted in Chapter 1, communication takes many forms and can involve one or a combination of our senses, including sight, hearing, smell, and touch. It can include both verbal, such as the spoken or written word, and nonverbal means, such as naturalistic gestures, facial expressions, or signs. The primary vehicle of human communication is language, and speech is the primary means of language expression for most individuals.

Language

Language is a socially shared code that is used to represent concepts. This code uses arbitrary symbols that are combined in rule-governed ways (Owens, 2020). Taken together, the characteristics of language are that it is:

- A socially shared tool
- An arbitrary code
- A rule-governed system
- A generative process
- A dynamic scheme

Let's discuss each aspect of language separately.

Language is a social tool for relating to others and for accomplishing a variety of objectives. As pointed out earlier, others must share the language code if communication is to occur. When an infant utters "ga da da ka," we cannot call this "language" because this "code" is not shared.

Many people are so accustomed to their own language that they fail to recognize its arbitrary nature. Is there anything in the sound combination or the written letters of the word *water* that resembles the wet stuff? No, words are arbitrary. Is the French word *l'eau* or the Mandarin *shui* any more or less moist? The equivalent of the English word *butterfly* is *kipepeo* in Swahili, *mariposa* in Spanish, and *farasha* in Arabic—four very different renditions for that graceful creature. Some words have no equivalent in other languages. For example, the Spanish word *salsa* and the Japanese word *sushi* have no one-word English equivalent, so in the United States we use the Spanish and Japanese words.

Each language, in addition to being composed of arbitrary but agreed-upon words, consists of rules that dictate how these words are arranged in sentences. In English, an adjective precedes a noun; for example, we say, "brown cow." In French, as in many other languages, this sequence is reversed, and French speakers say, "le vache brun" ("the cow brown"). The rules of a language make up its **grammar**. Interestingly, you do not have to be able to explain the rules to recognize when they have been broken. Take, for example, the sentence "The leaves of the maple green tree in the breeze swayed." You know intuitively that the sentence doesn't sound correct.

Language is **generative**; this means that you can create new utterances. As a speaker, you don't just quote or repeat what you heard before. Instead, you present your own ideas in an individual way. Imagine trying to have a conversation if all you could do was imitate your conversation partner.

Languages are also **dynamic**; they change over time. American English adds five or six new words each day, many from other languages. The word *texting* was added to the dictionary in 2010. Pronunciation, grammar, and even ways of communicating also change. For example, there was no texting as a form of communication in 1980.

All human languages consist of similar basic ingredients. The primary interrelated components have been labeled form, content, and use. See Figure 2.1.

Form

Form consists of phonology, morphology, and syntax. **Phonology**, or the sound system of English, consists of about 43 phonemes, or unique speech sounds. Although different languages use many of the same phonemes, variations exist. Spanish and Korean, to name only two, do not use the English *th*.

Speech sounds are not combined arbitrarily. **Phonotactic** rules specify how sounds may be arranged in words and syllables structured. Like rules of grammar, phonotactic rules are not universal. For example, *k* and *n* cannot be blended in spoken English. For this reason, the *k* in "knife" and "Knoxville" is silent for native English speakers.

Parents often assume that their infant's earliest "ma ma" or "da da" are uttered in reference to themselves. These sound combinations are not considered true words unless there is evidence that they are used meaningfully.

Pearson eTextbook
Video Example 2.1

Environmental changes influence the evolution of language. In this video, you learn about how the Internet is changing the English language.
www.youtube.com/watch?v=P2XVdDSJHqY

FIGURE 2.1 Components of language.

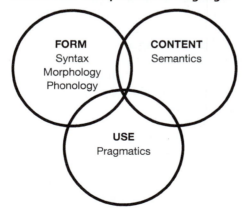

Sources: Data from Owens (2012) and Shadden and Toner (1997).

Individual sounds are called phonemes and are written using the International Phonetic Alphabet (IPA) rather than the letters or symbols of any individual language. For example, the English *th* which actually represents two sounds is written as either ð (*the*) or Θ (*thin*). Phonemes are usually placed between forward slashes, as in /ð/.

Morphology, the second aspect of form, involves the structure of words. A **morpheme** is the smallest grammatical unit within a language. Words contain both **free morphemes** and **bound morphemes**. A free morpheme may stand alone as a word. For example, *cat, go, spite, like,* and *magnificent* are all free morphemes. If you attempt to break them into smaller units, you lose the meaning of the word. In contrast, *cats, going, spiteful, dislike,* and *magnificently* each contain one free morpheme and one bound morpheme. The bound morphemes *-s, -ing, -ful, dis-,* and *-ly* change the meanings of the original words by adding their own meanings. The *-s* means more than one" Bound morphemes cannot be used alone and must be attached to free morphemes. A brief tutorial on English morphemes can be found at www.youtube.com/watch?v=jMfS4jLyTnE.

Syntax pertains to how words are arranged in a sentence and to the ways in which one word may affect another. In an English declarative sentence, the subject comes before the verb: "John is going to the gym." When we reverse the order of the subject and the auxiliary or helping verb *is*, we change the meaning of the sentence and end up with a question: "Is John going to the gym?" Other word orders such as "Gym going John is to" are meaningless in English. That takes us to *content*.

Content

Because language is used to communicate, it must be about something, and this is its content, meaning, or **semantics**. Semantics helps us differentiate sense from nonsense. In the previous example, because of syntax "Gym going John is to" is nonsense. Features of words also affect meaning. For example, "I sliced them some milk" doesn't make sense because milk is poured and drunk, not sliced. Put it in the form of cheese and now pouring it wouldn't make sense.

Use

While all aspects of language are important, it is the use or the purpose of communication that dictates form and content.

Use, or **pragmatics**, is the driving force behind all aspects of language. We speak for a reason. It is the purpose of our utterance that primarily determines its form and content. For example, if you are with a friend and are hungry, you might say, "Let's get something to eat." If the purpose were a simple biological drive, then simply "Eat" or "French fries" might suffice. But who and where you are, whom you are with, and the time of day also influence what you say. If you are at your home and you have invited a friend to dinner, you might say, "Dinner is ready." If you are working with someone as noon approaches, you might suggest, "Let's break for lunch."

Pragmatic rules vary with culture. For example, in the United States business meetings tend to be very task oriented. Very little time is spent on social exchanges; the work to be done has center stage. In Saudi Arabia, however, when two people meet for the first time for business purposes, they might spend the entire session talking about family and friends and not get to the meat of the business until the second meeting. The rules for business conversations in each of these societies are different.

A few general rules for speakers of American English are presented in Figure 2.2. These are not rules telling us what to do. Rather, they are a description of what we do most of the time.

Pearson eTextbook
Video Example 2.2
Pragmatics may be difficult to understand. This video about pragmatics includes a brief overview.
www.youtube.com/watch?v=0xc0KUD1umw

FIGURE 2.2 A sampling of pragmatic rules for speakers of American English.

1. Only one person speaks at a time. Each person should contribute to the conversation.
2. Speakers should not be interrupted.
3. Each utterance should be relevant.
4. Each speech act should provide new information.
5. Politeness forms reflect the relationship of the speakers.
6. Topics of conversation must be established, maintained, and terminated.
7. The speaker should be sensitive to successfully communicating the message, avoiding vagueness and ambiguity.
8. The listener should provide feedback that reflects comprehension of the message.

Bringing It Together

Let's look at one sentence and how all aspects of language come together.

Are you sure you don't mind walking?

- Syntax: 7 words, negative question, 2 clauses: You are sure + you don't mind
- Morphology: 9 morphemes, 7 free + 2 bound (*-n't, -ing*)
- Phonology: Some consonant clusters (/nt/, /nd/)
- Semantics: "Sure" indicates the listener person has made a decision on this issue, "mind" is used to mean "bothered by."
- Pragmatics: Indicates that another form of transportation may be available. It's an appropriate way to ask a question about feelings.

Any aspect or combination may be present in a child with typically developing language or a child with a language disorder.

CASE STUDY   Billy John *(continued)*

Recall that Billy John had immature language by preschool. There can be numerous causes, including his hearing and early failure to express an interest in socialization. Either or both can affect language development.

Speech

Speech is the process of producing the acoustic representations or sounds of language. Features such as articulation, fluency, and voice interact to influence speech production. The final product in the form of speech reflects the rapid coordination of movements associated with each of these features.

Articulation

Articulation refers to the way in which speech sounds are formed. How do we move our tongue, palate, teeth, and lips to produce the specific phonemes of a language? How do we combine these individual sounds to form words? For now, we'll skip the process because Chapter 8 explains the nature of speech sound production and describes the problems that may occur.

The component of speech that includes rate and rhythm is referred to as *prosody*. Prosodic features are known as suprasegmentals. *Supra-* means "above" or "beyond," so suprasegmental features go beyond individual speech sounds (or segmental units) and are applied to words, phrases, or sentences. Stress or emphasis and intonation are also suprasegmental features of speech production that are discussed later in this chapter.

Although most of the time we attempt to use a clear, sufficiently loud voice, sometimes our meaning may be more effectively communicated by a whisper, a whine, or a throaty rasp. When you are upset, your voice might sound angry to the point where someone says, "Don't use that tone of voice with me." Clearly, tone communicates information.

Here again, Billy John is likely to experience challenges. Cleft palate can result in a child's inability to seal off the oral chamber or mouth from the nasal chamber. Try this yourself. Say the sound of the letter *P* or "puh," not the letter name or "pee." Notice the pressure buildup needed to do this. It required closing off the nasal areas. If a child or adult had difficulty doing this, air would escape and sound production would be affected.

Fluency

Fluency is the smooth, forward flow of communication. It is influenced by the rhythm and rate of speech. Every language has its own rhythmic pattern, or timing. Do we pause after each word that we speak? Do we pause after each sentence? If we do, how long do the pauses last? What is our phrasing or grouping of words? You'll note that timing is not an isolated feature of speech. A word or syllable that is held tends to be emphasized and said more loudly.

The speed at which we talk is our **rate**. Overall rate can reveal things about us. It may provide clues about where we come from. For example, people from New York City usually speak more rapidly than those from rural Georgia. However, if you habitually speak very quickly, it may suggest that you are in a hurry, are impatient, or have a great deal to say. By contrast, slow speech may connote a relaxed or casual demeanor.

Voice

Voice can reveal things about the speaker as well as about the message. A person with a hoarse voice might (correctly or not) communicate to others that they smoke. A person with a soft, high-pitched voice might be communicating youth or immaturity. A deep, throaty voice might connote masculinity or authority.

Both the overall level of loudness and the loudness pattern within sentences and words are important. A generally loud voice may communicate strength; a soft one may suggest timidity. By stressing different words within a sentence, you are also conveying different meanings. Say the following sentence in each of the ways listed here, with the emphasis or increased loudness on the underlined word. Notice how the meaning changes:

I got an "A" on my Physics final.

I got an "<u>A</u>" on my Physics final.

I got an "A" on my <u>Physics</u> final.

I got an "A" on my Physics <u>final</u>.

Placing the stress on different syllables within certain words also changes the meaning. Stressed syllables often have long vowels, as in the first word in each of the following pairs:

record   record

recess   recess

present   present

You might have noticed that as you vary the stress, the pitch, duration, and pronunciation of different speech sounds may also change. The pitch tends to go up as the loudness is increased. Similarly, you are likely to prolong the syllable that receives stress.

Pitch is a listener's perception of how high or low a sound is; it can be physically measured as frequency or cycles per second, called *hertz*. **Habitual pitch** is the basic tone that an individual uses most of the time. For example, children have higher-pitched voices than adults. So our habitual pitch tells something about who we are.

Pitch movement within an utterance is called intonation. Say the following sentence by bringing your pitch down for the last word and then say it by raising your pitch at the end:

She wants to do the dishes.

A rising intonation can turn a statement into a question.

You'll notice that intonation influences meaning. You should also observe that as you alter intonation, your rhythm and loudness patterns also change.

Punctuation, font type and size, and upper case may contribute to the meaning of an e-mail or a text. These are attempts to indicate emphasis in written form.

The symbols /ɛ/, /ə/, and /ɪ/ represent phonemes, or speech sounds, to be described in more detail in Chapter 9.

Nonverbal Communication

Although most humans rely heavily on spoken communication, some researchers report that about two-thirds of human exchanges of meaning take place nonverbally. The term *nonverbal* encompasses both the suprasegmental aspects of speech that we described in the previous section and the **nonvocal** (without voice) and nonlinguistic (nonlanguage) aspects of communication.

Artifacts

The way you look and the way you have decided to show yourself and your personal environment communicate something about you. People make assumptions about our personalities and trustworthiness on the basis of our possessions, clothing, and general appearance. For example, I dress professionally when I present a workshop as a sign that I value both the audience and the topic.

Kinesics

Kinesics refers to the way we move our bodies, called *body language*. This includes overall body movement and position as well as gestures and facial expressions. Gestures such as a "brush-off" and facial expressions such as a frown have explicit meanings, and they support and contribute to the larger speech system. By contrast, signing may be a primary means of communication for someone who has deafness. American Sign Language is described in greater detail in Chapters 12 and 13.

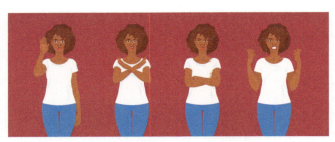

Gestures and facial expressions support and contribute to the speech system.

© Jet/Shutterstock

Speech-language pathologists recognize the heterogeneous nature of the U.S. population and strive to be sensitive to both verbal and nonverbal variations.

Tactiles are touching behaviors. Who touches whom and how and where on the body the touch occurs can reveal a great deal. Although children in our society learn that touching others is usually not appropriate and are told early on to "keep your hands to yourself," infants' earliest interactions normally include considerable parental and caretaker touch.

Proxemics

The study of the physical distance between people as it affects communication is called **proxemics**. Proxemics not only reflects the relationship between people but is also influenced by age and culture. Infants, children, people from Middle Eastern and Latin cultures, and those with strong emotional attachments, such as lovers, tend to interact in intimate or close proximity, very near one another.

Summary

Age, sex, education, and cultural background influence every aspect of communication. These natural variations in communication are not impairments. Differences reflect regional, social, cultural, or ethnic identity and are not a disorder of speech or language.

As we mature, our communication changes. The crying of an infant may become the call "Mommy" within a year. Table 2.1 offers a sampling of typical communication features at different life stages. We describe communication impairments in the next section.

Communication Through the Lifespan

The most complex and challenging task newborns face is learning the abstract code called "language" that those around them use to communicate. To do this, infants must first learn the rudiments of communication and begin to master the primary means of language transmission, called "speech." The early establishment of communication between children and their caregivers fosters the development of both speech and language, which in turn influences the quality of communication. This intricate pattern is fostered by physical, cognitive, and social development as a child matures. In a seeming reversal, language proficiency is critical to development of higher cognitive and social skills (Oller et al., 2001) as we mature.

The key to an infant becoming a communicator is being treated as one. The process of learning speech and language is a social one that occurs through interactions of children and the people in their environment. Although both speech and language depend on physical and cognitive maturation, neither is sufficient to account for the rapid developments in children's communication.

Speech and language are learned within routines and familiar activities that shape children's days and within conversations about food, toys, and pets and later about school, social life, and the like. A young child uses a variety of speech cues and patterns to break continuous speech into more readily interpretable chunks

TABLE 2.1

A Lifespan View of Typical Communication

Receptive Communication	Age Range	Expressive Communication							Nonverbal Communication	
		Language			Speech			Artifacts	Kinesics	Space/Time
		Form	Content	Use	Articulation	Fluency	Voice			
Quiets/turns to human voice; distinguishes speech sounds	Infancy	Prelinguistic sound making	No "true" speech; vocalizations; body movement focus on here-and-now	Obtain assistance; imitate and respond to others	Gurgles, coos, babbles	Rhythm and rate begin to resemble that of surrounding language toward end of year	Varies volume, rate, pitch	Toys, materials given to child; may "give" objects to others	Gestures precede meaningful spoken language	Close proximity/immediacy
Responds to some verbal commands	Toddler	Vocabulary growth from 4 to 300 words; moves from single word to short utterances	Familiar names, actions	Imitate, greet, protest, question	Simplified phonology		High (childish) pitch, more variability than adults	Toys; begins to construct things; start of imaginary play	Gestures slowly take second place to spoken language	Proximity decreases; begins to comprehend "now" and "later"
Comprehension far exceeds expression; enjoys stories, books; follows increasingly complex commands; comprehends simple humor	Preschool	Vocabulary grows from 1,000 to more than 2,000 words; uses complete sentences	Immediate to imaginary; includes past, present, and future	Greet, request, protest, inform, pretend, entertain	Almost all speech sounds correctly produced by the end of this period	Part-word, whole-word, and phrase repetition not uncommon	Adjusts to listener; often used effectively to enhance verbal communication	Tremendous variability; reflects social/cultural background	Gestures used to enhance verbal communication	Begins to understand personal space

(continued)

TABLE 2.1
(Continued)

Age Range	Receptive Communication	Expressive Communication						Nonverbal Communication		
		Language		Use	Speech			Artifacts	Kinesics	Space/Time
		Form	Content		Articulation	Fluency	Voice			
School-age	Reading skills improve; receptive language grows to 50,000 words by sixth grade, 80,000 words end of high school; comprehension becomes adult-like	Vocabulary grows to 25,000 to 30,000 words; slang important; written language more complex than spoken language	Very broad; includes distant as well as near and abstract concepts	May enjoy talking, sharing thoughts, raising and answering personal as well as abstract questions; narrative skills expand	Speech sounds correctly produced	Rate may be rapid; fluency is good	Pitch drops to adult levels with puberty; voice used to supplement verbal message	Clear indication of what is wanted; reflect peer group, gender	Gestures used in wide array of means to supplement speech	Becomes territorial; mature understanding of space and time
Early and middle adulthood	Comprehension increases	Education and occupation may be reflected in vocabulary	Full range of topics; written language continues in importance and sophistication	Instructing; directing others may be added if not there earlier	Mature articulation	Use of rhythm and rate to enhance message	Mature pitch; full-bodied vocal quality	Tremendous variety dependent on sociocultural and individual variables	Body movement and gestures continue to supplement verbal communication	Space may reflect relative "importance" in environment as well as cultural factors
Advanced age	Comprehension may decrease with hearing loss	Vocabulary may reflect "older" generation	May focus more on past than future	May have limited communication partners; speech may be major way to achieve companionship	Normally not impaired	Rate may slow	Pitch may increase; vocal quality may become "thinner"	Old/familiar items may become increasingly treasured	Body movement may be less forceful	May crave touch, as significant others become less available

Sources: Data from Owens (2020) and Shadden and Toner (1997).

Note: This is a sampling of communication behaviors. Variability within each age group is the norm.

(Sanders & Neville, 2000). For example, no words in American English begin with the "ks" (written /ks/) sound, but that same combination can signal the end of a word.

In different cultures, the type of child–caregiver interaction, the model of language presented to the child, and the expectations for the child differ, but each is sufficient for the learning of the language of the culture. Learning to become an effective communicator is a dynamic and active process in which children in our culture become involved in the give-and-take of conversations. Even the more formal educational processes of learning to read and write are initially social and occur within early book-sharing activities in the home involving children and caregivers.

Every person's speech and language continue to change until the end of life. Communication reflects the changes occurring in us and around us. Even the means of communication can change. Your grandparents began life without a computer or texting and had to learn these new means of communication as adults. You, in contrast, grew up with the Internet and cell phones. Many preschoolers now have tablets and Kindles.

Languages change, too. New words and phrases have entered American English within your lifetime, such as *bromance, automagically, alternative truth, PPE, adulting, unconscious bias,* and *metaverse.* Other cultures and languages have contributed *mullah, sushi, bodega,* and *tsunami.* A competent communicator continues to adapt to changes in the language and in the communication process.

> Communication is established very early between child and caregiver.

> Children become communicators because we treat them as if they already are.

> **Pearson eTextbook**
> **Video Example 2.3**
> Before we begin a discussion of disorders, it's helpful to ask "What's normal?" Here's a TED Talk video that addresses that issue.
> www.youtube.com/watch?v=Zz0Xcneakeg

Communication and Swallowing Disorders

Learning Objective 2.3 Demonstrate how communication disorders may be classified, including the names and frequency of occurrence of different types of communication disorders.

Now that you have an idea of the complexity and varied nature of communication, it should be easy to see that much can go wrong. Before we move on, take a minute to digest what you just read. Listen to people around you or online as they talk and exchange ideas. Notice some of the aspects of communication that we've discussed. Now, you're ready to resume. Let's expand on what we discussed in Chapter 1.

We can define communication disorders as consisting of disorders of speech (articulation, voice, resonance, fluency), oral neuromotor patterns of control and movement, feeding and swallowing disorders, language and/or literacy disorders, cognitive and social communication deficits, and hearing and processing difficulties. This definition does not confine itself to speech communication and includes other communication systems. That's a lot! Although communication disorders may be categorized on the basis of whether reception, processing, and/or expression is affected, the three dimensions are often intertwined, reflecting the integration of the processes. Figure 2.3 presents various systems for categorizing speech and language disorders. In similar fashion, swallowing disorders could be classified based on the type and severity of the impairment.

The ASHA website (www.asha.org) discusses various disorders that affect children and adults who may benefit from the help of an SLP or audiologist. Enter the disorder you wish to explore in the search box in the upper right of the website.

FIGURE 2.3 Possible speech, language, and hearing disorders.

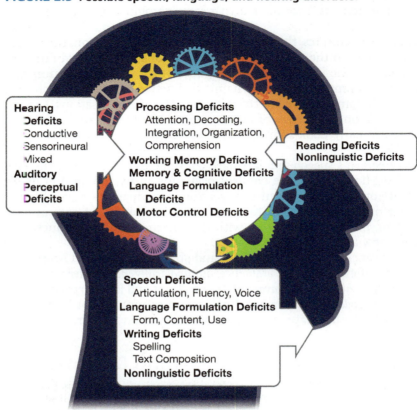

Speech communication disorders can have various causes that are congenital and/or acquired and severities ranging from mild to severe. Nonverbal and literacy impairments can further complicate communication impairments.

Etiology, the cause or origin of a problem, may be used to classify a communication problem. Disorders may be due to faulty learning, neurological impairments, anatomical or physiological abnormalities, cognitive deficits, hearing impairment, damage to any part of the speech system, or a combination.

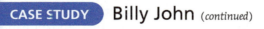 **CASE STUDY** **Billy John** *(continued)*

Billy John has both anatomical and physiological challenges. In addition, his language learning seems to have been affected.

Sometimes a dichotomy is made between **congenital** and **acquired** problems. Congenital disorders are present at birth; acquired ones result from illness, accident, or environmental circumstances anytime later in life. An individual may have a disorder that is congenital (meaning present at birth), acquired, or both. Finally, an individual's disorder may range from borderline or mild to profoundly severe. This variation is the reason many disorders are thought of as being on a spectrum of severity.

As mentioned in Chapter 1, typical variations in communication and swallowing are not disorders. For example, **dialects** are differences that reflect a particular regional, social, cultural, or ethnic identity and are not disorders of speech or language. Likewise, differences found in the speech and language of English learners (ELs) are not disorders.

Language Disorders

In this section, we give you an overview of different types of disorders. This will give you the basics for later, more in-depth discussions in the following chapters. Although we focus on form, content, and use, language disorders tend to cross these boundaries. A deficit in one area tends to affect the others.

Disorders of Form

As explained earlier, language form includes phonology, morphology, and syntax. An error in sound use, such as not producing the ends of words ("hi shi i too sma" for "his shirt is too small"), constitutes a disorder of phonology. This in turn might affect morphology if a child omits the plural -s or the past tense -ed. Syntactical errors include incorrect word order and run-on sentences (e.g., "I want to go mall and go skate and buy peanuts and you come with me 'cause I want you to but not Jimmy 'cause he's not big enough to go skate"). These errors in school-age children may affect both academic achievement and social well-being.

Disorders of form may be due to many factors, including sensory limitations such as hearing problems or perceptual difficulties found in learning disabilities. Limited exposure to correct models may also hinder a child's language development. For many children who are delayed in their production of mature language forms, the cause is not readily apparent. Neurological disorders caused by stroke or traumatic brain injury may result in a loss of access to language even though language remains intact.

Patterns that seem like errors at first are sometimes a reflection of a particular speech dialect or the influence of another language. An SLP must distinguish between dialectal or second-language variations and disorders.

Disorders of Content

Children and adults with limited vocabularies, those who misuse words, and those with word-finding difficulties may have disorders of content or semantics. Similarly, limited ability to understand and use abstract language, as in metaphors, proverbs, sarcasm, and some humor, suggests semantic difficulties. A persistent pattern of avoiding naming objects and referring instead to "the thing" is another indication of a disorder of content. Although limited experience or a concrete learning style may contribute to this problem in youngsters, among older people stroke, head trauma, and certain illnesses with cognitive impairment may result in word-retrieval problems and other content-related difficulties.

Disorders of Use

Pragmatic language problems may be related to limited or unacceptable conversational, social, and narrative skills; deficits in spoken vocabulary; and/or immature or disordered phonology, morphology, and syntax. Examples of impaired

Speech-language pathologists are concerned with both verbal and nonverbal disorders of communication.

Pearson eTextbook
Video Example 2.4
This video describes characteristics of individuals who stutter or have a fluency disorder. Note the behaviors that often accompany stuttering and imagine how they would affect overall communication. Might some characteristics be shared with other communication disorders?
www.youtube.com/watch?v=d a6xnm5feV4&index=4&list=PL EBC36C3D7AA1E348

It is not uncommon for an individual to have an impairment in more than one aspect of communication.

pragmatic language skills might include difficulty staying on topic, providing inappropriate or incongruent responses to questions, and constantly interrupting the conversational partner. Culture, group affiliations, setting, and participants described earlier in this chapter play a major role in judgments regarding pragmatic competence.

Speech Disorders

Remember, language is the code. Speech is the mode or means for most human communication. As mentioned earlier, disorders of speech may involve articulation (the production of speech sounds), fluency (rhythm and rate), or **voice** (pitch, loudness, and quality). They may affect people of all ages, be congenital or acquired, be due to numerous causes, and reflect any degree of severity.

Disorders of Articulation

Production of speech requires perception and conceptualization of the speech sounds in a language as well as motor movements to form these sounds in isolation and in connected speech. You must have both a mental/auditory image of the sound you are going to say and the neuromuscular skills to produce the sound. The cognitive and theoretical concepts of the nature, production, and rules for producing and combining speech sounds in language is known as *phonology*, which we know from the previous section is an aspect of language. The actual production of these sounds is called **articulation**.

It is not always easy to determine whether an individual's speech-sound errors indicate an impairment of phonology or articulation. To sort this out, SLPs identify the phonemes that are incorrectly produced and look for error patterns that may point to phonological disturbances. The sound system of a language is usually fully in place by age 7 or 8. Children with multiple speech-sound errors past age 4 may have *phonological* difficulties. The causes of phonological disorders are often not known but may result from faulty learning due to illness such as ear infections, hearing or perceptual impairments, or other problems in the early years.

An SLP is interested in a client's ability to move the structures needed in speech, such as the jaw, lips, and tongue. The causes of articulation disorders include neuromotor problems such as cerebral palsy, physical anomalies such as cleft palate, and faulty learning. When paralysis, weakness, or poor coordination of the muscles for speech result in poor speech articulation, the disorder is called **dysarthria**. In contrast, **apraxia of speech**, although also poor articulation due to neuromotor difficulties, appears to be due to planning and programming the speech mechanism, not muscle strength. Dysarthria and apraxia can affect both children and adults. Assessment and treatment of phonological and articulatory disorders are described in Chapter 10.

Disorders of Fluency

As we described earlier, fluency is the smooth, uninterrupted flow of communication. Certain types of fluency disruptions are fairly common at different ages. For example, many 2-year-olds repeat words: "I want-want-want a cookie." Around age 3, youngsters often make false starts and revise their utterances: "Ben took . . . he broked my crayon." Because this speech pattern is so common, it is sometimes referred to as **developmental disfluency**. Even typically fluent adults occasionally use **fillers** ("er," "um," "ya know," and so on), **hesitations** (unexpected pauses), **repetitions** ("g-go-go"), and **prolongations** ("wwwwell"). When these speech behaviors exceed or are qualitatively different from the norm or are accompanied by excessive tension, struggle, and fear, they may be identified as **stuttering**. Appropriate diagnosis and intervention when warranted are the tasks of an SLP (Yairi et al., 2001).

Fluency disorders are generally first noticed before 6 years of age. If remediation efforts are not made or are unsuccessful, this condition might continue and even worsen by adulthood. Adult onset of disfluency also occurs. Advancing age, accidents, and disease can all disrupt the normal ease, speed, and rhythm of speech. The causes of nonfluent speech are typically unclear; this is explored further in Chapter 8.

> Speech-language pathologists use several indices to differentiate developmental disfluency from early stuttering.

Disorders of Voice

As in other areas of speech, voice matures as a child gets older. From uncontrolled cries to carefully modulated whispers, shouts, and variations in pitch, the development of voice follows a predictable pattern. Although occasionally children are born with physiological problems that interfere with normal voice, as Billy John was, more common is the pattern of **vocal abuse**. It is characterized by excessive yelling, screaming, or even occasional loud singing that results in **hoarseness** or another voice disorder.

Habits such as physical tension and excessive yelling, coughing, throat clearing, smoking, and drinking alcohol can disrupt normal voice production. These behaviors may result in polyps, nodules, or ulcers on the vocal folds where voice production begins. Disease, trauma, allergies, and neuromuscular and endocrine disorders can also affect voice quality. For example, individuals with Parkinson disease, a progressive neurological disorder affecting the range of muscle movement, may have a soft voice with limited pitch and loudness variation.

Hearing Disorders

A hearing disorder results from impaired sensitivity in the auditory or hearing system. It may affect the ability to detect sound, to recognize voices or other auditory stimuli, to discriminate between different sounds, such as mistaking the phoneme /s/ for /f/, and to understand speech.

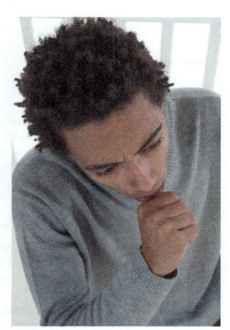

Vocal abuse such as coughing or yelling can lead to disorders of voice.
© Jean-Paul CHASSENET/123RF

CASE STUDY **Billy John** *(continued)*

Recall that Billy John's early intervention SLP was concerned that his cleft palate might have affected his hearing.

Deafness

When a person's ability to perceive sound is limited to such an extent that the auditory channel is not the primary sensory input for communication, the individual is considered to have deafness. Deafness may be congenital or acquired.

Universal neonatal hearing screening is mandated by law in many states. In this way, congenital deafness can be identified and addressed very early.

Total communication, including sign, speech, and speechreading, is often considered the most effective intervention for deafness. **Assistive listening devices (ALDs)**, **cochlear implants**, and **auditory training** may also be helpful. These are explained in Chapter 12.

Hard of Hearing

A person who is hard of hearing, in contrast to one who has deafness, depends primarily on audition for communication. Hearing loss may be temporary due to an illness, such as an ear infection, or permanent, caused by disease, injury, or advancing age. Hearing loss is usually categorized in terms of severity, laterality, and type. The severity of a hearing loss may range from mild to severe. It may be either bilateral, involving both ears, or **unilateral**, affecting primarily one ear. Finally, the loss may be **conductive**, **sensorineural**, or **mixed**. A conductive loss is caused by damage to the outer or middle ear. People with this type of loss usually report that sounds are generally too soft. A sensorineural loss involves problems with the inner ear and/or auditory nerve. This type of damage is likely to affect a person's ability to discriminate and consequently understand speech sounds, although they may "hear" them. Mixed hearing loss, as the name implies, is a combination of both conductive and sensorineural loss (see Chapter 12 for further discussion).

Auditory Processing Disorders

An individual with an auditory processing disorder (APD) may have normal hearing but still have difficulty understanding speech. Individuals with APDs struggle to keep up with conversation, to understand speech in less-than-optimal listening conditions (i.e., degraded speech signal, presence of background noise), to discriminate and identify speech sounds, and integrate what they hear with nonverbal aspects of communication (DeBonis & Moncrieff, 2008). These difficulties are sometimes traced to tumors, disease, or brain injury, but often the cause is unknown. APDs can occur in both children and adults. APDs may coexist with other disorders, including attention-deficit/hyperactivity disorder and speech-language and learning disorders (ASHA, 2005c). As you might guess, processing speech is a complex interaction involving language, cognition, and auditory mechanisms (Medwetsky, 2011).

Swallowing Disorders

Difficulty swallowing is called **dysphagia**, and stated simply it means difficulty moving food or liquid from your mouth to your stomach. In some cases dysphagia may be associated with pain, or swallowing may be impossible. Persistent dysphagia may indicate a serious medical condition. Although swallowing difficulties may occur at any age, dysphagia is more common in older adults. The causes of swallowing problems vary, and treatment depends on the cause. These causes are usually associated with other neuromuscular disorders. Our little friend Billy John had initial feeding and swallowing challenges related to his cleft palate.

How Common Are Communication Disorders?

Before we attempt to estimate the numbers of people who have disorders of communication and swallowing, we should examine the concept of normalcy.

What Is "Normal"?

A recent cartoon showed an empty room and a sign reading "Meeting of Members of Functional Families." The implication was that there are no functional, or "normal," families. Likewise, we could ask, "Is anybody normal?" If anything, variability is the norm. We humans are remarkable in our diversity. Just as no two snowflakes are identical, no two individuals, even twins, are exactly alike. Our faces, fingerprints, and manner of communication are unique.

Most measures of humans, such as the number of individuals at varying heights, will result in what is called a "bell-shaped curve" (see Figure 2.4). We see this phenomenon with test scores as well. Most people will cluster near the average or the *mean* and will be considered "normal," typical, or average. Higher or lower scores are above or below average. An individual performing in the lowest 5 to 10% would have a score considered to be significantly below average. If we are testing language ability, such a low score may indicate a language disorder.

Because the word *normal* suggests "without problems," we, the authors, prefer to use the term *typical* when we mean "like most others of the same age and

FIGURE 2.4 **The normal curve, percentile equivalents, and standard scores.**

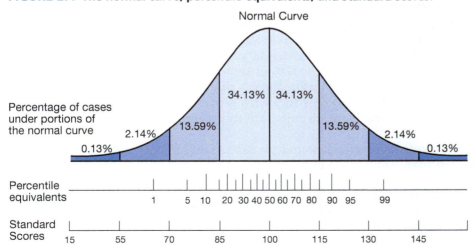

Sources: Based on Romero et al. (1998); Wiig and Secord (1992).

> **REFLECTION QUESTION 2.3**
>
> *Although we prefer the term* typical *rather than* normal*, what does "normal" mean to you? Does it matter to you? If so, how would you define "normal"?*

group." In addition, abnormal sounds harsh. Classifying people as *other-than-typical* requires clear definitions of speech and language disorders and a thorough analysis of a person's performance.

Many communication disorders are secondary to other disabilities. For example, children with a cleft palate have physical health problems as well as voice and articulation disorders. People with cerebral palsy typically have motor deficits beyond speech and swallowing. Children with learning disabilities are especially likely to have language difficulties but may also have articulation, voice, fluency, and/or hearing deficits. In addition, they may experience academic and social difficulties.

Estimates of Prevalence

Prevalence refers to the number or percentage of people within a specified population who have a particular disorder or condition at a given point in time. If you determined the prevalence of stuttering in the entire U.S. population, among first-grade children, college seniors, or older adults you would get different prevalence figures in each case. For this reason, prevalence statistics must specify the population on which they are based.

The terms *incidence* and *prevalence* are often confused. Incidence refers to the number of *new* cases of a disease or disorder in a particular time period. Prevalence is the number of *new and old* cases in a particular time period.

Current estimates suggest that about 17% of the total U.S. population have some communicative disorder. About 11% have a hearing loss and approximately 6% have a speech, voice, or language disorder, including nearly 8% of all children (Black et al., 2015). Many of those with hearing losses also have speech, voice, or language disorders.

The percentage of people with hearing loss increases with age. Overall, approximately 13% of the U.S. population over age 12 has a hearing loss (Lin et al., 2011). Between 1 and 2% of people under 18 years of age have a chronic hearing loss, compared with approximately 32% of those over age 75. Exposure to noise has contributed to the hearing loss in about a third of those affected.

Communication disorders vary with gender. For example, certain disorders, such as autism spectrum disorder, are four times as prevalent in males as in females.

Impairments of speech-sound production and fluency are more common in children than adults and more common among males than females. Speech disorders due to neurological disorders or brain and spinal cord injury occur more often among adults. It has been estimated that anywhere between 3 and 10% of Americans have voice disorders; the percentage is greater among school-age children and among people over age 65.

Language disorders occur in 8 to 12% of the preschool population; the prevalence decreases through the school years. Language deficits in older adults may be associated with stroke or cognitive impairment. It is likely that 5 to 10% of people over age 65 experience language disabilities related to these disorders.

It is estimated that 6 to 10 million Americans (about 3% of the population) have dysphagia. Although these figures may seem relatively low, it is likely that more, generally mild, cases are not reported (Tierney et al., 2000). The prevalence of dysphagia varies based on age, the definition that researchers use, and the population studied. For example, the prevalence of pediatric dysphagia among otherwise typically developing children has been reported to be 25 to 45% and to be higher for children with developmental disabilities (Arvedson, 2008; Bernard-Bonnin, 2006; Brackett et al., 2006; Lefton-Greif, 2008; Linscheid, 2006; Manikam & Perman, 2000; Rudolph & Link, 2002).

Among adult populations prevalence is higher in older adults (Barczi et al., 2000; Bhattacharyya, 2014; Cabré et al., 2014; Roden & Altman, 2013; Sura et al., 2012). In part, accurate data collection is complicated by the many disorders that can lead to dysphagia (Bhattacharyya, 2014). Estimates range from 13% of older adults living independently to 68% of long-term care facility residents (Kawashima et al., 2004; Serra-Prat et al., 2011).

Table 2.2 highlights some communication and swallowing disorders that may appear through the lifespan.

TABLE 2.2

Communication Disorders That May Manifest Themselves through the Lifespan

Age Range	Disorders	Receptive Communication	Expressive Communication	Swallowing
Infancy	Hearing impairment Fetal alcohol or drug-exposure syndrome Parental neglect/abuse Cerebral palsy	Limited response to sound/speech Limited response to others Atypical physical postures and movement Deaf infants vocalize normally for first 6 mos. Others may have little vocalization Passivity	Atypical birth and other early cries	May have difficulties with breast or bottle; later problems with solid foods
Toddler	Autism/pervasive developmental disorder may be identified (hypersensitive to stimuli) Intellectual disability not suspected earlier may now become apparent Brain injury due to falls	Comprehension of spoken language limited	Delay in first spoken word Utterances limited May use objects ritualistically	Rigid food preferences/dislikes Caution needs to be taken to prevent putting small objects in mouth that may be swallowed/choked on
Preschool	Delays that were suspected earlier may become more pronounced Fluency difficulties may emerge Specific language disabilities Middle ear problems common	Interactions with peers and others may be difficult	Inappropriate use of toys/objects Vocabulary may be limited, utterances short Alternative/augmentative communication may be recommended Excessive disfluency; delayed phonology and grammatical development	Food preferences may be more entrenched

(continued)

TABLE 2.2
(Continued)

Age Range	Disorders	Receptive Communication	Expressive Communication	Swallowing
School age	Language learning problems Attention-deficit/hyperactivity disorder Brain injury due to falls and other accidents	Difficulties in attending, following directions, speech and reading comprehension	Narrative and other pragmatic skills may be affected	Inappropriate eating habits may become established
Young adulthood	Brain injury due to bike, motorcycle, car, and other accidents most prevalent in these years	Comprehension affected, generalized confusion, abstract thinking impaired	Pragmatic skills affected Life plans altered Dysarthria and apraxia may affect speech intelligibility	Neuromotor injury may impact swallowing
Middle adulthood	Hearing often starts to decline Life-threatening illnesses such as cancer may be diagnosed Neurogenic problems may appear; multiple sclerosis, amyotrophic lateral sclerosis (ALS), Parkinson and Alzheimer diseases, stroke (aphasia)	Speech in noise may be difficult to comprehend Aphasia and Alzheimer disease may result in comprehension difficulties	Illness-related depression may affect expressive communication Dysarthria and apraxia may impair speech intelligibility Alzheimer disease and aphasia cause language difficulties	Eating/swallowing may be impaired initially following stroke; swallowing difficulties often present in degenerative neuromotor diseases (e.g., multiple sclerosis, ALS)
Advanced age	Hearing deficits common Neurogenic problems become progressively worse	Difficulty understanding speech may cause "tuning out"	Voice may be weak Word-finding problems Inappropriate speech Perseveration	Disinterest in food, swallowing impairments may lead to aspiration pneumonia

Sources: Data from Owens (2014) and Shadden and Toner (1997).

Note: This is a sampling of problems that may be seen. Variability within each age group is the norm.

Assessment and Intervention

Learning Objective 2.4 Describe in general the assessment and intervention process.

An SLP, perhaps you someday, has many responsibilities for the management of communication and swallowing disorders. At the top of the list would be assessment to ascertain the presence of a disorder and to describe the extent and intervention to ameliorate any disorder identified. Other responsibilities include prevention and advocacy and serving as a clinician counselor.

The Role of the SLP in Prevention

As an SLP, you'll be involved in prevention of communication disorders as well as assessment and intervention. The goal of ASHA is that SLPs can help eliminate the causes and onset of communication disorders and foster optimal communication. This can be accomplished through education and the identification of potentially harmful and unhealthy situations, such as smoking and noise abatement. Secondary to prevention is early identification and intervention to forestall more serious conditions. A key lifespan concept is *wellness* or the optimal level of communication competence at all stages of life. To this end, SLPs take part in classroom education, community forums, wellness fairs, and counseling activities. If you go to the ASHA website (www.asha.org) and type in "prevention" in the search box, you'll be able to read all the different ways in which SLPs are involved in prevention activities.

Assessment of Communication and Swallowing Disorders

Not everyone is assessed for communication disorders. Formal assessment occurs only after someone recognizes the possibility of a problem. Selection for assessment may come following referral by another professional or concerned adult, such as a pediatrician or parent, or from screening. Adults may also refer themselves if they feel they have a communication disorder or dysphagia.

The purpose of screening is to determine whether a problem exists. Children between the ages of birth and 36 months may be brought to special centers for screening for speech, language, hearing, motor, and other functions. Older children are screened in preschools and schools. In addition, every state in the United States requires that hearing screening tests be given to infants at their birthing facility or as soon after birth as possible.

Specialists in communication disorders may encourage referrals from other professionals and concerned individuals by publicizing the nature of the services that they provide.

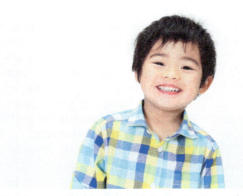

Children under the age of 3 may be brought to special centers for screening.
© Siro46/Shutterstock

Defining the Problem

A person who has been identified during screening may have a communication disorder. A screening is not a diagnostic evaluation. Screenings simply suggest which individuals should receive further evaluation.

Assessment of communication disorders is the systematic process of obtaining information from many sources, through various means, and in different settings to verify and specify communication and swallowing strengths and weaknesses, identify possible causes of problems, and make plans to address them. If a problem is identified, an SLP may make a **diagnosis**, which distinguishes an individual's difficulties from the broad range of possible problems. Although a diagnostic report might include a label such as *dysphonia*, it more importantly contains a complete description of this disorder that reflects the person's ability to communicate, variability of symptoms, severity, and possible causes. This process goes well beyond applying a label to a child's disorder. As an SLP, you won't be working with "labels"; you'll be helping to modify a person's behaviors, thoughts, and feelings.

Pearson eTextbook
Video Example 2.5

Many beginning students think of assessment as simply testing, but tests alone can't capture the subtle and dynamic aspects of communication. That requires personalizing the assessment. This TED-Ed video on standardized testing will familiarize you with the issues surrounding testing.

www.youtube.com/
watch?v=YtE0OsRWeYI

The World Health Organization (WHO; 2001) has proposed an *International Classification of Functioning, Disability, and Health* (ICF) that goes beyond the immediate causes and considers the social determinants of health. The comprehensive ICF framework considers four aspects of a disorder:

- Impairments in body structure and function
- Comorbid (co-occurring) deficits or health conditions
- Limitations in activity and participation
- Contextual (environmental and personal) factors

By shifting the focus from solely the individual with a disorder, the WHO ICF considers the social and environmental challenges faced by the individual.

Assessment Goals

The goals of assessment are listed in Figure 2.5. The primary goal of diagnosis is determining the nature of the disorder. Sometimes **diagnostic therapy** is suggested. In this case, the SLP will work with the client for a time and will obtain a clearer picture of the person's communication abilities and limitations in the process.

As mentioned earlier, communication impairments may involve hearing, speech, language, processing, and/or swallowing, or, more likely, some combination of these. During assessment, specifics of all of these are probed. Both the client's communicative strengths and limitations are noted. An SLP provides data reporting the consistency of behaviors and, where appropriate, indicates how the client compares with more typical individuals.

If a problem exists, an SLP will want to describe its severity. Exactly what determines a particular severity rating is related to several factors. Although published tests often suggest severity ratings depending on a client's performance scores,

FIGURE 2.5 Goals of assessment.

An SLP is charged with answering the following questions when assessing an individual:

1. Does a communication or swallowing problem exist?
2. What is the diagnosis of the communication or swallowing problem?
   a. What are the deficit areas? How consistent are they? Under what conditions do the deficits change?
   b. How severe is the problem?
   c. What are the probable causes of the problem?
   d. What are contributing factors that exacerbate or contribute to the problem?
3. What are the individual's strengths? How might these affect possible intervention?
4. What favorable environmental factors exist? How might these affect possible intervention?
5. What recommendations should be made?
   a. Is intervention recommended?
   b. What direction might intervention take?
6. What is the prognosis or likely outcome without and with intervention?

these must be used with caution. There is a broad range of typical communication behavior, and an SLP should not overrely on any single test.

Whenever possible, an SLP should try to ascertain the reason(s) for the communication and/or swallowing deficit, especially if the cause persists. The cause is referred to as the **etiology**. There may be **predisposing causes** that underlie the problem, such as genetic factors; **precipitating causes** that triggered the disorder, such as a stroke; and **maintaining** or **perpetuating causes** that continue or add to the problem. Whether the etiology is known or not, an SLP must thoroughly describe the client's communication behavior.

Recommendations for addressing the client's communicative and/or swallowing deficiencies are often the most-read portions of assessment reports. In making a plan, the first decision is whether intervention is warranted. If it is, then its nature and both causal and contributing factors must be described. Treatment recommendations can be thought of as a "working hypothesis" that may need to be altered as intervention proceeds. Assessment continues throughout treatment, in the forms of data collection and probes of behavior.

An SLP obtains background information about a client from a written case history completed by the client, parent, or significant other; an interview; and reports from other professionals.

In communication disorders, an SLP makes a **prognosis** regarding whether the problem will persist if no intervention occurs and what the likely outcome is if a course of therapy or other treatment plan is followed. A prognosis is an informed prediction of the outcome of a disorder, both with and without intervention, and is based, in part, on the nature and severity of the disorder; the client's responsiveness to trial therapy during assessment; and the client's overall communicative, intellectual, and personal strengths and weaknesses. The client's home and school environments are also important factors that can affect the outcome.

Assessment Procedures

Assessment may take many forms. Depending on the situation, the SLP may be a member of a team of professionals. The team may include educational and medical personnel and, in some cases, family members.

Ideally, the SLP will sample a broad variety of communication skills through multiple procedures in several settings. The focus should be on the collection of **authentic data**—that is, actual real-life information—in sufficient quantity to be able to make meaningful and accurate decisions.

Each client has individual needs. An SLP must attempt to determine which needs are paramount at a particular time and then develop a plan to meet these needs.

The need for the use of a variety of procedures should be readily apparent. How often as a student have you said that a test did not accurately measure what you know or what you can do? The same is true for individuals with communication disorders. By using multiple measures and reports, an SLP or audiologist tries to obtain the most accurate description of a child's communication possible. These methods may include:

- A case history filled out by a parent, family member, professional, or the client
- A questionnaire completed by a parent, family member, professional, or the client

Clinicians may differ in their judgments of the severity of a disorder. Use of objective criteria ensures more consistency in this determination.

Family members and clients are often eager to know the prognosis. They will ask such questions as "Will my child outgrow this problem?" or "How long will it take to correct this disorder?"

An SLP makes a determination about a client's current functioning and the nature of the problem from multiple sources and clinical intuition.

- An interview with a parent, family member, and/or the client
- A systematic observation of the client's communication and/or swallowing skills
- Testing with more than one assessment tool and including a hearing screening and an **examination of the oral peripheral mechanism**
- **Dynamic assessment**
- Communication sampling and analysis

CASE STUDY   **Billy John** (*continued*)

For Billy John, testing that includes an examination of the oral peripheral mechanism will be especially important.

Formal test results during assessment differ from baseline data. During formal testing, a wide range of communicative skills are evaluated. Baseline data reveal an individual's performance level with regard to a few selected potential targets.

Most tests are **norm-referenced**, meaning they yield scores that are used to compare a client with a sample of similar individuals. Norm-referenced instruments should be chosen carefully to fit the characteristics of each individual child. In contrast, a **criterion-referenced** test evaluates a client's strengths and weaknesses with regard to particular skills and does not make comparisons to other children. This more descriptive method is usually reserved for dynamic assessment and sampling.

Dynamic assessment includes probing to explore a client's ability to modify behavior by producing previously misarticulated sounds, learning a language rule, reducing disfluencies, and the like. The goal is to mesh more flexible nonstandardized approaches with more formal, structured methods found in most tests. For example, a test item might be repeated with additional information, such as the use of pictures previously not included in the test procedures. Dynamic assessment often takes the form of a *test–teach–test* paradigm to examine the "teachability" of a communication feature. The client's potential for learning is assessed by giving small amounts of assistance and determining the difficulty for the client with additional input.

Most clinicians also use a **speech** and/or **language sampling** technique when assessing the communication of both children and adults. Guidelines for sample collection and analysis are described in Chapter 4. With adult clients, sampling can be accomplished while reviewing the case history with clients or asking them to explain how they spent their day or to tell about their last vacation.

Although patients who have dysphagia may have a variety of complaints, they usually report coughing or choking or an abnormal sensation when trying to swallow. The evaluation often involves a team of specialists, including an SLP. A case history can be extremely important in identifying the cause(s). General health information should also be reviewed, including illnesses, current medications, and alcohol and tobacco use. A case history can help identify the location of the difficulty. Other evaluations may include a neurological assessment of neuromuscular control, motor and sensory assessment, a guided eating assessment including a variety of liquids and solids, an oral examination, and laboratory tests as needed to screen for infections and inflammatory conditions.

> **BOX 2.1**   **Evidence-Based Practice in Assessment of Individuals with Communication**

Disorders

Developmental Level

- Early identification may be especially important for young children with significant communication disorders.
- The form of communication varies with a child's age and developmental status and should be reflected in the communication features assessed.

Difference versus Disorder

- Multilingualism and dialectal variations in the home and other care environments affect the way in which language is learned and used and should be considered in an assessment.
- Bilingual clients should be assessed in both languages in order to provide an accurate picture of speech and language strengths and weaknesses.

Format

- Significant others who interact with the client on an ongoing daily basis should be included in the assessment process.
- Assessment and analysis should be multifaceted and in depth because the dividing line between typical and disordered speech and language is not always clear.
- Assessment materials and strategies should be appropriate to the culture and language of the client and family.
- The setting of the assessment should be appropriate to the developmental stage and/or overall health of the client and be comfortable for both the client and significant others.
- Assessment materials and strategies should reflect the developmental level or condition of the client.

Source: From Clinical Practice Guideline. Published by New York State Department of Health.

Evidence-Based Practice

Most ASHA assessment guidelines relate to specific disorders and are described in the following chapters. Still, some general guidelines can be deduced from these evidence-based analyses. These are included in Box 2.1.

Intervention with Communication and Swallowing Disorders

Each client brings their sense of self to the therapeutic situation. Most of this self-concept has grown out of interactions with family members and individuals in the immediate community. An SLP's failure to recognize and include these dimensions of an individual's social identity can negatively impact intervention (Demmert et al., 2006). In early intervention with children birth to 3 years of age, inclusion of family is required.

Intervention is influenced by the nature and severity of the communication disorder, the age and status of the client, and environmental considerations, as well as personal and cultural characteristics of both client and clinician. Despite this, some general principles and procedures can be identified.

Providing culturally responsive intervention is extremely important for children from culturally and linguistically diverse backgrounds. SLPs should integrate culturally based materials into intervention. If you want to learn more, I suggest you begin with ASHA's *Working with Culturally and Linguistically Diverse (CLD) Students in Schools* (ASHA, n.d.-b)

As mentioned in Chapter 1, ASHA has taken a proactive position stressing the need to integrate research and clinical practice (Kamhi, 2006a; Katz, 2003; Ramig, 2002; Wambaugh & Bain, 2002). ASHA's Code of Ethics requires clinicians to "provide services that are based on careful, professional reasoning" (Apel & Self, 2003, p. 6). Evidence-based practices (EBP) ensure that "clinicians abide by these ethical codes while best serving their clients" (Apel & Self, 2003, p. 6). ASHA has established the National Center for Treatment Effectiveness in Communicative Disorders and is currently coordinating a National Institutes of Health–funded effort to promote clinical research that will support EBP.

Objectives of Intervention

Regardless of the specific nature of a problem, intervention in speech-language pathology has as its overriding goal the improvement of the client's communication and swallowing skills:

1. The client should show improvement not just in a clinical setting; progress should generalize to their real-world environments, such as home, school, and work.
2. The client should not have to think about what has been learned; in large part, it should be **automatic**.
3. The client must be able to **self-monitor**. Although modifications should be automatic, they will still require monitoring. The client should be able to listen to and observe themself, and make corrections as needed without the therapist's being present.
4. The client should make optimum progress in the minimum amount of time.
5. Intervention should be sensitive to the personal and cultural characteristics of the client.

Target Selection

Even young and relatively low-functioning individuals are more responsive to therapy when they understand the goals.

The assessment report should provide recommendations for long-term goals and short-term objectives for communication intervention. The clinician, however, will have to decide which specific targets should be addressed and in what sequence. The client's personal needs and the potential for intervention to generalize to everyday use are most relevant in making meaningful choices. Likelihood of success and typical behavior of others of the client's age and gender might provide additional insights.

Baseline Data

Before beginning a program of intervention, an SLP obtains **baseline data**; that is, the SLP tries to elicit the target behavior(s) multiple times and under multiple conditions and records the accuracy of the client's responses. This gives the SLP information about the client's starting point. Baselines are essential in determining a client's progress and the success of a treatment program.

Behavioral Objectives

Once a clinician has obtained baseline data, they develop short-term objectives. These are the targets for each treatment session or for several sessions. A behavioral objective is a statement that specifies the target behavior in an observable and measurable way. To do this requires that the clinician identify what the client is expected to do, under what conditions, and with what degree of success. The letters ABCD might help you to remember the format for writing behavioral objectives:

A. *Actor.* Who is expected to do the behavior?
B. *Behavior.* What is the observable and measurable behavior?
C. *Condition.* What is the context or condition of the behavior?
D. *Degree.* What is the targeted degree of success?

For example, *John* [Actor] *will describe pictures* [Behavior] *using both the correct noun and verb* [Condition] *with 90% accuracy* [Degree]. "Degree" might also include a task to be accomplished, such as "in order to complete this week's written assignment" or "in order to talk with his grandmother on the phone." Goals and objectives enable an SLP to observe and measure progress in intervention (Roth, 2011). Poorly written objectives make it difficult to determine efficacy. Specific goals and objectives are required for individualized family service plans used with infants and toddlers and their families, individualized education plans used in the schools, and for third-party payers, such as insurance companies and government agencies.

Clinical Elements

Successful intervention is multifaceted and includes a variety of elements. This may include, but is not limited to, direct and incidental teaching, counseling, and inclusion of the family and family environment.

Intervention for communication disorders occurs in many settings. Broadening the base for treatment helps to ensure that what is learned in a clinical setting is transferred to a variety of real-world contexts.

Treatment Plan. As with writing goals and objectives, conscious selection of specific intervention techniques also allows for accountability. SLPs select what they believe and what evidence has shown to be the best intervention approach, types of materials, and logical steps to follow to take the client from where they are now to the objective selected. Successful intervention builds on what the client can do at present.

Direct Teaching. Part of the role of an SLP is being a teacher. Traditional clinical methods include explaining or reviewing the target and guided practice. **Behavior modification** training approaches have been shown to be successful for a broad variety of communication disorders. Behavior modification is a systematic method of changing behavior. During training, the SLP attempts to elicit the desired response from the client by providing a **stimulus**. The client is expected to *respond*, and the clinician **reinforces** this response if correct or provides corrective feedback if it is not.

Incidental Teaching. Behavior modification follows a highly structured format that an SLP directs. A low-structured or more client-led approach may also be used. In this method, the SLP follows the client's lead but teaches along the way. This is referred to as **incidental teaching**. The SLP manipulates the environment so that communication occurs more naturally. For example, imaginary play with a young child or a cooking or art project with one who is older may serve as situations in which therapy occurs.

Counseling. In addition to direct work with the client on a communication problem, an SLP can provide a supportive environment for the client and other key people in the client's life. A person with a communication disorder may experience a host of feelings including embarrassment, anger, depression, and inadequacy. Family members may have similar emotions regarding the client's communication and may also feel pity or guilt, perhaps blaming themselves for the problem.

Family and Environmental Involvement. An individual might spend 2 hours a week with an SLP and 110 awake hours alone and with other people, often family. Depending on the family circumstances, family members may be asked to help the client with specific activities at home to foster carryover to everyday situations. A spouse may be critical in assisting therapy for an adult who had a stroke or has a voice problem due to recent accident or illness. An SLP must recognize the significant others in the client's life, from infancy through advanced age, and engage them in productive ways. **Support groups** consisting of individuals who have similar difficulties often provide an avenue to practice what has been learned in therapy, to share feelings related to the disability, and to maintain communication skills once formal treatment has been terminated.

REFLECTION QUESTION 2.4

You probably envisioned SLPs and audiologists working with individual clients or small groups of clients, helping them change communication and swallowing behaviors. Did you imagine yourself being a counselor or working with parents or spouses? When might you wish to do either or both?

Measuring Effectiveness

An SLP determines readiness for dismissal from therapy largely by assessing its effectiveness. Did the client meet the long-term goals and short-term objectives? SLP-designed **post-therapy tests** similar to those used to determine baselines are normally used to answer this question. In addition, it is essential that the client has gained a degree of *automaticity* in the use of the communication target. Errors will occur, however, and the client should be able to *self-monitor* and self-correct when needed. If therapy has been effective, the client has been successful in *generalizing* learned skills to the out-of-clinic world.

Follow-up and Maintenance

After a client has been dismissed from therapy, an SLP must take steps to ensure that the progress that was achieved is not lost. This is done in two ways. Upon dismissal, the client or family should be encouraged to return when anyone feels a need. More reliable is the establishment of a regular follow-up schedule. The client may be contacted by telephone or email every 6 months for a period of 2 years or so after the termination of therapy. If warranted, retesting may be suggested and **booster treatment** may be provided, if needed.

Summary

Communication is an exchange of ideas; it involves message transmission and response. Human communication is remarkable and may take many forms. It is strongly influenced by culture and environment. Not only do people speak different languages, but within language groups, age, gender, socioeconomic status, geographical background, race/ethnicity, and other factors influence our communication.

The primary vehicle of human communication is language. It may be spoken, written, or signed and has been described in terms of form, content, and use. Form refers to the sound system, or phonology; word structure, or morphology; and syntax, or how the words are arranged in sentences. Content is semantics or meaning and use is the purpose or pragmatics of the communication. Communication is also transmitted by nonverbal behaviors and characteristics.

A breakdown can occur in any aspect of communication. When communication is unimpaired, we tend to take it for granted; but when it fails, we may feel frustrated and isolated. About 17% of the U.S. population currently experiences some limitation of hearing, speech, and/or language. An additional 3% may have dysphagia. See the ASHA website to learn more about various disorders at www .asha.org.

Assessment of communication and swallowing disorders requires an understanding of both in context. Communication behaviors can be viewed as occurring on a continuum from typical to disordered. With each case, an SLP must decide where the demarcation is.

Referrals and screenings are the primary ways in which individuals are selected for assessment. During assessment, an SLP verifies and defines the client's problem, identifies deficits and strengths, probes causality, makes a treatment plan, and provides a prognosis for improvement. This is achieved through multiple techniques, including sampling of communicative and swallowing behaviors in several settings.

Assessment and treatment function in a cyclical fashion, with one influencing the other. In many ways, an SLP is assessing the client each time the client is seen in therapy. Successful intervention often uses a team approach that involves family members as well as professionals. Provisions for follow-up ensure that the gains made in therapy are maintained. In the chapters that follow, techniques for assessment and treatment of specific communication and swallowing disorders are described.

As authors, we'd be doing a disservice if we don't correct a misconception that many people have about disorders. A disorder in one aspect of functioning, such as fluency, does not mean that the entire person is disordered. Our job as an SLP is not to remake our client but to help them function in the world, to give them the skills they need to succeed. In fact, many people with disorders are very successful in other ways. For example, people with dyslexia, a reading disorder, can be brilliant and creative, in part, because their brains function differently. So, we must not see the line between typical and disordered as a solid impenetrable barrier separating one group of people from another.

Pearson eTextbook
Video Example 2.6
This TED Talk video, entitled "The Creative Brilliance of Dyslexia" is a reminder of the danger in labelling our clients as "disordered."
www.youtube.com/
watch?v=CYM40HN82I4&
t=296s

Epilogue   Case Study: Billy John

When Billy John went to kindergarten, his SLP helped him transition from preschool and met with his school-based SLP to ensure that his speech, language, and swallowing program went with him. By age 5, his swallowing difficulties were minimal but his speech still included occasional nasal emissions (sounds through his nose) and his language was significantly below his peers.

Billy John received thorough speech and language services in school. Placed in a language-intensive classroom, he continued to improve. Now in third grade, he is reading at grade level but in the low normal range. Billy John still exhibits some speech difficulties, especially when talking loudly. Although he was initially shunned by some classmates, his personality and his ability in sports have won over the other children. Although not the star, he is popular in class.

Billy John's speech and language intervention will continue. He is scheduled for additional surgery in the summer, which will offer new challenges for him as he learns to adjust to a somewhat modified method of speaking. His language intervention will also continue, primarily focusing on literacy skills.

Reflections   from a School-Based Speech-Language Pathologist

I was so naive when I began in this field as an undergraduate. In my mind, it all seemed so simple. Give a test, find that the child had a disorder, then use a published program for intervention. My preconceptions were quickly overcome by the reality of working with individual children, no two of whom were the same. They didn't fit into nice, neat categories. And even when a child had been labeled by another professional as having this disorder or that one, children were not cookie-cutter copies of that category. Instead, each child had their own personality and abilities.

To my pleasant surprise I found that using my own skills to describe how a child communicates, deciding if a disorder exists and to what extent and creatively devising personalized interventions, was incredibly fulfilling. I don't need to reinvent the wheel with each child, but I do need to consider the unique character of each of them. It's what gives me joy.

Suggested Readings/Sources

Levinson, S. C. (2015). Turn-taking in human communication—origins and implications for language processing. *Trends in Cognitive Science, 20,* 6–14. www.cell.com/trends/cognitive-sciences/fulltext/S1364-6613(15)00276-4

Owens, R. E. (2020). *Language development, An introduction* (10th ed.). Pearson.

Ruben, B., & Stewart, L. (2019). *Communication and human behavior* (7th ed.). Pearson Education.

Tomasello, M. (2010). *Origins of human communication.* MIT Press.

3 Overview of the Anatomy and Physiology of Swallowing and Speech Production

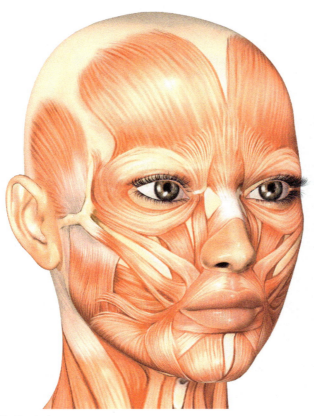

© ChastityQ/Shutterstock

Learning Objectives

When you have finished this chapter, you should be able to:

3.1 List and describe the principal structures and muscles of the respiratory system and differentiate resting tidal breathing from speech breathing.

3.2 List and describe the principal structures, muscles, and functions of the laryngeal system.

3.3 Briefly describe the structures and functions of the upper airway.

3.4 Explain the speech production process.

> ❝ During my freshman year at the State University of New York at Geneseo I switched my major from chemistry to communication sciences and disorders. My roommate shared that her cousin, a speech-language pathologist, worked in the area of "swallowing" and took coursework in the hard sciences during her undergraduate and master's programs. Because I had a strong interest in science and in helping others, I thought speech-language pathology might be a better fit for me than chemistry. My first course in the field was Language Development with Dr. Bob Owens (first author of this text), and I was immediately hooked! I was surprised, however, when I was struggling with the Anatomy & Physiology and Speech Sciences coursework during my undergraduate program and began to realize that

(continued)

when complex information was presented without context (e.g., patient information), I had difficulty with learning and retention. My experience was like many other students when studying the hard sciences in our field. To that end, we present anatomy and physiology of swallowing and speech production alongside a

case study embedded throughout the chapter. This is meant to provide a real-world context you may encounter during future clinical practicum experiences or during your career. We hope this helps you to understand and retain the information presented here.

—*Kimberly Allyn Farinella*

CASE STUDY   Jennifer

Jennifer was excited to begin training for an upcoming 5K run in her neighborhood to raise money for charity. Despite being an avid jogger and gym enthusiast, it had been a while since she trained due to recent shelter-in-place orders during the COVID-19 pandemic. Jennifer worked as a physical therapy assistant, so exercise was not only a hobby but also important in her career. She worked in a skilled nursing facility primarily with geriatric patients. Because she was 39 years old and healthy, she had decided to wait on getting the COVID vaccine. She wanted to ensure vulnerable individuals such as those she worked with received their doses of vaccine first. Several weeks after resuming her training routine, Jennifer came down with a fever, sore throat, dry cough, headache, and body aches. She thought she had the flu but knew the symptoms were consistent with possible COVID-19 disease. Symptoms were mild to moderate at first, and she wasn't worried. She didn't have any preexisting conditions that she was aware, and she was young and healthy.

Over the next few days, Jennifer started having difficulties breathing and decided to go to the emergency department. She was admitted to the intensive care unit for observation and monitoring. In less than 24 hours, Jennifer's symptoms worsened. She began experiencing severe dyspnea (shortness of breath), with oxygen saturation levels (SpO_2) less than 90% and a respiratory rate greater than 30 breaths per minute, requiring supplemental oxygen. Jennifer's best friend came to the hospital but was not allowed near her given the highly contagious nature of SARS-CoV-2.

Jennifer's condition continued to deteriorate, with SpO_2 continuing to drop and the disease progressing to pneumonia, followed by acute respiratory failure requiring **intubation** and mechanical ventilation. Jennifer remained sedated and mechanically ventilated for 12 days.

Her condition eventually improved, and she was successfully weaned from the ventilator and transferred to an acute care rehabilitation setting.

The SLP who evaluated Jennifer noted continued respiratory difficulties. When speaking, she had significantly reduced loudness levels and short phrases (one to three words at a time); a breathy-hoarse voice quality and wet, productive cough; and significant feeding/swallowing deficits and discoordination caused by deconditioning (changes in the body associated with a period of inactivity) of muscles used in swallowing and speech production. A nasogastric tube (thin tube placed through the nose that runs to the stomach) was inserted to provide Jennifer nutrition until her conditioning and swallow function improved.

The treatment plan focused on systematically training the respiratory, speech, and swallowing musculature to regain strength, endurance, and coordination in each of these systems, with the goal of recovery to premorbid (prior to onset of disease) states.

As you read this chapter and subsequent chapters in this text, think about:

- The role of the SLP on the clinical team serving patients on mechanical ventilation, and the extent of knowledge required in anatomy and physiology to successfully evaluate and manage such patients
- How breathing for life, breathing for speech, feeding/swallowing, and communicating following acute respiratory failure with and without mechanical ventilation is affected
- How understanding the normal structure and function of swallowing and speech production will allow the SLP to develop and execute an effective treatment plan to improve breathing, communication, and swallowing function for Jennifer and other patients

Swallowing and speaking are biological functions that are often taken for granted. When you drink your coffee or tea and eat a piece of toast or bowl of cereal in the morning, you are probably not aware of the complex physiologic functions involved in these basic, everyday activities. Similarly, you express your thoughts and ideas with little or no apparent effort. But for all its apparent simplicity, swallowing and speech production requires an incredibly complex coordination of biophysical events involving hundreds of muscles and millions of nerves. It is paradoxical that such complex physiological behavior involved in swallowing and speaking appear to be effortless. This natural paradox is necessary, however. Imagine being fully aware of every bite of food or sip of liquid you take each day, or what your jaw, lips, and tongue are doing when you speak; you would probably be unable to successfully eat or drink or utter a single word. Monitoring all the muscles, nerves, and organ systems during swallowing and speech are impossible intellectual feats.

For many individuals, however, swallowing and speech production are anything but effortless. Sometimes abnormalities or diseases of anatomical structures and physiological systems that support swallowing and speech processes interfere with the ability to eat, drink, swallow, or talk. The Case Study in this chapter describes a patient with severe complications after contracting SARS-CoV-2 (severe acute respiratory syndrome coronavirus 2), the virus responsible for COVID-19 disease. Knowledge of the anatomy and physiology of the biological systems involved in speech and swallowing is fundamental to understanding and successfully treating the many different communication and feeding/swallowing disorders diagnosed and managed by speech-language pathologists (SLPs). Even if you do not plan to work in a health care setting, having a strong foundation in normal structure and function of speech and swallowing systems is essential to becoming a successful SLP in any clinical setting.

Before you can fully appreciate disease states that result in failure of organ systems involved in swallowing and speech production, you must first understand the normal structure and function of the subsystems that support these processes. **Anatomy** is the study of the structures of the body and the relationship of these structures to one another. **Physiology** is a branch of biology that is concerned with the functions of organisms and bodily structures.

Three physiological subsystems are involved in swallowing and speech production:

- The **respiratory system** moves air into and out of the body like a mechanical pump for life-sustaining processes like gas exchange (delivery of oxygen to the body and elimination of carbon dioxide), coordination with swallowing, coughing, as well as providing the driving force for speech production.

- The **laryngeal system** or *larynx* is an air valve that serves to protect the lower airways from foreign substances and it functions as a sound generator for speech production.

- The **upper airway system** comprises the supralaryngeal structures of the pharynx (throat), velopharynx, and oral and nasal cavities. These structures serve important roles in feeding/swallowing, resonance (how sound generated by the larynx is modified), and articulation. You may see the upper airway system further subdivided into the velopharyngeal-nasal subsystem (velopharynx and nasal airways) and the pharyngeal-oral subsystem (middle and lower pharynx and oral cavity) elsewhere (Hoit et al., 2022). For purposes of simplicity, we use the term *upper airway system* in this text.

In this chapter, we discuss the basic structures, muscles, and physiology of the three subsystems involved in normal swallowing and speech production, so you may better understand abnormalities that occur in disease states such as the case of Jennifer. We also address changes in each of these three physiological subsystems across the lifespan.

The Respiratory System

Learning Objective 3.1 List and describe the principal structures and muscles of the respiratory system and differentiate resting tidal breathing from speech breathing.

The primary biological function of the respiratory system is to supply oxygen to the blood and to remove excess carbon dioxide from the body. This process is automatic and controlled by the respiratory centers located in the brainstem of the central nervous system. Although the primary function of respiration is to sustain life, it also serves as the driving source for speech production. Air is inhaled (inspired) into your lungs to become the potential energy source for sound production. The air is then exhaled (expired) in a controlled manner, to be modified by the laryngeal and upper airway systems to generate speech sounds. For feeding, most healthy individuals hold their breath when they swallow; this coordination of breathing and swallowing is necessary to ensure substances are not accidentally sucked down into your airways or lungs while you're eating or drinking.

Structures of the Respiratory System

The respiratory system includes the pulmonary apparatus and chest wall, located within the torso, or body trunk. The pulmonary apparatus consists of the pulmonary airways and lungs, which provide oxygen and remove carbon dioxide from the cells of the body (Hoit & Weismer, 2018). The pulmonary apparatus is surrounded and encased by the structures of the chest wall, which include the rib cage wall, the diaphragm, the abdominal wall, and the abdominal content. The pulmonary apparatus and chest wall are linked together by fluid membranes forming a single functional unit (Hoit et al., 2022). As such, movements of the chest wall are indirectly translated to movements of the pulmonary apparatus.

The pulmonary airways are a complex network of tubes that move air to and from the lungs and between different parts of the lungs (Hixon & Hoit, 2005). The lungs, known as the organs of breathing, are a pair of irregular cone-shaped spongy structures that surround the pulmonary airways. They are composed of highly elastic fibers that can change in size and shape, enabling us to breathe (Hixon et al., 2008).

The pulmonary airways have numerous subdivisions and branches that form an inverted pulmonary tree. The top part of this tree is the **trachea** (windpipe), a tube composed of 16–20 C-shaped cartilages interconnected by fibrous tissue and muscle that extends from the larynx down through the neck into the torso. The open end of each tracheal cartilage faces toward the back where the trachea is completed by the flexible wall it shares with the esophagus (muscular tube that carries food and liquid to the stomach) (Hixon et al., 2020; Zemlin, 1998). The trachea divides into two smaller tubes, the left and right main-stem bronchi, and each further divides into lobar bronchi (Figure 3.1a), which are the tubes that run to the five lobes of the lungs, two lobes on the left and three lobes on the right (Figure 3.1b). The left lung is smaller than the right to allow room for the heart.

FIGURE 3.1 Anterior view of the trachea and bronchi (a) and anterior view of the bronchi entering the right and left lungs (b).

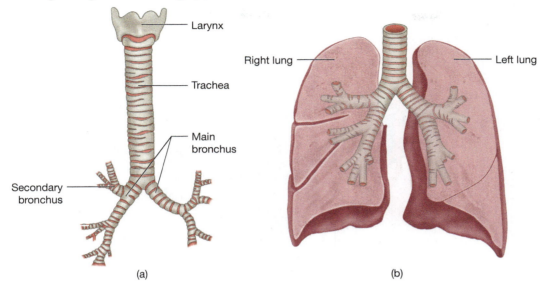

Larynx

Right lung

Left lung

Trachea

Main bronchus

Secondary bronchus

(a)   (b)

The five lobar bronchi each divide through more than 20 generations, each extending farther out through the lungs (Hixon et al., 2020).

Near the periphery of the lung, successive branches of the pulmonary airways lead to smaller and less rigid airway structures, the last of which are **alveoli**, the tiny air sacs where gas exchange occurs. Air contains approximately 21% oxygen; when you breathe in, the more than 300 million alveoli in your lungs pick up the oxygen and release the outgoing carbon dioxide when you exhale. The walls of the alveoli are very thin and allow oxygen and carbon dioxide to pass easily through very small blood vessels called capillaries (Figure 3.2). Oxygen leaves the alveoli and enters the bloodstream, oxygenating the tissues of the body as it travels. Body tissues release carbon dioxide as a by-product of metabolism; carbon dioxide travels through the bloodstream back to the alveoli where it is released (Hixon et al., 2020). Gas levels (oxygen and carbon dioxide) are regulated in arterial blood

---

CASE STUDY   Jennifer *(continued)*

Jennifer contracted SARS-CoV-2, which enters and replicates within the nasal mucosa and then travels to the conducting airways where it triggers an inflammatory response, manifesting in clinical signs and symptoms of COVID-19 disease. Infection often begins in the upper airway (nasal cavity, pharynx) epithelium, or thin, outer protective layer of tissue. However, in a subset of patients like Jennifer, the virus infects the lower airways, particularly the alveolar epithelium (the lining of the alveoli), causing diffuse damage that markedly impairs the ability of the alveoli to take in oxygen and release carbon dioxide. This leads to respiratory failure along with a host of other downstream negative effects (e.g., severe immune system reaction that can damage or kill tissue) (Brosnahan et al., 2020). When a patient is unable to breathe on their own to meet metabolic demand, mechanical ventilation may be necessary to provide and maintain adequate gas exchange and allow time for the lungs to heal, as was the case with Jennifer.

FIGURE 3.2 Blood supply of alveoli.

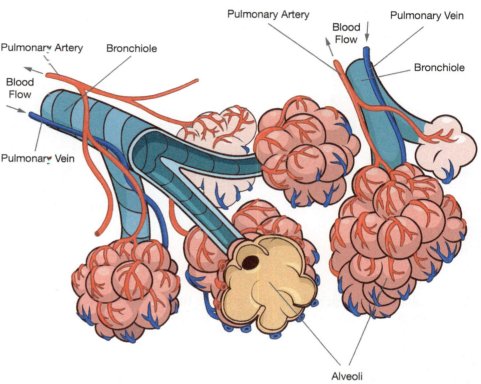

© Alexander_P/Shutterstock

by adjusting ventilation, that is, the amount of air inhaled (inspired) or exhaled (expired) (Hoit et al., 2022).

As previously mentioned, the chest wall encases the pulmonary apparatus and consists of four parts; the rib cage wall, the diaphragm, the abdominal wall, and the abdominal content. The rib cage wall is a framework of bone and cartilage that surrounds the lungs. It consists of the 12 pairs of ribs extending from the thoracic segment of the vertebral column (backbone) and attaching to cartilage connected to the flat center bone, or the sternum, along with the pectoral (shoulder) girdle at the top of the rib cage. The pectoral girdle is formed by the two clavicle (collar) bones in the front that attach at the back to the two flat, triangular bony scapulae (shoulder blades).

The **diaphragm**, which divides the upper (thorax or chest) and lower (abdomen or belly) cavities of the torso (body trunk), is dome-shaped and looks like an inverted bowl at rest. The left side of the diaphgram rests slighty lower than the right to accommodate the heart above and liver below. The diaghram is discussed in more detail in the next section given its importance as the primary muscle of inspiration.

The abdominal wall provides the framework for the lower half of the torso. It is oblong-shaped and consists of the vertebral column at the back, with 15 of the 32 vertebrae (i.e., five lumbar, five sacral, five coccygeal) that extend from approximately the bottom of the rib cage to the coccyx (tailbone) and the pelvic

FIGURE 3.3 Skeletal framework of the respiratory system.

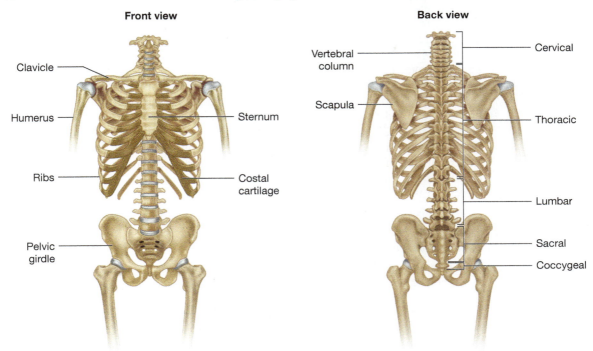

Front view

Clavicle

Humerus

Ribs

Pelvic
girdle

Sternum

Costal
cartilage

Back view

Vertebral
column

Scapula

Cervical

Thoracic

Lumbar

Sacral

Coccygeal

girdle (bony pelvis). The pelvic girdle is formed by the two large, irregularly shaped hip bones together with the sacral and coccygeal vertebrae (Hixon & Hoit, 2005; Hixon et al., 2008). Figure 3.3 depicts the skeletal framework of the respiratory system.

The abdominal wall is covered by two broad sheets of connective tissue; the one in the front is called the **abdominal aponeurosis** and the one in the back is the lumbodorsal fascia. The abdominal aponeurosis, along with the abdominal muscles (discussed later in this section), enclose and support the abdominal content, which include various internal structures like the stomach and intestines (Hixon & Hoit, 2005).

Muscles of the Respiratory System

The respiratory muscles can be divided functionally into muscles of inspiration (inhalation) and muscles of expiration (exhalation) or anatomically into muscles of the thorax and muscles of the abdomen. Inspiratory muscles are generally found above the diaphragm confined primarily to the thorax; expiratory muscles are located below the diaphragm and largely confined to the abdomen. Except for the diaphragm, all respiratory muscles are paired (i.e., located on both the right and left sides of the body).

Muscles of Inspiration

Inspiration, or inhalation, is the process by which we bring oxygen into our bodies. As already mentioned, the diaphragm separates the thorax (chest) from the abdomen and is the principal muscle of inspiration. The word *diaphragm* means "the fence between" (Hoit et al., 2022). The diaphragm is composed of a thin, flat, nonelastic central tendon and a broad rim of muscle fibers that course upward and insert into the edges of this central tendon (Hixon et al., 2020; Zemlin, 1998). The central tendon is in direct contact with each lung, as shown in Figure 3.4a. Figure 3.4b shows the relative position of the diaphragm at rest with its dome-shaped, inverted bowl-like appearance. When the diaphragm contracts during inspiration, it pulls the central tendon downward and forward and assumes a flattened configuration, enlarging the thorax vertically. Contraction of the diaphragm can also expand the circumference of the thorax by elevating the lower six ribs (Hoit et al., 2022). Because the lungs and thorax are held together as a unit by *pleural linkage* (i.e., by way of delicate, serous membranes that line the lungs and inner surface of the thoracic cavity), the lungs also expand when the thorax is expanded via contraction of the diaphragm.

> **CASE STUDY**   **Jennifer** *(continued)*
>
> Mechanical ventilation completely unloads the respiratory muscles and silences the respiratory control centers in the brainstem (Brosnahan et al., 2020), causing deconditioning, or muscle weakness and muscular atrophy. While Jennifer was able to eventually wean from the ventilator and breathe on her own, she did so with difficulty due to weakness of the diaphragm. The old saying "use it or lose it" is in fact true; if you have ever broken your arm or leg, think how it looked after the cast was removed, perhaps smaller and weaker due to muscle atrophy (or muscle wasting)?

FIGURE 3.4 Anterior view of the relationship of the diaphragm to the lungs (a) and anterior view of the diaphragm at rest (b).

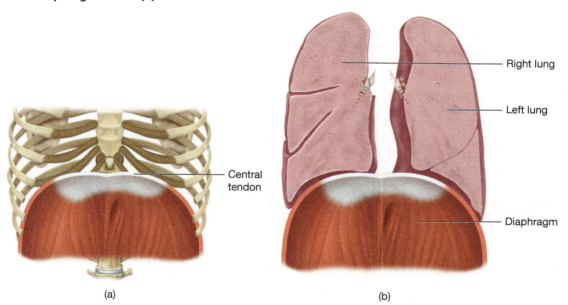

(a)   (b)

In addition to the diaphragm, numerous thoracic and neck muscles contribute to increasing the vertical dimension of the thoracic cavity, thereby contributing to inspiration. For example, *external intercostals*, as shown in Figure 3.5, which include 11 (paired) muscles located in the spaces between the outer portions of the ribs, elevate the rib cage when they contract, increasing the size of the thoracic cavity. Other muscles that serve to elevate the ribs and expand the thorax during inspiration include the *pectoralis major muscle*, *pectoralis minor muscle*, *serratus anterior muscle*, and *levatores costarum*. These muscles, with the exception of the *levatores costarum*, which are 12 small muscles located on the back of the rib cage wall, are illustrated in Figure 3.5.

The *sternocleidomastoid* is a prominent muscle positioned on the front and side of the neck (Figure 3.6). When the head is in a fixed position, contraction of the sternocleidomastoid raises the sternum and clavicle, thereby elevating the rib cage and assisting with inspiration. A similar action is performed by the scalene muscles, which are also muscles of the neck (Figure 3.6). Contraction of the scalene muscles raises the first two ribs, thereby assisting with inspiration (Hoit et al., 2022; Zemlin, 1998).

Muscles of Expiration

Expiration (or exhalation) allows for carbon dioxide to be expelled from the body and for speech to be produced. The *internal intercostal muscles*, illustrated in Figure 3.7, are 11 (paired) muscles that lie underneath the external intercostals in the internal portions of the rib interspaces. When they contract, they pull downward on the rib cage, thereby decreasing the size of the thorax, representing

FIGURE 3.5 **External intercostal muscles.**

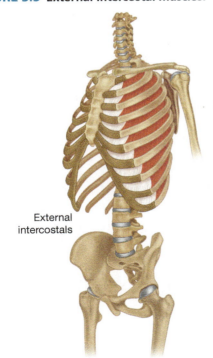

External
intercostals

FIGURE 3.6 **Anterior view of thoracic muscles.**

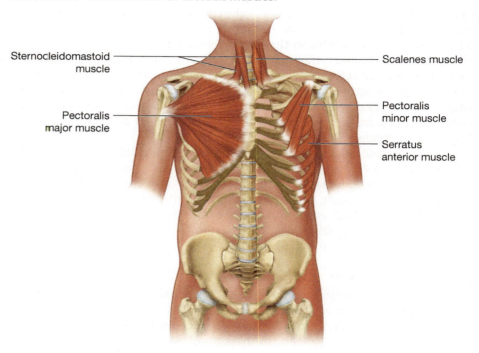

Sternocleidomastoid muscle

Scalenes muscle

Pectoralis major muscle

Pectoralis minor muscle

Serratus anterior muscle

FIGURE 3.7 **Internal intercostal muscles.**

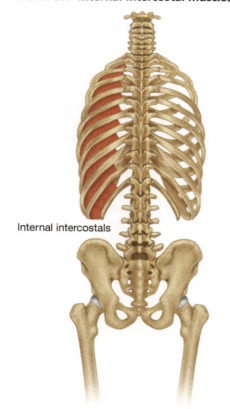

Internal intercostals

an expiratory action (Hoit et al., 2022). Recall that the external intercostal muscles are important during inspiration since their activation elevates the rib cage, increasing the size of the thorax.

The most important muscles of expiration are located on the front and sides of the abdomen. The *external oblique, internal oblique, transverse abdominis*, and the *rectus abdominis* are four paired muscles that encase a portion of the abdominal wall. Contraction of these abdominal muscles pull the lower ribs and sternum downward and force the abdominal wall inward (Hoit et al., 2022). During expiration, these muscles, depicted in Figure 3.8, assist the diaphragm's movement back to its relaxed dome-shaped configuration. Abdominal muscles are attached to the skeleton by means of the *abdominal aponeurosis*, the broad sheet of connective tissue that covers the front of the abdominal wall (Figure 3.8).

The Physiology of Tidal Breathing and Speech Breathing

Quiet breathing, or **resting tidal breathing**, is breathing to sustain life. As you are reading this chapter, you are using tidal breathing. The rate and depth of breaths taken during tidal breathing are determined by your body's oxygen needs and the amount of carbon dioxide in the blood and controlled by a network of

FIGURE 3.8 Anterior view of abdominal musculature. Muscles are cut to illustrate the different layers of muscle.

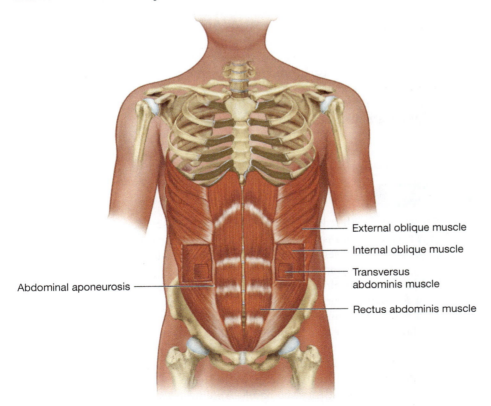

Abdominal aponeurosis

External oblique muscle

Internal oblique muscle

Transversus abdominis muscle

Rectus abdominis muscle

neurons in the brainstem that give rise to the continuous rhythmic pattern of breathing (Hixon & Hoit, 2005). Motor commands from the respiratory brainstem centers activate the diaphragm, the principal muscle of inspiration, and possibly also the external intercostal muscles to assist the diaphragm for a more forceful inspiration. When the diaphragm or other muscles of inspiration like the external intercostals contract, the chest wall expands, causing the lungs to also expand. **Alveolar pressure** (i.e., pressure within the lungs) decreases, creating a pressure gradient where pressure inside the pulmonary apparatus is below that of atmospheric pressure. Air then rushes into the lungs, equalizing alveolar pressure with atmospheric pressure (0 cm H_2O). Approximately 0.5 L of air is inhaled during quiet breathing.

When the resting tidal inspiratory cycle ends, expiration begins. Expiration results from the decrease in the size of the rib cage wall and compression of the lungs that increases the pressure within the lungs (Hixon & Hoit, 2005). Air rushes out of the lungs until equilibrium with pressure in the atmosphere is reached. Expiration during quiet breathing is a relatively passive process, meaning there isn't much need for expiratory muscular effort unless standing upright (Hixon et al., 2020). A respiratory cycle is defined as one inhalation followed by one exhalation. During resting tidal breathing, the duration of inspiration and expiration are relatively equal. Swallowing usually occurs during the expiratory phase of the breathing cycle, such that you expire, swallow (while holding your breath), and then continue to expire immediately after the swallow (Hoit et al., 2022).

Breathing for purposes of speech production differs from resting tidal breathing in several ways. First, contraction of the diaphragm produces rapid, forceful inspirations. Furthermore, the time spent inhaling is short relative to the time spent exhaling, which is much longer. You may inhale as much as 2 L of air during speech breathing depending on the specific demands of the utterance. Unlike expiration during quiet breathing, which is largely a passive process, active muscle contraction of both inspiratory and expiratory muscles is needed during speech. This prevents the air from quickly rushing out of your lungs so you can produce the appropriate amount of speech on one breath.

> Speech breathing differs from quiet breathing in many ways, but the oxygen and carbon dioxide ratio in the blood is the same for both types of breathing.

CASE STUDY   Jennifer *(continued)*

Jennifer struggled with reduced loudness and short phrases after she was weaned from the ventilator. This is consistent with weakened respiratory muscles for speech breathing purposes. Speech produced with adequate loudness requires inspiratory muscular effort to ensure speech starts at twice resting tidal breathing depth. Additionally, inspiratory and expiratory muscle activation is needed to maintain adequate loudness throughout the utterance and produce utterances of typical duration (about 10–12 words per breath group).

Jennifer would benefit from a muscle training exercise regimen to increase the strength and endurance of respiratory muscles to improve inspiration and expiration during speech breathing. Muscle training using an expiratory muscle strength training device, like the one shown in Figure 3.9, is one type of evidence-based intervention for patients who have weaned from a ventilator.

FIGURE 3.9 A patient works with an expiratory muscle strength training device to improve respiration, coughing, voice, and swallowing. This type of evidence-based behavioral intervention may be used with individuals who have weaned from mechanical ventilation.

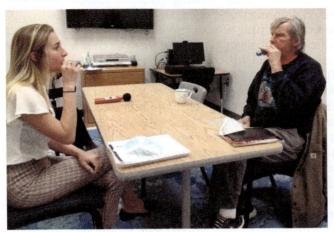

© Sarah Cullimore and Paul Marfechuk

Lifespan Issues of the Respiratory System

At birth, you had a quiet breathing rate between 30 and 80 breaths per minute. This is considerably higher than the adult quiet breathing rate of 12 to 20 breaths per minute By age 3, your tidal breathing rate had decreased to values between 20 and 30 breaths per minute. Watch preschool children and make note of their more frequent and deeper inhalations relative to adults. This change in rate occurs because at birth, newborns only have between 20 and 50 million alveoli (sites of gas exchange). Within the first couple of years of life there is a six- to eightfold increase in alveolarization (growth of alveoli) along with rapid growth of the lungs.

While lung growth slows and stabilizes by around 8 years of age, alveolarization continues through adolescence (Herring et al., 2014). As children grow, the structures of the respiratory system increase in size, and in turn lung capacity increases. Maximum lung function is achieved by around age 20 in females and by age 25 in males. Thereafter, a progressive decline in lung function occurs with aging (Sharma & Goodwin, 2006).

Breathing during vocalization in infants and toddlers is a period of emerging motor skill. For instance, the amount of air expired per breath increases as babies and toddlers get older and bigger (Hoit et al., 1990). As early as 18 months of age, inspirations that proceed vocalizations are quicker than those of tidal breathing, similar to adults (Boliek et al., 1997; Parham et al., 2011). Infants and toddlers are highly variable in their chest wall movements and lung volumes during speech breathing, unlike adults who are consistent in these movements during speech breathing across time (Hoit et al., 1990).

As young children get older, their control of speech breathing becomes more refined. By adolescence, breathing for speech is less variable and more adult-like.

Advanced age brings about stiffing (reduced compliance) of the chest wall and reductions in diaphragmatic strength (Sharma & Goodwin, 2006). However, changes in speech breathing appear more related to inefficiencies at the level of the larynx; older individuals tend to "waste air" as they are speaking. This usually begins in the seventh or eighth decade of life in healthy older individuals (Hoit & Weismer, 2018).

Maturation of swallowing and respiratory coordination during feeding occurs during the first year of life. Recall that the temporal coordination of respiration and swallowing in adults is exhale–swallow–exhale (Hoit et al., 2022). Swallowing usually starts in the mid-expiratory phase of respiration, and expiration resumes after the swallow. Continuing expiration after a swallow is regarded as an airway protective mechanism to prevent inhalation of residual material in the pharynx after the swallow.

As with speech breathing, the temporal pattern of breathing and swallowing in infants is more variable compared to adults, such that swallows are more likely to occur during inspiration. This is likely due to anatomical differences between infants and adults, as well as maturation of neural control mechanisms (Matsuo & Palmer, 2009). Infants rely on breastfeeding (or nipple feeding from a bottle) during the first few months of life; this form of feeding involves suck–swallow, or suck–swallow–breathe sequences usually repeated 8 to 12 times, followed by a rest period. Although infants can breathe while sucking, they hold their breath like adults during the swallow (Wilson et al., 1981).

Respiratory and swallowing coordination is affected by advanced age, with respiratory patterns characterized by increased inspiration both before and after the swallow in elderly individuals. This contributes to a lesser degree of airway protection (Matsuo & Palmer, 2009).

The Laryngeal System

Learning Objective 3.2 List and describe the principal structures, muscles, and functions of the laryngeal system.

From a biological standpoint, the larynx may be considered a component of the respiratory system. The primary biological function of the larynx is to prevent foreign objects from entering the trachea and lungs. Active closure of the laryngeal valve at multiple levels prevents foreign substances from entering the lower airways during swallowing. In addition, the larynx can impound air for forceful expulsion of foreign objects that threaten to enter the larynx or trachea (Hixon et al., 2020; Zemlin, 1998).

Structures of the Laryngeal System

The primary structure of the laryngeal system is the **larynx**, which is an air valve located within the front of the neck composed of cartilages, muscles, and other tissue (Figure 3.10). It is the principal sound generator for voice and speech production and is colloquially known as the "voice box." The larynx sits between

FIGURE 3.10 **Anterior view of the skeletal framework of the larynx.**

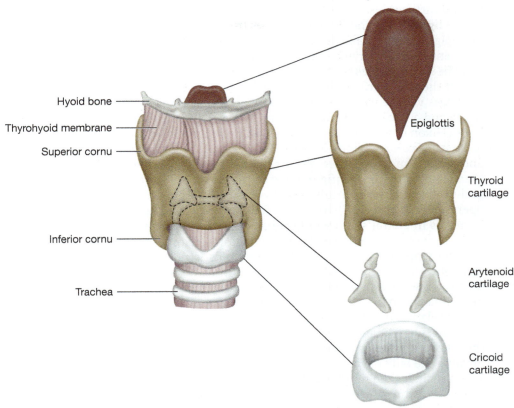

the trachea and pharynx and appears to be suspended from the **hyoid bone**, a U-shaped, free-floating structure (not attached to any other bone) that serves as the point of attachment for both laryngeal and tongue musculature.

The larynx consists of the thyroid, cricoid, and arytenoid cricoid cartilages connected to one another by joints, ligaments, and membranes. The **thyroid cartilage** is the largest laryngeal cartilage. It forms most of the front and sides of the laryngeal skeleton and protects the inner components of the larynx. The upper part has a V-shaped depression called the thyroid notch. It can be felt by palpating the front of the neck. Just below this notch is a jutting protrusion called the **thyroid prominence**, or Adam's apple (Hixon et al., 2020), which can be very prominent in some adult males. The back edges of the thyroid cartilage have two long upper horns, called the *superior cornua*, and two short lower horns, called the *inferior cornua*. The upper horns connect the thyroid cartilage with the hyoid bone, and the lower horns connect the thyroid and cricoid cartilages.

The *cricoid cartilage* is a ring-shaped structure that sits immediately above the first tracheal ring and directly below the thyroid cartilage. It forms the lower aspect of the laryngeal skeleton. On the upper sloping rim of the posterior border of each cricoid cartilage are the *arytenoid cartilages*. These paired cartilages are shaped like pyramids and have an apex (top), a base, and three sides. The base of each arytenoid cartilage has a forward pointed projection called the *vocal process* and a rounded broad projection extending toward the back called the *muscular process* (Hixon et al., 2020).

The epiglottis is a large leaf-shaped cartilage attached at its lower end to the thyroid cartilage just below the thyroid notch. Its midportion is attached to the body of the hyoid bone and its upper part is free, extending to the root of the tongue. The epiglottis has no role in speech production. Rather, it assists in preventing food from entering the larynx and lower airways during swallowing (see Figure 3.10).

The larynx houses the vocal folds, which are attached at the front near the midline of the thyroid cartilage and at the back to the vocal processes of the arytenoid cartilages via the vocal ligament. Each vocal fold is made up mostly of muscular tissue and a vocal ligament that run through it near its inner edge from front to back (Hixon et al., 2020). When viewed from above, the paired vocal folds appear to be ivory-colored bands of tissue. They abduct (move apart) during respiration and adduct (move together) during phonation. The space between the vocal folds is called the **glottis**. Configurations of the glottis are largely dependent on laryngeal muscle activity and adjustments of the arytenoid cartilages during vocal fold opening, or **adduction**, and vocal fold closing, or **abduction** (Zemlin, 1998). Increases in glottal size opening are associated with abduction of the vocal folds, while decreases are associated with adduction (Hixon et al., 2020).

The structural makeup of the vocal folds is not homogenous. Instead, it is recognized as having five different layers. The outermost layer is a thin, stiff epithelial tissue that gives the vocal folds their outer shape, followed by three layers of lamina propria (i.e., superficial layer made up of loose fibers that can be likened to soft gelatin; an intermediate layer that contains elastic fibers that are similar to soft rubber bands, and a deep layer that consists of collagen fibers similar to cotton thread); finally, an innermost layer of muscle fibers, with the *thyroarytenoid muscle* forming the bulk of each vocal fold. These five layers are subgrouped into the *body*, which includes the muscle fibers and the deepest layer of lamina propria, and the *cover*, consisting of the intermediate and superficial layers of lamina propria and the epithelium (Hixon et al., 2020).

Less prominent structures that lie above the vocal folds and attach to the thyroid cartilage at the front and attach to the front and sides of the arytenoid cartilages at the back are called the *ventricular folds*, or false vocal folds (Hixon et al., 2020). The ventricular folds move with the arytenoid cartilages but do not vibrate during phonation; the space between the ventricular folds is called the *false glottis* (Zemlin, 1998). During swallowing, both the vocal folds and ventricular folds adduct firmly to help seal off the entrance to the trachea to protect against foreign substances entering the larynx and pulmonary airways (Hixon et al., 2020).

Muscles of the Larynx

The laryngeal muscles are divided into three groups: intrinsic, extrinsic, and supplementary muscles (Zemlin, 1998).

The intrinsic muscles, with both points of attachment on the larynx itself, are critical for phonation and for modifying the pitch and loudness of the voice. Intrinsic muscles are the following:

- Thyroarytenoid
- Cricothyroid
- Posterior cricoarytenoid
- Lateral cricoarytenoid
- Arytenoid

FIGURE 3.11 Laryngeal muscles responsible for phonation and changing vocal fold length and tension.

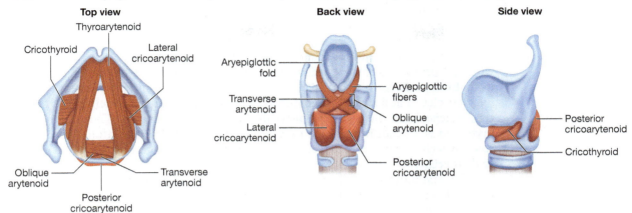

Figure 3.11 depicts the laryngeal muscles important for adducting and abducting the vocal folds and altering vocal fold length and tension. As mentioned, the *thyroarytenoid* muscle forms the bulk of each vocal fold. This muscle extends from the angle of the thyroid cartilage to the arytenoid cartilage.

Contraction of the longitudinal fibers of the thyroarytenoid muscle reduces the distance between the thyroid and arytenoid cartilages, resulting in a forward pull on the arytenoid cartilage rocking it toward midline, shortening (i.e., relaxing) the vocal folds. Tensing of the vocal folds by the thyroarytenoid muscle occurs when opposing intrinsic laryngeal muscles are also active (Hixon et al., 2020).

The thyroarytenoid muscle is often described as having two distinct bundles: the external thyroarytenoid muscle (thyromuscularis) and the internal thyroarytenoid muscle (thyrovocalis or vocalis), although this viewpoint is not universally accepted. There is some evidence to suggest the two subdivisions of the thyroarytenoid muscle have different types of muscle fibers, suggesting they function independently.

The thyromuscularis (lateral to the thyrovocalis or vocalis) is thought to be responsible for shortening or relaxing the vocal folds (closing the glottis), while contraction of the thyrovocalis or vocalis muscle, which makes up the main vibrating mass of the vocal folds, draws the thyroid and cricoid cartilages farther apart in front thereby tensing the vocal folds (Hixon et al., 2020; Sanders et al., 1998; Seikel et al., 2010).

The thyroarytenoid muscle therefore has differential actions depending on activation of other laryngeal muscles. This muscle is important for adjusting pitch, the perceptual correlate of *fundamental frequency* discussed later in this chapter. It is also associated with increases in loudness, particularly at lower pitch ranges (Hirano et al., 1970; Isshiki, 1964).

The *cricothyroid* muscle is a fan-shaped muscle with its fibers extending outward as they course from the cricoid cartilage to the thyroid cartilage. Two subdivisions of the cricothyroid muscle are recognized: the *pars oblique* and the *pars rectus*. When the cricothyroid muscles (pars oblique and pars rectus) contract, the distance between the front of the thyroid cartilage and the vocal processes of the arytenoid cartilages increases, thereby lengthening and stiffening (tensing) the vocal folds (Hoit et al., 2022). Increasing the length and tension of the vocal folds via the cricothyroid muscle results in an increase in what we commonly think of as a higher pitch.

The *posterior cricoarytenoid muscle* is a fan-shaped muscle located on the back surface of the cricoid cartilage (Hixon et al., 2020). The posterior cricoarytenoid muscle is the sole muscle of abduction or moving apart of the vocal folds. Contraction of this muscle rotates the vocal processes of the arytenoid cartilages away from the midline, separating the vocal folds and opening the glottis.

Muscles of adduction or moving together of the vocal folds include the *lateral cricoarytenoid* and the *arytenoid*, also called *interarytenoid muscles*. The lateral cricoarytenoid is a small fan-shaped muscle that brings the front portion of the vocal folds together, while the arytenoid muscles bring the back portion of the vocal folds together.

The arytenoid (or interarytenoid) muscles are complex structures located on the back surfaces of the arytenoid cartilages with two separate subdivisions: the *transverse arytenoid* muscle and the *oblique arytenoid* muscle.

Some muscle fibers of the oblique arytenoid muscle insert into the epiglottis and are given a separate name, the *aryepiglottic muscle*. Contraction of the aryepiglottic muscles pulls the epiglottis backward and downward, covering the upper opening of the larynx. This plays a key role in the protection of the pulmonary airways during swallowing (Hixon et al., 2020; Hoit et al., 2022).

Extrinsic laryngeal muscles support and stabilize the larynx, as well as serve a role in changing its position in the neck (Hixon et al., 2020). Extrinsic muscles are the following:

- Sternothyroid
- Thyrohyoid
- Inferior constrictor muscles

Extrinsic laryngeal muscles are shown in Figure 3.12.

Supplemental muscles generally have one point of attachment on the hyoid bone and are subdivided into the suprahyoid and infrahyoid groups. Muscles in the

FIGURE 3.12 **Extrinsic laryngeal muscles.**

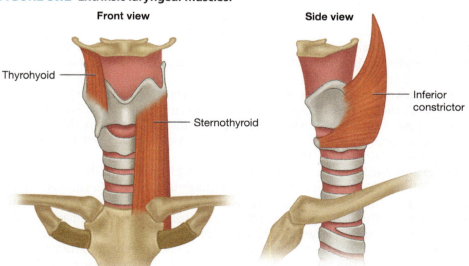

suprahyoid group are generally located above the hyoid bone and assist in laryngeal elevation. Those in the infrahyoid group are generally located below the hyoid bone and assist in laryngeal depression. Place your hand on your larynx and swallow. Note that your larynx is pulled upward and then lowered. This motion is a result of supplemental muscle contraction.

CASE STUDY   Jennifer *(continued)*

Like respiratory muscles that experience long periods of disuse, laryngeal muscles become deconditioned and weakened as the result of prolonged disuse also. Speech and voice behavioral therapies are necessary to recondition muscles during speech production (e.g., practicing speech, voice production drills with feedback from the SLP). Additionally, during endotracheal intubation for purposes of mechanical ventilation, a tube is inserted into the trachea via the mouth (or nose) (Figure 3.13).

Because this tube passes through the larynx on its way down to the trachea, damage (temporary or permanent) can occur to laryngeal structures and the vocal folds or alter vocal fold tissue, causing edema (swelling), hematoma (bruising), or ulceration (Yonick et al., 1990). Changes in Jennifer's voice quality noted by the SLP, specifically a breathy-hoarse voice following extubation (removal of the tube), are common and usually resolve without medical or behavioral intervention. This will depend on the nature of the problem (e.g., laryngeal edema vs. arytenoid cartilage dislocation, a much less common intubation-related injury, vs. voice quality changes associated with muscle deconditioning).

FIGURE 3.13 Mannequin connected to mechanical ventilator via endotracheal tube (tube inserted into the mouth and passing through the larynx and vocal folds on the way down to the trachea) to move air in and out of the lungs.

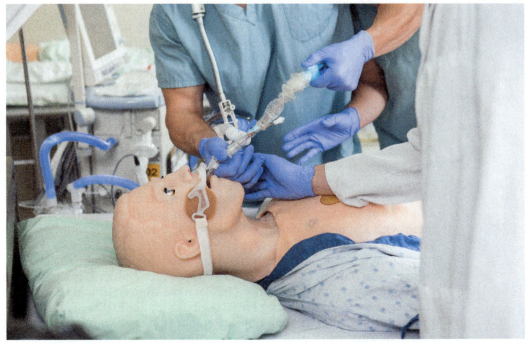

© Tyler Olson/123RF

Lifespan Issues of the Laryngeal System

The laryngeal system also goes through significant changes as a function of age. In a newborn, the larynx is small and positioned very high in the neck. The high position of the larynx near the hyoid bone allows the newborn to breathe and nurse simultaneously, while protection of the airway is maintained. As the infant grows, the larynx begins to move downward in the neck; by age 3, the larynx has descended to the middle of the fifth cervical (neck) vertebrae (bone). It reaches its final position in the region of the seventh cervical vertebrae sometime between 10 and 20 years of age (Hixon et al., 2014).

The laryngeal cartilages increase in size, particularly during the first 18 months of life, and become less pliable with age (Kent, 1997; Tucker &Tucker, 1979). For the most part, growth of the laryngeal cartilages involves an increase in size and weight while maintaining their basic configuration (Kahane, 1978, 1982). The hyoid bone ossifies (turns to bone) by 2 years of age. Much later in life, laryngeal cartilages begin to show signs of ossification (Aronson, 1990b).

The vocal folds are approximately 4 to 6 mm long in a newborn. By age 6, they increase to about 8 or 9 mm in length. The increase in length of the vocal folds is equal in boys and girls until puberty. During puberty, the vocal folds increase to approximately 12 to 17 mm in girls and 15 to 25 mm in boys. Between 12.5 and 14.5 years of age is when a noticeable decrease in fundamental frequency (vocal pitch) occurs in males, often accompanied by pitch breaks (Hixon et al., 2020; Hollien et al., 1994). However, some acoustic studies show a male–female difference in fundamental frequency by age 5 to 8 years, reflecting possibly learned characteristics associated with gender (Bent & Holt, 2017; Glaze et al., 1988). By adulthood, females' vocal folds are about 21 mm in length and males' are about 29 mm in length (Kent, 1997). The sex difference in adult vocal fold length accounts for the fact that men typically have lower-pitched voices compared to women.

The structural composition of the vocal folds undergoes significant change during development. In a newborn, the vocal folds' makeup is homogenous, with undifferentiated lamina propria (Hirano & Sato, 1993); the adult multilayered lamina propria is present by about 16 years of age. The vocal ligament appears sometime between 1 and 4 years of age (Kent, 1997).

With advancing age, laryngeal cartilages begin to ossify, although the female larynx, unlike that of males, never completely ossifies; these changes are most evident during singing and manifested as a reduced vocal range (Kent, 1997). The vocal folds begin to lose muscle tissue (**atrophy**) while the more superficial layers of vocal fold tissue thicken and lose their elasticity (Xue & Hao, 2003). As a result, the vocal folds become stiffer and less flexible with age. Age effects are realized in men as an increase in pitch, likely due to muscle atrophy and loss of mass of the folds. Women, in contrast, experience a decrease in pitch with age much later in life, possibly due to age-related increases in edema (swelling) of the vocal folds (Ferreri, 1959; Honjo & Isshiki, 1980). Women who have completed menopause have lower fundamental frequencies compared to women who have not (Stoicheff, 1981); however, postmenopausal women using hormone replacement therapy (HRT) have higher fundamental frequencies compared to those not using HRT (Hamdan et al., 2018). Transgender women using hormone therapies do not experience increases in fundamental frequency before or after menopause (Kim, 2020). Transgender care is discussed in more detail in Chapter 9.

The Upper Airway System

Learning Objective 3.3 Briefly describe the structures and functions of the upper airway.

The upper airway extends from the opening of the mouth to the vocal folds comprising the oral cavity, nasal cavities, and the pharyngeal cavity, as shown in Figure 3.14. Together they form the *vocal tract*, which is a resonant acoustic tube that shapes the sound energy produced by the respiratory and laryngeal systems

FIGURE 3.14 Schematic of the human vocal tract.

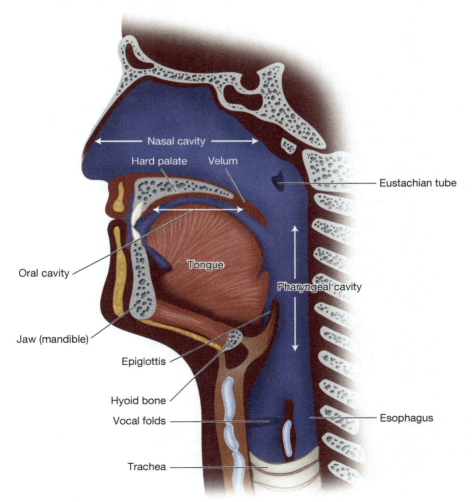

into all the English speech sounds (Kent, 1997). Structures important for swallowing and speech production such as the teeth, tongue, and velum (soft palate) are housed within these cavities.

Structures of the Upper Airway System

The skeletal framework supporting the upper airway system consists of the first six cervical (neck) vertebrae and 22 skull bones that form the cranium (braincase that houses and protects the brain) and facial skeleton (forehead, eyes, nose, mouth, and upper pharynx). There are eight cranial bones, some of which are paired and include the temporal bones (sides of the lower braincase) and parietal bones (sides of the upper braincase). Unpaired cranial bones are the frontal bone (front of the upper braincase), occipital bone (back of the lower braincase), sphenoid bone (double-winged structure behind the eyes that forms the base of the front of the cranium and the back wall of the nasal cavities), and the ethmoid bone (complex, delicate bone structure that forms the upper sidewalls of the nasal cavities and the upper part of their medial wall) (Hixon et al., 2020; Hoit et al., 2022).

The 14 facial bones, most of which are paired, include the maxillary bones that form the upper jaw, hard palate (or roof of the mouth), and front floor of the nasal cavities; the palatine bones that form the back of the roof of the mouth and back of the floor of the nasal cavities; the inferior nasal conchae that form the lower sidewalls of the nasal cavities; the lacrimal bones, the smallest of the facial bones, that form part of the orbits and articulate with the inferior nasal concha, ethmoid, frontal, and maxillary bones; nasal bones that form the bridge of the outer nose; and zygomatic bones that form the prominences of the cheeks and are also called cheekbones. Unpaired facial bones are the vomer bone that forms the lower part of the medial wall of the nasal cavities and the mandible or lower jaw (Hixon et al., 2020; Hoit & Weismer, 2018).

Some of these bones are shown in Figure 3.15a. Except for the *mandible* or lower jaw, the bones of the face and cranium are fused tightly together by sutures. The mandible articulates with the right and left temporal bones by means of a complex joint known as the *temporomandibular joint (TMJ)*. On each side of the mandible toward the back is an upward projection called the *ramus*. The upper part of each ramus has two projections; the one at the front is called the *coronoid process* and the one at the back is called the *condylar process*, or *condyle*, which along with the temporal bone forms the lower bony part of the TMJ. Movements of the mandible are mediated through the condyloid processes of the TMJ and enable the mandible to move up and down, forward and backward, and side to side, which is important for chewing (Hoit & Weismer, 2018).

Additional boney structures depicted in Figure 3.15b are the mastoid, styloid process, and zygomatic arch, which are all parts of the paired temporal bones (sides of the lower braincase). A projection of bone from the base of the mastoid called the *mastoid process* provides attachment for the sternocleidomastoid and other neck muscles. The styloid process is a sharp pillar of bone that serves as the site of origin for several muscles important for chewing, swallowing, and speech production (Zemlin, 1998).

Teeth

Adults have a total of 32 teeth that are held within the *alveolar processes* (thick spongy projections) of the mandible (lower jaw) and *maxilla* (upper jaw) inside the oral cavity. The obvious biological function of teeth is chewing food, but the teeth play a minor role in the production of some English speech sounds.

FIGURE 3.15 **Anterior (a) and lateral (b) views of skull bones.**

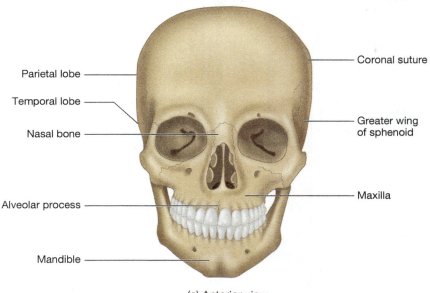

Coronal suture

Parietal lobe

Temporal lobe

Nasal bone

Greater wing of sphenoid

Alveolar process

Maxilla

Mandible

(a) Anterior view

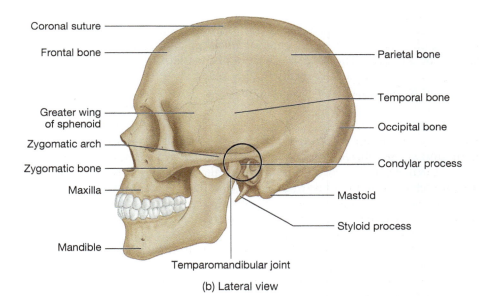

Coronal suture

Frontal bone

Parietal bone

Temporal bone

Greater wing of sphenoid

Occipital bone

Zygomatic arch

Zygomatic bone

Condylar process

Maxilla

Mastoid

Mandible

Styloid process

Temparomandibular joint

(b) Lateral view

Horizontal bones of the maxilla form the bony hard palate, comprising the front two-thirds of the roof of the mouth. Figure 3.16 shows the structures of the bony hard palate and the relationship of the maxillary teeth.

Oral Cavity

In the field of speech-language pathology, scientific jargon is a necessity but can be a bit much at times. For instance, your mouth is termed the *oral cavity*, and the front entryway of your mouth (or oral cavity) is called the *oral vestibule*. This area

FIGURE 3.16 Inferior view of an adult bony hard palate and teeth.

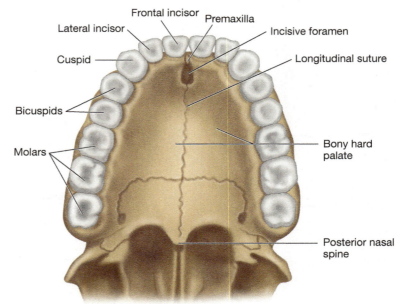

includes the lips, cheeks, front teeth, and front portions of the alveolar processes of the maxilla and mandible. The anterior *faucial pillars* (palatoglossal arches) form the back of the cavity. The hard palate (roof of the mouth) and velum make up the top of your mouth, and the floor is mainly made up of the tongue (Hixon et al., 2020; Hoit & Weismer, 2018). See Figure 3.17.

Tongue

The principal structure within the oral cavity important for swallowing and speech production is the *tongue*. The tongue is a muscular hydrostat, meaning it has no bone or cartilage, much like an elephant's trunk. It provides its own structural support through contraction of its muscles but also has a "soft skeleton" of connective tissue that surrounds and separates its different components (Hixon et al., 2020; Kent, 1997). It can be functionally divided into five parts: the *body*, or central mass; the *root*, which forms the front wall of the pharyngeal cavity; the broad surface called the *dorsum*; and the *blade* that makes up its front surface and lies just behind the *tongue tip* (Kent, 1997).

The tongue is made up of four intrinsic muscles and four extrinsic muscles. Intrinsic tongue muscles are confined to the tongue itself and include the *superior longitudinal*, *inferior longitudinal*, *vertical*, and *transverse* muscles.

The *superior longitudinal muscle* pulls the lateral margins of the tongue up, forming a trough-like shape. Contraction of the *inferior longitudinal muscle* shortens the tongue and pulls the tongue tip downward. The tongue can be narrowed and elongated or broadened and flattened by contraction of the *transverse* and *vertical* muscles, respectively.

The extrinsic tongue muscles originate from structures outside the tongue and insert on various locations within the tongue, blending with intrinsic muscle fibers.

FIGURE 3.17 **Front view of the soft palate and uvula.**

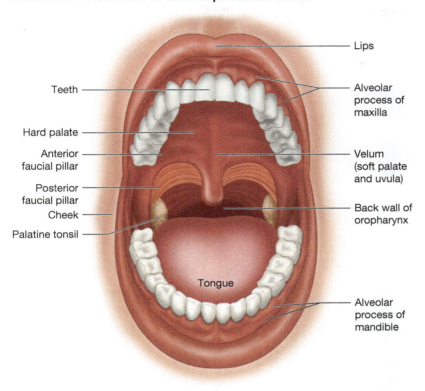

Lips

Teeth

Alveolar process of maxilla

Hard palate

Anterior faucial pillar

Velum (soft palate and uvula)

Posterior faucial pillar

Cheek

Back wall of oropharynx

Palatine tonsil

Tongue

Alveolar process of mandible

They are the *styloglossus, palatoglossus, hyoglossus,* and *genioglossus* muscles. The extrinsic muscles are responsible for changing the position of the tongue in the oral cavity. Figure 3.18 shows the locations of some of the intrinsic and extrinsic tongue muscles.

Pharynx

The *pharynx* (throat) is a highly mobile tube made up of tendon and muscle that starts at the base of the skull where it is widest and extends down to the larynx, narrowing in length on its way down. It is open at the front and connects from top to bottom with the nasal cavities, oral cavity, and the entrance to the larynx. At its lower end, the pharynx is continuous with the esophagus where its front and back walls are in direct contact. During swallowing and regurgitation, this contact is broken (Hixon et al., 2008; Hoit et al., 2022). The pharynx has three cavities designated from top to bottom as the nasopharynx, oropharynx, and laryngopharynx. Muscles of the pharynx that influence its size and shape are located within these three cavities and include the *superior constrictor, middle constrictor,* and *inferior constrictor* muscles, which are muscles that constrict the pharynx; the *salpingopharyngeas* and *palatopharyngeas* muscles pull both upward and inward on the pharynx; and finally, the *stylopharyngeus* muscle pulls upward and outward on the pharynx (Hixon et al., 2020; Hoit et al., 2022).

FIGURE 3.18 Intrinsic and extrinsic muscles of the tongue.

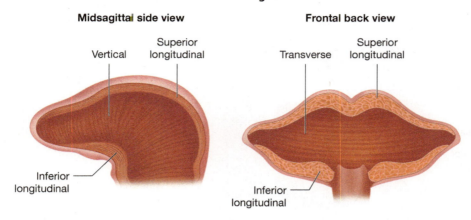

Midsagittal side view

Vertical · Superior longitudinal · Inferior longitudinal

Frontal back view

Transverse · Superior longitudinal · Inferior longitudinal

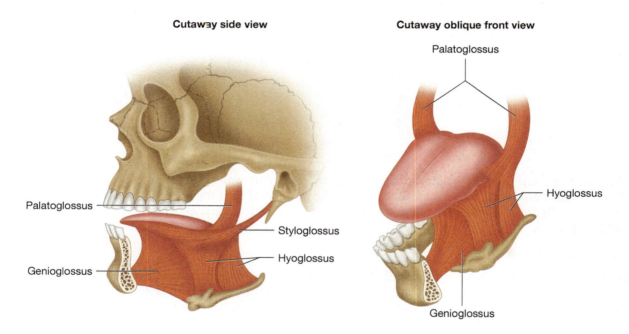

Cutaway side view

Palatoglossus · Genioglossus · Styloglossus · Hyoglossus

Cutaway oblique front view

Palatoglossus · Hyoglossus · Genioglossus

Velum

The *velum*, or soft palate, located in the pharynx is an important structure for both speech and swallowing. You can see a portion of your velum (which means "curtain") by looking into a well-illuminated bathroom mirror. You will see a structure projecting downward called the **uvula** (which means "little grape"); the uvula is the termination of your velum. Muscles of the velum include the *palatal levator (levator veli palatini)*, *palatal tensor (tensor veli palatini)*, *uvulus*, *glossopalatine*, and *pharyngopalatine* muscles. Most of these muscles act to effectively raise or lower the velum. The *palatal levator* muscle, which forms much of the bulk of the velum, pulls the velum upward and backward; the *uvulus* muscle shortens and lifts the velum; the *glossopalatine* muscle pulls the velum down and forward; and the *pharyngopalatine* muscle pulls the velum down and backward. See Figure 3.19.

FIGURE 3.19 Muscles of the velum.

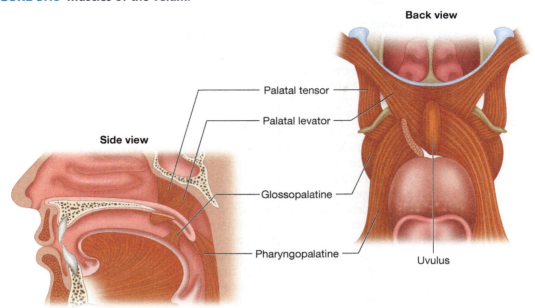

Back view

Side view

Palatal tensor

Palatal levator

Glossopalatine

Pharyngopalatine

Uvulus

The *palatal tensor*, or *tensor veli palatini* muscle, is now known to have a minimum effect on the velum, although it does play an important role in opening the eustachian (auditory) tube, permitting air pressure in the middle ear to equalize with atmospheric pressure (Hoit et al., 2022).

When you breathe through your nose, the velum hangs like a curtain from the posterior aspect of the bony hard palate. During swallowing and speech production, the velum elevates and decouples (separates) the nasal cavity from the pharyngeal cavity, leading to **velopharyngeal closure**, or contact of the velum with the posterior and lateral pharyngeal walls (Kuehn & Henne, 2003). Failure to separate these cavities during swallowing would result in food passing through the nasal cavity.

During speech production, velar elevation is necessary to prevent air from escaping through the nose and to allow sufficient air pressure to build up in the oral cavity for production of pressure sounds (e.g., /p/, /b/). Any air that escapes through the nose during speech can result in a nasal-sounding resonance (quality).

CASE STUDY   Jennifer *(continued)*

While structures of the upper airway are important in speech production, as is discussed below, these structures are also important for swallowing (discussed in greater detail in Chapter 11). Difficulties effectively and safely moving food and liquid from the mouth to the stomach after extubation are common in critical care patients, as seen with Jennifer. Oropharyngeal muscle deconditioning and atrophy (wasting) from disuse can occur with lengthy periods of intubation, along with diminished sensation and proprioception (awareness of position or movement) of upper airway structures contributing to feeding and swallowing deficits postextubation (Rassameehiran et al., 2015).

Lifespan Issues of the Upper Airway System

The bones of the skull grow rapidly during the first years of life and reach adult size by about 8 years of age. At birth, the newborn has 45 separate skull bones that ultimately fuse into 22 bones by adulthood. Once they fuse together, the cranium appears to be one solid bone.

The bones of the lower portion of the face grow at a much slower rate than the bones of the skull. These lower facial bones do not reach maximum adult size until about 18 years of age. Because of these different growth patterns of the skull bones and the facial bones, the face can grow downward and forward relative to the cranium (Kent, 1997).

Dentition in the infant begins to emerge at about 6 months of age. This first set of teeth is temporary and is usually referred to as primary, or deciduous, dentition. Emergence of the primary dentition is usually complete by 3 years of age. At approximately 5 years of age the primary teeth begin to fall out, and the permanent, or secondary, teeth begin to appear. The emergence of the secondary teeth is usually complete by 18 years of age.

The tongue of the newborn almost fills the oral cavity and is oriented primarily in the horizonal plane. During the first few years of life, the posterior third of the tongue gradually descends into the pharyngeal cavity and continues to do so until about age 5. Growth of the tongue continues throughout childhood and puberty, with occasional growth spurts along the way; it reaches its adult size by about 16 years of age (Kerr et al., 1991). In general, growth of the tongue shows a similar pattern of growth with the mandible (lower jaw) and the lips (Kent, 1997). With advancing age, tongue movements during swallowing are slower and have decreased range of motion when compared to younger adults (Sonies et al., 1984; Steele & Van Lieshout, 2009).

At birth, the epiglottis is in contact with velum, which facilitates simultaneous nursing and (nasal) breathing; around 4 to 6 months the epiglottis and velum separate (Kent & Murray, 1982; Sasaki et al., 1977). The pharynx is approximately 4 cm long in the newborn and lengthens rapidly downward, assisting the descent of the larynx. The pharynx is approximately 12 cm long by adulthood (Tourne, 1991).

In the first few months of life, the velopharynx is open during cry and non-cry vocalizations, causing the infant to sound nasalized; that is, sound energy is directed through the nasal cavity rather than through the oral cavity (Hixon et al., 2020; Kent, 1981). As early as 2 months of age, infants can close the velopharynx for syllable productions, but this closure is not consistent (Thom et al., 2006). At some point between 6 months and 3 years of age, children consistently achieve airtight velopharyngeal closure for production of oral speech sounds. Adult patterns of velopharyngeal closure are achieved by age 3 and are generally maintained throughout the lifespan (Hixon et al., 2014). Aging has been shown to have minimal impact on velopharyngeal function as it relates to speech production (Hoit et al., 1994; Zajac, 1997).

Finally, the oral cavity gradually increases in length and cross section with age, continuing into advanced age (Israel, 1968, 1973). The bones of the oral cavity and oral vestibule may become more fragile, and muscles may lose bulk and power with advancing age (Fremont & Hoyland, 2007). Saliva thickens and changes in composition in older individuals (Hoit et al., 2022), which can cause dry mouth and negatively impact feeding and swallowing and speech production.

The Speech Production Process

Learning Objective 3.4 Explain the speech production process.

Up to this point, we have focused on the basic anatomy and physiology of the respiratory, laryngeal, and upper airway systems and their healthy structure and function, and how diseases such as COVID-19 alter each of these subsystems. Now we turn to the normal process of speech production, which is considered an adaptation to each organ system's biological functioning (e.g., breathing for life, airway protection, feeding/swallowing). We discussed how resting tidal breathing differs from speech breathing. We now explore how the subsystems work together for speech production to occur.

Speech begins with sound produced by vocal fold vibration, or **phonation**. Phonation is initiated by approximating or adducting the vocal folds and closing the glottis. Recall that laryngeal muscles important in vocal fold adduction include the *lateral cricoarytenoids*, *arytenoids*, and *thyrovocalis* portions of the *thyroartenoid* muscles, while vocal fold abduction (movement of the folds away from midline) occurs primarily by contraction of the *posterior cricoarytenoid* muscles. Once the vocal folds are closed, air pressure generated by the respiratory system, called *alveolar pressure*, increases beneath the vocal folds. Once vocal fold vibration is established, laryngeal muscular contractions are not needed; rather, movements of the vocal folds are passive during vibration and maintained by the steady source of energy generated by the respiratory system (Hoit et al., 2022).

The air pressure generated by the respiratory system from below displaces the lower edges of each vocal fold laterally (apart). This is followed by lateral displacement of the middle and upper edges of each vocal fold until the vocal folds are fully separated, opening the airway (frames 1, 2, 3, and 4 of Figure 3.20). Following maximum opening of the folds, the vocal folds' natural elastic restoring forces cause the lower edges of the folds to begin to move inward toward the midline, followed by the middle and upper edges, until the vocal folds collide with each other, closing off the airway (frames 5, 6, and 7 of Figure 3.20). This pattern of movement of the vocal folds during vibration is called *vertical phase difference*; the entire process is repeated in a cyclical fashion at the average **fundamental frequency** of vibration, or the number of cycles (i.e., opening and closing of the vocal folds) per second (Story, 2002).

Earlier theories of vocal fold vibration (i.e., Van den Berg, 1958) described the importance of the "Bernoulli effect" as the primary mechanism responsible for sustained vocal fold vibration. The "Bernoulli effect," based on Bernoulli's principle, states that high air velocity through a narrow opening (the glottis) creates a negative pressure that sucks the vocal folds together; afterward, air pressure

FIGURE 3.20 Anterior view of the vocal folds during one cycle of vibration. Air from the lungs creates pressure beneath the vocal folds (1, 2, and 3). This pressure causes them to separate (4). The natural elastic restoring forces of the vocal folds and the time delay with respect to the upper and lower portions of the vocal folds causes them to begin to close (5 and 6). The vocal folds close the glottis to end the cycle, and the next cycle begins (7).

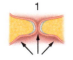 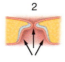 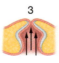 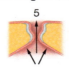 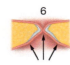 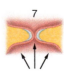

1   2   3   4   5   6   7

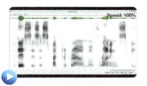

Pearson eTextbook
Video Example 3.1

This video contains a spectrogram, or visual representation of the acoustic characteristics of speech sounds, while the speaker is talking. Notice the wide, dark horizontal bands of acoustic energy. These are the vowel formant frequencies that correspond to the resonant frequencies of the vocal tract.

Air-filled cavities are acoustic resonators. The frequency or frequencies at which a filled cavity will resonate are determined by the volume of the cavity, the area of the opening of the cavity, and the length of the opening of the cavity.

---

builds up below the closed vocal folds and then blows the vocal folds apart; the process then repeats itself. We know now that the "Bernoulli effect" has almost no role in vocal fold vibration (cf., Story, 2002; Van den Berg, 1958). Rather, the self-sustaining vibration of the vocal folds, once set in motion by the respiratory system, is due to the pattern of vertical phase difference of the vocal folds (i.e., separation of the inferior margins of the vocal folds before the superior margins), combined with the changes in air pressure and air flow right above the glottis that transfers energy to the vocal folds during continued cycles of vibration (Hoit et al., 2022; Kent, 1997).

Recall that the vocal tract is made up of the upper airway structures of oral, nasal, and pharyngeal cavities. For each vibratory cycle, the air in the vocal tract is set into vibration and sound is produced. The sound that results from vocal fold vibration is complex, consisting of a fundamental frequency, or the lowest-frequency component that corresponds to the rate of vocal fold vibration and approximately 40 additional higher frequencies called **harmonics**. The harmonic frequencies are whole-number multiples of the fundamental frequency. For example, when the fundamental frequency is 100 Hz, the second harmonic is 200 Hz, the third is 300 Hz, and so on. Figure 3.21 is a stylized spectrum of the complex sound produced by vocal fold vibration. A spectrum represents the frequencies of a complex sound along the horizontal (*x*) axis, and their relative *intensity* (perceptually known as loudness) is represented on the

FIGURE 3.21 A spectrum illustrating a fundamental frequency of 200 Hz and related harmonics (a) and a spectrum of a fundamental frequency of 100 Hz and related harmonics (b).

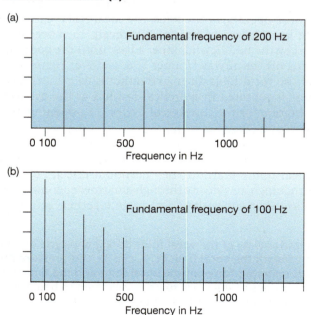

vertical (*y*) axis. Note that the relative intensity decreases systematically with increases in harmonic frequency.

The vocal tract is an acoustic resonator that will modify the quality of the sound produced by the larynx. In any acoustic resonator some frequencies are reduced or attenuated and other frequencies are enhanced, depending on certain physical aspects of the resonator. In speech, these vocal tract resonances are called *formants*, and their frequencies are called *formant frequencies*. Formants are identified by the formant number; the first formant (F1) is the lowest frequency; the second formant (F2) is the next highest frequency; and the third formant (F3) is immediately after F2 (Kent, 1997).

Movement of the tongue, lips, and larynx will change the shape of the vocal tract, and in turn modify the sound emanating from the larynx. Produce the vowels /i/ (as in the word *bee*) and /u/ (as in the word *boot*). Try to sense how your tongue and lips change position during production of these two vowels. Changes in the position of your lips and tongue in turn change certain physical characteristics of the vocal tract that directly affect the quality of the sound that emanates from your mouth.

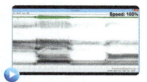

Pearson eTextbook
Video Example 3.2

This is a spectrogram, or visual representation of the acoustic characteristics of the vowels /i/, /a/, /u/, and the /r/ colored vowel, "er." Recall that the wide, dark horizontal bands of acoustic energy are the vowel formant frequencies. Generally, the first vowel formant (F1) varies as a result of tongue height, and the second vowel formant (F2) varies as a result of front or back positioning of the tongue in the oral cavity. Most /r/ colored sounds like "er" show a lowering of the third formant (F3).

> **REFLECTION QUESTION 3.3**
>
> *Different languages share some of the same vowel sounds, like /i/ and /u/, yet acoustic analyses have shown that /i/ and /u/ have different formant frequencies in different languages. Why might this be the case?*

Figure 3.22 represents how changes of vocal tract shape influence which frequencies are enhanced and which are attenuated. A complex sound is produced by vocal fold vibration (a), and the vocal tract acts as a filter attenuating some frequencies and enhancing others (b). The sound that emanates from the mouth during vowel production (c) is related directly to the general shape of the vocal tract determined largely by tongue position. Note that for the /u/ vowel low frequencies are enhanced, whereas high frequencies are somewhat attenuated. For the /i/ vowel low frequencies are somewhat attenuated, whereas high frequencies are enhanced.

During consonant production, your tongue is sometimes used to momentarily occlude your vocal tract for the production of stop sounds such as /t/, /d/, /k/, and /g/. Production of sounds such as /s/ and /sh/ require your tongue to form a constriction in the vocal tract that will produce frication noise when air is passed through the constriction.

Our discussion here relates to the acoustic stage, where the speech sound wave (acoustic product) is produced (Hoit et al., 2022). You can make measurements of acoustic features in your own voice and speech using the browser-based acoustic analysis package WASP2 (Huckvale, 2020). Just type WASP2 into your browser's search bar and launch the program. There is a cheat sheet that explains how to use each of the functions.

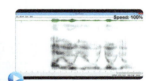

Pearson eTextbook
Video Example 3.3

This is a spectrogram, or visual representation of the acoustic characteristics of the vowels and semivowel (glide) /j/ (or "y" as in "you"), in the sentence "I owe you a yoyo." Semivowels (glides) are associated with rapidly changing formant frequencies due to quick movements of the tongue. In this spectrogram, the semivowel /j/ ("y") is represented by large formant transitions of the second formant, or rising and falling pattern of F2.

FIGURE 3.22 **Spectra of glottal sound source (a) that sets the air in the vocal tract (b) into vibration. The vocal tract filters the glottal sound source differently for the vowels /i/ and /u/, as seen in the radiated spectra (c).**

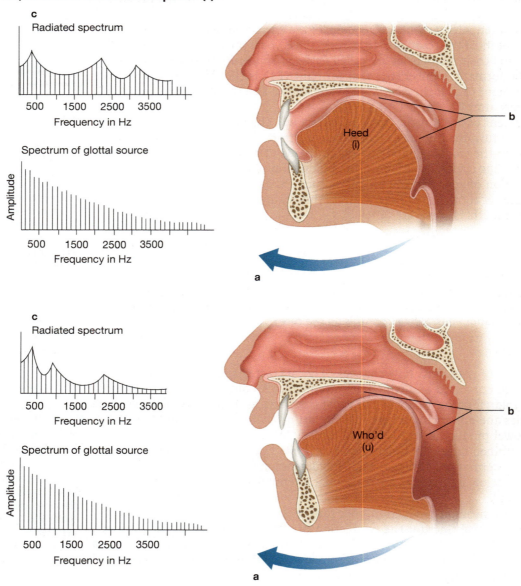

Summary

This chapter provides a general overview of the anatomy and physiology of the organ systems involved in swallowing and speech. The study of the structures and function used for swallowing and speech is extensive and complex, and you will be repeatedly exposed to this content, in greater depth, as you move through your academic program of study. It is important to remember that although anatomy is static, these structures are capable of dynamic movement that result in biological, life-sustaining functions, as well as the nonbiological, unique human processes of speech.

The study of anatomy and physiology is essential for an SLP. Knowledge and understanding of the respiratory, laryngeal, and upper airway systems will assist you in the evaluation and treatment of individuals with swallowing and communication disorders resulting from direct or indirect breakdown within these systems, especially when providing care for critically ill patients alongside doctors, nurses, respiratory therapists, and other rehabilitation professionals.

Epilogue   Case Study: Jennifer

Jennifer is still receiving physical therapy and speech-language therapy in the outpatient setting for continued difficulties with diminished physical endurance and reduced vocal loudness, especially during dual-motor tasks (e.g., walking and talking at the same time). She also struggles with mild memory and attention difficulties; she sees a counselor to manage new onset of mild depression and post-traumatic stress resulting from separation from loved ones for an extended period while in the hospital. Jennifer was able to return to work part time and is making positive gains in her physical and mental functioning with each therapy session. She hopes to continue building her endurance and return to jogging and her gym workouts over the next year.

Reflections   from a Medical Speech-Language Pathologist: Carolyn Abraham

1. *Why did you become a speech-language pathologist?*

   I had a lot of interests that matched up with speech pathology as a whole. I was interested in voice disorders, hearing loss, linguistics, and language acquisition. When I first started school, I was not sure the direction I was going to go, but I liked the variety in the field and knowing I had options.

2. *Did you always want to be a speech-language pathologist?*

   I started my undergraduate education as an elementary education major. I soon realized that I wanted to work one on one with people and discovered speech-language pathology.

3. *What clinical setting do you work in, and what types of patients do you primarily evaluate and treat?*

   I currently work in an outpatient rehabilitation clinic. I specialize in swallowing disorders but also assess and treat voice, cognitive-communication, and language deficits. The types of patients I am involved with include those with head and neck cancers, cardiopulmonary diseases, and neurological injuries and lung transplant recipients.

4. *Why did you choose to become a medical speech-language pathologist versus a school-based SLP or private practitioner?*

   I found the adult medical world fascinating. I preferred rehabilitating over habilitating. Patients are motivated and know what they've lost and are eager to strive toward goals.

5. *What coursework during your undergraduate and graduate programs do you feel was most important for your area of expertise?*

   The foundations from my neuroscience, neurogenic speech and language disorders, swallowing and voice disorders as well as my clinical practicum set me up for success. In both undergraduate and graduate school, I found speech science challenging; in reflection I now know that what I do all day is applied speech science.

6. *What is the best part of your job?*

   Many of my patients require feeding tubes while they are rehabilitating. I love being able to get patients swallowing better, and they begin to eat more and more by mouth. The best part is when a patient is able to eat by mouth safely and get their feeding tube removed.

7. *How has COVID-19 changed your work as a speech-language pathologist, for better and for worse?*

   COVID-19 has added a lot of logistical challenges to many of the therapies I provide. For swallowing interventions, patients have to remove their masks, which puts me at an increased risk. I typically wear an N95 mask and eyewear regardless. Prior to swallow studies, patients are required to have a negative COVID test. The use of teletherapy has also increased, making services even more accessible to patients.

8. *What advice to you have for students considering the field of speech-language pathology, particularly those considering working in a medical setting?*

   There are so many facets of medical speech pathology. Many times, people assume it's only hospital care, but there is a whole continuum and so many medical options such as home health, acute rehabilitation, vocational rehabilitation, and medical clinics. Seek out opportunities to observe across the continuum. Think broadly and make sure your education supports your personal goals.

Suggested Readings/Sources

Hixon, T. (2006). *Respiratory function in singing: A primer for singers and singing teachers.* Redington Brown.

Hixon, T., & Hoit, J. (2005). *Evaluation and management of speech breathing disorders: Principles and methods.* Redington Brown.

Hixon, T., Weismer, G., & Hoit, J. (2020). *Preclinical speech science: Anatomy, physiology, acoustics, and perception* (3rd ed.). Plural Publishing.

Hoit, J., Weismer, G., & Story, B. (2022). *Foundations of speech and hearing: Anatomy and physiology* (2nd ed.). Plural Publishing.

4 Childhood Language Disorders

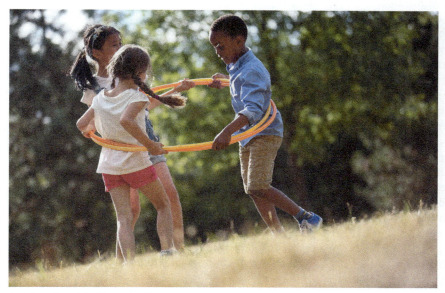

© Robert Kneschke/Shutterstock

Learning Objectives

When you have finished this chapter, you should be able to:

4.1 Describe language development through the lifespan.

4.2 Characterize language disorders and associated disorders.

4.3 Explain the process of assessment in language disorder.

4.4 Describe the overall design of language intervention.

> Language disorders, as you'll see, come in may shapes and sizes. I've spent much of my professional life working with children and adults who are just beginning to communicate, getting them started and after much consultation with family and teachers, mapping out language that will work best for the child.
>
> Initially, intervention may be getting a child to communicate by any means, crafting situations in which communication works for the child. For example, a child who enjoys "floaty" toys in the tub may now be required to point to the storage basket to have the toys dumped in. Children who have not been required to communicate or have had every need anticipated may resist at first.
>
> I recall being confronted by a 4-year-old sister, arms akimbo, who challenged, "You're making my little sister work!"
>
> "Yes, we are."
>
> Her sister, a late starter, went on to use single words and then to combine them into short phrases, such as *no eat, go up, ride bike, more juice*, and the like. She eventually began to use short sentences, such as *Daddy go car*. At this point, the structure of language became very important. By first grade, although still experiencing language difficulties, she was ready to begin school with some assistance and continued language intervention.
>
> —*Robert Owens*

Language disorders are a complex group of both disorders and delays with a wide range of characteristics, levels of severity, and causes. Some children may exhibit disorders in which language is inappropriate, inefficient, or ineffectual; others use language that is seemingly immature. A word of

CASE STUDY   Jayden

Just like other new parents, Jayden's mom and dad awaited their first child with heightened anticipation. He was born full term, with no complications, and seemed healthy. Although he had some difficulties nursing and seemed uninterested in eating, these problems were attributed to his being a generally fussy baby who seemed unable to be comforted.

As Jayden developed, he met physical developmental milestones but seemed to lag slightly in social and cognitive development. The pediatrician assured his parents that there is wide variability across infants and that boys often develop more slowly than girls. His mother described him as irritable and quick to cry. He often had temper tantrums, especially when it was time to eat, bathe, or go to bed. Because of these increasing behavior outbursts, Jayden's parents took him from the home less often than they had previously.

When Jayden had not spoken by 18 months, his parents took him to a speech-language pathologist

(SLP) for an evaluation. They were surprised by the many questions the SLP asked concerning Jayden's early social development. She explained speech and language development to them, especially the early acquisition of intent to communicate, which is expressed initially in gestures.

Although the SLP did not diagnose Jayden as having autism spectrum disorder (ASD), she recommended that he be enrolled in a social play group for late talkers and strongly suggested that they should have him evaluated at a local hospital by an ASD team, if only to rule it out as a cause of his delay and his increasing acting-out behavior.

As you read the chapter, think about:

• Other explanations beyond the ASD label that might explain Jayden's disorder
• Possible evaluative procedures that could be used to measure Jayden's language
• Possible targets that the intervention team might choose to help Jayden develop and use language

advice before we begin: It might be helpful to review the parts of language, such as syntax and semantics, mentioned in Chapter 2 because disorders can affect all aspects of language.

The term *language disorders* applies to a heterogeneous group of developmental and/or acquired disorders that principally affect the use of spoken or written language for comprehension and/or production and may involve the form, content, and/or function of language. Consider the following comments about this definition of language disorders:

• Individuals with language disorders are very different from each other. The disorder may occur at any time within the lifespan, and individuals vary in terms of symptoms, manifestations, effects, and severity over time. The communication context, content of the communication, and learning task are also contributing factors to language disorders.

• The disorder may be a result of atypical development and/or may be acquired as a result of accident, injury, or other environmental factors.

• Deficits and/or immaturities may exist in one or more means of communication. For example, preschoolers with language disorders are often less able to recognize and copy letters. They are also less likely to write and draw, to pretend to read, and to ask questions during parental reading

(Marvin & Wright, 1997). In short, young children with language disorders are at risk for literacy difficulties when they later attend school (Nathan et al., 2004).

- One or more aspects of language—form, content, and use—may be affected. For example, as a group, children with language disorders use shorter, less elaborate sentences than typical children their age (Greenhalgh & Strong, 2001).

It is unclear whether most children with language disorders exhibit disorders in other areas of development as well, but language deficits persist at least through the primary school years for many children (Tomblin et al., 2003). In the classroom and even on the playground, children with language disorders, especially boys and those with severe receptive language deficits, may be reticent to speak and may lack social maturity and exhibit behavioral problems (Hart et al., 2004; Huaquing Qi & Kaiser, 2004).

It's estimated that at the time of school entry, approximately 10% of children will have severe enough language disorders to hinder academic progress. In a study of over 12,000 children, it was reported that the prevalence of language disorders was 9.92% (Frazier Norbury et al., 2016). Even this figure may be low.

According to a recent national report by the U.S. Social Security Administration's Supplemental Security Income Program, children in low-socioeconomic (SES) families are more likely than the general population to exhibit all types of disabilities (McNeilly, 2016). Although approximately 21% of children live in low-SES households, 26% of children with speech and language disorders live in these same households.

Noticeably absent from our definition of language disorders are language differences, such as those found in some dialectal speakers and in English learners (ELs). Differences do not in themselves constitute a disorder and do not require clinical intervention by an SLP, although elective assistance is possible at the client's or family's request.

You can find easy-to-read guides to language disorders and other communication disorders at the American Speech-Language-Hearing Association website at www.asha.org. Go to the lower portion of the page and select "Public" at the right, and then select "Speech and Language Disorders and Diseases."

Box 4.1 presents a conversation between a teacher and a child with a language disorder. Notice the child's repetition and confusion. For example, the child misunderstands the question about who walks the dog and responds with a reference to a leash.

BOX 4.1   **Example of a Conversation with a Child with a Language Disorder**

Teacher: Does your family have a pet?

Child: Yeah.

Teacher: Tell me about this pet.

Child: Got a pet.

Teacher: Um-hm, tell me about the pet.

Child: Got a pet.

Teacher: Yes, and I really want to hear about him.

Child: Got with my . . . ah, go with my . . . Dad go with . . .

Teacher: Your dad walks the pet.

(continued)

Child: No, me.

Teacher: Oh, you and your dad walk the pet.

Child: No, me.

Teacher: Oh, just you walk the dog.

Child: No, me.

Teacher: I'm confused.

Child: Me dog.

Teacher: Oh, it's your dog. Who walks your dog?

Child: With one of them things, you know.

Teacher: What things? Who walks your dog?

Child: With them things like this.

Teacher: Yes, you use a leash.

Theoretically, all speakers of a language should be able to communicate. Some differences may be so great as to impair communication but not qualify as a disorder.

To guide you through this complicated topic, this chapter briefly looks at typical language development followed by a discussion of language disorders. As an SLP, you'll need to know both. Of necessity, this discussion is an overview, with details left for further study. You'll have additional courses in both development and disorders.

Language Development Through the Lifespan

Learning Objective 4.1 Describe language development through the lifespan.

As you already know, language is complex; thus, any attempt to describe its development is also very complicated. In the following sections, we cover only the highlights of child and adolescent development and relate these to some of the disorders to be discussed later in the chapter. An outline of language development is presented in Table 4.1.

TABLE 4.1

Language Development Through the Lifespan

Age	Accomplishments	
3 months	Responds vocally to partner.	
8 months	Begins gesturing.	
12 months	First word spoken. Words fill intentions previously signaled by gestures.	
18 months	Begins combining words on the basis of word-order rules.	
2 years	Begins adding bound morphemes. Average length or mean length of utterance (MLU) is 1.6–2.2 morphemes.	
3 years	More adult-like sentence structure. MLU is 3.0–3.3 morphemes.	
4 years	Begins to change style of talking to fit conversational partner. MLU is 3.6–4.7 morphemes.	
5 years	Ninety percent of language form learned.	
6 years	Begins to learn visual mode of communication with writing and reading.	
Adolescence	Able to participate competently in conversations and telling of narratives. Knows multiple meanings of words and figurative language. Uses a gender style, or genderlect, when talking.	

Source: Based on Owens (2020).

Pre-Language

Much of your first year of life was spent learning to communicate. Parents talk to a newborn as if the child understands what the adults are saying. Later on, as children begin to comprehend language in limited ways, parents and caregivers modify their style of talking to maximize comprehension and participation by the child.

Shortly after birth, you became actively involved in a reciprocal process with your family. Sensitive mothers vary their rate of speech based on their infants' rate of responding (Hane et al., 2003). To maintain attention, a parent or caregiver exaggerates their facial expressions and voice and vocalizes more often. In turn, the infant responds with eye contact or sound making, called *vocalizing*.

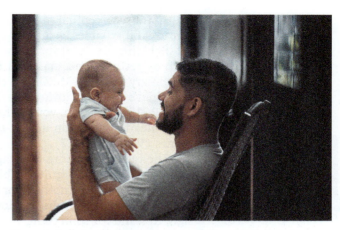

Parents talk to their newborn as if the child already understands what they are saying.

© Pollyana Ventura/E+/Getty Images

As an infant you were a full partner in this interaction, and your behavior was influenced by the communication behavior of your caregivers. Gradually, your babbling became more speechlike and mature, containing syllables rather than individual sounds.

Children become communicators because even as newborns they are treated as if they are communicators.

During the first 3 months, caregivers' responses teach children the "signal" value of specific behaviors, and infants learn a stimulus–response sequence. If they signal—by crying, for example—caregivers respond. In addition, they learn that a relatively constant stimulus or signal, such as a bottle, results in a predictable response, such as feeding. The bottle "signals" feeding as words will do later.

By 3 to 4 months, rituals and game playing have emerged. Rituals, such as feeding and diaper changing, provide children with predictable patterns. As they learn that interactions can unfold in predictable ways, they begin to form expectations of events and to participate more. In addition, games such as "Peekaboo" and "I'm Gonna Get You" have many of the aspects of communication. There is an exchange of turns, rules for each turn, and particular slots for words and actions.

Games and rituals share many characteristics with conversations.

At about 8 to 9 months, you developed **intentionality** in your interactions, primarily through gestures. For the first time, your behavior was meant to influence the other person. The intention to communicate is signaled in gestures accompanied by eye contact with a partner, the use of consistent sound and intonational patterns for specific intentions, and persistent attempts to communicate. These intentional vocalizations or sounds are different from the sounds infants use in solitary activities like play (Papaliou & Trevarthen, 2006).

Early intentions, such as attracting attention, are established in gestures, and first words fill these same functions, often with the accompanying gesture.

As an infant, you probably said your first meaningful word at around 12 months. Real words are produced by infants with or without accompanying gestures to accomplish communication purposes, such as requesting, that were previously filled by gestures.

To develop spoken language, children must be able to store sounds, use this information for later comparison and identification, and relate these sounds to meaning. During the first year, an infant learns the sound patterns of the native language. Better speech perception at 6 months of age is related to better word understanding, word production, and phrase understanding later (Tsao et al., 2004).

An infant's perceptual ability is usually tuned to their native language's speech sounds and syllables by 8 to 10 months of age.

Babbling is important in the emergence of first words, although other factors, such as gestures and maternal education, may be important in later lexical or vocabulary growth (McGillion et al., 2017). The frequency of various phonemes in a child's babbling influences the words that a child first begins to say (Edwards et al., 2015). This said, young children seem to operate at a holistic or whole-word level, meaning children do not seem to build a word bit by bit from various phonemes (Vihman, 2017).

The task of learning language and learning to represent and to symbolize is strongly related to cognitive abilities. **Representation** is the process of having one thing stand for another. For example, in play a hand towel might be used as a blanket for a doll. **Symbolization** is using an arbitrary symbol, such as a word or sign, to stand for something.

Even minimal exposure to multiple languages enhances an infant's communication skills, including those of children who are effectively monolingual (Liberman et al., 2017). This may be because infants growing up in a multilingual environment have different social experiences that may affect early communication skills. Different social experiences may provide children with the opportunity of taking another person's linguistic perspective early in the language development process.

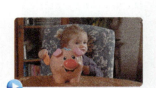

Pearson eTextbook
Video Example 4.1

This video features a conversation between a mother and her 1-year-old daughter. Note how the child attempts sounds and words and the way in which her mother prompts her to do so.

Toddler Language

By 18 months you, like many other children, probably could produce approximately 50 single words and were beginning to combine words in predictable ways. Within a few short months, three- and four-word combinations appeared. Accompanying the increases in utterance length and vocabulary is a decrease in the use of babbling, or sound making.

CASE STUDY   Jayden *(continued)*

Recall that Jayden at 18 months of age was not saying any words.

Use

People who are unfamiliar with young children's language often think that children either imitate all first words or use them only to name. In fact, single words are used to make requests, comments, inquiries, and more.

As mentioned, words are acquired first within the intentions that the child is able to express in previously acquired gestures. Several early intentions are presented in Table 4.2. Note all the uses or intentions expressed in the conversation presented in Box 4.2.

Content and Form

Vocabulary growth is slow for the first few months, but then increases rapidly. Although the ability to comprehend words develops gradually, it is highly context dependent at first (Striano et al., 2003). Eighteen-month-olds are capable of learning associations of new words and the things to which they refer in as few as

TABLE 4.2

Examples of Early Intentions of Children

Intention	Example
Wanting demand	Says the name of the desired item with an insistent voice. Often accompanied by a reaching gesture.
Protesting	Says "No" or the name of the item while pushing it away, turning away, and/or making a frowning face.
Content questioning	Asks "What?" or "That?" or "Wassat?" while pointing and/or looking at an item.
Verbal accompaniment	Speech accompanies some action, such as "whee-e-e" when swung or "uh-oh" when something spills.
Greeting/farewell	Waves hi or bye with accompanying words.

Note: A fuller list can be found in Owens (2020).

BOX 4.2 **Example of Toddler Language**

Stacy and her mother are talking while they are coloring. Note that the language concerns the task. Stacy's mom keeps her utterances short and cues Stacy to respond by asking questions. Stacy participates by talking about the task, often incorporating part of the previous utterance into her own:

Mom: What are you making?

Stacy: Doggie.

Mom: Are you making a doggie? Oh, that's nice, Stacy.

Stacy: Where more doggie?

Mom: Is there another doggie underneath?

Stacy: Yeah.

Mom: Where? Can you find the picture? Is that what you're looking for, the picture of the doggie? Where's a doggie?

Stacy: A doggie. Color a doggie.

Mom: Okay, you color the doggie.

Stacy: Mommy color crayon.

Mom: Mommy has crayons. Mommy's coloring. What's mommy making?

Stacy: Doggie.

Mom: A doggie.

Stacy: Okay.

Mom: All right, I'll make a doggie. Is this the doggie's tail?

Stacy: Doggie's tail. More.

Mom: More doggie?

Stacy: Okay.

Mom: Can Stacy color? Hum?

Stacy: More doggie there. More doggie daddy.

Mom: More doggie daddy?

Stacy: Want a more doggie. More doggie. Put more doggie there.

Mom: Okay, you color the doggie on this page. What color's your doggie?

Stacy: Blue. Color this page, mommy.

---

three exposures (Houston-Price et al., 2005). By age 2, a toddler has an expressive vocabulary of about 150 to 300 words. Two-year-olds with larger vocabularies also use a greater range of grammatical structures (McGregor et al., 2005).

Each toddler has their own **lexicon**, or personal dictionary, containing words that reflect that child's environment. In general, toddlers' definitions are not the same as those of adults because they are based on each child's limited experience.

The frequency of caregiver child-directed speech is an important predictor of lexical development (Hansen, 2017) but quantity is only part of the picture. More important is the quality of caregiver speech. For example, among 24-month-old Black children from low-SES backgrounds, the quality of *wh-* questions used by fathers is associated with toddlers' vocabulary and later verbal reasoning skills (Rowe et al., 2017).

Interestingly, expressive language use also affects expressive vocabulary development (Ribot et al., 2017). In other words, using language increases vocabulary.

Early word combinations follow predictable patterns. Some individual words are joined with other individual words, such as "Throw ball." Neither word may be combined with other words. In contrast, some words are combined with several others, as in "Eat cookie," "Eat cracker," "Eat candy," and the like. Finally, other words are used flexibly in several different combinations, as in "Mommy drink," "Drink juice," and "More drink." A child's short utterances represent a complex interaction of syntactic or word order knowledge, cognitive ability, communicative goals, and the structure of the conversation (Valian & Aubry, 2005).

> Adult and toddler definitions are very different. Toddler definitions are based almost exclusively on experience, whereas adult definitions are based more on meanings shared with others.

Preschool Language

For preschoolers, most communication occurs within the framework of conversations with parents or caregivers. With increased memory, children with typically developing language (TDL) expand their conversational skills to include recounting the past and remembering short personal stories. This memory and recall are aided by the child's increased language skills.

> Language learning is a lengthy process that involves identifying patterns, hypothesis testing, and refinement.

A high percentage of preschool children's utterances differ only slightly from utterances produced previously. For example, a child might say, "Doggies are yucky," "Kitties are yucky," "Cows are yucky," and the like, substituting different words in the same frame (Lieven et al., 2003).

From interaction with others, children with TDL notice patterns and use these to produce ever more complex language. This process takes time and begins one utterance at a time. Caregivers in each child's environment provide feedback and models for further growth (Chouinard & Clark, 2003). For example, in a **reformulation**, an adult might respond to "Tommy come 'morrow my birthday" with "Yes, tomorrow your cousin Tommy is coming to your birthday party with all the other kids."

Individual children differ. Some children—maybe you—are risk takers who attempt new structures and make mistakes. Other, more cautious children may make few errors because they attempt to produce new structures infrequently (Rispoli, 2005).

Use

In conversations with caregivers, preschool children introduce topics and maintain them for an average of two to three turns. It is often easier for a preschool child to introduce a new topic than to continue an old one, as in the following example:

Child:	I got a new bike.
Partner:	What color is it?
Child:	Red.
Partner:	Did you ride it on your birthday?
Child:	Mommy saw a spider.

In conversations, preschool children begin to consider that the listener needs to know certain information and the amount of information needed and that there is a need to change conversational style when speaking to younger children. Style of talking is also reflected in role playing and narration or storytelling. Four-year-old children can tell simple sequential stories, usually about past events.

Content

Children's expressive vocabularies grow to approximately 300 words by age 2, then mushroom to 900 and 1,500 at ages 3 and 4, respectively (see Box 4.3). They may comprehend two or three times that many words in context.

Words are learned quickly through a process called **fast mapping**, in which the child infers the meaning from context and then uses the word in a similar manner. Fuller definitions evolve over time.

In addition to single words, preschool children acquire words and phrases that are used to join other words and create longer units of language. These include locational terms such as *in, on,* and *under*; temporal terms such as *first* and *last*; quantitative terms such as *more than*; qualitative terms such as *bigger than*; familial terms such as *brother*; and conjunctions such as *and, if, so, but,* and *because*.

In part, semantic development reflects cognitive development. For example, 4-year-olds demonstrate categorization skills that seem to indicate more advanced procedures for storage of learned information than are seen in younger children.

Adult-like forms of many sentences evolve during the preschool years.

BOX 4.3   **Example of Preschool Language**

G and B are young 4-year-olds. They are playing with firefighter hats, dishes, and dolls. Notice how different this sample is from the toddler language in Box 4.2. Each child supports her portion of the conversation. The syntax seems adult-like, but the content is pure preschool. The rapid change of topics gives this sample a nonsensical quality. With no adult to maintain a cohesive topic structure, this is a free-for-all with only one or two turns on each topic before it shifts:

G: And I gonna wear both of these.

B: At the same time? No, I'm wearing this one.

G: I'm wearing this one.

B: And then I do this.

G: You wear this and I'll wear this.

B: Two colored cups. You drink out of this one. I drink out of the big one. I'm putting the box up there.

G: Okay, I will have this and you have this.

B: Stay up there.

G: She doesn't look too happy.

B: Uh-oh. Why did I spill it?

G: Mine will only stand.

B: Mine sat.

G: All done with supper. What kind of spoon is this?

B: A plastic one, what else? Now it's time for me to make my own dinner.

G: Time for me too. I have to use this. My baby has to go to bed now. We have to first change their diapers.

B: No we don't.

G: Come here, look.

B: There's a button. I want something to drink.

G: Okay, I'll give you some. Look at this. Watch this. I'm gonna try and make this stand. Do you think this is a girl or a boy?

B: A boy.

G: Oh, cause the boy has the pants on and the girl has the dress on.

B: Happy birthday to you.

G: Grab everythin' up. I'm grabbing most of the doll stuff.

As a child's vocabulary increases, categorization will become increasingly important for storage and word finding.

Interestingly, among both monolingual English and EL preschoolers, expressive language skills are related to vocabulary growth (Ribot & Burridge, 2018). The most important factor seems to be a child's conversational experience with adults, which impacts cognitive functioning more than other factors such as SES (Romeo et al., 2018).

When they try using novel words, children are also influenced by the response behaviors of others and by the interaction involved in building a conversation together (Tolins et al., 2017). The partner's level of acceptance, overall demeanor, and cooperative effort help the child build a lexicon.

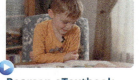

Pearson eTextbook
Video Example 4.2

This video features a conversation between a mother and her 4-year-old son. Note how much his grammar has improved from the level of his 1-year-old sister. He uses sentences and is able to construct a story from a familiar book.

Form

During the preschool years, changes in language form are very dramatic. Beginning with two- to four-word sentences when you were age 2, you probably acquired 90% of adult syntax by age 5. For English-speaking preschoolers, language becomes more complex as it becomes longer. We can describe children's language development by calculating the average, or **mean length of utterance (MLU)**, in morphemes. The calculation of MLU is discussed later in this chapter. Some MLU values are presented in Table 4.1.

The simple constructions found in the utterances of 18- to 24-month-olds form the basis for a more elaborate grammar, and by age 3 most children's utterances contain both a subject and a verb. This basic structure is elaborated with the addition of articles, adjectives, auxiliary verbs, prepositions, pronouns, and adverbs.

In addition, adult-like negative, interrogative, and imperative sentence forms evolve. For example, a toddler negative consisting of *No cookie* is modified by words such as *no, not, can't, don't*, and *won't* being placed between the subject and verb, as in *Mommy can't catch me*. Other negatives such as *wouldn't, couldn't, is not*, and *isn't* are added later.

Similarly, interrogatives or questions go from single words—such as *Doggie?* and *What?* or *Wassat?*—to more complex questions that ask *what* and *where*; followed developmentally by *who, which*, and *whose*; and, finally, *when, why*, and *how*, and a more mature form in which the verb or auxiliary verb and the subject are reversed from the statement "She is happy" to form "Is she happy?" or "Why is she happy?" Repeatedly hearing caregiver questions can have a beneficial effect on a preschooler's development of adult-like questions (Valian & Casey, 2003).

Early sentences consist of only one clause. A clause, like a sentence, has both a subject and an accompanying verb. By the end of preschool, children with TDL are joining two or more independent clauses together to form compound sentences. Late preschoolers can also attach dependent clauses to independent clauses to form complex sentences such as *I didn't like the big dog that barked at grandpa last night*. "That barked at grandpa last night" is a clause but not a sentence and cannot stand alone, so it's called a dependent clause and must be attached to an independent clause, which can stand alone and can be a sentence. These structures appear infrequently in preschool; they develop slowly and are refined throughout the school-age years.

Several bound morphemes are added during the preschool years. These include the progressive verb ending *-ing*, as in *jumping*; plural *-s*, as in *cats*; possessive *'-s* (or *-s'*), as in *mommy's*; and the past tense verb ending *-ed*, as in *talked*. As might be expected, it takes children some time to acquire the use of these morphemes, and it is not uncommon to hear words such as *eated, goed, sheeps*, and *foots*. The learning of some low-frequency endings is still underway for many children into ages 5 and 6 (Tomas et al., 2017).

> **REFLECTION QUESTION 4.1**
>
> *At what ages would you say children are able to participate in communication, comprehend language, or hold up their end in a simple conversation? On what would you base these decisions?*

School-Age and Adolescent Language

When children begin to attend school, they start the long process of establishing their identity independent of their family. Most communication now occurs in conversations outside the home. In part, the status of adolescents within their own social grouping is determined by communication skills.

The means of communication change in school as children learn to read and write. In turn, this skill enables children to use computers, tablets, and cell phones, and it opens a whole new world of information. This development is discussed in Chapter 6.

Reading and writing development is related to **metalinguistic skills**, which enable a child to consider language in the abstract, to make judgments about its correctness, and to create verbal contexts, such as in writing. Younger children are unable to make such judgments, especially without a supporting nonlinguistic context. I once asked a 3-year-old if the sentence *Daddy painted the fence* was correct. Her reply was laughter and the response, "No, daddy painted my closet."

Five-year-olds with TDL use very adult-like language form, although many of the more subtle syntactic structures are missing. In addition, these children have not acquired some of the pragmatic skills that are needed to be truly effective communicators.

As children learn language, they form models or *constructs* that are used for various language tasks. Up through early elementary school, children depend on a single form for various language tasks (Anthony et al., 2014; Bornstein et al., 2014; Language and Reading Research Consortium, 2017). As language becomes more complex and develops new uses, such as literacy, this model becomes more multidimensional.

Over the next few years, language development slows and begins to stabilize, but it will be nonetheless significant. Many complex forms and subtle linguistic uses are learned in the adolescent period. The preschool emphasis on development of language form becomes less prominent and semantic and pragmatic development blossom.

Conversation continues to be the primary locus of communication, and children and adolescents learn to be more effective and efficient communicators. Interactional lessons from the family form a basis for the deepening relationships with peers (Whitmire, 2000). In contrast, a child such as Jayden in our Case Study may be at a real disadvantage given his lack of conversational skill.

Use

During the early school-age years, children's language use changes in two ways: Conversational skills continue to develop, and conversational narratives expand and gain all the elements of mature storytelling. Children with TDL learn effective

Even with the development of writing, conversation is still the predominant use for language.

ways to introduce new topics and to continue and to end conversations smoothly and appropriately. While in a conversation, they make relevant comments and adapt their roles and moods to fit the situation. In addition, school-age children learn to make even more and increasingly subtle assumptions about the level of knowledge of their listeners and to adjust their conversations accordingly.

Within conversation, teens demonstrate more affect or emotion and discuss topics infrequently mentioned at home. The number of turns on a topic increase greatly. Although interrupting increases, it evolves into behaviors, such as asking pertinent questions, that serve to move the topic along.

Narratives, both in conversation and in writing, gain the elements needed in our culture to be considered satisfying. American English narratives contain an introductory setting statement and a challenge or challenges that the characters—often the speaker—overcome. Events are organized both sequentially and by cause and effect.

Content

Vocabulary continues to grow, but number of words is only the most superficial measure of semantic change. First-graders with TDL have an expressive vocabulary of approximately 2,600 words but may understand as many as 8,000 root English words, such as *happy*, and possibly 14,000 when various derivations are included, such as *unhappy* and *happily*. Aided in school, this receptive vocabulary expands to approximately 30,000 words by sixth grade and to 60,000 words by high school. As a bright young adult, you may have close to 100,000 words in your receptive store.

Definitions become more dictionary-like, which means they become less experiential or less based on individual experience and more shared, more categorical (as in *An apple is a kind of fruit*), and more precise. Multiple word meanings are also acquired. The ability to provide definitions is related to the acquisition of metalinguistics, mentioned previously (Benelli et al., 2006).

With vocabulary increases, children find new ways to organize their language for storage and retrieval. Words with similar meanings (i.e., *rich-wealthy*), category membership (i.e., *pets*) or thematic clustering (i.e., *associated with birthday party*) aid memory by minimizing cognitive energy while maximizing navigation between words (Stella et al., 2018). The resultant neural networks consist of several types of relationships operating simultaneously.

School-age children also learn to understand and use **figurative language**. Unlike literal meanings, figurative language does not always mean what it seems to mean. For example, *idioms* are expressions that often cannot be understood literally, such as "hit the road" or "off the wall." Figurative language enriches communication, requires higher language functions of interpretation, and correlates with adolescent literacy skills (Dean Qualls et al., 2003). Some forms are not comprehended until adulthood.

Form

Following the rapid development of language form in preschool, there is a gradual slowing, although development continues. Many forms continue to develop into adolescence.

By age 5, children with TDL use most verb tenses with common verbs and auxiliary or helping verbs, such as *would, should, must*, and *might*; possessive pronouns (*his, hers, yours*); and the conjunctions *and, but, if, because, when*, and *so*.

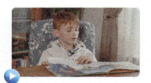

Pearson eTextbook
Video Example 4.3
This video features a conversation between a mother and her 7-year-old son. As with the other children in this section, he is being raised as a bilingual German-English speaker. Note that the child easily holds up his end of the conversation, making relevant and appropriate comments and displaying a range of intentions.

They still have some difficulty with multiple auxiliary verbs, as in *should have been*. Five-year-old children also have limited use of the comparative *-er*, as in *bigger*, and superlative *-est*, as in *biggest*; relative pronouns used in complex sentences (I know *who* lives next door); gerunds (We go *fishing*); and infinitives (I want *to eat* now).

Many syntactic structures appear slowly, and children may struggle with acquisition well into the school years (Eisenberg et al., 2008). During the school years, children gradually add passive sentences, such as *The cat is chased by the dog*, in which the entity performing the action is placed at the end rather than the beginning of the sentence; reflexive pronouns, such as *myself, yourself, himself*, and *themselves*; conjunctions, such as *although* and *however*; and variations of compound and complex sentences. It frequently takes a child several years of practice to gain complete control of these linguistic structures. And children may use some forms, such as the conjunctions *though* and *although*, correctly in speech before they fully understand the relationships expressed (Cain et al., 2005).

Morphological development focuses on derivational suffixes—word endings that change the word class, such as adding *-er* to a verb to make a noun, as in *paint/painter*—and prefixes. Development of prefixes, such as *un-, ir-*, and *dis-*, will continue into adulthood.

Language Disorders

Learning Objective 4.2 Characterize language disorders and associated disorders.

Across children with language disorders, prelinguistic development is a relatively stable measure and predictor of later language development. In other words, children who lag behind in early communication development are likely to have later language disorders (Määttä et al., 2016). Children identified as late-talkers at 24 to 31 months are likely to have a weakness in language-related skills in late adolescence (Rescorla, 2009).

Let's make some general statements about language disorder before we get more specific. Children with expressive vocabulary delays at 24 months of age are at increased risk for later speech/language problems and need for SLP services. Late-talkers have an ongoing weakness in language that continues through the preschool years and into early adulthood (Rescorla & Turner, 2015). Children with TDL and those with language disorders have similar but divergent developmental paths. Although both groups have more rapid language growth in preschool, language growth of those with TDL appears to slow at age 7 while those with language disorders do so at age 5 (Schmitt et al., 2017). These facts do not bode well for Jayden, a late-talker who may have ASD.

Children with language disorders have poorer academic attainment (Schoon et al., 2010), fewer social relationships (Durkin & Conti-Ramsden, 2007), less independence (Conti-Ramsden & Durkin, 2008; Howlin et al., 2000), peer neglect, and bullying—chronic stressors that can lead to social-emotional

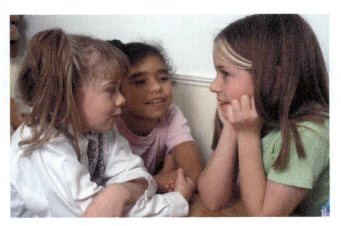

Children with TDL and those with language disorders have similar but divergent developmental paths.

© Angela Hampton/Angela Hampton Picture Library/Alamy Stock Photo

problems (Barkley, 2006; Tomblin, 2014) and poorer employment (Clegg et al., 2005; Howlin et al., 2000) than their peers with TDL. A nationwide longitudinal study in the United Kingdom found that when compared to peers with TDL, children with language disorders had poorer outcomes in literacy and in mental health as well as in employment, even at 34 years of age (Law et al., 2009).

As we saw, language is extremely complex, so it would seem logical to assume that language disorders would be also. So many things can go wrong at so many junctures that each child with a language disorder represents a unique set of circumstances.

Although language disorders are found across children, some children are more susceptible. The biggest risk factors for language disorder include (Brignell et al., 2018; Harrison & McLeod, 2010; McNeilly, 2016; Zambrana et al., 2014):

- Being male
- Having ongoing hearing problems
- Having a more reactive temperament
- Coming from a low SES background
- Exhibiting poor early communicative skills
- Having a family history, suggesting a genetic and/or environmental link in some cases
- Having a low IQ

The risk of being a late-talker at 24 months is strongly associated with being a boy, low SES, not being an only child, older maternal age at birth, moderately low birth weight, low-quality parenting, receipt of no day care or for less than 10 hours a week, and hearing and attention problems (Harrison & McLeod, 2010; Scheffner Hammer et al., 2017).

Researchers are also identifying important genetic factors that account for variance in children's conversational language skills (DeThorne et al., 2008). For example, a family history of writing and reading difficulties greatly increases the odds for late-onset and persistent language disorder (Zambrana et al., 2014).

The effect that any disorder has on communication and on language development varies with the severity of the disorder and the age of the child. As individuals mature, the communicative requirements change. It's easy to assume from these data that children with language disorders perform like younger children with similar language skills. That would be incorrect and would overlook the struggles of these children.

In this section, we discuss several types of language disorders. Of necessity, we discuss groups of children under different categories. Although categories are helpful for discussion of shared characteristics, they are not the same as individuals. Each of us and each child with a language disorder is unique.

Broad Groupings

We can roughly divide children with language disorders into two broad groups: those children with seemingly unexplained language problems and those who have other co-occurring or comorbid conditions, such as ASD, that affect their language development and use. Our discussion begins with children who seem to exhibit only language disorders with no associated disorders. Then we look at language disorders co-occurring with other disorders.

TABLE 4.3

Categories of Language Disorders

Categories	Disorders
Language disorders in the absence of other disorders	Developmental language disorder (DLD) Social communication disorder (SCD)
Language disorders associated with other disorders	Autism spectrum disorder (ASD) Intellectual developmental disorder (IDD) Learning disability Brain injury Late language emergence (LLE) Childhood schizophrenia Selective mutism (SM) Otitis media (middle ear infection) Cochlear implants Disorders due to exposure to drugs and alcohol in utero Disorders due to abuse and neglect

Unfortunately, we are unable to cover all possible language disorders. Table 4.3 presents the language disorders we do discuss.

Some concomitant disorders have been omitted because of the small numbers of children or the paucity of research data. In others, such as Tourette syndrome, language difficulties are tangential. In addition, hearing impairment and deafness have also been excluded because these individuals are more thoroughly discussed in Chapter 12. Children may also exhibit language disorders as a result of localized brain injury, which is discussed in Chapter 7.

Language Disorders in the Absence of Other Disorders

According to one study, the prevalence of language disorders with no know origin nor association with other existing disorders is 7.58% of all children (Frazier Norbury et al., 2016). These children will be the bulk of those you might see as a school-based SLP. The two disorders found in this category are developmental language disorder and social communication disorder. Because there are no co-occurring disorders, SLPs diagnose children as having these disorders.

Developmental Language Disorder

Developmental language disorder (DLD) is defined by what it is not. There is no obvious cause and DLD seems not to affect nor be affected by anatomical, physical, or intellectual problems. The language problems of children with DLD are not the result of other co-occurring disorders.

These children are underidentified or identified late, if at all, especially if they are not male, White, or from well-educated high-SES families (Catts et al., 2012; Frazier Norbury et al., 2016; P. L. Morgan et al., 2016; Wittke & Spaulding, 2018). A general lack of awareness of DLD results in inadequate service delivery (McGregor et al., 2020). DLD is replacing an older term, specific language impairment (SLI), although you may encounter SLI in texts and journals.

Children with DLD seem typical in other ways except language. They have a seemingly unexplained deficit in language abilities despite appropriate environmental stimulation and cognitive abilities and no neurological disorders (Bishop et al., 2017; Leonard, 2014; National Institute of Deafness and Other Communication Disorders, 2017). Although intelligence ranges across the scale, many children with DLD are in the low normal range for nonverbal or nonlanguage intelligence (Gallinat & Spaulding, 2014).

An analysis of several studies identified five risk factors, not causes, that are predictive for the majority of children with DLD, including (Rudolph, 2017):

Pearson eTextbook
Video Example 4.4
The "DLD and Me" site, sponsored by Boys Town National Research Hospital, has a number of videos on DLD. Go to the website at www .dldandme.org/topics/videos/

- Late language emergence
- Maternal education level
- Five-minute Apgar score (a health measure used with newborns)
- Birth order
- Biological sex

Lifespan Issues. A majority of children with DLD is likely to experience the following:

- High risk for reading disorders (Catts, 2004; Catts et al., 2014)
- Low academic achievement and increased risk for stopping education at the high school level (Tomblin, 2014)
- Peer relationship difficulties (Durkin & Conti-Ramsden, 2007)
- Heightened risk for peer victimization and bullying (Redmond, 2011)
- Increased risk for being identified as having attention deficit hyperactive disorder
- Increased social anxiety (Brownlie et al., 2016)

In addition, the majority of children with DLD are perceived more negatively by both teachers and peers (Segebart DeThorne & Watkins, 2001).

Given that communication is fundamental to the initiation and maintenance of successful relationships, it's not surprising that children with DLD often have peer problems. In addition, these children have increased emotional difficulties (St. Clair et al., 2019). These challenges may arise from deficits in both language and **social cognition**, the ability to process, store, and apply information about other people and social situations. Thus, forty percent of 7- and 8-year-old children with DLD report physical bullying in school compared with 10% of children with TDL (Redmond, 2011). Children who are victimized report higher levels of sadness and fear. These children withdraw and engage in more individual play and outlier behaviors (Hart et al., 2004; Liiva & Cleave, 2005). Their reticence is characterized by staring at other children but not reacting, doing nothing even when there are many opportunities, and demonstrating fear of approaching other children.

Because language and literacy play an increasingly larger role in adolescent independent functioning, teens with DLD are less independent than their peers with TDL (Conti-Ramsden & Durkin, 2008). As these teens transition into adulthood, parents and caregivers express concern about several aspects of their behavior (Conti-Ramsden et al., 2008). Young adults with a history of language disorder enter adulthood less socially confident than their peers with TDL (Durkin et al., 2017; Wadman et al., 2008). For many children with DLD, brain imaging indicates brain symmetry in the left and right hemispheres, unlike the usual asymmetry of left-side predominance in language processing regions (Ors et al., 2005).

Further investigation using magnetic resonance imaging suggests that many children with DLD exhibit different patterns of brain activation and coordination, reflecting less efficient patterns of functioning, including reduced activation in the brain areas critical for communication processing (Ellis Weismer et al., 2005; Hugdahl et al., 2004). In general, children with DLD have increased integration of the parietal lobe and decreased integration of the frontal lobe on encoding and decreased integration of the parietal lobe on decoding.

Many but not all children with DLD show marked deficits in working memory abilities (Archibald & Joanisse, 2009) and executive function. **Working memory (WM)** is an active process that allows limited information to be held in a temporarily accessible state while cognitive processing occurs (Cowan et al., 2005). Tasks that are particularly demanding from either a storage and/or a processing perspective result in fewer resources being available for other aspects of the task. Children with WM deficits, such as those with DLD, exhibit learning difficulties (Swanson & Beebe-Frankenberger, 2004). Relative to age-matched TD peers, many children with DLD show several significant limitations in WM mechanisms and in processing speed. These deficits can, in turn, have a negative impact on language learning and functioning.

Executive function, located in the frontal lobe of the brain, is the organizing and directing function of the brain. These functions will vary depending on the cognitive task. Preschool children with DLD demonstrate executive function deficits in both visual and linguistic tasks and in problems with both inhibition control and cognitive flexibility (Pauls & Archibald, 2016; Yang & Gray, 2017). Many children with DLD also have difficulty controlling auditory attention in both quiet and noisy situations (Victorino & Schwartz, 2015).

Language Characteristics. DLD is a persistent language disorder. Therefore, it's likely that a child with DLD will become an adult with poor language skills, especially in language form.

Children with DLD begin to use single words and to combine words later than children with TDL. Language growth is similar to but less advanced and growth slows even more in preadolescence (Rice, 2012, 2017).

Among school-age children and adolescents with DLD, there is a deficit in the ability to detect regularities in language, such as verb endings and sentence structure. In contrast, children with TDL use these patterns to determine the underlying language rules. This problem stems, in part, from reduced auditory WM. If a child has difficulty mentally holding a sentence to process it, they have little cognitive energy left to notice patterns that represent underlying rules. In addition, to compensate for reduced WM, children with DLD may shorten their own sentences by omitting smaller, less essential units, such as morphological endings.

In conversation, where most language is learned, many things are occurring at once that require both of these abilities in order to focus on language. Children with DLD have deficits in their ability to recognize to express emotions (Brinton et al., 2007). Social perception skills, such as understanding the thoughts and emotions of others, affect children's communication abilities.

Children with DLD often have vocabulary disorders, seen in their smaller receptive vocabulary (Rice & Hoffman, 2015). Both semantic and phonological deficits contribute to word-learning difficulties (Gray, 2005). In short, children with DLD have limited semantic knowledge, which, in turn, contributes to their frequent word errors (McGregor et al., 2002). In part, these semantic issues may reflect a difficulty inhibiting similar-sounding words while processing language (Mainela-Arnold et al., 2008).

A relationship exists between executive function and word learning. Preschoolers with DLD perform more poorly than peers with TDL on measures of both executive function and novel word learning (Kapa & Erikson, 2020). Compared to peers with TDL, school-age children with DLD demonstrate more effortful cognition during language comprehension. This contrasts with the more automatic word processing of children with TDL (Montgomery et al., 2018).

Language comprehension and processing are active processes based on the auditory message, contextual information, and stored world and word knowledge. Not surprisingly, school-age children with DLD exhibit significant deficits in spoken sentence comprehension. Much of this difference can be explained by memory-based deficits, but we still need more research (Montgomery et al., 2016).

The comprehension and production of complex syntactic structures is restricted in the majority of children with DLD (Frizelle & Fletcher, 2014a, 2014b; Riches et al., 2010). This limitation is related to memory difficulties, especially with sequence-specific information (Hsu & Bishop, 2014; Marton et al., 2006).

Morphological endings and shorter words, such as pronouns, are especially difficult. As small units of speech, morphemes receive little stress and may be difficult for a child to identify. Thus, children with DLD often make errors with verb endings, pronouns, and auxiliary verbs (Goffman & Leonard, 2000; Redmond & Rice, 2001). These children exhibit an ongoing maturational lag in language form compared to age-matched and language-matched peers with TDL (Rice et al., 2009).

In summary, we can say that children with DLD have difficulty (1) learning language rules, (2) registering different contexts, and (3) constructing word–meaning associations. The result is difficulty in morphological and phonological rule learning and in vocabulary development. Pragmatic problems result from inability to use effective forms to accomplish their intentions.

Social Communication Disorder

With this disorder, you might be asking, "Isn't all communication social?" The answer, of course, is yes. We can define social communication as "social interaction, social cognition, pragmatics (verbal and nonverbal), and receptive and expressive language processing" (Adams, 2005, p. 182). That's a mouthful. In general, it's the ability to communicate with a variety of partners in various situations not only through language but through nonlinguistic means, such as facial expression and eye contact (Curenton & Justice, 2004; Inglebret et al., 2008).

These behaviors vary by culture and also with situations and partners. For example, lack of eye contact may signal disinterest in general American culture but be considered polite in other cultures, such as Korean or Japanese.

Social communication disorder (SCD) is persistent difficulty in the social use of verbal and nonverbal communication and may include problems in all those areas. Given that many children with ASD exhibit interactional difficulties, there might be some confusion. As we'll see later, one characteristic of ASD is the presence of restricted and repetitive interests and behaviors (RRIBs). Children with SCD do not exhibit RRIBs (Cholemkery et al., 2016; Swineford et al., 2014; Timler, 2018a).

SCD is a relatively newly identified disorder, recognized only in 2013 in the fifth edition of the *Diagnostic and Statistical Manual of Mental Disorders* (DSM-5) of the American Psychiatric Association. The presence of SCD can limit effective

Pearson eTextbook

Video Example 4.5

In this video is another description of DLD that includes children with the disorder.

www.youtube.com/ watch?v=tQ-s02HWLb0

communication and social participation, negatively affect relationships, and lead to academic and vocational problems.

The causes of SCD may be many and varied and reflect related disorders. Causes may be biological or may reflect neurological conditions, mental disorders and/or overall developmental delays.

Precise estimates of the prevalence of SCD are difficult to determine because of the somewhat ambiguous definition and the validity of the assessment criteria (Swineford et al., 2014). Pragmatic language disorders occur in about 7.5% of kindergarten children (Ketelaars et al., 2009) but many are undiagnosed. The rate is much higher (23%–33%) among children previously diagnosed with language disorders (Ketelaars et al., 2009). Pragmatic disorders are 2.6 times as prevalent in boys as in girls.

Lifespan Issues. A young child with SCD may not respond differentially to the faces of others or to games or sound-making activities. As infants, these children may prefer aloneness and not respond to or imitate others. They may not initiate interactions or gesture to express their intentions.

Given the social nature of language development, a child with SCD may be slow to develop language. At age 4, when children with TDL are becoming aware of their own and others' ability to think and reason, children with SCD may fall behind in emotional understanding and expression. Because delayed development may mirror a number of disorders or simply reflect typical individuality, it is difficult to diagnose SCD in young children. Diagnosis is rare before age 4. Children with mild SCD may not be diagnosed until adolescence.

As preschool and school-age children, those with SCD may become socially isolated. The lack of both language and social skills makes them less desirable play and study partners. Their poor language skills, especially the pragmatics of conversation and storytelling, result in difficulties with literacy. They may be inflexible in conversation and talk *at* rather than *with* their peers. As teenagers, children with SCD may be bullied by other students because of their lack of social skills.

Language Characteristics. In general, the characteristics of SCD include problems with communication for social purposes. These include deficits in interactional skills, social cognition, pragmatics, and language. Interactional skills include adjusting your communication style to your partner. For example, around age 4, we begin to talk differently with younger children than we do with adults. Children with SCD may have difficulty adjusting their language to different communication partners, especially in politeness and role recognition. Cooperative tasks such as play and conflict resolution may be difficult.

Social cognition includes understanding and regulating our emotions as they affect others and involves something called theory of mind (ToM). ToM is an evolving notion in children that others have a mind and emotions that differ from their own and that these must be considered in communication.

The pragmatic aspect of language includes using language to accomplish our intentions and clearly signaling our intention to our conversational partner. This is accomplished through linguistic and nonlinguistic means such as body language. Children with SCD may experience difficulty interpreting the intentions of others and encoding their own intentions. Conversations may be incoherent, with frequent abrupt topic shifts. Events may be related in a confused manner. As mentioned, nonlinguistic behaviors may be inappropriate or odd, sending confusing messages that may not match the words spoken. Children with SCD may also have difficulty interpreting the gestures, facial expressions, and other body language of others.

Common language characteristics of SCD include (American Speech-Language-Hearing Association [ASHA], 2019):

- Inappropriate and inadequate greetings
- Lack of flexibility in changing language and communication style for different settings or partners
- Difficulty producing and comprehending narratives
- Awkward engagement in all aspects of conversation, such as initiating or entering a conversation, maintaining the topic, and turn taking
- Poor repair of communication breakdowns
- Inadequate, ineffective, or confused verbal and nonverbal signals used to regulate conversational interactions
- Misinterpretation of the verbal and nonverbal signals of others
- Difficulty understanding ambiguous or figurative language and information not explicitly stated

Not all communication is explicit. As a participant, you sometimes must infer a speaker's meaning. When a partner says, "Do you think it's warm enough in here?" they may be subtly asking you to turn up the heat. Children with SCD may be very literal in their interpretations of such indirect comments.

Language Disorders Associated with Other Disorders

The following discussion begins with children with language disorders co-occurring with ASD. We then proceed through learning disability, intellectual developmental disorder, neurocognitive disorders such as traumatic brain injury, language disorders associated with maltreatment and neglect, and finish with some less frequent disorders.

Autism Spectrum Disorder

According to DSM-5, for a child or an older individual to be diagnosed as having **autism spectrum disorder (ASD)**, they must have all of the following:

- Persistent problems in social communication and interaction across different contexts. Deficits do not result from general developmental delays, such as those in intellectual disability. Problems are seen in all of the following:
  - Social-emotional reciprocity
  - Nonverbal communicative and social interaction behaviors
  - Developing and maintaining relationships appropriate for maturity level
- Restricted, repetitive patterns of behavior, interests, or activities characterized by two or more of the following:
  - Stereotyped or repetitive motor movements, use of objects, or speech
  - Excessive reliance on routines, ritualized patterns of behavior, or resistance to change

- Highly fixated and restricted, abnormally intense interests or focus
- Hyper- or hyposensitivity and reactivity to environmental input or unusual interest in sensory information

Taken together, these characteristics limit and impair daily functioning. Think of our friend Jayden at the beginning of the chapter as we discuss ASD.

What the characteristics mean are that many but not all children with ASD have abnormal social interactions and failure in the give-and-take of conversation; poorly integrated verbal and nonverbal communication, including eye contact and body language; difficulty adjusting to different social situations and stereotypical motor patterns; and echolalia, or repetition of others' speech, repetitive use of objects, and repetition of certain expressions. For example, when the teacher says, "It's time to clean up," the child may "echo" or repeat the phrase over and over again. In general, the more severe the symptoms, the poorer the individual's language and overall development (Pry et al., 2005).

Motor patterns of behavior may include rocking and a fascination with lights or spinning objects. In addition, a child may insist on certain routines or be preoccupied with specific objects, foods, or clothing. Paired with these preferences, a child with ASD may have an adverse reaction to other sounds or textures. One child in a camp situation had approximately a half-dozen outfits consisting of exactly the same articles of clothing. Another would eat only foods of certain colors and textures. Recall Jayden's behaviors.

ASD is much more common than previously believed. In the United States, according to the Centers for Disease Control and Prevention (CDC; 2018c), ASD affects approximately 1 in every 44 children. These data are similar to that reported in Asia, Europe, South America, and Canada. ASD is four times as common in males as in females who tend to have less restricted and repetitive behavior compared to males of similar age and severity (Knutsen et al., 2019). Although 44% of children identified with ASD have average to above-average intellectual ability (CDC, 2022), approximately 25% of children with ASD also exhibit intellectual developmental disorder (IDD) (Chakrabarti & Fombonne, 2001; Fombonne, 2003).

At present, many researchers are trying to identify the early signs of ASD. Early identification can lead to early intervention. The Autism Spectrum Disorder Foundation website (www.myasdf.org) provides some possible early warning signs. Select "About Autism" and then "Identifying the Disorder."

The primary causal factors in autism are biological. The incidence of ASD is highest among males and those with a family history of autism. The family pattern suggests a genetic basis for the disorder. For example, at least 15% of children with ASD have a genetic mutation not inherited from either parent (Sebat et al., 2007; Zhao et al., 2007). This is even higher for those with more severe forms of the disorder. In addition, between 2 and 6% of children with ASD also have fragile X syndrome, a genetic mutation of the X chromosome associated with IDD (Belmonte & Bourgerone, 2006). In addition, approximately 20% of children with Down syndrome also have ASD (DiGuiseppi et al., 2010; Oxelgren et al., 2017; Warner et al., 2014).

The average medical expense for a family of a child with ASD is $4,110–6,200 annually (CDC, 2022). Intensive behavioral intervention for a child may cost an additional $40,000–60,000 per year (Amendah et al., 2011).

Differences in processing incoming information also suggest a neurological basis for ASD. Individuals with ASD experience difficulty in analyzing and integrating information, resulting in a tendency to fixate on one aspect of a complex stimulus—often some irrelevant, minor detail. Although more research is still needed, cross-sectional neuroimaging to date reveals abnormalities in primary sensory areas of the brain (Lainhart, 2015).

Overall cognitive processing by children with ASD has been characterized as a *gestalt*, in which unanalyzed wholes are stored and later reproduced in identical fashion. The storage of unanalyzed information may account for the way in which individuals with ASD become quickly overloaded with sensory information. Storage of unanalyzed wholes also might hinder memory. It's difficult to organize information on the basis of relationships between stimuli if those stimuli remain unanalyzed.

Lifespan Issues. Neural studies suggest that the eye and face detection processing of children with autism may be delayed, explaining in part the early failure to bond with caregivers (Grice et al., 2005). In addition, infants with autism show no difference in brain response to familiar and unfamiliar faces, supporting the notion of a facial processing disorder (Dawson et al., 2002).

At present, children with ASD are identified by the time they are 2 or 3 years of age. Although early intervention (EI) is critical to maximizing outcomes for children with ASD, EI is often difficult to obtain because of the late age of most diagnoses. Although no babbling or gesturing by 12 months is an early sign, it's not possible at this time to make a definitive diagnosis prior to 24 months of age (Woods & Wetherby, 2003). Although symptoms are present in early childhood, they may not manifest fully until social demands exceed a child's limited capacities.

Parental behavior can result in more promising outcomes. Positive emotional behavior or affect by the mother and her use of multimodal initiations and responses are associated with more positive affect, vocalizations, gaze to face, and multimodal bids or responses among infants with ASD (Schwichtenberg et al., 2019). Multimodal behaviors include facial expressions, gestures, and speech.

School-age children and adolescents with ASD may be included in regular education classes or be in special classes, depending on the severity of the disorder. In some children, the severity of ASD lessens with age. For example, a young child with ASD whose behavior is disruptive may have fewer outbursts as a teenager.

People with milder forms of the disorder may be able to live on their own and hold competitive employment. Unfortunately, the vast majority of people with severe ASD require lifelong supervision and care; many have adult life patterns similar to those of adults with ID.

CASE STUDY   **Jayden** *(continued)*

Jayden was diagnosed with ASD and enrolled in a special preschool. He received speech and language services in the classroom daily, and his parents continued intervention at home under the direction of an SLP. Intervention was primarily in the form of play. By age 5, Jayden signed approximately 50 single words and spoke about 10 words with a variety of purposes, primarily to request.

Language Characteristics. As a group, children with ASD demonstrate significant delays in language and communication, especially in pragmatics (Tager-Flusberg et al., 2005). A communication problem is often one of the first indicators of possible ASD. At 18 months, Jayden was not speaking.

Between 25 and 60% of individuals with severe ASD remain nonspeaking throughout their language life. Some autistic children who use speech and language demonstrate immediate or delayed echolalia, which is a whole or partial repetition of previous utterances, often with the same intonation. For example, a child named Mickey would say little during the day but store things said to him and repeat them in sequence before he went to sleep at night. In contrast, another child, Adam, would echo immediately. Without his preschool SLP's use of sign, Jayden may have also remained nonverbal or minimally verbal.

For some children, echolalia might either be a language processing strategy or signal agreement with the previous utterance. Even when echolalia decreases, other problems, especially those related to pragmatics, persist in the child's language. Most children with ASD who learn to talk go through a period of using echolalia (Prizant et al., 1997).

Even those with high-functioning ASD (HFA) have difficulty with the nonverbal aspects of communication. I remember a college student with HFA relating that he couldn't trust what people said because their body language and gestures didn't make sense. Although we find a reliance on gestures by children with other language disorders, those with ASD exhibit a deficit in both oral language and nonverbal communication (Perrault et al., 2018).

ASD affects pragmatics and semantics more than language form. Syntactic errors seem to represent a lack of underlying semantic relationships. Prosodic features or suprasegmentals, such as stress, intonation, loudness, pitch, and rate, are often affected, giving the speech of children with ASD the sometimes-mechanical quality mentioned. Individuals with ASD often have peculiarities and irregularities in the pragmatics of conversation. The range of intentions is often very limited and may consist solely of demands and, in severe cases, unintelligible vocalizations. Recall that most of Jayden's speech served a requesting function or purpose.

Some individuals incorporate entire verbal routines, called *formuli*, into their communication. For example, a child might repeat part or all of a television commercial to indicate a desire for the item that had been in the advertisement. A formula represents the person's attempt to overcome the difficulty of matching the content and form of language to the communicative context. Adults with mild ASD who have good language skills might still misinterpret some of the subtleties of conversation.

As with any other disorder, ASD offers a challenge to parents. The National Institute of Mental Health website (www.nimh.nih.gov) has a helpful parents' guide to ASD. Select "Autism Spectrum Disorder" at the right, then "Brochures and Fact Sheets" at the top. There are several other disorders you can also explore on this site.

Pearson eTextbook
Video Example 4.7

The Oregon Speech-Language & Hearing Association has a number of videos on working with children with ASD. Go to the website at www.oregon speechandhearing.org, scroll down to "Short Film Series," and select "Visit our channel."

You can also find one of their videos at this link: www.youtube .com/watch?v=4rivpFzwMl8

Intellectual Developmental Disorder

Previously termed *mental retardation* and commonly called **intellectual disability** in educational circles, **intellectual developmental disorder** is the designation found in DSM-5. The simpler term *intellectual disability* can be confusing because medically it applies to other cognitive impairments, such as dementia and traumatic brain injury. So, for these reasons, we use IDD.

IDD is a neurodevelopmental disorder characterized by intellectual difficulties as well as difficulties in conceptual, social, and practical areas of living. The disorder has three aspects (American Psychiatric Association [APA], 2013):

- Deficits in intellectual functioning confirmed by clinical evaluation and individualized standard IQ testing
- Deficits in adaptive functioning that significantly hinder an individual's independence and ability to meet their social responsibilities
- Onset during childhood, hence the word *developmental*

In recognition that IQ is only one factor, the focus is on the types and intensities of supports needed by an individual to lead a normal and independent life. In general, a child with IDD is affected in all areas of conceptual or intellectual development and social and daily living skills. Approximately 2.5% of the population are individuals with IDD, which in practical terms is intellectual functioning significantly below the general population or below an IQ of approximately 70. Nonetheless, the designation of IDD reflects several different components of functioning.

Children with IDD differ in severity and other factors, such as amount of home support, living environment, education, type of IDD, mode of communication, and age. Some individuals are nonverbal and need round-the-clock care whereas some adults function well in society, have employment, and are married. The range of severities of IDD are presented in Table 3.4. Although these classifications are based on daily living skills, the criteria are somewhat non-specific and for that reason older classification based on IQ is included.

As we move from mild to profound IDD, we find an increase in co-occurring disorders. Children with profound IDD often have multiple disorders. The most frequent co-occurring disorders are cerebral palsy and seizure activity. In addition, children with severe to profound IDD more often have chromosomal syndromes, such as Down syndrome and fragile X syndrome, which are discussed later in this section.

Several websites provide more information on IDD. The National Institute of Child Health and Human Development website (www.nichd.nih.gov/health/topics/idds/conditioninfo) is a good place to begin your research of intellectual and developmental disabilities.

Causes of IDD are almost as varied as individuals. Two large categories of possible causal factors are biological and socioenvironmental. These factors may be complicated by cognitive limitations that can affect the processing of incoming and outgoing information such as speech and language. Biological factors include the following:

- Genetic and chromosomal abnormalities
- Maternal infections during pregnancy
- Toxins and chemical agents
- Nutritional and metabolic causes
- Gestational disorders affecting development of the fetus
- Complications from pregnancy
- Complications from delivery
- Brain diseases

Socioenvironmental factors include a stimulation-impoverished environment, poor housing, inadequate diet, poor hygiene, and lack of medical care. The effect of each of these factors varies with each child.

In the United States, SES is a determinant of health. In general, those with a low-SES background have poorer health overall, poorer nutrition, and poorer access to education and health care, and a higher incidence of disabilities (Graham, 2015). The prevalence of mild to moderate IDD among children of color from low-SES backgrounds is more than twice as high as that among children from middle- or high-SES backgrounds (Bhasin et al., 2006; Boyle et al., 2011; Van Naarden Braun et al., 2015). That said, race and ethnicity are not causal factors as much as factors related to low SES. In addition, these same children are less likely to receive educational services (Gary et al., 2019). Severe IDD is more random in relation to race/ethnicity and SES.

IQ is not the entire picture. For some individuals with IDD there may be other cognitive processing differences. Incoming sensory information, such as sounds, are processed by first attending to a stimulus, then perceiving differences and likenesses, organizing and storing the information, and finally retrieval from memory. When compared to peers with TDL, some individuals with IDD do not rely on organizational strategies that link words and concepts to one another. Nor do they spontaneously rehearse information for easy retrieval. Information stored poorly can lead to memory or retrieval problems. To some extent, memory is affected by the type of input. In general, individuals with IDD have more difficulty with auditory input, especially linguistic, than with visual input.

> Individuals with intellectual disability may process incoming sensory information differently from those without disability.

Incoming language information undergoes several types of decoding. Simultaneous synthesis occurs all at once and extracts overall meaning. Successive synthesis is more linear, occurring one at a time. Although individuals with IDD exhibit some difficulty with both types, those with Down syndrome have much greater difficulty with successive processing, possibly reflecting poor auditory working memory.

Lifespan Issues. Some newborns and infants with IDD are identified early because of obvious physical factors, such as syndromes or anatomical anomalies, at-risk indicators such as low birth weight or poor physical responses, or delayed development. Intervention may begin at home or in special EI programs in which a child is seen by a team of medical and educational specialists. It is best for the child if intervention begins as soon as possible. EI focuses on sensorimotor skills such as eye–hand coordination, physical development, and social and communicative abilities. An individualized family service plan specifying services is written in collaboration with caregivers.

Some children with IDD are not identified until age 2 or 3. These youngsters, along with those previously identified, will likely attend a special preschool. They may receive intervention services, such as physical therapy, special education, or speech-language therapy, in either the home or school.

Depending on the severity of a school-age child's IDD, they may either attend a regular education class and receive special services or receive education in a self-contained, special classroom. Education and training will focus on academic skills, daily living and self-help activities, and vocational needs, depending on the abilities of the child.

Only children with the most profound IDD accompanied by other disabilities reside in developmental centers. Generally, children who cannot reside at home live in community residences with 8 to 10 other children their age and with house parents.

Very few individuals with intellectual disability live in large institutions. Since the 1970s, a philosophy called *deinstitutionalization* has been responsible for the movement of individuals with IDD into small community residences.

Mike, a man with profound IDD and cerebral palsy, lived at home with his older parents as an infant and preschooler. As he matured and his parents aged, Mike was placed in a community residence with other young adults with IDD. He received daily care at this center and was able to continue his education at the same school. Most of his training involved daily living skills and use of assistive communication.

In adulthood, living and working arrangements vary widely. People with milder IDD often live in the community and work competitively in minimally skilled jobs. More severely involved individuals may live with family members or in community residences containing a small group of similar adults. They may work in a special workshop or be enrolled in a day treatment program in which education and training continue to be the focus.

Language Characteristics. Children with IDD vary greatly in their communication abilities. For example, children with Down syndrome (DS) and fragile X syndrome (FXS) have moderate to severe delays in communication development in all areas of language (Roberts et al., 2001). In phonology, boys with FXS make errors similar to those of younger, typically developing youth, whereas those with DS have more significant phonological differences than might be expected by delayed development alone (Roberts et al., 2005). In contrast, boys with FXS produce longer, more complex utterances than do boys with DS (Price et al., 2008).

Boys with FXS perform differently in conversation than boys with Down syndrome. Although both groups make more off-topic responses than boys with TDL, those with FXS use more repetitive speech (Roberts et al., 2007). Boys with ASD and boys and girls with FXS co-occurring with ASD have more off-topic language and more repetitions than those with TDL and FXS without ASD (Martin et al., 2018).

Late school-age children and adolescents with FXS are less likely to signal noncomprehension than younger, cognitively matched children with TDL (Thurman et al., 2017). Likewise, although capable of requesting clarification when communication breaks down, children with IDD are less likely to do so within conversations.

Boys who have FXS with and without ASD and boys with DS produce shorter, less complex utterances than do boys with TDL (Price et al., 2008), although the utterances of boys with FXS are more complex than those of boys with DS. In general, children with FXS show significant syntactic growth during the preschool years but seem to plateau or, in some cases, to decline during early school age (Komesidou et al., 2017). Longitudinal studies indicate that language challenges persist for both boys and girls with FXS (Brady et al., 2020).

For many individuals with IDD, language is the single most important limitation. For approximately half of the population with IDD, language comprehension and/or production is below the level of cognition. This might be indicative of cognitive processing problems that accompany IDD. For example, those with DS exhibit auditory working memory deficits (Seung & Chapman, 2000).

In initial language development, individuals with ID follow a similar but slower developmental path than that of typically developing children. Even so, these children often produce shorter, more immature language forms (Boudreau & Chapman, 2000). In later development, the paths begin to differ more from typical development. All areas of language exhibit some delay and disorder in children with IDD.

Learning Disabilities

Learning disability (LD) is an educational term defined in the Individuals with Disabilities Education Act (IDEA; 2004), a U.S. federal education law. DSM-5 uses the medical term *specific learning disorder (SLD)*, and there is considerable overlap (Cortiella & Horowitz, 2014). Given the wording in IDEA and the common usage in education, we use the more general term *learning disability* or *LD*.

IDEA defines **learning disability** as:

- Involving one or more of the basic psychological processes
- Affecting the understanding or use of spoken and/or written language
- Manifested in the imperfect ability to listen, think, speak, read, write, spell, or do mathematical calculations
- Not primarily the result of visual, hearing, motor disabilities, intellectual disability, or emotional disturbance or of environmental, cultural, or economic disadvantage.

Schools often use terms such as *dyslexia* to describe specific learning problems. **Dyslexia** refers to difficulties with accurate or fluent word recognition, poor spelling, and deficits in coding abilities (International Dyslexia Association, 2015).

> Children with learning disabilities have difficulty learning and using symbols for speaking, listening, reading, and writing.

Approximately 5–15% of school-age children have LD. It's estimated that about 80% of these children also have a reading disorder (APA, 2018). LD is a neurodevelopmental disorder that becomes evident during the school-age years and will most likely persist into adulthood. Learning disabilities affect males four times as frequently as they do females.

A good place to begin your online exploration of LD is the Learning Disabilities Association website at www.ldaamerica.us. If you select "For Teachers" or "For Professionals," you will find a wealth of information on intervention. The site also offers links to several other sites. Simply select "Resources."

Pearson eTextbook
Video Example 4.8

You can find an introduction to and overview of LD and how these disabilities affect language in this video from the Learning Disabilities Association of Toronto District (LDATD).

www.youtube.com/ watch?v=GoM5HcfQBwE

The characteristics of LD fall into six categories: motor, attention, perception, symbol, memory, and emotion. Few children exhibit all the characteristics described. Motor difficulties may include either hyperactivity or hypoactivity. Hyperactivity, or overactivity, is more prevalent, especially among boys. This results in difficulty attending and concentrating for more than very short periods. Children with hypoactivity may be deficient in their sense of body movement, definition of handedness, eye–hand coordination, and space and time conceptualization.

For example, one of the authors has a slight learning disability that is characterized by poor coordination and language issues such as word recall and perception: "I was once told it was so funny how I mispronounced words on purpose. It was not being done on purpose."

Attentional difficulties include a short attention span, inattentiveness, and distractibility. Irrelevant stimuli may capture the child's attention, and overstimulation easily occurs. Some children become fixed on a single task or behavior and repeat it compulsively, a process called *perseveration*.

Perceptual difficulties of children with LD involve interpretation of incoming stimuli, although this is not a sensory disorder like deafness and blindness.

Children with perceptual disabilities often confuse similar sounds, similar-sounding words, and similar-looking printed letters and words. In addition, children with LD may have difficulty both in determining where to focus their attention and in integrating sensory information from different sources, such as vision and hearing. As the above-mentioned author notes, "If a restaurant has a TV in the bar area, I ask to sit with it at my back or it will capture my attention to the detriment of any conversation."

Some children with LD have particular difficulty in comprehending printed symbols and producing written symbols. It's estimated that as many as 80% of children with LD have some form of reading problem and that the incidence of these problems in the overall population may range from 5 to 17% (Sawyer, 2006).

Memory difficulties affect short-term retrieval, as in remembering directions, and long-term retrieval, as in recalling names, event sequences, and words. Some children exhibit word-finding problems that result in blocks and the use of fillers ("Ah, ah, you know . . . ") or circumlocutions.

Emotional problems are usually a factor that accompanies LD, and not a causal factor. They are a reaction to the frustration that these children feel. Although most children with LD have normal intelligence, they perform poorly on language-based tasks, and their parents or teachers may tell them that they are not trying or that they're lazy or stupid. Emotional outbursts may result in children being described as aggressive, impulsive, unpredictable, withdrawn, and/or impatient. These youngsters may exhibit poor judgment, unusual fears, and/or poor adjustment to change.

The fact that LD occurs more frequently in families with a history of the disorder and in children who had a premature or difficult birth suggests possible biological causal factors. A central nervous system dysfunction may involve a breakdown along the neural pathways that connect the midbrain with the frontal cortex, an area that is responsible for attention, regulation, and planning of cognitive activity.

Although not a causal factor, socioenvironmental factors may account for at least some of the behaviors seen in children with LD. For example, misperceptions by a child affect interactions, which influence the child's development, especially language development. Language difficulties, in turn, affect the child's interactions.

Information processing difficulties are characterized by an inability to use certain strategies or to access certain stored information. In general, children with LD exhibit poor ability to attend selectively or have difficulty deciding on the relevant information to which to attend. As we have seen, discrimination is also extremely difficult. Information that is poorly attended to and poorly perceived will be poorly organized. The cognitive organization of children with LD reflects this confusion. In short, the organization is too inefficient for easy retrieval, so memory is less accurate and retrieval is slower.

Several websites discuss LD. The Learning Disabilities Association of America website (www.ldaamerica.org) has a brief checklist of symptoms for parents. Simply go to the site, select "Parents" at the bottom left, and follow "New to LD." This will take you to common behaviors seen with LD.

Those who have hyperactivity and attentional difficulties but do not manifest other characteristics of LD, especially perceptual difficulties, may be labeled as having **attention-deficit/hyperactivity disorder (ADHD)**. Children with ADHD have an underlying neurological disorder in executive function that regulates

LDs are not caused by emotional disorders; rather, emotional problems result from misperception and from frustration.

behavior; as a result, they may be impulsive. Although ADHD is not a learning disability, children with ADHD often experience problems in social relations that are explained in part by their accompanying pragmatic problems with language use (Leonard et al., 2011). Children with ADHD may not be identified on language testing that ignores pragmatics.

Possibly because of difficulties attending, children with ADHD are less accurate in their interpretations of speech (Nilsen et al., 2013). These difficulties could lead to more miscommunication.

Lifespan Issues. As preschoolers, children with LD may exhibit little interest in language or even in books. When a child reaches school, the linguistic demands of the classroom are often well above their language abilities. The result is often academic underachievement.

Most learning disabilities are not discovered until children go to school, although some children may be enrolled in special preschool programs or may receive therapy services because of poor motor coordination, hyperactivity, or failure to develop language typically. When they reach school, with its accompanying demand for language skills, many children with LD require the services of special educators, SLPs, and reading specialists. Some children might not be identified in early grades. For example, very bright children may "learn" to read by memorizing word shapes rather than using phonics-based word-attack skills, as discussed in Chapter 6.

Children with LD often receive special services while being included in regular classrooms. They can be successful if the teacher makes some adaptation, such as repeating instructions or allowing for a quiet work space, to accommodate their needs.

Some children with LD seem to outgrow aspects of their disability. For example, hyperactivity seems to lessen in some adolescents. Other adolescents succeed well enough to continue their education and graduate from college. We know adults with LDs who are chemists, engineers, teachers, and speech-language pathologists, although some have lingering vestiges of LD that require lifelong adaptations.

Other adults continue to have difficulty. Matt received special services throughout his school years and finished high school. His language difficulties were complicated by a volatile temper and frequent misinterpretations of the communicative intentions of others. After being fired from a series of jobs, Matt hit on the idea of informing his new boss that he was "partially deaf" and needed all instructions and feedback repeated face to face. He no longer flies off the handle when given a simple directive by his supervisor and is gainfully employed. Harry, on the other hand, is in his 50s but has never held a job that required either reading or writing.

Language Characteristics. All aspects of language, spoken and written, are usually affected in children with LD. These children experience difficulty with the give-and-take of conversation and with the form and content of language. Deducing language rules is particularly difficult, resulting in delays in morphological rule acquisition and in the development of syntactic complexity. As a result, overall oral language development may be slow and frequent communicative breakdown is possible. Word-finding problems may exist, resulting in the child needing more time to respond verbally.

Attentional, discriminatory, and memory deficits, along with both receptive and expressive symbol use problems, can result in many communication breakdowns.

Pearson eTextbook
Video Example 4.9
In this TED Talk, a young woman with LD presents her challenges and triumphs.
www.youtube.com/watch?v=mwRnPF_NPbk

> **REFLECTION QUESTION 4.2**
>
> *What types of challenges did the woman face?*
>
> *If you understand the underlying cause for a type of language disorder, you can often predict the aspects of language that will be difficult. Let's take two different disorders with similar outcomes. Children with DLD and those with LD both tend to omit morphological endings but for different reasons. With limited capacity, children with DLD tend to not remember endings. Those with LD often misperceive morphological endings or do not notice them at all.*

Brain Injury

Impaired brain functioning, which can happen to any of us, can result from **traumatic brain injury (TBI)**, cerebrovascular accident or stroke, congenital malformation, convulsive disorders, or encephalopathy, such as infection or tumors. According to the CDC (2021), in the United States, TBI is the leading cause of disability and death in children and adolescents. At greatest risk for brain injury are those age 0–4 and 15–19. Based on emergency department data, an average of 564,000 children sustain brain injury annually. Of these, 62,000 require hospitalization. Cerebrovascular accidents and a fuller discussion of TBI in adults are presented in Chapter 7.

Approximately a million children and adolescents in the United States are living with TBI-related injury (CDC, 2022). Damage, which may be either localized or diffuse, is the result of external force, such as a blow to the head from an auto accident, a fall, or firearms. Individuals with TBI differ greatly from one another as a result of the site and extent of the injury, the age at onset, and the age of the injury. In general, the smaller the damaged area, the better the chance of recovery. Some individuals recover fully; others remain in a vegetative state. People with TBI exhibit a range of cognitive, physical, behavioral, academic, and linguistic deficits, any of which may be long term.

Cognitive deficits include difficulties in perception, memory, reasoning, and problem solving. Deficits vary and may be permanent or temporary and may partially or totally affect functioning ability. Children with TBI tend to be inattentive and easily distractible. All aspects of cognitive organization—categorizing, sequencing, abstracting, and generalization—may be affected. Children with TBI have difficulty perceiving relationships, making inferences, and solving problems. They struggle to formulate goals, plan, and achieve their ends. Memory is also affected, although long-term memory before the trauma is often intact.

Psychological maladjustment or "acting-out" behaviors, called *social disinhibition*, may occur, in which a person is incapable of inhibiting or controlling impulsive behavior. Other characteristics of TBI may include a lack of initiative, distractibility, inability to adapt quickly, perseveration, low frustration levels, passive-aggressiveness, anxiety, depression, fear of failure, and misperception.

Lifespan Issues. After a cranial accident, some children with TBI may be unconscious for a few minutes or much longer. Upon regaining consciousness, a child usually experiences some disorientation and memory loss. Memory loss may involve only the time of the immediate accident or may be more extensive, including long-term memory loss. TBI may be accompanied by physical disability and personality changes.

Neural recovery over time is often unpredictable and irregular, and the variables that affect recovery of children with TBI are extremely independent. In general, a better recovery is signaled by a shorter, less severe period of unconsciousness following the injury, a shorter period of amnesia, and better posttraumatic abilities.

The age of the injury can be an inaccurate prognosticator. In general, the older the injury, the less chance of change, although this can be complicated by the delayed onset of some deficits, making neural recovery unpredictable and irregular over time.

When stabilized, a child with TBI begins a long recovery process that can take years. Within the first few months, they might experience spontaneous recovery when large gains in ability are made.

Young children often recover quickly but experience difficulties learning new information and may exhibit severe, long-lasting problems. For example, young children with TBI may perform within average limits on standardized language tests but show differences later in more complex language skills, such as reading comprehension and pragmatics (Cermak et al., 2019; Haarbauer-Krupa et al., 2018). Older children and adolescents have more to recover from their memory but less new information to learn.

Although the brains of younger children are more malleable or more adaptable than those of older people, this does not mean that younger children will always recover more fully. In addition to recovering the language lost, younger children may still have much language to learn, a task that is possibly made more difficult by the brain injury.

Language Characteristics. Language problems may be evident even after mild cognitive injuries. Some deficits remain long after the injury, even when general improvement is good. For example, individuals with severe TBI and resultant deficits in executive function or ability to focus the brain demonstrate problems with pragmatics (Douglas, 2010). More specifically, these individuals have difficulty regulating the amount and manner of conversational participation as well as the relevance of their contributions. A child with TBI may lose the central focus or topic in conversation. Utterances are often lengthy, inappropriate, and off topic and fluency is disturbed, especially if there are accompanying motor problems.

Language comprehension and higher functions such as figurative language and dual meanings are also often impaired, although language form is relatively unaffected. Semantics, especially concrete vocabulary, is also relatively undisturbed, although word retrieval, naming, and object description difficulties may be present. Narration, especially maintaining story structure and providing enough information, may also pose a problem.

Even individuals who have made a seemingly full recovery may lack subtle cognitive and social skills. For example, although Jane had been injured in an auto accident but made a seemingly full recovery, she began to exhibit learning problems later when she attended elementary school. Unfortunately, her lack of success in school translated into disciplinary problems later on.

Other Language Disorders

Although we've touched on some of the most prevalent language disorders, we have by no means exhausted the discussion. Other forms of language disorder include but are not limited to:

- Children who are late-talkers
- Those with childhood schizophrenia, selective mutism, or middle ear infections (otitis media)

- Children who have received cochlear implants
- Those who have been exposed to alcohol and drugs in utero
- Those who have experienced abuse and neglect

Although child health is an important factor among late-talkers, most early language delay is due to environmental factors such as poverty and/or homelessness. Another factor may be preterm birth and/or low birth weight.

Childhood schizophrenia, a serious psychiatric illness that causes strange thinking, odd feelings, and unusual behavior, is uncommon, occurring in approximately 1 of every 14,000 children younger than 13 years of age. Approximately 55% of children and adolescents with schizophrenia have language abnormalities, including language delay, especially in pragmatics (Mental Health Research Association, 2007; Nicolson et al., 2000).

Selective mutism (SM) is a relatively rare disorder in which a child does not speak in specific situations, such as school, although they may speak normally in others. From 0.2 to 0.7% of all children may have SM at some time, and girls are nearly twice as likely as boys to be affected (Bergman et al., 2002; Kristensen, 2000).

Many young children suffer from chronic otitis media. In general, the cumulative effect of recurrent otitis media can be a significant factor in delayed language development (Feldman et al., 2003).

Those who receive cochlear implants develop language in a manner similar to typically developing children. Although children implanted later have an initial advantage of maturity that enhances language growth, those who receive implants at an earlier age begin to develop spoken language at an ever-increasing rate that soon eclipses the rate for children receiving implants later in childhood (Ertmer et al., 2003).

Children with FASD and drug exposure have many learning problems similar to those of children with learning disabilities.

Annually in the United States, approximately 40,000 infants, 1 in every 500 to 600 live births, are born with fetal alcohol spectrum disorder (FASD). Of these, as high as 8,000 are born with fetal alcohol syndrome (FAS), the most severe form (American Academy of Pediatrics, 2022). Alcohol interferes with embryonic development, and infants with FASD often have low birth weight and exhibit central nervous system problems. Later, these children demonstrate hyperactivity, motor problems, attention deficits, and cognitive disabilities. The limitations noted at birth remain with the child for life and can result in poor academic achievement and antisocial behavior. Children with FASD exhibit language problems characterized by delayed development of language, echolalia or inappropriate repetition, and comprehension problems. Children with FASD and those with fetal drug exposure are behind their peers in reading and other academic tasks.

Prenatal cocaine exposure (PCE) is a continuing problem in children's language development, even into adolescence (Lewis et al., 2013). As a group, children with PCE have mild but persistent deficits in syntax and phonological processing, which in turn adversely affects reading ability. In addition, caregiver variables, such as low maternal vocabulary, more psychological symptoms, and a poor home environment, are also contributing factors.

Finally, each year in the United States 1 in 7 children, approximately 900,000, are maltreated sufficiently for the neglect and/or abuse to be reported to the authorities (U.S. Department of Health and Human Services, 2022). Although neglect and abuse are rarely the direct cause of communication problems, the context in which they occur directly influences a child's development. Poor maternal health, substance abuse, poor or nonexistent pediatric services, and poor nutrition can all affect brain development and maturation.

In general, maltreated children demonstrated consistently poorer language skills with respect to receptive vocabulary, expressive language, and receptive language (Lum et al., 2015). Maltreated and abused children are less talkative and have fewer conversational skills than their peers. Their utterances and conversations are shorter, with less complex language, than are those of nonmaltreated children (Eigsti & Cicchetti, 2004). Although all aspects of language are affected, it is in pragmatics that children who have been neglected or abused exhibit the greatest difficulties.

REFLECTION QUESTION 4.3

Why is pragmatics or language use so frequently the aspect of language disorder seen in several disorders? Is it related to the nature of pragmatics and how it differs from other aspects of language?

So many disorders are associated with language disorder that they probably all have begun to look similar to you. In actual practice, SLPs treat each child as an individual, not as a member of a category. Of importance is each child's behavior and language features, not group characteristics.

Although this section has focused on disorders, it does not address all the factors that may be related to language disorder. Factors such as SES, nutrition, child and maternal health, and maternal sensitivity to and stimulation of a child are also important. For example, most children and mothers who are homeless exhibit language deficits for a variety of reasons (La Paro et al., 2004; O'Neil-Pirozzi, 2003). Approximately 580,000 people experienced homelessness on an average night in the United States, an increase of 12,751 people, or 2.2%, from 2019 (U.S. Department of Housing and Urban Development, 2021). Unfortunately, Black children, children from low-SES households, and children who are ELs are less likely to receive services when compared to White, middle class, English-speaking children (Morgan et al., 2016).

Aspects of Language Affected

In addition to the etiological categories we have just described, language disorders can also be characterized by the language features affected. For example, a child may have difficulty with word recall and conversational initiation or may possess a limited vocabulary and seem to talk nonstop. Another child may have poor syntax and very short sentences or withdraw from conversational give-and-take. Figure 4.1 presents the most common language features associated with language disorders. In evaluations, SLPs assess many language features to determine where to begin intervention.

To understand the range of responsibilities of an SLP in various disorders, check the ASHA website (www.asha.org). Enter "scope of practice" in the search field and then select the communication disorder you want to explore.

FIGURE 4.1 Most common language characteristics of children with language disorders.

Pragmatics

Difficulty answering questions or requesting clarification

Difficulty initiating and maintaining a conversation or securing a conversational turn

Poor flexibility in language when tailoring the message to the listener or repairing communication breakdowns

Short conversational episodes

Limited range of communication functions

Inappropriate topics and off-topic comments; ineffectual, inappropriate comments

Asocial monologues

Difficulty with stylistic variations and speaker–listener roles

Narrative difficulties

Few interactions

Semantics

Limited expressive vocabulary and slow vocabulary growth

Few or decontextualized utterances, more here-and-now; more concrete meanings

Limited variety of semantic functions

Relational term difficulty (comparative, spatial, temporal)

Figurative language and dual-definition problems

Conjunction (*and, but, so, because,* etc.) confusion

Naming difficulties may reflect less rich and less elaborate semantic storage or actual retrieval difficulties

Syntax/Morphology

Short, uncomplex utterances

Rule learning difficulties

Run-on, short, or fragmented sentences

Few morphemes, especially verb endings, auxiliary verbs, pronouns, and function words (articles, prepositions)

Overreliance on word order over word relationships

Difficulty with negative and passive constructions, relative clauses, contractions, and adjectival forms

Article (*a, an, the*) confusion

Phonology

Limited syllable structure

Fewer consonants in repertoire

Inconsistent sound production, especially as complexity increases

Comprehension

Poor discrimination of units of short duration (bound morphemes)

Impaired comprehension, especially in connected discourse such as conversations

Reliance on context to extract meaning

Wh- question confusion

Overreliance on nonlinguistic cues for meaning

Assessment

Learning Objective 4.3 Explain the process of assessment in language disorder.

An SLP's first task in assessment is to distinguish between children who have a disorder and those who do not. Accurate diagnosis is a prerequisite to ensuring appropriate intervention and also that scarce financial and personnel resources, especially in schools, are allocated in the most beneficial way.

Assessment and intervention overlap and are parts of the same process.

As with other diagnostics, language assessment is a systematic process of discovery and information gathering. Good clinical practice requires that the boundary between assessment and intervention be permeable. A portion of any good assessment is attempting to determine possible avenues for intervention. In turn, each intervention session should contain some assessment of a child's current skill level.

Assessment should be sufficiently broad and deep and come from a variety of sources so that all areas of possible concern are identified and described as accurately as possible. For example, preschool children born preterm perform very differently when measured on standardized tests and through language sampling (Imgrund et al., 2019). These findings support the importance of using both methods of assessment in the evaluation of young children's language skills.

Ideally, the language assessment would occur within a team that might include a psychologist, special educator, you as SLP, audiologist, and medical personnel. Standardized testing is no substitute for assessing language in real-life contexts. For example, observing WM in communication tasks can offer valuable insight into cognitive functioning beyond measures of WM out of context (Gray et al., 2019).

Assessment of English Learners and Nonmainstream Dialectal Speakers

Children who are ELs accounted for approximately 10.2% of the students enrolled in U.S. public schools, rising to 15–22% in Texas, Nevada, and California (National Clearinghouse for English Language Acquisition, 2018). In preschool Head Start programs, the percentage of children who use a language other than English is approximately 30% (Office of Head Start, 2016). These percentages are predicted to rise nationwide (Silverman & Doyle, 2013).

In addition, many children speak nonmainstream American English (NMAE) dialects that differ from the mainstream American English dialects that teachers use for instruction. For example, Black children make up approximately 17% of the children enrolled in public schools (Fry, 2007). The language of NMAE speakers and those with language disorders are qualitatively different. In general, language disorder results in a more restricted range of language on than does dialect (Oetting, 2019).

Any assessment of children with culturally and linguistically diverse backgrounds must recognize the possible risk for language disorder. For example, children from low-SES backgrounds with poorer maternal education have an increased incidence of language disorder (Schuele, 2001). The task of an SLP is to differentiate language disorder from language difference.

ELs and children with dialectal differences are more likely to be identified as needing special education services (de Valenzuela et al., 2006). This is most likely related to performance on standardized tests, many of which may not be appropriate for these children. Clearly, there is a critical need to develop language assessment measures and/or procedures that are appropriate.

Assessment of ELs poses a challenge for SLPs, especially when the SLP is a monolingual English speaker. Deciding whether a child has a language disorder or a language difference can be difficult. We do not have tests in most languages, few SLPs speak languages that infrequently occur in the United States, and tests normed on bilingual children are almost nonexistent. ELs with language disorders have significantly poorer performance than typically developing ELs on most measures of language except vocabulary (Paradis et al., 2013).

Diagnostic methods for children from culturally and linguistically diverse backgrounds vary widely, and no single measure or procedure is adequate (Dollaghan & Horner, 2011). Although grammatical ability of EL preschoolers seems to be related to lexical vocabulary in that language, there does not seem to be a relation between vocabulary and grammar skills across languages (Simon-Cereijido & Méndez, 2018). These data would lend support to testing in both languages.

A comprehensive assessment can reduce potential misdiagnosis of language disorders in children who are ELs (Dragoo, 2017; Peña & Halle, 2011; U.S. Department of Education, 2016). Thus, there is a critical need for development and use of measures to assess all aspects of language (Wright Karem et al., 2019).

Diagnosis should include published tests in both languages, if possible; spontaneous and elicited language samples in various settings with differing partners; and dynamic assessment procedures that are more open-ended and include descriptions of a child's use of both English and the child's first language. In dynamic assessment, an SLP modifies procedures to explore the optimal strategies to enhance a child's performance. Dynamic assessment can provide a systematic way to measure learning processes and learning outcomes (Peña et al., 2014).

For children speaking NMAE, the challenge is to differentiate dialectal differences from language disorders. Although some tests have separate norms for speakers of some dialects, the sample group may be too small to truly represent the language experience of any given child. The Diagnostic Evaluation of Language Variation (DELV; Seymour et al., 2018) has been developed for and normed on NMAE speakers. For other measures, an alternative procedure is **dialectal scoring** (Oetting et al., 2019), which accounts for language variations. Dialectal scoring potentially decreases the number of dialectal speakers who may be misdiagnosed as having a language disorder (Cleveland & Oetting, 2013; Oetting & Garrity, 2006).

Referral and Screening

For any individual, referral for a communication evaluation may occur at any point in their lifespan. Children, such as those with identifiable syndromes or those who are at risk for developing language disorder, might be referred at birth or in early infancy; those with LD might go undetected until they begin school; and those with TBI may be referred at the age when injury occurs. Although parents can be effective referral sources for children with more severe language problems, they are less reliable in identifying mild disorder (Conti-Ramsden et al., 2006). Instead, referral may come from a teacher or health care professional, such as the family physician.

In a public school, an SLP may decide to test a child on the basis of results of screening testing or teacher referral. Screening tests, used to determine the presence or absence of language problems, are routinely administered to all kindergarten and first-grade students. Screening tests must be chosen and administered very carefully. Even though a test is generally considered nonbiased, some items should be interpreted with caution because they may be problematic for children with differing cultural or linguistic backgrounds (Qi et al., 2003).

Children who are late-talkers but appear to have recovered by age 4 are at modest risk for continuing difficulties in elementary school. This risk is no greater than that for other 4-year-olds who have similar language performance at age 4. This indicates that the language of all children in the low normal range at age 4 should be monitored in an ongoing way, including periodic screening (Dale et al., 2014).

Surveys and parental questionnaires are also effective diagnostic tools. They compare favorably with other language measures and are part of a thorough, well-rounded assessment (Patterson, 2000; Rescorla & Alley, 2001; Thal et al., 2000).

In some settings, an interdisciplinary team of child specialists may handle referral and subsequent evaluation. The nature of many of the disorders mentioned

Information from referrals, questionnaires, and interviews provides needed background from which to begin investigating for possible language disorder and determining what that disorder entails.

previously may necessitate input from a pediatrician, a neurologist, an occupational therapist, a physical therapist, a developmental psychologist, a special education teacher, an audiologist, and/or an SLP. An interdisciplinary assessment that includes families as active participants and collaborators has been shown to be effective with young children with ASD (Prelock et al., 2003).

Case History and Interview

Administering a case history questionnaire and conducting a parent or teacher interview are the first steps in a formal information-gathering process. In addition to asking questions about birth and development, an SLP asks more specific questions relevant to language disorder. Questions relate to language development, the language environment of the home, and possible causes for language disorder. Possible questions are presented in Figure 4.2.

Observation

Language is heavily influenced by the context in which it occurs. It is helpful, therefore, to observe a child using language in as many contexts as possible. For example, a school-based SLP might observe in the classroom while a clinic-based

FIGURE 4.2 Possible questions for questionnaires/interviews when a language disorder is suspected.

Language Use

How does your child . . .

  Ask for information?

  Describe things in the environment?

  Discuss things in the past, future, or outside of the immediate context?

  Express emotions or discuss feelings?

  Request desired items?

  Request attention?

  Direct your attention?

Conversational Skills

How does your child . . .

  Initiate conversations or interactions with others? What are the child's frequent topics?

  Join in when others initiate?

  Get your attention before saying something?

  Take turns easily while talking? Are there long gaps between your utterances and the child's responses?

  Demonstrate an expectation that you will respond when they speak?

  Act if you do not respond?

  Ask for clarification when confused?

  Respond when asked to clarify?

  Demonstrate frustration when not understood?

  Relay sequential information or stories?

  Respond when you say something?

  Express emotions?

Are your child's responses meaningful, mismatched, off-topic, or irrelevant?

Form and Content

Does your child . . .

  Know the names of common events, objects, and people in the environment?

  Seem to rely on gestures, sounds, or immediate environment to be understood?

  Speak in single words, phrases, or sentences? How long is a typical utterance? Does the child leave out words?

  Use words such as *tomorrow, yesterday,* or *last night*?

  Follow simple directions?

How does your child . . .

  Talk about past, present, and future events?

  Put several sentences together to form complex descriptions and explanations?

Source: Based on Owens (2014).

FIGURE 4.3 Possible behaviors to observe during an assessment of language disorder.

With whom the child communicates

Purposes for the child's communication

Effectiveness of the child's communication:
 Obvious patterns of breakdown

Maturity of the child's language:
 Utterance length
 Verb usage
 Complexity

Relative amounts of initiative versus responsive communication

Relative amounts of nonsocial versus social communication

Responsiveness of caregiver

Turn allocation, relative size of child's and caregiver's turns

SLP might observe on a home visit, in a waiting room, or during a free-play period between the mother and child. Subsequent testing and sampling can provide additional observational periods.

Behaviors that are observed vary with the age of the child and the reported disorder. In addition to observing a child's communicative behavior, an SLP is also concerned with a child's interests, topics, style, and methods of communicating. With young children, an SLP will also want to note parental sensitivity to a child's communication attempts and parental responding to these attempts. Figure 4.3 presents some behaviors that might be observed during an assessment.

An SLP must remain focused during observation. This requires that they define very carefully the behaviors and/or language features that are observed and fully describe the events preceding and following them. Hypotheses about a child's language disorder are formed during observation. These are either confirmed or negated during the remainder of the assessment and further modified throughout intervention. For example, I observed one adolescent with IDD scream "Don't hit me" repeatedly. The teacher determined that the girl was not being abused. I hypothesized that this occurred when she was asked a question, but the behavior was inconsistent. It was further hypothesized that the type of question influenced the response. This hypothesis was confirmed later in the assessment through careful data collection in which over time the type of question was modified systematically.

Testing

SLPs should consult test manuals carefully and select tests that are sensitive and specific to language disorders. Although standardized, norm-referenced tests are appropriate for determining whether a problem exists, they are less useful in identifying specific language deficits. More descriptive measures, such as language sampling, allow an SLP to explore a child's strengths and weaknesses. In addition, descriptive results can provide useful information for intervention planning.

After building rapport with a child, an SLP can begin testing. It is best to use a series of testing tasks to ensure that many features of language are assessed. For example, one study found that a combination of tasks using children's books, such as shared story retelling in which a familiar story element is altered and comprehension questions, were effective in identifying 96% of children with language disorders (Skarakis-Doyle et al., 2008). At the very least, receptive and expressive aspects of language form, content, and use should be tested or sampled in some way.

Tasks should be varied, based on their potential effect on different children. Some children can remain on a given task, whereas others are highly distractible. Others may be reticent to talk or be withdrawn.

Test methodology varies widely. Children may be asked to form syntactically similar sentences, to make judgments of correctness, to reconfigure scrambled sentences, or to imitate exactly what they hear. They may have to supply definitions, form sentences, or point to words named. All these tasks require different language skills. Unfamiliar tasks may unintentionally prejudice the results against the child. Examples of language test tasks are presented in Figure 4.4. Testing is an atypical situation for most children. Typical language use is most likely to be displayed in language sampling.

During testing, an SLP probes a child's performance to try to identify possible effective intervention procedures. Of interest are strategies that either increase

FIGURE 4.4 Examples of language test tasks.

Test Procedure	Example
Grammatical completion	I'm going to say a sentence with one word missing. Listen carefully, then fill in the missing word. *John has a dish and Fred has a dish.* *They have two _____.*
Receptive vocabulary	Look at the pictures on this page. I'm going to name one, and I want you to point to it. *Touch (Show me) the officer.*
Defining words	I'm going to say some words. I want you to tell me what each word means or use it in a sentence in a way that makes sense. For example, if I said "coin," you might respond "money made from metal" or "I put my coin in the vending machine."
Pragmatic functions	I'm going to tell you a story and ask you to imagine what the person in the story might say. *Mary lost her money and she must call home for a ride after band practice. She decides to borrow a quarter from her best friend, Julie. Before practice begins, she sits down next to Julie and says _____.*
Sentence imitation	I'm going to say some sentences, and I want you to repeat exactly what I say. Let's try one. *We are going to play ball after school tomorrow.*
Parallel sentence production	Here are two pictures. I'll describe the first one, and then you describe the second one, using the same type of sentence as I use. For example, for this picture I would say, "The girl is riding her bike," and for this one you would say, "The man is driving his car."
Grammatical correctness	I'm going to say a sentence, and I want you to tell me if it is correct or incorrect. If it is incorrect, you must correct it. For example, if I say, "Thems is going to the dance," you would respond, "Incorrect. They are going to the dance."

production or result in more correct production of a certain language feature (Peña et al., 2001). Sometimes called **dynamic assessment**, this probing is invaluable in providing direction for subsequent intervention. Dynamic assessment and techniques that ask children to demonstrate skills that represent realistic learning demands are especially well suited for children with multicultural or bilingual backgrounds (Peña et al., 2006; Ukrainetz et al., 2000).

Test scores should be interpreted cautiously. For example, the omission of some morphological endings by children who are ELs is similar to the error pattern of children with DLD (Paradis, 2005). This can lead to misdiagnosis. In addition, children with language disorders aren't always identified by low scores (Spaulding et al., 2006).

REFLECTION QUESTION 4.4

Did you think initially that testing alone would be sufficient for assessing a language disorder? Can you think of some reasons why testing may not give a total picture of a child's communication?

Sampling

Tests do not address all aspects of language. Language is influenced by context. It follows that the context of test taking influences the language a child produces. For some children, especially young children, children of color, and those with disabilities, test structure decreases performance (Eisenberg et al., 2001). In addition, there may be few choices for tests that assess an individual child's communication.

CASE STUDY **Jayden** (*continued*)

Jayden used sign, speech, and an iPad, and his language progressed to two- to three-word sentences that he used for very limited purposes.

Language sample analysis (LSA) is an additional way to assess a child's language. LSA offers several advantages (Timler, 2018b). Among them is that LSA is flexible, can be repeated as often as needed, and in some cases, may be the only way to capture some concerns.

In sampling, an SLP engages a child in conversation or other naturalistic tasks in an attempt to "stretch" language performance and, in the process, reveal possible language difficulties. For example, the SLP might attempt to get longer, more complex language by asking a child to explain how to do something or to relate a familiar event. When we look at samples from young children with ASD, we find that the most severe communication impairments are not as common in naturalistic settings as in standardized assessments such as tests (Bacon et al., 2018). Although young children engaged in free play produce more utterances than those telling stories, they produce more complex utterances while telling stories and in conversation (Southwood & Russell, 2004). A variety of language tasks, such as conversation, narration, explanation, and interview, can be included in the sample.

Narratives or stories are especially helpful for exhibiting deficits in school-age children because of the demands on a speaker. In addition, narratives tend to elicit a large number and variety of syntactic structures. The personal narratives of children with language disorders are often so disordered that these stories negatively impact the social interactions of these children (McCabe & Bliss, 2004–2005). The shorter personal narratives of children with language disorders often omit key information and violate chronological sequences of events. With adolescents, posing peer conflict resolution problems or asking for explanations of how to accomplish a task is an effective method for eliciting grammatically complex utterances (Nippold et al., 2007). Figure 4.5 presents two very different types of language samples.

Whenever possible, it is best to collect at least two samples of the child interacting with different partners, locations, and activities or topics (Owens, 2014). For example, parent and teacher perceptions of specific social behaviors in children with ASD do not always agree (Murray et al., 2009). This disparity indicates that specific social behaviors may be context dependent and would suggest collecting data in different communication contexts. Typical performance may also be enhanced if parents or teachers interact with a child in familiar settings. An experienced SLP can also be an excellent conversational or play partner for the child.

The SLP records the language sample(s) and later carefully transcribes the child's exact words. MP3 players, cell phones, and tablets can be used effectively to collect language samples.

The amount of language collected may vary with the child and the aspect of language that is of concern. For example, most SLPs collect 50 utterances or less, which takes approximately 7 minutes to collect (Pavelko et al., 2016; Pavelko & Owens, 2017, 2019). Longer samples of up to 30 minutes have been suggested for very young children (Hadley et al., 2018).

LSA may consist of several quantitative and qualitative measures. Values such as *mean length of utterance (MLU)* in morphemes, the average number of clauses

FIGURE 4.5 **Examples of different types of language sampling.**

Open-Ended	Structured
Clinician: I'll play with this farm set, and you can too, or you can pick another toy.	*Clinician:* Well, here's the puppy. What should we say to him?
	Child: Hi puppy. [GREETING]
Child: Want farm.	*Clinician:* Hi Timmy. I'm hungry. We need to get someone to help us get those cookies.
Clinician: Oh, you want the farm. We can share. I wonder what we should do first.	*Child:* You help. Want cookie. [REQUESTING]
	Clinician: I wonder how I can reach it.
Child: Open door. Animals come out.	*Child:* Get chair. [HYPOTHESIZING]
Clinician: Okay.	*Clinician:* Oh, get on the chair. Should I (mumble).
Child: You be horsie and I man.	*Child:* Yeah. [DOES NOT REQUEST CLARIFICATION]
Clinician: Oh, the farmer.	*Clinician:* You want me to (mumble)?
Child: Farmerman chase horsie in barn.	*Child:* What's that? [REQUESTS CLARIFICATION]
Clinician: Oh, he did. I better run fast.	*Clinician:* Which do you want, the cookie or the chair?
Child: Man go fast in barn.	*Child:* Want cookie. No chair. [CHOICE MAKING]

per sentence, and the number of different words used within a given period of time or number of utterances can be compared to the values for typical children of the same age or developmental level (Johnston, 2001). MLU has been shown to be both a reliable and valid measure of general language development through age 10 for children with DLD (Pavelko & Owens, 2017; Rice et al., 2006).

LSA might also provide information on the percentage correct for a language feature, such as past tense *-ed*. More descriptive measures might be the variety of intentions expressed by the child, the conversational styles used, and the types of repair the child uses when the conversation breaks down (Yont et al., 2000). With some children, the SLP might carefully note the number of different words or lexical diversity of the sample (Charest et al., 2020).

Being as thorough as possible, an SLP attempts to analyze the sample for all aspects of form, content, and use appropriate for the particular assessment. For example, with ELs an SLP might consider **code switching** (the movement between two languages), dialect, English proficiency, and contextual effects in addition to aspects of both languages (Gutierrez-Clellan et al., 2000).

Although LSA may seem very open-ended, it need not be. Methods such as *Systematic Analysis of Language Transcripts* (SALT; Miller & Iglesias, 2015), *Computerized Language Analysis* (CLAN; MacWhinney, 2022), and *Sampling Utterances and Grammatical Analysis Revised* (SUGAR; Owens & Pavelko, 2021) are designed for use with computers. Others, such as *Developmental Sentence Scoring* (DSS; Lee, 1974) and *Index of Productive Syntax* (IPSyn; Scarborough, 1990), have been adapted to computer analysis. These methods vary in their software but also in the aspects of language analyzed

For school-age children experiencing literacy difficulties, an SLP may also want to collect samples of written language. These are discussed in Chapter 6.

Intervention

Learning Objective 4.4 Describe the overall design of language intervention.

As you might guess, the complexity of language necessitates using multiple intervention methods. Different intervention approaches target specific aspects of language and employ a variety of procedures. Within limits, we explore these diverse approaches to remediation of language disorders.

All aspects of language are interrelated. Changes in one area affect others. For example, learning to use the past tense *-ed* might increase the quality of personal narratives because we usually tell of what happened in the past. In intervention, an SLP should not take such changes for granted and focus solely on one aspect of language. Intervention goals should focus on stimulating the language acquisition process beyond the immediate target (Fey et al., 2003).

Similarly, SLPs should use a variety of intervention techniques. For example, children with ASD can improve social skills better through a combination of peer training and written cues than by either method alone (Thiemann & Goldstein, 2004). The most effective intervention approach for older school-age children and adolescents with deficits in syntax is an integrated one in which naturalistic stimulation approaches are supplemented with deductive teaching procedures. In a deductive method, children are presented with a rule that guides the use of a morphological marker, such as past tense *-ed*, along with models of the inflection (Finestack & Fey, 2009).

Increasingly, SLPs are including other individuals from a child's environment in the training. Recall the SLP working with Jayden worked with him directly and also worked through the preschool teacher and Jayden's parents.

Without training, day care providers fail to fine-tune their language for individual children's needs (Girolametto et al., 2000). In early intervention and in preschool, parents are usually an integral part of their child's language program. Working through parents and other caregivers is different than direct intervention by the SLP with the child, although this is also a program component. Teaching adults to be language teachers can offer a challenge. Various techniques such as a Teach-Model-Coach-Review instructional approach have been shown to be effective (Roberts et al., 2014).

SLPs can help preschool teachers implement intervention both through activities such as dramatic play, art, and storybook reading and through language instruction processes (Pence et al., 2008). Preschool staff being trained to respond to children's initiations, to engage children, to model simplified language, and to encourage peer interactions has a significant effect on children's language production (Girolametto et al., 2003). Even peers can serve as effective tutors or models for children with language disorders (McGregor, 2000).

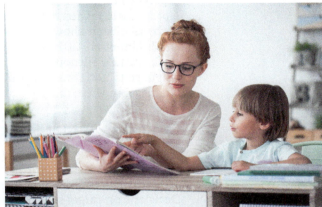

Preschool teachers can learn from SLPs how to implement intervention through activities such as dramatic play, art, and storybook reading.

© Ground Picture/Shutterstock

With the aid of an SLP, these and other care providers, such as parents, may learn how to be better language partners for children. Despite the many demands on and restrictions faced by mothers and children who are homeless, it is possible to teach homeless parents, even those with limited language skills, to use facilitating language strategies during interactions with their preschool children (O'Neil-Pirozzi, 2009).

With school-age children, the SLP can use a variety of intervention models, including individual and group sessions both within and outside the classroom. Teachers and aides can also be trained to help children participate. Ideally, the SLP would also teach the entire class on occasion, being mindful of the needs of children with language disorders.

Considerations for Children with Culturally and Linguistically Diverse Backgrounds

According to federal law and American Speech-Language-Hearing Association guidelines, intervention for language disorders must be responsive to the cultural and linguistic backgrounds of children and their families (ASHA, 2008, 2017; IDEA, 2004). Population variability is likely to impact the cultural validity of language intervention, especially for young children and their families (Cycyk & Huerta, 2020).

Cultural congruency is the synchrony of intervention strategies and techniques with the cultural values, beliefs and behaviors of a community and is important in providing appropriate and effective services. In short, language interventions that match parental, caregiver, and community expectations will have more successful outcomes than those that do not (García Coll et al., 2002; Griner & Smith, 2006; Larson et al., 2020). For example, parents and caregivers may question being asked to assist or providing intervention in the home for very young children. Some intervention techniques, such as the use of play or conversation as a vehicle for teaching, may not fit cultural norms or expectations. It's important to note that what may seem second nature to an SLP may seem very foreign to some families.

Although SLPs may be focused on English with children who are ELs, maintaining the heritage language is frequently as important for the family and community. Continued development of the heritage language depends on rich and frequent exposure and opportunities for practice that usually occur in the home (Pham & Tipton, 2018). Intervention in both home and school languages and support of both have been shown to have positive effects (Goodrich et al., 2013; Gorman, 2012; Lim et al., 2019; Restrepo et al., 2013; Riquelme & Rosas, 2014; Rosa-Lugo et al., 2012). Although optimal, intervention in both English and the heritage language is not always feasible, especially if the SLP does not speak the heritage language. In these cases, community resources or the use of translators may help.

Language Target Selection and Sequence of Teaching

The criteria for target selection will vary with the child, the affected aspects of language, the child's disorder, and the needs of the environment.

The goal of intervention is the maximally effective use of language to accomplish communication goals within everyday interactions. Although most SLPs would agree on this overall goal, less unanimity exists on the route to achieving it. Decisions on target selection and training vary with each child and each SLP.

Using the same assessment results, SLPs might differ in the targets they select. One SLP might use language acquisition knowledge as a general guide. Another might begin intervention at the point of communication breakdown and frustration for the child. A more classroom-based approach might suggest training for language used within the class. Still another approach might be to begin with language features that are just emerging.

Decisions must also be made about where to begin once the target is selected. Some SLPs prefer to begin with receptive language training and progress to expressive. Others might start with expressive training.

Expressive training may be bottom-up, in which the SLP begins at the symbol level and works toward conversational goals; top-down, in which training is placed within a conversational framework; or a combination of the two. Obviously, the child's abilities are an important determinant of the method selected. To the best extent possible, training should be placed within meaningful communicative contexts.

Evidence-Based Intervention Principles

The needs of children with language disorders suggest several principles that should guide intervention services. These principles, presented in Figure 4.6, recognize the need to target a child's language abilities in their entirety rather than to focus exclusively on one deficit area. The interrelatedness of all areas of language and the importance of communication context on the form and content of language necessitate a more holistic approach.

As a profession, speech-language pathology stresses the importance of evidence-based practice. This is a combination of scientific evidence, SLP experience and

FIGURE 4.6 **Principles of language intervention.**

1. The goal of intervention should be greater facility of language use in conversation, narration, exposition, and other textual genres in hearing, speaking, reading, and writing.
2. Deficit areas are rarely, if ever, the only areas of language that should be targeted in an intervention program.
3. Select intermediate goals that stimulate a child's language acquisition process rather than goals that focus solely on deficit areas.
4. Select specific goals of intervention based on a child's readiness and need for the targeted goals.
5. Manipulate the context to create more opportunities for the language target to occur.
6. Exploit different genres and modalities to develop appropriate contexts for intervention targets.
7. Manipulate clinical discourse so targeted areas are more noticeable and important in various contexts.
8. Systematically contrast a child's language performance with more mature adult usage by recasting a child's utterances.
9. Provide good models of easily comprehended, well-formed phrases and sentences.
10. Use a variety of verbal and nonverbal strategies to elicit and modify a child's language and to give a child practice in using language to accomplish their communication needs.

client needs and wishes. Although a lack of direct empirical evidence should not automatically rule out a new teaching method, it should be grounds for suspicion (Cirrin & Gillam, 2008). Box 4.4 presents recommended practices for language disorders.

BOX 4.4 **Evidence-Based Practice for Childhood Language Disorders**

General

- Intervention is effective for the vast majority of children.
- Benefits accrue from beginning intervention as early as possible.
- Multiple measures provide the most accurate and valid language assessment.

English Learners

- No single measure is adequate for assessment.
- Maintaining the home language enables parents, who may not speak English, to support language development.

Presymbolic Children

- Interactive language intervention in which parents are trained to provide intervention at

home is effective. Long-term and standardized measures have not been applied.
- Intervention gains in both receptive language and expressive syntax are best for children receiving both SLP and parent-implemented intervention.

Children with Autism Spectrum Disorder

- Effective interventions are characterized by early intervention and intensive and individualized instruction.
- Both structural behavioral approaches and naturalistic approaches are effective in replacing challenging behavior with social interactions, although no method works with all children with ASD.
- Approximately two-thirds of children make significant measurable gains with intervention.

(continued)

- The Picture Exchange Communication System (PECS), in which a picture is used to request items, demonstrates only small to moderate gains in communication and small to negative gains in speech. Gains may be enhanced if others, such as peers with TDL, are taught to be responsive listeners.
- Although video-modeling is an effective strategy for teaching some social interactional behaviors, we still need exploration of the efficacy of other methods.

Preschool

- Speech and language intervention are most effective for children with phonological or expressive vocabulary difficulties.
- Parent-implemented language interventions have a significant, positive impact on both receptive language and expressive syntactic skills.
- Intervention of more than 8 weeks results in better outcomes than shorter intervention.
- Seventy percent of preschool children with language impairments make significant measurable gains with intervention.

School-Age and Adolescent

Syntax and Morphology

- Moderately large to large effects follow use of imitation, modeling, or modeling plus evoked production strategies.
- Computerized input strategies alone have not demonstrated extensive benefit as yet.

Semantics and Vocabulary

- A paucity of research exists and we do not yet have evidence on the best possible technique for effective vocabulary instruction for children in the early elementary grades.

- Collaborating with teachers on large-group instruction and slowed presentation rate can positively impact vocabulary development.
- Interactive conversational reading strategies may be somewhat helpful for improving receptive and expressive vocabulary.
- There do not seem to be clear differences in outcome between the various methods used to assist children with word finding.

Language Processing

- Computer intervention using modified speech stimuli or speech and language games does not improve performance.

Pragmatics and Discourse

- Direct instruction on topic initiation and group entry behaviors can yield moderately large to large effects for students with social communication deficits.
- It is possible to teach social skills to adolescents with ASD, although the data are not sufficient to identify the most effective method of intervention.

Method of Intervention

- We can tentatively conclude that preschool and early elementary children with LI show greater improvement with collaborative (teacher and SLP) teaching, classroom-based language intervention model than they do in more traditional pull-out intervention.
- Recast sentences are an effective responsive method for grammatical intervention. In a recast, the SLP modifies the elements in the child's utterance to make it more correct or mature, to change the form of the sentence, or to offer another variation.
- Computer/Internet programs that target cognitive learning rather than specific skills training are effective for working memory and executive function.

Sources: Based on Bedore (2010); Burgess and Turkstra (2006); Cirrin and Gillam (2008); Cleave et al. (2015); Dollaghan and Horner (2011); Goldstein and Prelock (2008); Johnson and Yeates (2006); Justice and Pence (2007); Law et al. (2004); Peijnenborgh, Hurks, et al. (2016).

Intervention Procedures

Remember that as an SLP, wherever you may work, you are *teaching* communicative skills. SLPs are teachers in the broadest sense. Throwing out questions or cues and hoping for the right response or providing the answer when the child is incorrect is not teaching. Teaching is a systematic analysis of what a child is lacking that results in their failure to succeed.

As an SLP, you need to break any learning task into the sequential steps required to move from where the child is now to where you want the child to be. Decisions on sequencing should be determined by the complexity of the task, its cognitive and linguistic requirements, and the learning characteristics of the individual child. The SLP enhances teaching by anticipating the types of support that a child is likely to need for success and the types of errors the child is likely to make (Schuele & Boudreau, 2008).

A few basic tenets of good teaching behavior include, but are not limited to, the following:

- *Model the desired behavior for the child.* Modeling may include multiple exposures, called focused stimulation or priming, that occur before the child is required to produce the language feature (Leonard, 2011). This might be followed by the child imitating the SLP. In a variation called parallel sentence production, an SLP provides a model of the type of utterance desired. The child is not expected to imitate the model but to provide a similar type of sentence. For example, you might describe a picture by saying "The girl is throwing the ball" and then ask the child to describe a second picture of a boy catching a ball. The need for modeling decreases as the language feature is learned. Older elementary school children and adolescents may also benefit from an explanation of the targeted behavior and a rationale for why its correct use is important.

- *Cue the child to respond.* Carefully selected cues, such as the use of the word *yesterday* to signal a past-tense response, serve as aids for the child in conversation. Cues may range from very specific, such as *say, imitate,* or *point to,* to more general conversational cues, such as *I wonder what I should say now* to elicit a specific linguistic structure in context or *Maybe Carol can help us if we ask* to elicit a question:

  - Cues may be either verbal or nonverbal. Verbal cues attempt to elicit the language feature by providing a linguistic framework; nonverbal cues use the context of an event to evoke the feature.

  - The SLP should rate each type of cue or prompt from least to most intrusive and supportive (Timler et al., 2007). As intervention proceeds, the SLP works to minimize prompting whenever possible, so the child can become more independent.

- *Respond to the child in the form of reinforcement and/or corrective feedback.* Reinforcement varies from very direct and obvious forms, such as "Good, that was much better," to more conversational responses, such as "That sounds like fun. Tell me more." Conversational responses come in many varieties, including imitating the child, imitating but expanding the child's utterance into a more mature version, replying conversationally, and asking for clarification, to name a few. With some children, especially those with vocabulary deficits, the relationship of the response to the content of the child's utterance has more effect on the child's language than the structural input of the clinician's feedback. In other words, respond to the meaning of what the child said:

  - *Natural reinforcers flow from the training target.* The most obvious example is one in which a child obtains a desired object upon responding to the cue "What do you want?" Conversational responses are natural and reinforcing.

SLPs are teachers of language. They must plan their behaviors well to teach without overly relying on less natural strategies, such as drill and the use of edible reinforcers.

- ▪ Corrective feedback may range from a gentle reminder to an instruction. For example, an SLP might recast a sentence. If the child says, "Boy eating cookie," and the target is use of the auxiliary verb *be*, the SLP might recast the sentence as "He *is* eating" or "The boy *is eating* the cookie." Children with DLD and low MLU scores benefit most from responses in which the child is prompted to attempt the structure prior to the adult's recast (Yoder et al., 2011).

- ▪ In general, as a language feature is produced more correctly by a child, an SLP relies less on these direct forms. When a language feature is correct most of the time, conversational feedback, such as "What?" or "I don't understand," may be sufficient to cause the child to self-correct the few errors made.

- • *Plan for generalization of the learned feature to the everyday use environment of the child.* SLPs can help with generalization by selecting training targets that are highly likely to occur in the child's everyday communication and by including elements of the everyday use environment in the training, such as familiar locations, people, and objects. Parents are often included in the training of young children, whereas teachers may be involved in the intervention of school-age children and adolescents.

  Although it may seem counterintuitive, with some intervention targets, such as verb endings, children with language disorders tend to generalize rules better if they are presented with a wide variety of verbs rather than a restricted set that they hear over and over (Plante et al., 2014). In addition, these children produce more utterances that generalize the learning.

Pearson eTextbook
Video Example 4.10
In this video is an example of a technique called "sentence recasts," or reformulating the child's utterance.
www.youtube.com/
watch?v=SNOk2nxBOhl

Specific examples of each teaching method are presented in Figure 4.7.

Not all teaching strategies have similar effects. For example, imitation can result in rapidly achieving production of grammatical targets (Eisenberg et al., 2020). The technique is not recommended, however as the sole method of intervention, in part because of poor long-term learning effects and poor generalization.

Initially, it might seem that the SLP's mere presentation of repeated examples of the language target is sufficient for learning to occur. This is an implicit approach that assumes a child will deduce the underlying language rule. **Explicit instruction** tries to make a child consciously aware of the underlying language pattern. In a study with 5- to 8-year-old children with DLD, Finestack (2018) demonstrated that children are more likely to acquire, maintain, and generalize novel grammatical forms when taught with explicit instruction. This methodology does not preclude using a more conversational approach with periodic reminders of the rule or why we're learning a language target.

In short, intervention that includes explicit instruction is more beneficial than implicit techniques alone (Bangert et al., 2019; Finestack, 2018; Finestack & Fey, 2009; Motsch & Riehemann, 2008). That said, research indicates that combining implicit and explicit approaches is beneficial when teaching children with significant weaknesses in language (Bolderson et al., 2011; Calder et al., 2018; Kulkarni et al., 2014; Smith-Lock et al., 2013).

Effective language intervention should enhance language and social skills in real-life interactions (Timler et al., 2007). Success occurs when the newly taught language feature generalizes to a child's everyday environment. Children learn to use language through interactions with many individuals and in varying situations.

FIGURE 4.7 Examples of teaching methods.

Method Modeling	Example
Focused stimulation	I'll pretend to make a cake first. Watch to see if I make a mistake. I'm *putting* the eggs in the bowl and *taking* them to the table. I'm *cracking* the eggs. Now I'm *beating* the eggs. Next, I'm *sifting* the flour. I'm *adding* the flour to the eggs and *mixing* them. Now I'm *measuring* the sugar and *pouring* it into the mix . . .
Cuing	
Direct Verbal	
Imitation	Say "I want cookie."
Cloze	This is a _____. She should say _____.
Question	What should I say now? What's this? Which one's this?
Indirect Verbal	
Pass it on	I wonder if Joan knows the answer. How could we find the answer? [TARGET IS FORMATION OF QUESTIONS]
Nonverbal	Not giving child all the materials needed to complete a task.
(Inherent in the activity)	Not explaining how to accomplish an assigned task. Playing dumb.
Responding	
Direct Reinforcement	Good, I like the way you said that. Much better than the last time.
Indirect Reinforcement	
Imitation	*Child:* I go horsie. *Clinician:* I go horsie.
Expansion	*Child:* I go horsie. *Clinician:* I'm going to go on the horsie.
Extension	*Child:* I go horsie. *Clinician:* Yes, cowboys go on horses, too.
Corrective Feedback	Remember, when we use a number like two, three, or more, we say /s/ on the word. Listen. One cat. Two cats.

Lastly, it's important to recall that these are children. Children's active participation is a significant factor in effective language therapy. The level of a child's active engagement is directly related to their language gains (Schmitt, 2020). In addition, more active involvement results in more stable generalization. Ideally, intervention consists of motivating participatory activities in various contexts.

Intervention Through the Lifespan

Targets of intervention vary with the age and language skills of a child. An infant in an early intervention program would have different training targets than an adolescent with mild LD. In contrast, an infant may be receiving some of the same training as an adolescent who has profound IDD and is functioning below age 1 year.

Early intervention, especially for children with IDD and ASD, can have a very positive benefit. Initial training may target presymbolic communicative skills and cognitive abilities, such as physical imitation, gestures, and understanding of object uses. Parents may be trained to treat their child's behaviors as having some communicative value or to interpret consistent behaviors as attempts to communicate. An SLP may attempt to establish an initial communication system by using an augmentative and alternative communication system (AAC) such as gesturing, a communication board, or an electronic device. AAC is discussed in more detail in Chapter 13.

Early symbolic training may focus on receptive understanding, vocabulary acquisition, semantic categories, word combinations, and an array of early intentions. The beneficial effects of treatment for children with delayed language extend beyond the trained targets into other areas of linguistic and overall development. Within a framework of play, shared attention, and naturalistic language teaching, the use of manual signs along with verbal models appears to facilitate development of expressive sign and word communication in some young children with ID (Wright et al., 2013).

CASE STUDY   Jayden *(continued)*

Jayden's parents continue to use signs to inform him about routine changes such as dinnertime. His own use of signs seems to have decreased his frustration and acting-out behaviors. Jayden prefers to be alone, and even in his preschool class he rarely interacted with other children, seeming to prefer the company of adults.

Children at the preschool language level usually work on language form in both conversations and narratives. Longer utterances, bound morphemes, and early phonological processes may be intervention goals. Vocabulary will continue to be targeted.

Intervention with school-age children may focus on pragmatic skills in conversations and semantic targets, such as figurative language, multiple meanings, abstract terms, and more advanced relational terms, such as conjunctions. Academic skills, including summarizing a reading and different types of writing and note taking, may also be targeted. SLPs may use computerized programs to supplement more face-to-face intervention. Computer use should mesh well with the SLP's overall clinical philosophy and the child's individual needs. Language enhancement can be infused into the curriculum. SLPs may work with the child on both spoken and written language. It is also important for children with language disorders to learn to navigate the curriculum and understand classroom expectations.

Language intervention doesn't end with childhood. Adolescents may continue to exhibit language disorders and be in need of services. Adults with severe ASD or

In schools, SLPs provide individual, group, and classroom language intervention.

ID will most likely require continued intervention for language and communication deficits and a range of educational and vocational needs. Individuals with LD may require additional support in postsecondary education (Downey & Snyder, 2000; Olivier et al., 2000).

With adolescents, an SLP might focus on multiclausal or complex sentences, variations in the verb, and expository text, which includes persuasive speech and writing, explanations of how to do something, and compare and contrast activities (Scott, 2014). A middle school SLP will need to collaborate with classroom teachers and reading specialists, have knowledge of the Common Core State Standards and the language demands of the classroom, and understand later language development and the reasons for speakers and writers using complex syntax (Nippold, 2014).

Summary

In this chapter, we discussed several types of language disorders. Although language disorders are very complex and multifaceted, we have only touched the surface in this chapter. The number of associated disorders, the language features that are affected, and the individual differences among children result in each child's language being very individualistic. Recall Jayden. We weren't as interested in a label for his disorder as we were with a description of his language and its use. It is very important to remember that each child is a unique case. Given this fact, assessment becomes a search to find and describe a child's individual language abilities. This is accomplished through referral, collection of a case history, interviews, observation, testing, and language sampling.

As a result of the assessment process and through repeated assessment probes during intervention, an SLP attempts to find the most efficient and effective method for teaching new skills. The SLP identifies targets for intervention and trains these through a combination of techniques in various settings with the aid of additional language facilitators.

Obviously, every SLP needs thorough training and extensive experience with language disorders to serve children with a variety of disabilities. As an SLP, you want to gain a firm foundation of speech and language development, take several courses in language disorders in both children and adults, and complete at least one clinical experience with both populations.

Epilogue   Case Study: Jayden

Now age 10, Jayden prefers to use an iPad to communicate even though his speech has greatly improved. Along with his use of two- to three-word sentences, his vocabulary has expanded to about 350 words, mostly nouns and verbs. Although still mostly used for requesting, he will ask the occasional question or make a comment. Jayden is much more social than in preschool and gets along well with his classmates, although he still seems to prefer being alone.

At the moment, Jayden has a keen interest in dinosaurs and beyond his 350 words are another 50 or so that relate to dinosaurs, including *tyrannosaurus rex* and *paleontology*. He will read anything related to dinosaurs but his progress is slow and labored. In addition, he has demonstrated a real skill at drawing dinosaurs.

Reflections from a Preschool-Based Speech-Language Pathologist

[We] have a district-run preschool for children with extra needs. . . . I'm in the classrooms every day and I do individual and group intervention there and in the speech room. I've trained the teacher and the aides in how to maximize communication with children. I also work with parents who are invited to work with me and/or observe therapy. With some parents I've had to explain that when I play with their child, play is the vehicle for change, not the goal of intervention. It's a subtle distinction.

Most of the children I work with have language needs but a few also have apraxia of speech. Two children are using AAC devices and one has feeding and swallowing issues. It's a diverse caseload and was a real education for me. Now, I feel at ease but each year a new cohort of kiddos poses new challenges for me. My job is taxing but also fun and enjoyable.

Although I'm sad when the children transition into kindergarten, I do get to see some in school later. Many are still receiving speech and language services but a few have transitioned into regular classrooms with no services.

I get my rewards from seeing children grow and change, which they do quickly at this age. And working closely with parents has its own rewards. Sometimes we focus on therapy and their child but, when possible, I also just let them talk about having a child with special needs and their hopes for the future. They're grateful for that opportunity and for what I do for their children.

Suggested Readings/Sources

Nelson, N. W. (2010). *Language and literacy disorders: Infancy through adolescence.* Pearson.

Owens, R. E. (2018). *Early language intervention for infants, toddlers, and preschoolers.* Pearson.

Owens, R. E. (2023). *Language disorders: A functional approach to assessment and intervention* (6th ed.). Plural.

Reed, V. A. (2018). *An introduction to children with language disorders* (5th ed.). Pearson.

5 Speech Sound Disorders

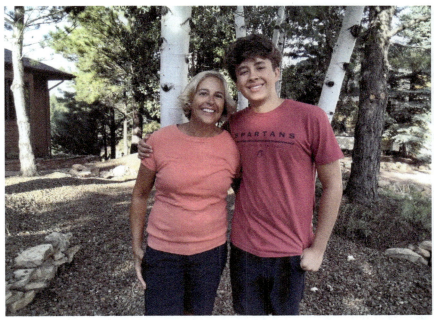

John with his mom, Anne
© Anne M. Vonesh

Learning Objectives

When you have finished this chapter, you should be able to:

5.1 Explain how speech sounds (vowels and consonants) are classified.

5.2 Outline the sequence of speech sound acquisition across the lifespan.

5.3 Discuss the types of speech sound disorders in children.

5.4 List the risk factors associated with speech sound disorders in children.

5.5 Describe the goals and procedures in speech sound assessment.

5.6 Describe approaches and techniques to treat speech sound disorders, including supportive evidence.

> " When I first arrived for work in the clinic at Northern Arizona University (NAU), I was asked to take a look at a soon-to-be 3-year-old male who was nonverbal and suspected of having childhood apraxia of speech. Because I had just returned from my postdoctoral fellowship at Mayo Clinic in Rochester, Minnesota, with Edythe Strand, renowned expert in CAS, I was not surprised by the request on my first day. CAS can be a difficult disorder to understand, diagnose, and treat, and few SLPs have sufficient experience to feel confident with diagnosing it. John did in fact have severe CAS; his family diligently brought him to speech therapy three times per week for 30-minute sessions. He practiced a small set of functional vocabulary words and phrases such as "eat," "up," "I want," and "I need." He practiced those few words and phrases for over a year until all vowels and consonants were mastered within each target word. John continued with therapy at the NAU Speech-Language-Hearing Clinic off and on until he was 10 years old. Now, at age 16 (pictured above), and no evidence of ever having a speech sound disorder, he serves as a volunteer for online webinars demonstrating speech production techniques for SLPs learning to work with children with motor speech disorders. John represents my greatest success story and the most rewarding clinical experience in my career. He is a constant reminder for why I chose the field of speech-language pathology.
>
> —*Kimberly Allyn Farinella*

CASE STUDY Daniel

Daniel, a bright, energetic 5-year-old boy bilingual in English and Spanish, was struggling to make friends in kindergarten. Because his speech was difficult to understand, he was quiet and shy at school and became frustrated when he was not understood. His kindergarten teachers also had a difficult time understanding him. Daniel would sometimes use gestures or act out what he wanted to say to get his message across to them. Other times, he would just shut down. Kindergarten speech-language screenings conducted by the speech-language pathologist (SLP) identified Daniel as a child struggling with speech production skills. He was recommended for comprehensive testing of his speech to determine or rule out a speech sound disorder.

As you read the chapter, think about:

- The importance of administering the speech evaluation in both languages
- Possible explanations for Daniel's speech difficulties
- Phonological patterns (processes) Daniel was exhibiting in his speech
- Specific treatment approaches the SLP may use with Daniel
- The need for a highly trained interpreter during speech therapy sessions if the SLP is not multilingual

Speech sound disorders (SSDs) in children refer to difficulties related to how speech sounds are used in the language (i.e., phonology), and how sounds of the language are produced (i.e., articulation). Causes of SSDs include impairments in the phonological representation of speech sounds, including knowledge of the rules that govern sound combinations; an inability or difficulty perceiving (i.e., hearing) speech sounds, thereby affecting the ability to acquire and produce those sounds; structural abnormalities (e.g., cleft of the hard and soft palates) that affect the integrity of the speech production mechanism; and/or motor speech disorders such as dysarthria and childhood apraxia of speech that affect motor control pathways governing speech sound production.

Speech sound disorders can be mild in severity, such as when the impairment affects a single sound (e.g., distortion of /r/), to more severe, as when the child deletes all sounds in the final positions of words, making it difficult to understand what the child is saying. To understand SSDs, it is first necessary to have a general understanding of the speech sound system, as well as knowledge of speech sound development. Therefore, our discussion begins here with how speech sounds are produced and classified, followed by a brief overview of normal speech sound acquisition. We then distinguish between phonological and articulation impairments and discuss their potential causes. Finally, we describe assessment techniques and evidence-based intervention approaches in the Case Study, in the context of a bilingual child, Daniel.

Understanding Speech Sounds

Learning Objective 5.1 Explain how speech sounds (vowels and consonants) are classified.

Although the written alphabet contains 26 letters, spoken English has about 44 different speech sounds or phonemes, which are combined to form spoken words, phrases, and sentences. For example, the word *cat* contains three phonemes /kæt/. Note that phonemes and letters are not the same. The word *that* also has three phonemes /ðæt/. Phonemes, or sounds that distinguish meaning in a person's speech, are generally written between two slashes, as in /p/ and /k/. Since /p/ and /k/ are different phonemes, they create different words and convey different meanings, like /pɪt/ *pit*, /pan/ *pan*, and /pɛt/ *pet* or /kæt/ *cat*, /kan/ *can*, and /kʌp/ *cup*.

Some phonemes are universal and found in all languages; other phonemes are used in only a few languages. For example, the tongue clicks used in some African languages are not used as phonemes in English. In general, the more phonemes two languages have in common, the more similar the languages sound.

The phonemic symbols for standard American English speech sounds are available at the Dyslexia Reading Well website at www.dyslexia-reading-well .com/44-phonemes-in-english.html. However, there are many websites with helpful charts that have audio and video recordings of standard American English speech sounds that are easily found using an online search.

In addition to phonemes, which are the building blocks of speech, *phonotactic* rules exist that specify acceptable sequences and locations. For example, the "ks" combination is never used at the beginning of an English word, but it is fine at the end, in words such as *books*. Many Polish and Russian names are difficult for English speakers to pronounce because these Slavic languages permit consonant combinations that are not found in English.

Classification of Speech Sounds

Phonemes are often categorized as either **vowel** or **consonant**. Very generally, vowels are produced with a relatively open or unobstructed vocal tract, and consonants are made with some degree of constriction.

Consonant phonemes may be classified according to which articulators are used (place of articulation), how the sound is made (manner of production), and whether they occur with laryngeal vibration (voicing). Vowels are typically described according to tongue and lip position and relative degree of tension in these articulators. These methods of characterizing phonemes are described next.

All spoken languages have vowels and consonants. The intelligibility of an utterance is determined largely by the consonants, whereas the sound energy comes primarily from the vowels.

Classification of Consonants by Place, Manner, and Voicing

Consonants are characterized by the degree of constriction or closure somewhere along the vocal tract, referred to as the *manner* of consonant production. The location of this point of closure or constriction refers to the *place* of consonant production. For instance:

- Consonants in which the location or place of constriction occurs at both lips are called **bilabial** sounds, literally meaning "two lips." Say "mom" and feel where your lips are for the /m/ sounds.

- **Labiodental** consonants are made with the bottom lip and upper teeth in contact, like /f/ in the word *off*.

- **Interdental** consonants are produced with the tongue between the teeth and are sometimes called **linguadental**, as in the "th" sound like in the word *the*.

- **Alveolar** sounds are made when the tongue tip is touching the alveolar or upper gum ridge, as in the way we say the /t/ or /s/ sounds.

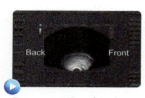

Pearson eTextbook
Video Example 5.1

In this video of ultrasound images of the tongue, the tongue tip and tongue blade elevate during production of alveolar consonant sounds, /t/, /d/, and /n/. Contrast this with production of velar consonant sounds /k/, /g/, and "ng" where the tongue body raises upward to contact the velum.

- In **palatal** consonants, the center of the tongue is near the hard palate as in the "y" sound like in *yawn*.
- The rear of the tongue approaches the velum or soft palate in the production of **velar** consonants such as /k/ and /g/.
- When the constriction occurs at the level of the vocal folds, the phonemes produced are called **glottal**, like the /h/ in *hat*.

As previously mentioned, the degree of constriction or closure is used when classifying consonant sounds by *manner*. For instance:

- Complete closure of the vocal tract in which airflow is completely blocked results in the **stop consonants** (/p/, /b/; /t/, /d/; /k/, /g/). In the production of stops, air pressure is built up behind the point of constriction, momentarily stopped, and then released, as in the /p/ sound.
- **Fricatives** (e.g., /s/, /z/; /f/, /v/) are produced with a narrow passageway for the air to pass through, creating a friction-like noise.
- **Affricates** (e.g., "ch" and "j") begin as stops and then are released as fricatives.
- The **nasals** (/m/, /n/, /ŋ/, "ng") are the only sounds produced with an open velopharyngeal port so that the sound energy comes through the nose as opposed to the mouth.
- **Glides** (e.g., /w/) occur when the articulatory posture changes gradually from consonant to vowel.
- **Liquids** include /l/ and /r/ and are produced with an open vocal tract and therefore are considered vowel-like consonants.

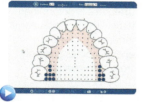

Pearson eTextbook
Video Example 5.2

In this video, electropalatagraphy is used to show where the tongue contacts the hard or soft palates during production of stop consonants /t, d, k, g/ and the nasals /n/ and "ng."

Voicing refers to what the vocal folds are doing during consonant sound production. For instance, if the vocal folds are vibrating during sound production, the consonant is said to be voiced. If the folds are not vibrating, the consonant sound is voiceless. The nasals, glides, and liquids are all voiced. The stops, fricatives, and affricates may be voiceless (e.g., /k/, /s/, "ch") or voiced (e.g., /g/, /z/, "j"). Consonants that have the same place and manner (e.g., /p/, /b/) but differ regarding voicing are called cognate pairs.

Can you describe the place, manner, and voicing features of the consonant sounds in the words *spinach and mushroom flatbread pizza*.

Classification of Vowels by Tongue and Lip Position and Tension

Vowels are produced when the sound energy produced by the vibrating vocal folds is modified and resonated by the opened vocal tract. The exact sound that is made depends on which part of the tongue is elevated (front, center, or back), its relative height (high, mid, or low), and the amount of tension (tense or lax) in the articulators. Whether the lips are rounded (pursed) or retracted (pulled back into a sort of smile) also influences the sound that is produced.

Figure 5.1 is a diagram of American English vowels. In the figure, the higher vowel of the front and back paired vowels and /ɝ/ are relatively tense; all other vowels are lax. High and mid back vowels and the back central vowels are produced with the lips somewhat rounded. All other English vowels are unrounded.

FIGURE 5.1 Classification of American English vowels by height and frontness/backness of the tongue.

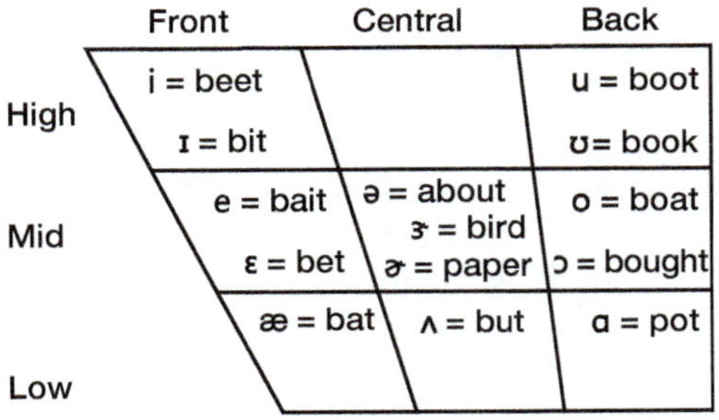

Source: Data from Introduction to Phonetics and Phonology, Pramod Pandey, Centre for Linguistics, SLL&CS, Jawaharlal Nehru University.

All English vowels are typically voiced and not nasal. Exceptions occur when you whisper and when nasal resonance occurs for any number of reasons, including proximity to a nasal phoneme such as /m/ or /n/.

When two vowels are said in close proximity, they produce a special type of phoneme called a **diphthong**. In English, the vowels in the words *sigh*, *now*, and *boy* are diphthongs. *Sigh* contains /aɪ/, *now* contains /aʊ/, and *boy* contains /ɔɪ/. Check out the interactive International Phonetic Association chart at the Seeing Speech website at www.seeingspeech.ac.uk. You can listen to the sounds of the International Phonetic Alphabet (IPA) while seeing the movements of the articulators imaged with ultrasound, magnetic resonance imaging, and animated form.

Speech Sound Acquisition Through the Lifespan

Learning Objective 5.2 Outline the sequence of speech sound acquisition across the lifespan.

Although you gained early control of most of the muscles needed for speech, it took you longer to refine their movement and produce all the sounds of your language. Even so, most children can produce all speech sounds by early elementary school.

Speech Sound Emergence

Newborns produce predominantly reflexive sounds, such as fussing and crying, and vegetative sounds, such as burps and hiccups. Noncrying, vowel-like sounds usually accompany feeding or are produced in response to smiling or talking by caregivers. These vowel-like productions contain some *phonation* or vibration at the larynx, but the infant has insufficient ability to produce full speech sounds.

By 2 months of age, infants develop nondistress sounds called either "gooing" or "cooing." During this early stage of speech production, infants produce back consonant sounds similar to /g/ and /k/ along with vowel-like sounds.

By 3 months of age, infants vocalize in response to the speech of others. Infants are most responsive if their caregivers respond to them.

Between 4 and 6 months of age, infants begin to imitate the tone and pitch signals of their caregivers. Most infant imitative and nonimitative vocalizations

Daniel (*continued*)

Background/case history collected by the speech-language pathologist (SLP) from Daniel's parents revealed he is a simultaneous bilingual speaker, having exposure to Spanish and English equally since infancy. Daniel's mom and dad are both native speakers of Spanish and originally from Mexico. The SLP also learned of a history of speech delay on the paternal side. Daniel's uncle received speech therapy as a young child for being a "late-talker" and continued in speech therapy throughout elementary school.

Once the SLP received parental permission to conduct a comprehensive assessment, a bilingual SLP was requested by the school to complete the evaluation. The *Bilingual Input-Output Survey* (BIOS), an informal survey that is part of the *Bilingual English Spanish Assessment* (BESA),

was completed by Daniel's parents. Questions from this survey help to determine the level of language input (languages the child hears) and output (languages the child uses). The survey determined that Daniel's mom primarily communicates with him in English while his dad speaks to him mostly in Spanish. Daniel watches YouTube on his iPad in English about 2 hours per day. When he is with his grandparents after school three times per week for 1–2 hours, he is exposed only to Spanish. Daniel attends an English-speaking full-day kindergarten Monday through Friday. Calculations on the BIOS determined Daniel's total Spanish input to be 40% and English input to be 60%. His Spanish output was calculated at 60% and English output calculated at 40%.

are single-syllable units of consonant-vowel (CV) or vowel-consonant (VC) construction. These sound units that begin around 4 months are called **babbling**. Babbling is random vocal play, and even infants who are deaf babble. During babbling, infants experiment with sound production. During this time, you may hear raspberries, trills, and more sounds near the front of the mouth (Bleile, 2020).

With maturity, longer sequences and prolonged individual sounds emerge. Children produce increasingly more complex combinations. Sounds are now more like adult speech sounds. As muscle control moves to the front of the oral cavity, we see strong tongue projection in 4- to 6-month-olds. Initially, back consonants predominate in babbling, but by 6 months bilabial sounds, such as /m/ and /p/, are produced more frequently. With age, children's babbling increasingly reflects the syllable structure and intonation of the caregivers' speech.

The consonant-vowel syllable becomes one of the predominant building blocks in first words.

At about 6 or 7 months, infants' babbling begins to change to **reduplicated babbling** which contains strings of consonant-vowel syllable repetitions or self-imitations (CV-CV-CV), such as *ma-ma-ma*. Hearing ability appears to be very important. Children with deafness continue to babble, but the range of consonants decreases, and few reduplicated strings are produced.

In contrast to babbling, reduplicated babbling more closely approximates mature speech in its resonant quality and timing. The child is beginning to adapt the speech patterns of the environment. Regardless of the language, infants' vocalizations and later first words have similar phonological patterns. For example, stops (/p, b, t, d, k, g/), nasals (/m, n/, "ng"), and approximants (/w/, "y") constitute approximately 80% of the consonants in infant vocalizations and in the first 50 words of Spanish-, Korean-, and English-speaking children.

Between 8 and 12 months, children begin to imitate sounds, but only sounds they have produced spontaneously on their own. Gradually, infants begin to use imitation to expand and modify their repertoire of speech sounds. At about the same time, they begin using gestures, with or without vocalizations, to communicate.

In the second half of the first year, children begin to recognize recurring patterns of sounds in specific situations. The child may even produce sounds in these situations. For example, a child might begin to say *M-m-m* during feeding if this sound is modeled for them. In response to caregiver conversations, infants may begin to experiment with **jargon**, or long strings of syllables with adultlike intonation.

Word production depends on sound grouping and sound variation. Children adopt a problem-solving or trial-and-error approach to word production. The resultant speech is a complex interaction of the ease of production and perception of the target syllable and its member sounds.

Toddler Speech

At around 12 months of age, you probably produced your first recognizable word. Sometimes a child's word is easily recognizable to others, but some words may be modified by the child for ease of production.

When faced with a difficult word, children adopt similar strategies. Armed with the CV structures of babbling and the CV-CV-CV strings of reduplicated babbling, children attempt to pronounce the adult words they encounter. It is therefore not surprising that many words are reduced to variations of a CV structure or another simplification. These adaptations, called phonological patterns (the preferred term) or processes, are presented in Table 5.1.

Toddlers often omit final consonants, resulting in a CVC word being produced as CV, as in *cat* pronounced as *ca*. Syllables in multisyllabic words may be repeated,

> Protowords, or phonetically consistent forms are sound patterns that function as "words" for the infant; they are a child's first attempt at consistent use of a sound to represent or "stand for" something else. When my son was very young, his protoword for the color red was "ai-yai-ya."

TABLE 5.1

Phonological Patterns (Processes) of Young Children

Pattern	Explanation	Example
Final consonant deletion	Reduces CVC structure to more familiar CV	*Cat* becomes *ca*
		Carrot becomes *cara* CVCVC → CVCV
Weak syllable deletion	Reduces number of syllables to conform to the child's ability to produce multisyllable words	*Telephone* becomes *tephone*
		Vacation becomes *cation*
Reduplication	Syllables in multisyllable words repeat	*Baby* becomes *bebe*
		Mommy becomes *mama*
Consonant cluster reduction	Reduces CCV+ structures to the more familiar CV	*Tree* becomes *te* *Stay* becomes *tay*
Assimilation	One consonant becomes like another, although the vowel is usually not affected	*Doggie* becomes *goggie*
Stopping	Fricatives (/f/, /v/, /s/, /z/, and others) are replaced by stops (/b/, /p/, /d/, /t/, /g/, /k/)	*Face* becomes *pace* *This* becomes *dis*
Fronting	Velars are replaced with more anteriorly produced sounds	*Go* becomes *do* *Ring* becomes *rin*

as in *water* produced as *wawa*. If the syllables are not duplicated, only the consonants may be, as in *doggie* becoming *goggie*. Consonant blends might be shortened to single consonants, as in *stop* becoming *top*. Finally, one type of sound might be substituted for another. For example, all initial consonants in words might be pronounced as the same consonant, as in, *Go bye-bye* becoming *Bo bye-bye*.

Preschool Speech

Development of individual sounds depends on the location in words, frequency of use, and the influence of other speech sounds.

Most of the phonological patterns described for toddlers have disappeared by age 4. Consonant blends consisting of two or more adjacent consonants, as in *strong*, continue to be difficult for some children, and simplification strategies, resulting in *tong*, may continue into early elementary school. Children who experience continuing phonological difficulties may persist in the use of more immature phonological patterns.

Children continue to master new speech sounds throughout the preschool period. The acquisition process is a gradual one and depends on the individual sound, its location in words, its frequency of use, and its proximity to other speech sounds. A sound may be produced correctly in single words but not in connected speech.

We can make a few generalizations about speech sound acquisition by young children:

- Phoneme acquisition is a gradual process.
- Speech sounds produced in the early word stages are similar regardless of language environment or number of languages the child is exposed to (Gildersleeve-Neumann et al., 2008).
- Vowels are easier to master than consonants; vowel development is mostly complete by age 3 (Pollack & Berni, 2003).

CASE STUDY **Daniel** *(continued)*

Speech sound assessment was conducted in both English and Spanish. Speech production errors were similar in both languages. Daniel produced about 50% of consonants correctly in English and Spanish. Daniel's speech was characterized by final fricative deletion (e.g., "mou" for *mouse*; "ma" for *mas/more*); substitution of /t/ for /k/ and /d/ for /g/ (e.g., "bota" for *boca/mouth*; "dato" for *gato/cat*; "tup" for *cup*; "do" for *go*); substitution of /p/ for /f/ (e.g., "tapé" for *café/coffee*; "op" for *off*); substitution of /t/ for "ch" (e.g., "titen" for *chicken*; "yete" for *leche/milk*); substitution of "y" for /l/ (e.g., "yete" for *leche/milk*; "peyo" for *pelo/hair*; "yite" for *like*) and /w/ for /r/ (e.g., "wat" for *rat*). He could produce the Spanish alveolar tap /ɾ/

(e.g., /aɾo/ for *carro/car*); however, the Spanish trill "r" (/r/) was not observed. Clusters were reduced to singleton sounds (e.g., "pato" for *plato/plate*; "tee" for *tree*). Three-syllable words were reduced to two syllables (e.g., "pato" for *zapato/shoe*); "nana" for *banana*).

Parents indicated on the *Intelligibility in Context Scale* (McLeod et al., 2012) that Daniel is sometimes intelligible regardless of the language spoken. **Stimulability** testing revealed he could correctly produce /k/ and /g/ sounds when provided with explicit teaching from the SLP. Daniel was determined to have a severe impairment in his speech sound production skills, and speech therapy was recommended.

- Children acquire most consonants by age 5 (McLeod & Crowe, 2018).
- Many sounds are first acquired in the initial position in words.
- Consonant clusters (e.g., con*sid*er; *street*) are not mastered until age 7 or 8, although some clusters appear as early as age 4.
- Some sounds are easier than others to produce and are acquired early by most children. As a group, stops (/p, b, t, d, g, k/), nasals (/m, n/ and "ng"), and glides (/w/, "y") are acquired first.
- Sounds that are more difficult to produce are acquired later, including fricatives (e.g., /s/, /z/), affricates (i.e., "ch"; "j"), and liquids (i.e., /r, l/).
- Much individual difference exists.

Shriberg (1993) examined speech sound mastery in 64 children ages 3–6 years with delayed speech production skills based on spontaneous speech samples and categorized 24 speech sounds into early-developing, middle-developing, and late-developing groups. This information, referred to as the "early 8," "middle 8," and "late 8," is presented in Figure 5.2. While based on children with speech sound delay, the data were determined to adhere fairly closely to speech sound acquisition data from children without delay (e.g., Sander, 1972; Smit et al., 1990). Additionally, the early, middle, and late speech sound data were more recently replicated in monolingual English-speaking children 3–4 years of age without delay with similar results (Fabiano-Smith & Goldstein, 2010).

More recent data examining acquisition of consonant phonemes in 27 languages determined that children across the world acquire most of the consonants in their language (over 90%) by 5 years of age, although individual variability exists (McLeod & Crowe, 2018). Typical children acquiring English in the United States were determined to have mastered all but four consonants by age 5 (Crowe & McLeod, 2020). While differences were determined between Shriberg's early-8, middle-8, and late-8 consonants (Figure 5.2) and the findings from Crowe & McLeod (Figure 5.3), some similarities were noted. Specifically, Shriberg's (1993) early-8 consonants were within Crowe and McLeod's (2020) early-13 consonants and their late-4 consonants were within Shriberg's late-8 consonant group.

Some sounds, however, are mastered earlier or later depending on the language. For instance, /s/ is mastered in typical Spanish-speaking children between 5;0 and 6;11 (years; months) of age. In monolingual English-speaking children, /s/ is mastered between 4;0 and 4;11. On the other hand, "ch" is mastered earlier in monolingual Spanish-speakers (3;0–3;11) compared to monolingual English-speakers (4;0–4;11) (McLeod & Crowe, 2018). As always, individual differences across speakers exist.

FIGURE 5.2 **Early-, middle-, and late-developing English speech sounds.**

The sound ʒ ("zh" in *measure*) was excluded from Shriberg's analysis because young children use this sound infrequently in spontaneous conversation.	
Early 8	/m, b, j ("y"), n, w, d, p, h/
Middle 8	/t, ŋ, k, g, f, v, tʃ ("ch"), dʒ ("j")/
Late 8	/ʃ ("sh"), ð ("th" in *the*), s, z, θ ("th" in *thin*), l, r/

Sources: Based on Fabiano-Smith and Goldstein (2010); Shriberg (1993).

FIGURE 5.3 **Early-, middle-, and late-developing English speech sounds by age (years; months).**

Early-13 (2;0–3;11)	/b, n, m, p, h, w, d, g, k, f, t, ŋ ("ng"), j ("y")/
Middle-7 (4;0–4;11)	/v, dʒ ("j"), s, tʃ ("ch"), l, ʃ ("sh"), z/
Late-4 (5;0–6;11)	/r, ʒ ("zh" in mea<u>s</u>ure), ð ("th" in <u>the</u>), θ ("th" in <u>thin</u>)/

Source: Based on Crowe and McLeod (2020).

While one language can influence the other (known as cross-linguistic effects) such as when /z/ is substituted for /s/ in Spanish productions even though there is no /z/ consonant in Spanish, phonological skill development in Spanish-English bilingual speakers is comparable to age-matched monological English- and Spanish-speaking children (Goldstein et al., 2005).

CASE STUDY **Daniel** *(continued)*

Based on the research findings, it is clear that Daniel is delayed in his mastery of English and Spanish consonant sounds. He is only producing 50% of consonant sounds correctly, whereas bilingual Spanish- and English-speaking children his age have mastered over 90% of consonants in their ambient languages.

Despite the difficulties Daniel is having learning the speech sounds of his ambient languages, his parents should be encouraged to continue speaking to him in both languages as they are currently. They should continue to let him respond in either language or a combination of both languages. Development of a child's competency in their home language or languages plays an important role in their cultural identity, well-being, and sense of self (De Houwer, 2015; Puig, 2010). Additional benefits of children learning multiple languages include enhanced cognitive abilities (e.g., working memory), improved social relationships (e.g., with grandparents) and greater community participation (e.g., Adesope et al., 2010; Park & Sarkar, 2007).

School-Age Speech

By early elementary school, your phonological system probably resembled that of an adult. A few children will still have difficulty with multiple consonant clusters, such as *str* and *sts*, as in *street* and *beasts*, respectively. By age 8, children have acquired consonant clusters, such as *str*, *sl*, and *dr*.

Phonology and Articulation

The distinction between phonology and articulation is often difficult to understand. Articulation refers to the actual production of speech sounds; phonology is knowledge of speech sounds within a language and the ways in which they are combined.

The correct use of speech sounds in a language requires knowledge of the sounds of the language and the rules that govern their production and combination, called *phonology*. Speech also requires neuromotor coordination to actually say sounds, words, and sentences—termed *articulation*.

To help you understand this distinction, visualize learning a new language such as French. You will be exposed to new words and sound combinations and begin to grasp the nature of that language's sound system or phonology. But you must also be able to form the words with your lips, tongue, and so on. You might find this very difficult because your neuromotor pathways have been trained to make English words; the inability to coordinate your muscles to produce the words correctly is a problem of articulation.

Types of Speech Sound Disorders in Children

Learning Objective 5.3 Discuss the types of speech sound disorders in children.

Phonological impairments are disorders of conceptualization or language rules. Remember that phonology is concerned with classes of sounds and sound patterns within words. For example, English has both open and closed syllables at the ends of words. An **open syllable** is one that ends in a vowel—for example, *hi*; a **closed syllable** ends in a consonant (*hat*). A child who uses only open syllables and deletes all final consonants is likely exhibiting a disorder of phonology. In this example, the child would say *hi* correctly but produce *hat* as *ha*.

Articulation impairments are disorders of production and are therefore motor based. A child whose only speech error is incorrect production of the /s/ phoneme has a disorder of articulation. Errors typically associated with articulation disorders include:

- Substitutions: when one phoneme is replaced with another. For example, a person who says "shair" for *chair* would be substituting *sh* for *ch*
- Omissions: the deletion of a phoneme, as in "chai" for *chair*
- Distortions: when a nonstandard form of a phoneme is used
- Additions: as in "chuh-air" for *chair*

Distinguishing SSDs as impairments in phonology or articulation can be difficult, especially in young children. For instance, the young child who deletes all final consonants and is said to have a phonological disorder may in fact be unable to motorically produce final sounds. Remember, final sounds are more difficult than initial sounds to produce and acquire. The child's use of only open syllables may in fact be due to an immature or impaired motor system, thus representing a disorder of articulation. It's possible that this same child has an impaired phonological system, along with delayed motor speech skills. In this case, the SSD represents an impairment in both phonology and articulation.

Young children are learning to acquire the rules of the phonological system at the same time their speech motor abilities are developing. As we talk more about specific patterns and types of errors later in this chapter, think about how such errors could represent impairments in phonology or articulation, especially in young children. In general, however, rule-based errors represent a disorder of phonology, while errors on vowels and prosody, and difficulties with speech production related to weakness, incoordination, or extraneous movements, represent motor-based impairments.

Speech Sound Disorders of Unknown Origin

A classification system proposed by Shriberg and colleagues (2010) to better understand speech sound impairments of unknown origin considered eight possible subgroups of children. Three subtypes were considered forms of speech delay and

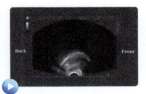

Pearson eTextbook
Video Example 5.3

This video shows ultrasound images of the tongue of a 7-year-old child's pre- and post-treatment production of "r" and "er" at the beginning and middle position of open syllables. Notice the low position of his tongue at pre-treatment resulting in distortion errors, and then a raising of the tongue post-treatment. Also notice the difference in his productions of "r" and "er" pre- and post-treatment.

were believed to be the result of (1) a family history of speech or language problems, (2) a history of early and frequent ear infections that involve fluid buildup behind the middle ear, or (3) a personality that makes it more difficult for the child to master speech sound production skills. Children in these subgroups are expected to successfully normalize their speech with treatment.

The next three subtypes of speech disorders of unknown origin are believed to result from motor speech impairments (i.e., childhood apraxia of speech; dysarthria), and are less likely to remediate easily with treatment. The last two subgroups represent children who exhibit distortion errors of later-developing sounds (i.e., /s/ and /r/, respectively), perhaps because they tried to master these sounds when they were not yet ready. As a result, they habituated and maintained an incorrect production pattern of these sounds through their school-age years, resulting in a persistent SSD.

Defining subtypes of SSDs of unknown origin in this manner represents only one perspective on the issue, and there is no agreement yet on how best to accomplish this classification. There is also no agreement on how to differentiate a speech sound delay from a SSD given the wide range of behaviors in young children. Trying to determine a specific cause or causes for the child's speech sound impairment is important in ultimately choosing the most effective treatment approach for the child (Bernthal et al., 2017).

Lifespan Issues

Approximately 75% of preschool children will normalize their speech sound errors by age 6 with or without treatment (Shriberg et al., 1999), and the majority will normalize by age 8. A small percentage, however, will continue to exhibit residual articulation errors past this age despite intervention. These errors can persist into adulthood and usually involve substitution or distortion of /r/, /s/, /z/, or /l/. Such errors may have a negative impact on an individual's academic or professional accomplishments, as well as on personal relationships. Although speech sound production can be modified at any stage of life, speech production patterns become habituated and increasingly difficult to change as we get older.

Risk Factors Associated with Speech Sound Disorders

Learning Objective 5.4 List the risk factors associated with speech sound disorders in children.

The causes of SSD in most children are not readily identifiable; however, a number of risk factors for SSD have been identified by researchers. Figure 5.4 lists the factors determined to increase a child's risk of developing an SSD. Understanding these risk factors will allow you as the SLP to make informed decisions about candidacy for treatment or ongoing monitoring of a child with increased risk. Note that risk factors are not predictors of a disorder, and the presence of risk factors in a child may not ultimately lead to the child having an SSD.

Male Sex

Speech sound delay tends to be more common in preschool-age boys (e.g., Campbell et al., 2003; Everhart, 1960), with a 1.5:1 to 3:1 male-to-female ratio (cf., Shriberg & Kwiatkowski, 1994; Shriberg et al., 1999). One possible reason for this is the slower

Most children with disordered articulation and phonology do not exhibit an identifiable physical reason for the problem. The majority will normalize their speech sound errors by age 8.

While there is no known cause for the majority of children who present with SSD, there are several known causes in some children, including structural functional abnormalities, intellectual impairment, autism spectrum disorder, hearing loss, and motor speech disorders secondary to neurological impairment.

FIGURE 5.4 Risk factors for SSDs in children.

Male sex

History of middle ear infections with fluid buildup

Hearing status

Diminished speech sound perception and discrimination ability

Oral-motor/feeding difficulties

Family history of speech or language disorders

Low maternal education

rate of maturation of certain cognitive processes (i.e., attention, planning) in boys compared to girls (Naglieri & Rojahn, 2001). Also, brain areas that control the ability to perform certain fine motor and tactile tasks have been found to be different in males and females (Rescher & Rappelsberger, 1996). This might explain male–female differences in early speech acquisition skills, given that speech production is a fine motor skill dependent on tactile feedback. And while males are at greater risk for early speech sound delay, other factors combined with male sex, including family history of speech-language delay and low maternal education (i.e., mother did not graduate from high school), pose an even greater risk for speech sound delay in early childhood (Campbell et al., 2003).

CASE STUDY **Daniel** *(continued)*

For Daniel, risk factors for SSD include being male and having a family history of speech production difficulties. Otherwise, he has no known cause(s) for his speech sound production difficulties (e.g., structural functional abnormalities, hearing loss).

Lifespan Issues

Until about age 6, girls tend to acquire speech sounds at a slightly earlier age compared to boys (Smit et al., 1990). Recent studies have also shown that girls use gestures coupled with speech combinations sooner than boys (approximately 16 months of age for girls vs. 19 months of age for boys; Özçalskan & Goldin-Meadow, 2010). Many tests for articulation and phonology have separate normative data for males and females to account for differences in speech sound acquisition rate in early childhood. However, the differences between boys and girls ultimately disappear as children get older (Bernthal et al., 2017).

Hearing Status/Hearing Loss

There is continued debate and mixed research findings about the association between ongoing middle ear infections accompanied by a buildup of fluid and SSD in children. Because the transmission of sound is blocked by the fluid in the middle ear, hearing loss may occur, subsequently impacting speech sound acquisition (Bernthal et al., 2017). Longitudinal studies have shown no to minimal

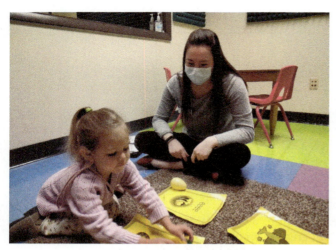

Graduate student clinician working with a 4-year-old child who was recently fitted with bilateral cochlear implants and can hear for the first time.

© Jocilyn Benninger

associations between middle ear disease with fluid buildup and SSD, however. Still, researchers recommend children with a history of middle ear infections undergo hearing screening to optimize their language and learning environment (Roberts et al., 2004).

Children older than 6 months of age identified as having hearing loss are at greater risk of speech and language difficulties (Yoshinaga-Itano et al., 1998). Because hearing is the primary way in which we acquire the speech sounds of a language, it is not surprising that children who are hard of hearing or deaf exhibit SSD. Hearing loss not only impairs a child's ability to hear others but also affects the ability to monitor their own speech production, which is necessary to adequately acquire the sounds of a language. It must be recognized that phonology will not be impaired alone, but all aspects of speech, including voice quality, pitch, rate, and rhythm, will similarly be affected.

Although an exact relationship between type and degree of hearing loss and speech cannot be made, certain patterns are frequently observed. Common omission error patterns in individuals who are deaf include final consonant deletion, initial consonant deletion, and deletion of /s/ in all contexts (Calvert, 1982).

> **REFLECTION QUESTION 5.1**
>
> *How does speech differ for someone who has congenital deafness versus someone who became deaf later in life? Why?*

Lifespan Issues

The age at onset and the degree and type of hearing loss influences the nature of the SSD. Individuals who are born deaf or with severe hearing impairment typically have more significant speech deficits compared to those who lose hearing later in life. Speech deteriorates over time for those who are initially hearing and become hard of hearing or deaf later in life. Speech sound production can be enhanced using hearing aids for individuals with some hearing, as well as appropriate training. (See Chapter 12.) Even the best speech of many adults with deafness is nearly unintelligible to others.

Structural Functional Abnormalities

Rapid and accurate movements involving the jaw, lips, tongue, hard and soft palates, and teeth are necessary for articulatory precision; however, usually only gross abnormalities of these structures can negatively impact speech intelligibility. Individuals are remarkably adept at compensating for most structural abnormalities, even partial or complete surgical removal of the tongue. Severe deformity of the hard and soft palates as a result of clefting is far more detrimental to speech production, however, as discussed later in Chapter 9.

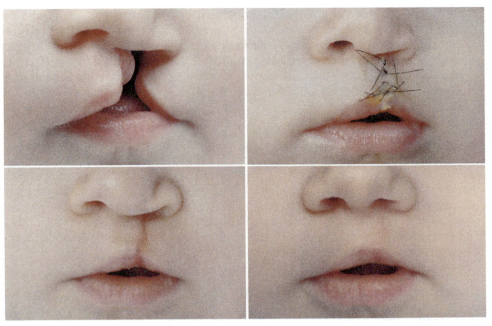

Unilateral complete cleft of the lip extending to and through the floor of the nostril.
© malost/Shutterstock

Lifespan Issues

Many children born with **craniofacial anomalies**, or congenital malformations of the head and face such as a cleft (i.e., abnormal opening) of the lip and palate, struggle not only with speech sound acquisition but also with feeding and even breathing. Clefts of the lip are typically surgically closed at 2½ to 3 months of age, while clefts of the hard and soft palates are closed between 7 and 18 months of age. Additional surgeries are usually necessary later to treat continued difficulties with velopharyngeal closure (discussed in more detail in Chapter 9). High-pressure consonants including stops (e.g., /k, g/), fricatives (e.g., /s, z/), and affricates (e.g., "ch") are often problematic for individuals with cleft palate; distortions of these particular sounds can persist into adolescence and even adulthood. Correct articulation can be expected in about 25% of preschoolers with repaired cleft palate who receive care early on from a qualified team of professionals (Peterson-Falzone et al., 2010). See Chapter 9 for more details about individuals with cleft palate.

Dysarthria

The dysarthrias are a group of motor speech disorders caused by neuromuscular deficits that result in weakness or paralysis and/or poor coordination of the speech musculature. Dysarthrias typically affect respiration, phonation, resonance, and articulation. They are described in more detail in Chapter 10.

Approximately 90% of children with **cerebral palsy (CP)** exhibit some form of motor speech impairment, ranging from very mild dysarthria to having no understandable speech (Mei et al., 2014). CP is a nonprogressive neuromotor disorder caused by brain damage that occurred sometime before, during, or soon after birth for the majority of children diagnosed with CP (Rosenbaum et al., 2007). The location and severity of brain damage predict dysarthria type(s) and degree of communication impairment. Newer research suggests that for some children with CP, a genetic condition may be responsible and not brain damage (Chopra et al., 2022). Articulatory difficulties and reduced speech intelligibility are common problems for children with CP (Mei et al., 2014).

Lifespan Issues

In CP, the general motor and speech signs are present from early childhood onward. Approximately a third of individuals with CP have average to above-average intelligence. Others exhibit varying degrees of cognitive deficits. Accompanying deficits may include epilepsy, visual processing deficits, and/or hearing impairment (Cummings, 2008). Although the condition itself does not get progressively worse, gross motor function, such as walking, can deteriorate over time (Haak et al., 2009). The symptoms of dysarthria also appear to change, becoming more severe in some cases with increasing age (Schölderle et al., 2016).

Childhood Apraxia of Speech

Childhood apraxia of speech (CAS) is a neurological SSD that affects the ability to plan and program the movement sequences necessary for accurate speech production. It is not the result of neuromuscular weakness. Before speech is produced, the motor plan/program that specifies all the necessary parameters for accurate production of that utterance (e.g., positioning and timing of the articulators, amount of muscle activation) is accessed in the brain. This enables speech to be produced rapidly yet accurately. If we had to think about how each structure needed to move (i.e., lips tongue, jaw, vocal folds, respiratory muscles) and with how much force every time we spoke, we might need several minutes to produce a sentence rather than the several seconds that is typical.

Because children with apraxia of speech have impaired motor planning and programming capabilities, they are unable to learn the motor plans/programs necessary for rapid, accurate speech production in the same fashion as unimpaired children. As a result, their connected speech is often highly unintelligible, segmented or choppy, disfluent, and lacking in prosodic variation.

Children with severe apraxia of speech with average intellectual and receptive language abilities are often aware that speech is difficult and may initially be unwilling to try to talk because they know they will fail. It is therefore important that you as an SLP build a trusting relationship with the child. It is essential that a child at least attempt to imitate words with an SLP to determine if they do in fact have CAS (Strand, 2019). Specific treatment for children with CAS is discussed later in this chapter.

Although there are no definitive neurological or behavioral markers of CAS, the American Speech-Language-Hearing Association has proposed the following speech characteristics to help guide SLPs in properly diagnosing CAS (ASHA, 2007):

- Inconsistent errors on consonants and vowels in repeated productions of syllables or words
- Lengthened and disrupted transitions between sounds and syllables
- Inappropriate prosody, especially in the realization of word or phrasal stress

In addition, children with CAS often have limited consonant and vowel repertoires, may exhibit groping and/or trial-and-error behaviors, frequently omit sounds or inappropriately add sounds, and produce single words better than they produce running speech (Murray et al., 2014). Although most consider CAS to be a motor-speech disorder because speech is necessary to learn language and linguistic sound representations, children with CAS have concomitant expressive language and phonological impairments also.

Lifespan Issues

Children can be diagnosed with CAS as early as 3 years age; however, to make this diagnosis correctly the child needs to attend and focus on the clinician and attempt multiple repetitions of word stimuli (Strand et al., 2013). Standardized assessments are available; however, no one test has been shown to be completely reliable or valid with regard to diagnosing CAS (McCauley & Strand, 2008). Strand's 10-point checklist (Shriberg et al., 2011) provides the 10 speech and prosodic features (e.g., distorted substitution errors; syllable segregation; vowel distortions; increased difficulty with multisyllabic words) that are frequently associated with CAS; any combination of at least four out of the 10 features in three speech tasks indicates the presence of motor planning/programming deficits. Children with severe CAS may initially be nonverbal. Therefore, children may need to rely on other means to help communicate effectively (i.e., augmentative or alternative communication) as they are learning to speak.

Children with average intellectual and receptive language abilities have a good prognosis for verbal communication. However, they may continue to have poor intelligibility throughout the school-age years. They will likely also have difficulties with phonological awareness skills, reading, writing, and spelling. Children with CAS continue to exhibit phonological patterns well past the age at which these should have resolved. They may continue to have difficulties with certain classes of sounds and/or production of multisyllabic words (e.g., umbrella) into adolescence and young adulthood. The Apraxia Kids website (www.apraxia-kids.org) provides the latest research in the area of CAS for parents and caregivers of children with CAS.

The most readily apparent difficulties in individuals who persist with motor planning/programming difficulties are prosodic abnormalities. Even if speech is intelligible, they may continue to have a segmented (choppy) speech pattern and/or incorrect word and sentence stress. CAS is a speech diagnosis that changes with maturation and with treatment (Strand, 2019). A child may present early on with a primary diagnosis of CAS, but this may change with age. Some children present with a primary diagnosis of phonological impairment but may also exhibit some mild motor planning/programming difficulties. As the SLP, you will correctly differentially diagnose the child to best determine the treatment approach and speech targets (Murray et al., 2015; Strand & McCauley, 2008). Table 5.2 may be helpful for differential diagnosis of SSDs in children.

Language and Dialectal Variations

If you are a native speaker of American English and go to another country, such as Greece, to live, you will learn Greek to communicate with those around you. When you speak in Greek, your speech will reveal your American background. You will speak Greek with an "American accent." This is not a speech disorder.

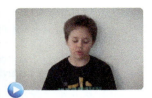

Pearson eTextbook
Video Example 5.4
Speech Errors Associated with Childhood Apraxia of Speech

This is John when he was 10 years old; notice how he is struggling to produce multisyllabic words, especially when those words contain "r" sounds.

A person whose speech reflects a regional or foreign language influence may also have a speech disorder. However, the regionalism or foreign dialect itself is not a disorder.

TABLE 5.2

Differential Diagnosis of Phonological and Motor Speech Impairments

	Phonological Disorder	Motor Speech Disorder: Apraxia	Motor Speech Disorder: Dysarthria
Speech sound errors	Consonant substitution and omission errors are common. Vowels are not affected.	Consonant substitution, distorted substitutions, omissions, and additions are common; vowel errors are also common.	Consonant distortion errors due to imprecise articulation are common; vowels may also be affected.
Consistency	Errors are generally consistent; patterns can readily be determined (e.g., fronting, stopping). Single word productions may be better than connected speech.	Errors may be inconsistent; patterns are not usually present early on; patterns may be present as child gets older, but are inappropriate for child's age (e.g., use of fronting at age 9). Unusual patterns may be observed (e.g., initial consonant deletion, backing of front sounds). Errors may quickly improve with practice, even during the evaluation session. Single word productions are better than connected speech. Individual sounds may be produced correctly in isolation, but production of those same sounds in words may be difficult.	Errors are generally consistent, although single word production is often better than connected speech. Improvements with practice will not occur immediately; even with treatment, articulatory imprecision will likely always be present to some degree.
Prosody	Normal	Prosodic abnormalities are pervasive and often persist even after articulation has normalized following intensive treatment. Segmentation (choppy) of speech, equal and excess stress, lengthened intersegment durations, and incorrect word and sentence stress are common.	Prosodic abnormalities are common and may include equal and excess stress, explosive loudness, slow rate, short phrases, or reduced pitch and loudness variability, depending on dysarthria type.
Strength of the oral musculature	Normal	Normal or near normal. Low tone at rest may be observed but has minimal impact on speech production.	Weakness or paralysis of the oral articulators may be present.
Coordination of the oral musculature	Normal	Coordination difficulties are common, and trial-and-error groping (articulators searching for correct position) may be present during speech or nonspeech movements.	Discoordination during speech and nonspeech tasks is common in certain types of dysarthria.

Similarly, if you are from Georgia and move to Massachusetts, you will bring your Georgia regionalism with you. Again, this is not a disorder but a dialectal difference to those in your new environment. Many Americans take pride in their regional and linguistic backgrounds and cherish the cultural diversity that characterizes this country.

In assessing speech sound production skills, an SLP must guard against over- and underdiagnosis, especially with bilingual and minority dialect speakers (McLeod et al., 2017; Yavas & Goldstein, 1998). The SLP must differentiate between disordered speech production and that which is simply different due to foreign language or dialect influences. This can be accomplished by doing the following:

1. Recognize cultural differences.
2. Obtain a thorough and culturally sensitive case history (McLeod et al., 2017).
3. Evaluate speech sound production competence in all relevant languages whenever possible.
4. Select appropriate assessment tools (see McLeod & Verdon, 2014).
5. Use nonstandard assessments often, with the help of bilingual assistants.
6. Use dynamic assessments, which involves systematic assessment of stimulability of sounds in a test–teach–retest format (Glaspey & Stoel-Gammon, 2007).
7. Describe phonological patterns (Scarpino & Goldstein, 2012).
8. Diagnose SSDs that exist (Ebert & Pham, 2017; Yavas & Goldstein, 1998).

The SLP then plans and engages in intervention as appropriate. If dialect differences are targeted, the SLP must assess the client's attitude toward their dialect and the individual's motivation for accent reduction. Some dialectical differences of the speech of individuals from various linguistic and regional backgrounds are presented in Table 5.3.

Characteristics of Speech Sound Production in Dialectal Variation

It is impossible to describe all the variations in articulation and phonology that reflect non-English or dialectal influences. The first language may interfere with languages that are learned later. For example, in Spanish /d/ and /ð/ are **allophones**, or variations of the same phoneme, whereas in English these are two separate phonemes, as can be seen in the words *dough* and *though*. Native Spanish speakers, however, may substitute the /d/ and /ð/ and pronounce both words the same way; these reflect dialectical differences and are not errors (Yavas & Goldstein, 1998).

Visit Portland State University's "Multilingual Topics in Communication Sciences and Disorders" for useful information to help you when working with multilingual individuals in clinical practice: www.sites.google.com/pdx.edu/multicsd/home.

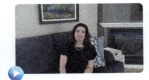

Pearson eTextbook
Video Example 5.5
Reflections from a Bilingual SLP

In this video, an expert bilingual SLP explains how she chose the field of speech-language pathology and what is necessary to become a bilingual SLP.

Lifespan Issues

Some adults for whom English is a second (or third or fourth) language choose to modify their foreign accent. Often this desire is based on professional considerations. Teachers of English to speakers of other languages and SLPs may contribute to the improvement of English expression and comprehension. However, for adolescents and beyond the articulatory patterns of a first language are often firmly established and are difficult to eliminate. The goal, then, is not to make a non-native speaker sound like a native, but rather to improve intelligibility and thereby the person's communicative effectiveness.

TABLE 5 3

Sample Phonological Characteristics of American English Dialects and Non-English-Language Influences on Spoken English

Rule	Example
African American English	
Final cluster reduction	*presents → presen*
Stopping of interdental initial and medial fricatives	*they → dey*
	nothing → noting
Deletion of *r*	*professor → puhfessuh*
Appalachian and Ozark English	
Addition of *t*	*once → oncet*
Addition of initial *h*	*it → hit*
Addition of vowel within clusters	*black → buhlack*
Cantonese	
Final consonant deletion	*dog → do*
/l/ for "ɹ" in all word positions	*ring → ling*
/f/ for /v/	*very → feli*
/d/ for voiced "th"	*that → dat*
Spanish	
Substitution of /d/ and /ð/	*they → day*
Devoicing of *z*	*lies → lice*
Affrication of /ʃ/	*shoe → chew*

Sources: Based on Cheng (1991); Goldstein and Iglesias (2017); Yavas and Goldstein (1998).

Speech Sound Assessment

Learning Objective 5.5 Describe the goals and procedures in speech sound assessment.

Comprehensive assessment by an SLP is necessary to determine whether treatment is needed and, if so, what type of treatment will be most beneficial. Formal and informal measures specifically designed to assess speech sound impairments are discussed in the following sections. The goals of speech sound assessment are as follows:

- Describe the speech sound system and determine if it deviates from normal to the extent that treatment is necessary.
- Identify phonological patterns if they are present.
- Determine the impact of speech sound errors or error patterns on communicative effectiveness and participation.
- Identify factors that may relate to etiology or maintenance of the speech sound impairment.
- Determine the intervention approach or approaches to be used and the behaviors to be targeted during therapy.
- Make a prognosis about the likelihood of change with and without treatment.

- Monitor change over time to determine the effectiveness of treatment; update the treatment plan/approach/target behavior as needed; or discharge from treatment, if appropriate (Bernthal et al., 2017).

In addition, the case history, interview, hearing screening, and structural functional examination may provide insight into the etiology of a disorder and contribute to predictions of improvement. Collection of baseline data from which to measure change over time with or without intervention is an integral part of the initial assessment. Typical assessment procedures are briefly described and explained in the following sections, with Daniel's case providing context where appropriate.

> Speech sound disorders sometimes occur with other impairments like social/pragmatic or receptive and expressive language deficits.

Case History

The SLP will obtain background or case history information from the child's caregiver(s) in an interview or by using a questionnaire (or both). Information is collected about the child's early communication history (e.g., when the child first babbled or spoke their first words), medical history (e.g., pregnancy complications), social history (e.g., family members), and educational history (e.g., attending day care or preschool) (Bleile, 2020).

For multilingual children, the case history should also include a comprehensive language profile including the age at which the child was exposed to each language, the amount of exposure and use of each language each day of the week, and the individuals who speak each language with the child, such as parents, siblings, friends, grandparents, and teachers (McLeod et al., 2017). A number of comprehensive language developmental profiles exist (see McLeod et al., 2017); the one completed by Daniel's parents in the Case Study was the BIOS (Peña et al., 2014).

Description of the Speech Sound System

As an SLP, you will obtain data on several aspects of speech sound production. Single-word tasks, such as those typical of many standardized tests of articulation and phonology in our field, are the most efficient way to collect data about the use of phonemes (consonants, vowels, and tones, if appropriate) across word positions in a language (or languages), as well as word shapes, and prosody. Connected speech samples, like those obtained during play interactions with a child, provide additional information about sound accuracy, overall intelligibility, and prosody (McLeod & Crowe, 2020).

> While the prevalence of SSD is similar in monolingual and multilingual populations (Hambly et al., 2013), multilingual children are at greater risk of being over- and underidentified for speech-language and special education services (e.g., MacSwan & Rolstad, 2006).

Speech Sound Inventory

Determining a speech sound inventory for the child in all languages is useful when determining the phonological abilities of children, particularly those who are bilingual (Fabiano-Smith, 2019). Using the speech samples obtained (e.g., single-word tests, connected speech samples), SLPs determine if the child produced a particular sound at least two times, whether in the correct context or not (independent analysis), and organize the inventory by place and manner of production (Fabiano-Smith, 2019).

CASE STUDY **Daniel** *(continued)*

Table 5.4 shows the speech sound inventory for 5-year-old Daniel in standard orthography.

TABLE 5.4

Consonants Produced by Daniel, According to Place and Manner

	Bilabial	Labiodental	Interdental	Alveolar	Post-Alveolar	Palatal	Velar	Glottal
Stops	p, b			t, d				
Fricatives				s, z	"sh"		x	h
Affricates					"ch", "j"			
Nasals	m			n		"nya"	"ng"	
Liquids				ɾ				
Glides						"y"		

Note: Other consonants may be present in his speech sound inventory but were not observed during the evaluation.

Speech Sound Accuracy

Using both single-word tasks and connected speech samples, the SLP can count the number of opportunities for consonant production (or CV productions if the child exhibits vowel errors), and then count the total number of consonants the child produced correctly relative to the adult target (relational analysis). Percent accuracy for consonants correct can be derived by dividing the total number of consonants produced correctly by the total number of opportunities for consonant production multiplied by 100 (Fabiano-Smith, 2019). Published criterion references for percent consonants correct (PCC) have been established for monolingual English-speaking children, as well as bilingual English (predominantly exposed to English) and bilingual Spanish-speaking (predominantly exposed to Spanish) children (Fabiano-Smith & Goldstein, 2010; Fabiano-Smith & Hoffman, 2018; Shriberg & Kwiatkowski, 1982).

Syllable and Word Structure

A list of the CV patterns that have been produced in words suggests their complexity. The SLP might list the word and syllable shapes that are most characteristic of a client's speech, as well as the reductions or simplifications that have occurred. Figure 5.5 provides a list of some of the words in Daniel's connected speech samples during play and picture description tasks in standard orthography.

Error Analysis (Substitutions, Omissions, Distortions, Additions)

In all cases, the SLP needs to identify sounds that the child produces incorrectly. Using both single-word standardized assessments and transcriptions of connected speech samples obtained during play and picture description, the SLP will report errors as either **substitutions**, **omissions**, **distortions**, or **additions** in syllable/word positions. A list of published standardized assessments we use in our clinic is provided in Table 5.5.

FIGURE 5.5 Words in Daniel's connected speech samples in standard orthography.

ma (mas)	dato/gato	yite (like)
mou (mouse)	tapé (café)	titen (chicken)
do (go)	tup (cup)	pato (plato)
op (off)	yete (leche)	nana (banana)
bota (boca)	peyo (pelo)	pato (zapato)

Word shapes produced include CV (do), CVCV (bota), VC (op), CVC (tup), and CVCVC (titen).

The word shapes that were reduced are:

CVC → CV   (mouse → mou)
CCVCV → CVCV   (plato → pato)
CVCVCV → CVCV   (banana → nana)

For Daniel, errors might be recorded as follows:

t/k (I, M) (meaning *t* was substituted for *k* in the initial and medial positions; i.e., at the beginning and middle of a word)

p/f (M, F) (meaning *p* was substituted for *f* in the medial and final positions)

pl/p- (I) (meaning *l* was deleted from the *pl* consonant cluster in word initial position)

For multilingual children, it is essential to examine sound errors to determine if they are related to cross-linguistic effects (i.e., sounds specific to one language being used as substitutes in the other languages) (Fabiano-Smith, 2019). For instance, a bilingual child who speaks Spanish with a Puerto Rican dialect may delete the final *s* in "dos" (*two*) and say "doh." This would not be scored as an error because syllable-final *s* is often deleted in this dialect. Production of "flor" (*flower*) as "flo" would be considered an error because syllable-final deletion of *r* is not a feature of the Puerto Rican dialect of Spanish (Yavas & Goldstein, 1998).

TABLE 5.5

Published Standardized Assessments

Test Name	Age Range (years; months)
Arizona Articulation and Phonology Scale, Fourth Revision (Fudala & Stegall, 2017)	1;6–21;11
Bilingual English-Spanish Assessment (BESA; Pena et al., 2014)	4;0–6;11
Clinical Assessment of Articulation and Phonology–Second Edition (CAAP-2; Secord & Donohue, 2014)	2;6–11;11
Contextual Probes of Articulation Competence: Spanish (Goldstein & Iglesias, 2006)	3;0–8;11
Diagnostic Evaluation of Articulation and Phonology (DEAP; Dodd et al., 2006)	3;0–8;11
Goldman-Fristoe Test of Articulation–3 (GFTA-3; Goldman & Fristoe, 2015)	2;0–21;11
Hodson Assessment of Phonological Patterns–3 (HAPP-3; Hodson, 2004)	3;0–7;11
Structured Photographic Articulation Test–Featuring Dudsberry–Third Edition (SPAT-D 3; Tattersall & Dawson, 2016)	3;0–9;11

Sources: Based on Bernthal et al. (2017); McLeod et al. (2017).

It is important to account for dialectical differences so they are not mistaken for an SSD (Goldstein, 2007; Yavas & Goldstein, 1998). If you are not a bilingual SLP, or if you do not speak the language or the languages of the individual you are evaluating, there are many available resources online that can help you learn about the specific dialects of various languages (e.g., visit the ASHA website at www.asha .org/practice/multicultural/Phono/).

Phonological Error Pattern Analysis

Many research studies have shown that targeting an error pattern (e.g., final consonant deletion) rather than an individual sound has the advantage of encouraging generalization of learning to similar sounds and phonological contexts (Gierut, 1998). Therefore, if a child has numerous errors it is helpful to determine the type and frequency of phonological error patterns (refer back to Table 5.1). An SLP may analyze phonological pattern information based on single-word tasks (e.g., standardized single-word assessments), as well as connected speech samples (e.g., conversations, play interactions, picture description tasks).

CASE STUDY   **Daniel** (*continued*)

Daniel exhibits the following phonological error patterns in both English and Spanish (refer again to Table 5.1):

- Velar fronting (t/k; d/g)
- Stopping (p/f; t/ch)
- Gliding for liquids (y/l; w/r)
- Weak syllable deletion (nana/banana; pato/zapato)
- Consonant cluster deletion (p/pl; t/tr).

Daniel's deletion of final fricatives (e.g., /s/ deleted in the words *mouse* and *mas*) may or may not be a dialectical variation. When evaluating bilingual children, it is useful to obtain a recording of an adult speaker (like the child's parent) or age-matched peer in the community who speaks the same language and dialect and compare the child's speech to the adult or peer as a comparative measure (McLeod et al., 2017).

If the child's only phoneme error was /l/ → /w/ (I), this would not be indicative of a phonological pattern; it is a *single* sound substitution, an error of articulation. If, however, the child produced /l/ → /w/ (I, M) and /r/ → /w/ (I, M), this *pattern* could be described as gliding for liquids because /l/ and /r/ are liquids and they were produced as the glide /w/.

Determining a child's ability to use speech to participate in their environment, called *communicative participation*, enables the SLP to develop treatment goals that have a positive impact on the child in their everyday environment. Communicative participation can be determined through child and caregiver interviews or published questionnaires available free online.

REFLECTION QUESTION 5.2

When evaluating a child you suspect of having an SSD, why is it important to include informal measures of speech sound assessment (e.g., PCC) and not rely solely on formal, single-word standardized tests?

Intelligibility

Speech **intelligibility** refers to how easy it is to understand an individual. Poor intelligibility has a negative impact on communicative effectiveness. Intelligibility depends on such factors as the number, type, and consistency of speech sound errors. The person's voice, fluency, rate, rhythm, language, and use of gesture also contribute to ease of understanding their speech, and these should be noted. Other factors beyond the speaker include the listener's hearing acuity, familiarity with the speaker, and experience listening to disordered speech, as well as environmental noise, message complexity, and environmental cues.

A number of different rating scales to quantify perceptions of intelligibility are available. One example is the *Intelligibility in Context Scale* (ICS; McLeod et al., 2012a), which is a rating scale that is completed by the parent about their child's intelligibility in a number of different communicative settings. It is available online for free in 60 different languages (www.csu.edu.au/research/multilingual-speech/ics). In general, highly unintelligible speech signals a more severe SSD.

Daniel's parents indicated on the ICS that he is sometimes intelligible when using either English or Spanish. Children should be intelligible 100% of the time by age 5 (Hustad et al., 2021), regardless of the language or languages spoken.

Highly trained interpreters ensure objectivity during speech sound assessment. Formal training for interpreters includes knowledge about children's speech and language development, speech and language impairments, multidisciplinary diagnostic processes, testing protocols, and transcription of grammatical and phonological features (Blumenthal, 2007).

Stimulability

Assessment should always include trial therapy. **Stimulability** is the ability of an individual to produce the target phoneme when given focused auditory and visual cues. Typically, an SLP will say, "Look at me. Listen to me. Now say exactly what I say: 'cup.'" The SLP will first prompt correct production of the error phoneme or pattern within the word in which it was misarticulated. If the client does not correctly imitate the SLP, the prompt is moved to the syllable or phoneme level.

Although stimulability is often a positive prognostic indicator, research studies suggest a more complex relationship. Children who are stimulable may respond more quickly to correction of the target sounds and may also be more likely to self-correct without therapy than those who are not stimulable. Those sounds for which a child is not stimulable are highly unlikely to change without treatment. However, among children in therapy, those with low stimulability scores often make more progress, especially with untreated sounds, than do those who are more stimulable.

Stimulability testing is a form of dynamic assessment (i.e., test–teach–retest). The use of dynamic assessment with multilingual children is considered a culturally sensitive approach because it allows identification of the child's skills, learning potential, and learning process, which aids in selection of effective teaching methods for use in treatment (Lidz, 1991).

Treatment for Speech Sound Disorders

Learning Objective 5.6 Describe approaches and techniques to treat speech sound disorders, including supportive evidence.

If the results of an assessment suggest that treatment is appropriate, an SLP must determine how to proceed. Initial questions to be answered include the following:

- Where will therapy occur? (Clinic, school, or home setting?)
- How frequently will the client be seen? (Once or twice a week or three, four, or five times weekly?)
- How long will the sessions be? (The typical range is 20 to 60 minutes.)
- Will therapy be one-to-one or in a group or classroom setting?

It is not necessary for SLPs to know many different languages or dialects to work effectively with culturally and linguistically diverse populations. Rather, SLPs must receive training to develop knowledge of cultural diversity, language acquisition, and language use by multilingual individuals to provide services effectively (McLeod et al., 2017).

Answers to these questions will be related to the facilities that are available, as well as to the needs of the client. In addition to such administrative-type decisions, an SLP must determine the following:

- What are the treatment targets?
- What treatment approach appears most suitable?

Target Selection

A major goal of therapy is to help the child to be more easily understood in their everyday speaking environments (i.e., home, school). Selecting sound or word targets for immediate use in social contexts will allow the child to increase communicative participation more quickly and effectively. See ASHA's website for an example of a person-centered functional treatment plan aimed to improve speech production in the child's immediate communicative environments at www.asha.org/siteassets/uploadedFiles/ICF-Speech-Sound-Disorder.pdf.

A second factor in target selection is the likelihood of success. An SLP might initially choose targets that the child can master relatively quickly, which are typically the sounds the child was stimulable for during the assessment. If the child can readily produce the target sounds when prompted to imitate the SLP when provided increased visual and auditory cues (e.g., "Watch me, and do what I do"), this is a favorable sign.

Some research studies have demonstrated that greater generalization (transfer) to untreated sounds occurs when the sound targets are more difficult—that is, not stimulable, later-developing, and more phonetically complex (Gierut, 1998). It is up to an SLP to determine whether early success on a few targets or more long-term progress on multiple sounds is best for an individual child.

When selecting treatment targets for bilingual children with SSDs, it is recommended that the SLP choose phonological error patterns exhibited in all languages spoken by the child, specifically the ones that affect intelligibility greatly in both languages (Yavas & Goldstein, 1998).

CASE STUDY **Daniel** (*continued*)

For Daniel, intervention in both English and Spanish would be warranted. His difficulties are not the result of cross-linguistic effects of one language on another but, rather, a disorder of speech sound production across both languages based on his error profile. Additionally, treatment goals to reduce the occurrence of velar fronting, stopping, weak syllable deletion, and consonant cluster reduction (excluding "r" clusters) to increase his ability to be understood might be best initially. Later-developing sounds ("r" and the Spanish trill "r") might be better addressed later in treatment to maximize success and minimize frustration. Recall that Daniel was stimulable for the /k/ and /g/ sounds, so these sounds should come along more readily once treatment begins. The monolingual SLP can work with parents or a trained interpreter to generate a functional list of target words in Spanish to target during treatment sessions, along with functionally relevant English words. Highly trained interpreters are recommended to help the monolingual SLP work with Daniel during treatment sessions. This ensures accurate instructions are provided to teach correct production of sounds or sound patterns in Spanish to obtain the desired treatment outcome (McLeod et al., 2017).

Treatment Approaches

A variety of therapy approaches and techniques exist. An SLP might target one or two phonemes or multiple phonemes at a time. Therapy might focus on phonological error patterns, emphasize motor speech production, or target the nonsegmental aspects of speech such as rate, rhythm, and stress and intonation. Most SLPs adjust their approach to suit each client and combine procedures to provide individually tailored therapy. Highlights of select phonological- and motor-based treatment approaches are described briefly in Box 5.1.

BOX 5.1 **Evidence-Based Phonological- and Motor-Based Treatments for Children with SSD**

Phonological-Based Treatment Approaches

- *Minimal pair contrasts*, the contrasting of phonemes in pairs of words. This is accomplished by presenting the child with two pictured words that differ by one phoneme; one pictured word contains the child's sound/error pattern and the other is the correct form (e.g., *pig–big*). These production exercises involve having the child produce both words in sentences and asking the child if the sentences make sense (e.g., "The *big* lives on the farm"). This approach has been shown to be effective, especially for children with mild to moderate phonological impairment (Williams, 2000a).

- The *cycles approach* targets multiple phonological patterns over an extended period of time and is effective for children who are highly unintelligible. Three to six cycles of phonological intervention involving 30 to 40 hours of instruction are reportedly necessary for a child to become intelligible. Research has shown that children with severe phonological impairments can become intelligible in less than 1 year using the cycles approach (Hodson, 2007), and the approach can be modified for use with toddlers (Hodson, 2011).

- The *multiple oppositions approach* contrasts several target sounds with a comparison sound. This approach is effective for children who substitute one sound for multiple sounds, which results in production of the same word for different words (e.g., "tip" is produced for *chip, trip, ship,* and *kip*). This approach has been shown to be effective for children who are highly unintelligible, particularly during the early stages of treatment.

- The *complexity approach*, based on the work of Judith Gierut and colleagues, has shown that targeting later-acquired sounds and/or consonant clusters leads to increases in treated and in untreated sounds, both within and across sound classes. Also, using phoneme pairs that are maximally contrasted (i.e., differ by major class distinctions) and that compare two new phonemes (vs. including the child's error sound) also results in greater system-wide changes.

Motor-Based Treatment Approaches

- The **traditional motor** and **sensory-motor approaches** are highly effective for children who have only one or a few sounds in error (e.g., /l/, /r/) and for whom language skills are within normal limits.

- *Dynamic temporal and tactile cueing* (*DTTC*) has been shown to be effective for children with severe childhood apraxia of speech. This intensive treatment involves speech production practice sessions two times per day (30 minutes each), 5 days per week for a total of 6 weeks. Replication studies examining the effectiveness of DTTC when used fewer times per week (i.e., two times per week for 60 minutes) showed positive results for some but not all research participants. More research is needed to determine the long-term effectiveness of DTTC.

- The *Lee Silverman Voice Treatment* has been shown to be effective in young children with spastic CP. Improvements in loudness and speech intelligibility have been shown to last even after treatment ends.

Sources: Based on Bernthal et al. (2017); Fox and Boliek (2012); Gierut (2007, 2009); Gierut et al. (1996); Hodson and Paden (1991); McLeod and Baker (2017); Murray et al. (2014); Strand (2019); Williams (2000).

Phonological-Based Treatment Approaches

Children who have multiple speech sound errors and are highly unintelligible may benefit from phonological-based treatment that focuses on targeting phonological patterned errors opposed to individual sounds. By targeting a phonological pattern, such as final consonant deletion, many sounds can be practiced at one time, thereby increasing the child's speech sound inventory and improving speech intelligibility more rapidly. The primary purpose of phonological-based approaches is to help the child establish the adult phonological system, including the entire inventory of speech sounds used to contrast meaning, as well as the phonotactic rules, or the correct ways in which sounds are combined to form syllables and words (Bernthal et al., 2017). Specific examples of phonological-based treatment approaches are described briefly in Box 5.1.

What treatment approach or approaches might you recommend for Daniel and why?

Motor-Based Treatment Approaches

Motor-based treatment approaches focus on discrete motor skills, often with progression from the simplest to the most complex movements. Error sounds may be targeted one at a time or combined using a core vocabulary approach to focus on a small set of target words instead of individual sounds. Speech production practice may also involve production of error sounds in nonsense words, structured phrases, sentences, or conversational speech.

Vowel sounds and prosody as well as consonant sounds may be targeted. Various ways to establish correct production of an error sound may be used, including phonetic placement (e.g., using a tongue blade to push the articulators into position) or sound shaping (i.e., using a sound the child can produce to help produce the new sound).

When a sound is mastered in the therapy setting, speech assignments are provided to allow the client daily practice of their new skills and promote generalization outside the therapy setting. Instruction on self-monitoring of correct speech sound production and/or monitoring by others in a child's environment may also be introduced.

Motor-based treatment approaches, specifically phonetic placement and sound shaping, are frequently used when children are working on correct production of the "r" sound, which was the case for Daniel later in his treatment journey.

Some motor-based approaches begin with auditory discrimination training or oral-motor exercises. However, no evidence supports the use of oral-motor exercises, so these are not recommended. The utility of auditory discrimination training is also not well established and more research is needed (Kamhi, 2006b).

Success of treatment is determined by the application of what has been learned in a clinical setting to everyday life. Incorporating functional activities that mimic a child's real-life speaking environment ensures new skills acquired during treatment will be more easily transferred outside of the treatment setting.

> **REFLECTION QUESTION 5.3**
>
> *How do you produce the "r" sound and how does this compare to your classmates? Can you produce the Spanish trill "r"?*

Generalization and Maintenance

Once a client has achieved an acceptable level of correct sound production, an SLP must ensure retention and habituation of the new speech sound production pattern. Many SLPs introduce self-monitoring exercises from the very beginning of therapy. Doing so helps clients understand that they are ultimately responsible for their own success. Once an SLP believes that a client is ready for dismissal from therapy, follow-up sessions may be scheduled at progressively longer intervals. If the progress has been maintained over time, the treatment was effective.

Summary

Producing the sounds of a language during speech is a complex process. It involves an inner conceptualization of phonemes and phonotactic rules so that in our "mind's ear" we know how the language we are speaking should sound. Speech production also requires the neuromotor ability to move our articulators to form the desired sounds in a smooth, rapid, and automatic fashion. As children develop spoken language, they typically employ phonological patterns that simplify adult forms. If these persist beyond the expected ages, they may present difficulties.

Hearing disorders, motor-based disorders of neurological origin, and structural abnormalities may contribute to SSDs. Foreign language background and regional dialects contribute to variations in speech. Speech assessment includes a detailed description of the child's speech sound system, as well as investigation of risk factors and possible etiology of the SSD. Accessing the many available resources online will help when assessing multilingual children. Intervention strategies may include contrasted phonemes in word pairs, speech production drill practice, and use of a core vocabulary for production practice. Knowledge of a family's worldview about disability and treatment services will help to ensure treatment is provided in meaningful and relevant ways for families of culturally and linguistically diverse backgrounds. The general goal is improved intelligibility in spontaneous speech to increase communicative participation in everyday life.

Epilogue   Case Study: Daniel

Within 12 months, Daniel's speech intelligibility improved to 90% in connected speech, although speech sound errors and error patterns continued to persist. By the middle of second grade, Daniel had normalized all speech production errors in both languages and was dismissed from therapy.

Reflections   from an SLP and Parent of a Child with Concerns about Speech Sound Development

1. *How long have you been a speech-language pathologist, in what setting do you work, and in what areas do you specialize?*

   I have been a speech-language pathologist for 10 years. I've worked in the school setting for 8 of those years and early intervention/private practice for 2 years. I've been in the middle school setting for the past 6 years and I consider adolescent language to be a particular area of passion and

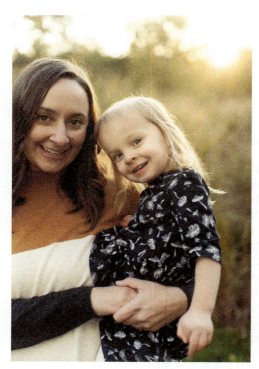

Emily (SLP and parent) and her daughter Eliza.

© Emily Flores

interest. I enjoy practicing neurodivergent-sensitive social-language intervention, higher-level language (e.g., syntax, vocabulary, written language) intervention, and functional communication intervention for my students with complex communication needs. I love being a school-based SLP for many reasons, one of which is being able to tie my services directly into reading, writing, and curriculum content.

2. *Did you ever wonder what you might think or how you might feel if one of your own children presented with speech developmental concerns?*

It has definitely been something I have thought about prior to having children, likely because the prevalence of speech/language disorders is relatively high. Being in this profession, I have had exposure to a very wide range of parent responses to their children's challenges and this has shaped how I have thought about what it would be like to have a child with speech development concerns. In my current setting, I encounter many parents that struggle with accepting their children for who they are, including both their strengths and needs, almost to the detriment of the child in some cases. While I can absolutely understand where these parents are coming from (and also acknowledge that they are doing what they feel is best for their child), my middle school students are extremely perceptive. Words and attitudes have significant weight, so having a message of "There are many things you need to fix about yourself" has the potential for impacting their self-esteem and feelings of self-worth. As they get older, it gets closer to sounding like, "You're not good enough because you're not like neurotypical children." Being an adolescent has enough challenges in these realms already, as it is a typical part of this stage of growing up. Having this lens, before having a child of my own with speech/language difficulties, I have decided that I would want to strive for balance between pushing my child to meet their potential but also recognize that words and attitudes bear weight on how you view yourself.

3. *What did you think and feel before, during, and after the speech-language evaluation process for your child?*

The biggest thing that comes to mind when I consider my thoughts and emotions through the evaluation process was my consistent gut feeling that there was indeed a delay but feeling brushed off when talking about it with family and friends. Having spent some time in early intervention, I felt that something was off around my daughter's first birthday. The most difficult part was hearing from (very well-intentioned) friends and family members messages that downplayed my concerns. "You're just sensitive because you're an SLP," "younger siblings always take longer to learn how to talk," "you have a skewed sense of things since you're in your profession," "you worry too much," were among some of the thoughts I was given, and few were even given by SLP colleagues. I am lucky enough to have a husband that was supportive and understanding of my early concerns, as well as my mother, who is an SLP as well. They both helped me trust my gut and initiate the evaluation process. Once we received the evaluation along with a few speech diagnoses, I felt validated and relieved that I did not choose to wait longer.

4. *What are your thoughts and feelings about the speech treatment process so far (if treatment has started)?*

It has truly been eye-opening being on the other side. My 3-year-old is already, even at this young age, aware that talking is harder for her than it is for other kids. She will electively avoid talking in situations where she feels like people will not understand her and this is heartbreaking to watch as both a parent and an SLP. Having formal intervention has already begun to help her find confidence in trying things that are difficult. I already love my profession, but this has continued to increase my respect for our field and the impact speech-language pathologists are able to make on peoples' lives.

The stakes are high when I am treating clients/students, but they feel even higher when you're a parent. This has helped me gain insight and empathy for the families I serve. It is impossible to understand the anxiety, fear, guilt, and stress that a parent with a child with a disability might feel until you have actually lived through it. I now take this knowledge into every IEP [individualized education plan] meeting, parent conversation, and treatment session I participate in.

I have also learned that there are many very important things we can do as SLPs to make our clients and their families feel comfortable, respected, and seen. Beyond the obvious need for delivering high-quality speech therapy, rapport and communication go a very long way. We have been incredibly fortunate to have a compassionate speech-language pathologist who makes it a priority to treat our daughter with kindness, patience (recognizing when to push and when to let go), and respect (using activities she is interested in, building her up to feel success vs. failure in sessions). My 3-year-old daughter asks every day if we can go see her SLP and I feel that is something worth striving for. Her SLP also takes the time to check in with me and actively listens to my concerns. These practices have built a positive connection to therapy for my child and have had a positive impact on her progress.

5. *What advice might you give to other parents who might be concerned about their child's speech sound production skills?*

Trust your gut and don't wait if you feel something may be "off." Recognize that, as a parent, you are the ultimate expert of your child. But also recognize that sometimes you can't do it all on your own. I felt that by having another SLP work with my daughter, I was failing as both an SLP and as a mom. That could not have been farther from the truth. It can be incredibly difficult to change lanes from parent to therapist. Seeking out help from other professionals has been very effective in helping my child make progress but has also been empowering for me as a mom.

Suggested Readings/Sources

Fabiano-Smith, L. (2019). Standardized tests and the diagnosis of speech sound disorders. *Perspectives of the ASHA Special Interest Groups, 4,* 58–66.

Kahmi, A. (2006). Treatment decisions for children with speech-sound disorders. *Language, Speech, and Hearing Services in Schools, 37,* 271–279.

McLeod, S., & Baker, E. (2017). Children's speech: An evidence-based approach to assessment and intervention. Pearson Education.

McLeod, S., Verdon, S., & International Expert Panel on Multilingual Children's Speech. (2017). Tutorial: Speech assessment for multilingual children who do not speak the same language(s) as the speech-language pathologist. *American Journal of Speech-Language Pathology, 26,* 691–708.

6 Developmental Literacy Disorders

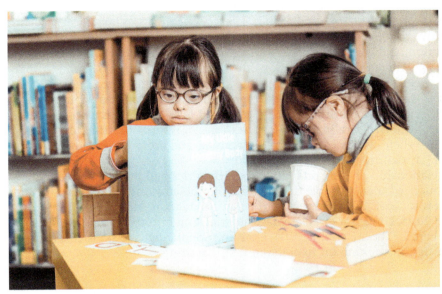

© Yakobchuk Viacheslav/Shutterstock

Learning Objectives

When you have finished this chapter, you should be able to:

6.1 Explain important aspects of reading and their development.

6.2 Characterize reading problems through the lifespan.

6.3 Detail assessment and intervention for reading disorder.

6.4 Explain important aspects of writing and their development.

6.5 Characterize writing problems through the lifespan.

6.6 Detail assessment and intervention for writing disorder.

"" Many years ago, I co-taught a course for future teachers in cognition and learning. When it came time to choose topics for papers, every reading teaching student chose dyslexia, a language disorder found in written language. My response was to say that I couldn't allow them to write a paper on something they had studied in depth previously.

The students were confused and replied, "We teach children who are having difficulty reading, not children with reading disorders."

Speech-language pathologists (SLPs) were just beginning to work with children with literacy disorders and it hadn't dawned on me that if SLPs didn't work with these children, their written language needs would not be addressed. As in so many areas of communication, SLPs have a crucial role in disorders of reading and writing.

Several years later, the special nature of what SLPs do in literacy disorders and the connection of these disorders to spoken language was made very clear by a young first-grader. His teacher came to me, saying she was concerned that he didn't seem to comprehend the simple stories they were beginning to read. After we spoke more, I asked her to inquire of him what he had done over the weekend. He responded in single words, such as "Picnic" and "TV."

Using a wordless picture book, I tried to elicit a simple narrative from him. He was unable to link events in a sequence and again responded in single words. With little oral narrative ability, he had no basis for comprehending written narratives. That's where we as SLPs become involved.

—*Robert Owens*

Modern democracy is based on the premise that we are an informed people. In the beginning of the American republic, the best informed were those who were literate. Even in our digital age, being informed means being literate. Using the Internet, texting, and accessing the vast stores of knowledge available requires literacy skills.

Literacy is the use of visual modes of communication, specifically reading and writing. The interrelatedness of aspects of literacy is illustrated by the correlation between reading and spelling ability. Poor readers tend to be poor spellers. But literacy is more than just letters and sounds. Literacy encompasses language; academics; cognitive processes, including thinking, memory, problem solving, planning, and execution; and is related to other forms of communication.

Although there is a clear relationship from mid-elementary through high school between oral language and reading comprehension (Tosto et al., 2017), reading and writing are not just speech in print. In addition to the obvious physical difference, reading and writing lack the give-and-take of conversation, are more permanent, lack the paralinguistic features (stress, intonation, fluency, etc.) of speech, have their own vocabulary and grammar, and are processed in the brain in a different manner (Kamhi & Catts, 2005).

The relationship of early oral language difficulties and literacy problems may be more nuanced than a simple transference of problems from one mode of communication to another. There seems to be an interaction between a child's early reading abilities, conversational language abilities, and history of language difficulties (Segebart DeThorne et al., 2010). Conversational language skills contribute a small but significant amount to children's early reading.

CASE STUDY   Liam

Liam grew up in a midwestern suburb and attended public schools. He's the youngest of four children and the only male. As a preschooler, he seemed to care little for books. Liam's language developed more slowly than his sisters', but his parents assumed that he would be fine and that he didn't talk much because his sisters talked for him. Still, his mom enrolled him in preschool to encourage his development. Liam scored low on his kindergarten readiness test and, although admitted to kindergarten, was later recommended to repeat the experience because of a lack of preacademic skills needed for first grade. His parents reluctantly agreed.

When he began school, Liam adjusted well, but he quickly began to fall behind other children in both reading and writing. An evaluation at the end of first grade resulted in Liam's being labeled as having a learning disability (LD). He read slowly and had several misread words. When he had finished a short passage, he was only able to provide the briefest of explanations of what he had read. Liam's independent writing contained frequent misspellings and often consisted of a single sentence. For example, in response to the cue *Tell me what you like about having a dog*, he wrote "I lik my dods play."

It was recommended that Liam remain in a regular classroom and receive additional instruction in literacy from a reading specialist and an SLP. At home, his parents worked closely with him on his reading and written assignments.

Through most of elementary school, Liam saw a reading specialist and an SLP several times each week.

As you read the chapter, think about:

- Possible explanations for Liam's reading problems
- Possible ways in which the evaluative team could explore different aspects of reading
- Possible explanations for Liam's later success

As in other forms of communication, use of literacy presupposes that you can encode and decode and, more importantly, that you are able to comprehend and compose messages for others. In other words, literacy rests on a language base—and so do literacy disorders.

As you might guess, many of the disorders mentioned under both childhood and adult language disorders (Chapters 4 and 7) figure prominently in literacy disorders. In fact, as many as 60% of children with language disorders may experience difficulties with literacy (Wiig et al., 2000). Children with language disorders may be unprepared for literacy learning because they lack emerging literacy skills and a strong oral language base. When compared to children developing typically, preschoolers and kindergartners with language disorders may be less able to recognize and copy letters and less likely to pretend to read or write, to engage in daily emerging literacy activities, or to engage adults in question–answer activities during reading and writing. As a consequence of poor literacy skills and failure to develop, children with literacy disorders often have less exposure to written text, which further hinders development and a child's ability to learn (Mol & Bus, 2011).

Academic demands increase as children mature, so literacy disorders don't disappear. You couldn't have read and understood this text as a first-grader. As adults, those who experienced literacy deficits in childhood may continue to struggle with reading and writing. I know an intelligent man in his 60s who has continually worked as a manual laborer because his lack of literacy skills has disqualified him from any positions requiring reading and writing.

Literacy deficits vary in complexity and severity. Maybe you are a college student with a literacy problem who has been able to succeed academically by adjusting to, compensating for, or overcoming deficits in your reading or writing. The authors of this text have worked with college students who have had to overcome literacy difficulties.

Although primary responsibility for teaching reading and writing still rests with the teacher and other educational specialists, an SLP is interested in children's language deficits and the ways in which those deficits influence the acquisition of literacy. In recognition of the special skills that SLPs bring to this area, the American Speech-Language-Hearing Association (ASHA; 2001d, 2010) recommends that SLPs play a role in literacy intervention.

As a consequence, SLPs are involved in literacy intervention from preschool through adulthood. According to ASHA, SLPs have the following responsibilities:

- Educate both teachers and parents in the relationship between oral language and literacy.
- Identify children who are at risk of having literacy difficulties.
- Make referrals to good literacy-rich programs.
- Recommend assessment and treatment in emerging literacy skills when needed.

Of necessity, the concerns of SLPs will differ with the maturational level and emerging literacy or literacy abilities of children.

Because children and adolescents with language disorders are at high risk for literacy disabilities, emerging literacy, reading, and writing assessment should be a portion of any thorough language evaluation, when appropriate. An SLP is concerned with establishing and improving reading and writing skills and helping children and adolescents develop the strong language base needed for both. Assessment and intervention for literacy are also vital parts of any thorough rehabilitative strategy for adults with neurological disorders (see Chapter 7).

As with most other communication disorders mentioned in this text, in literacy disorder SLPs often work as part of a team, collaborating with teachers and reading specialists to design literacy-based programs for vocabulary, language, and thinking skills (Silliman & Wilkinson, 2004). By working with teachers and applying evidence-based strategies, SLPs help children with developmental literacy disorders develop skills needed for meaningful participation in the classroom (Al Otaiba et al., 2018). Effective collaboration includes curriculum planning, naturalistic language facilitation, and careful teaming of personnel (Hadley et al., 2000). Other members of a literacy intervention team may include a reading specialist, school psychologist, and parent(s).

REFLECTION QUESTION 6.1

Many professionals recognize that literacy is not just speech in print form. If this is the case, why is oral language considered so important as a good literacy base?

In the remainder of the chapter, we discuss literacy and associated skills, disorders, assessment, and intervention, first with reading and then with writing. As you'll see, many language disorders discussed in Chapter 4 also affect literacy acquisition.

Reading

Learning Objective 6.1 Explain important aspects of reading and their development.

In the United States, only about 35% of fourth-graders can read at grade level proficiently (National Center for Education Statistics [NCES], 2022). Among children of color (e.g., Black, Latino/a) and those living in poverty, this rate is 15–21%. These statistics are even more alarming when we realize that 67% of students with disabilities read below even a basic level (National Assessment of Educational Progress, 2022).

Several steps are involved in reading and reading comprehension. Both language and the written context play a role in word recognition and in the ability to construct meaning from print (Gillam & Gorman, 2004).

The first step in reading is **decoding** the printed word, a process that initially consists of breaking or segmenting a word into its component sounds and then blending them together to form a word that is recognizable to the reader. At your level of literacy, visual recognition of a word is generally enough. Individual words take on meaning based on the grammar and context surrounding them. In addition, the reader interprets the print of the page based on their linguistic and conceptual knowledge (Whitehurst & Lonigan, 2001). We interpret what we read based on what we know. This is called comprehension. Given these processes, it shouldn't surprise you that a child with an oral language disorder might have reading problems as well. Figure 6.1 is a model of the dynamic process of text interpretation.

Reading comprehension is multidimensional. Comprehension consists of a complex interplay of linguistic input, general world knowledge, and working memory; making inferences in spoken and written discourse has been reported as

FIGURE 6.1 Reading comprehension.

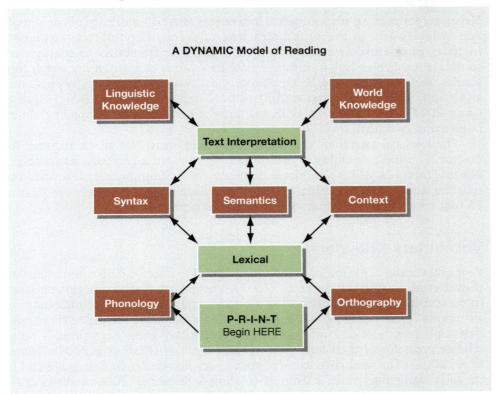

Beginning with print, a reader uses letters and their corresponding speech sounds to decode words that they then recognize based on the reader's lexical or vocabulary memory. The reader combines words with other words and uses syntax, semantics, and context to interpret and comprehend the meaning.

Source: Based on Gillam and Gorman (2004).

difficult for individuals with a variety of types of language disorders (Catts et al., 2006; Humphries et al., 2004; Moran & Gillon, 2005; Nation et al., 2004). As an active reader, you use self-monitoring, semantic organization, summarization, interpretation, mental imagery, connection with prior knowledge, and metacognition or your knowledge about these processes.

In summary, we can say that reading consists of decoding and comprehending text. Although phonological skills are essential for decoding, other areas of language are needed for comprehension (Nation & Norbury, 2005). The reader uses language and experience to interpret the message conveyed by the author. This may give you some idea of why language and literacy go hand in hand. Let's look briefly at three aspects of reading that are of particular interest to SLPs: phonological awareness, vocabulary knowledge, morphological awareness, comprehension, and inferencing.

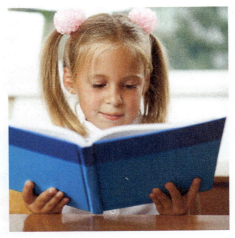

A reader uses language and experience to interpret an author's message.

© Milles Studio/Shutterstock

Phonological Awareness

Necessary for reading, **phonological awareness (PA)** is knowledge of the sounds and syllables and of the sound structure of words. Phonological awareness includes **phonemic awareness**, which is the specific ability to manipulate sounds, such as blending sounds to create new words or segmenting words into sounds. As you might guess, better phonological awareness, specifically phonemic awareness, is related to better reading skills (Cupples & Iacono, 2000; Hogan & Catts, 2004). In addition, PA skills also are the best predictor of spelling ability in elementary school.

Phonological awareness consists of many skill areas. Not all are required for reading. The auditory ability to determine a word when a phoneme or syllable is deleted (*cart − t = car*), to **blend**, or create a word from individual sounds and syllables, and to compare initial phonemes for likeness and difference are areas of PA that are particularly important for the development of reading.

Vocabulary Knowledge

Poor oral vocabulary knowledge is strongly linked to poor reading comprehension (Elwer et al., 2013; Nation et al., 2007). Vocabulary knowledge aids children in correcting their partial decoding attempts and may influence phonological awareness (Dyson et al., 2017; Tunmer & Chapman, 2012). Despite these relationships, preschool or kindergarten oral vocabulary knowledge alone is not a reliable predictor of their later word reading abilities (Duff et al., 2015; Muter et al., 2004). The predictive value of vocabulary knowledge in first grade and in the later elementary years is stronger (Nation & Snowling, 2004; Ricketts et al., 2007, 2016).

Morphological Awareness

Morphological awareness is understanding the effects bound morphemes have on root words, such as adding *un-* to *happy*. Although phonological awareness skills are essential for learning to read and write, recent findings suggest that by 10 years of age or even earlier, awareness of and knowledge about the morphological structure of words is a better predictor of decoding ability (Deacon et al., 2013, 2017; Mann & Singson, 2003; Wolter et al., 2009). In fact, morphological awareness is an important factor in literacy performance in early elementary school (Wolter & Pike, 2015). As you moved through the elementary grades and into middle school, morphologically complex words made up an increasing proportion of the words you encountered.

Comprehension

Several levels of text comprehension exist. At the basic level, a reader is primarily concerned with decoding. Meaning is actively constructed from words and sentences and from personal meanings and experiences. Above this level is **critical literacy**, in which a reader actively analyzes and synthesizes information and is able to explain the content. A reader bridges the gaps between what is written and what is meant (Caccamise & Snyder, 2005). At the highest level, **dynamic**

It does seem easy to confuse terms. Simply put, phonological awareness is an alertness of phonology; so, yes, it contains the elements of phonology.

Pearson eTextbook
Video Example 6.1

Phonological awareness provides the basis for reading. Hearing and recognizing sound differences is important. This video is a quick introduction from public broadcasting.

www.ny.pbslearningmedia.org/resource/3485d17a-eaf0-492c-974c-cfe4b28c1444/phonological-awareness-phoneme-awareness-k-1-introductory-video/

literacy, a reader is able to interrelate content to other knowledge through reasoning. Dynamic literacy is comparing and contrasting, integrating, and using ideas to raise problems and solve them (Westby, 2005).

A reader's mental representation of meaning is composed of the text and the mental model the reader creates through the comprehension process. Comprehension occurs as a reader combines textual material, text grammar, and their own world knowledge and experience.

An important factor in comprehension is *inferencing*. Inferencing is the ability to understand a message in a context where some elements are not explicitly known (Trabasso & Wiley, 2005; van Kleeck, 2008). Active readers engage with the text and infer meaning from the material on the page.

Reading is a goal-directed activity. For example, a reader may be gathering information to be used in a problem-solving task. Knowing what to do and how to do it is called **metacognition**, and two aspects of it are important for reading. One aspect is self-appraisal, or knowledge of one's own cognitive processes. The other is **executive function**, or self-regulation, and includes the ability to attend; to set reasonable goals; to plan and organize to achieve each goal; to initiate, monitor, and evaluate performance in relation to the goal; and to revise plans and strategies based on feedback. As you read, you form hypotheses about the material, then predict and either confirm or do not confirm your predictions.

Studies with twins indicate that both genetics and the environment are important for reading achievement (Harlaar et al., 2008). In contrast, genetic factors alone seem to play a role in the relationship between early speech and reading (Hayiou-Thomas et al., 2010).

> Each reader must interpret what they read in light of personal experiences and knowledge. In other words, our comprehension will differ based on our own unique self.

Inferencing

Inference construction within spoken and written narratives and texts is an important social and educational tool. Inferencing is understanding meaning that is not explicitly stated, as in the request for more heat in "Do you think it's chilly in here?" Constructing inferences can facilitate the coherent representation needed for comprehension (Cain et al., 2001; Virtue et al., 2006; Virtue & van den Broek, 2004). Some children with language disorders tend to find inferencing challenging.

Reading Development through the Lifespan

You may believe that literacy development begins with reading and writing instruction in school. Actually, literacy development begins much earlier and continues throughout our lives. Significant relationships exist between emergent literacy vocabulary knowledge and later reading. Infant vocabulary comprehension and expression is a significant predictor of later vocabulary, phonological awareness, reading accuracy, and reading comprehension (Duff et al., 2015).

Emerging Literacy

Reading development begins within social interactions between a child and caregiver(s) at around age 1, as parents or other caregivers begin to share books with toddlers. Book sharing is usually conversational in tone, with the book serving as the focus of communication. Here's an example:

> *Adult:* This is a book about a . . .
>
> *Child:* Bear.
>
> *Adult:* Yeah. And you found him right here. What do bears say?
>
> *Child:* Grrrrrrr.
>
> *Adult:* Um-hm, they growl. Grrrrrrr. Let's see, can you find his eye?

Reading the book is secondary to the conversation.

As children mature, some caregivers engage in **dialogic reading**, an interactive method of reading picture books. When reading, adults encourage their children to become actively involved in the reading process by asking questions and allowing opportunities to become storytellers. The development of English narrative abilities is enhanced for children from Spanish-speaking homes who are exposed to English through home literacy (Bitetti & Scheffner Hammer, 2016).

By age 3, most children in the United States are beginning to develop **print awareness**. Early print awareness consists of knowledge of the meaning and function of print, basic concepts concerning the direction print proceeds across a page and through a book, and recognition of some letters. Later-developing skills include recognizing words as discrete units, being able to identify letters, and using terminology, such as *letter*, *word*, and *sentence*. Children with good language skills seem to enjoy reading activities more than children with poor language and will pretend to read at an early age.

By age 4, children begin to notice phonological similarities and syllable structure in words they hear. This is the beginning of phonological awareness. Four-year-olds also appreciate both sounds and rhymes. Children who have been exposed to a home literacy environment and to print media have better phoneme awareness, letter knowledge, and vocabulary (Foy & Mann, 2003). Children from disadvantaged socioeconomic backgrounds, and those with language disorder and impoverished literacy experiences, may be in danger of not developing these skills (McGinty & Justice, 2009).

Phonological awareness may arise from children's need to store words in their brain with increasingly more detailed representation. This becomes necessary as children's vocabulary grows, and there are more and more words, some very similar in sound, to store.

Early childhood settings have great potential as sources of emergent literacy experiences for children at risk. Unfortunately, in publicly funded preschool classrooms serving at-risk children in the United States, the overall quality of literacy instruction is low (Justice et al., 2008). Although many preschool teachers have only limited training in emergent literacy, they can learn to facilitate development of emerging literary skills by using a higher rate of utterances that include print/sound references and decontextualized language (Girolametto et al., 2012).

Although similar language skills contribute to reading across the age span, the relative importance of each changes with literacy stage (Skebo et al., 2013). The best predictors of kindergarten reading status are oral language, alphabet knowledge, and print concept knowledge, such as how print proceeds across the page and that print stands for words and letters have sounds. Potential reading difficulties for children with language disorders can be estimated in preschool using these predictors (Murphy et al., 2016). By middle school, overall language predicts both decoding and reading comprehension at middle school and decoding at high school. Vocabulary predicts reading comprehension at high school. In contrast, among children with speech sound disorders, vocabulary predicts both decoding and reading comprehension at early elementary school, while among children with typically developing language (TDL), phonological awareness predicts decoding.

Inferencing abilities emerge during the preschool years (Filiatrault-Veilleux et al., 2016; Florit et al., 2014; Reed et al., 2015). By age 4 years, children demonstrate some ability to infer the problem and the goal of the character in a story (Makdissi & Boisclair, 2006). By knowing the goal, a reader can understand the motivation of the characters. Children at age 4 can also predict what will happen next (Filiatrault-Veilleux et al., 2016). Between ages 5 and 6, children are able to make inferences concerning the consequences of events, to attempt to solve the problem, and to predict the next event of a story (Kendeou et al., 2008).

In kindergarten additional variables seem to predict reading success by second grade, including rapid automatized naming (RAN) and caregiver education level (Catts et al., 2001). RAN is the ability to quickly name a series of items in a category, such as types of clothes or food. Although poor performance on PA tasks is found in children with reading disorders and those with developmental language disorder (DLD), difficulty with RAN is more characteristic of children with reading disorders only (De Groot et al., 2015).

In general, children develop the skills associated with reading more rapidly at earlier ages than in later ones. Development gradually plateaus and is followed by slow refinement.

In first grade, children are introduced to reading instruction and learn the sound–letter correspondence called **phonics**. A child reads words and links them with meanings stored in memory. Most of the child's effort goes into decoding, leaving little cognitive energy for either comprehension or interpretation. This is one reason we don't assign *War and Peace* to first-graders.

Phonology (sound) and orthography (letters) are important for early reading, but as reading matures grammar and meaning contribute more. Later, developing knowledge of morphology may aid students in breaking words apart, recombining them, and creating new words (Berninger et al., 2001).

As a child's reading improves, reading becomes more automatic or fluent, especially with familiar words. Fluency is aided by the use of grapheme–phoneme patterns in the child's memory and by analogy, the process of relating unfamiliar words to familiar ones based on similar spelling. For example, *lion* and *lionize* have similar elements.

By third grade, there is a shift from *learning to read* to *reading to learn* (Snow et al., 1999). As language continues to improve, so does comprehension, with a resultant increase in reading fluency.

Mature Literacy

Although all reading begins with the printed word, mature readers like you use very little cognitive energy for determining word pronunciation. At a higher level of processing, a person uses both language and experience to understand text, monitoring automatically to ensure that the information makes sense.

A skilled reader then predicts the next word or phrase and glances at it to confirm the prediction. Printed words are processed quickly, automatically, and below the level of consciousness most of the time. In less than a quarter of a second, your brain retrieves all the information from a word or phrase that it needs to confirm the prediction and form another prediction of the next word or phrase. This process is presented in Figure 6.2.

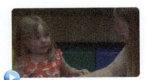

Pearson eTextbook
Video Example 6.2
Emerging Phonological Awareness and Phonics

In this video, a young girl demonstrates phonics and emergent phonological awareness.

FIGURE 6.2 Model of mature reading.

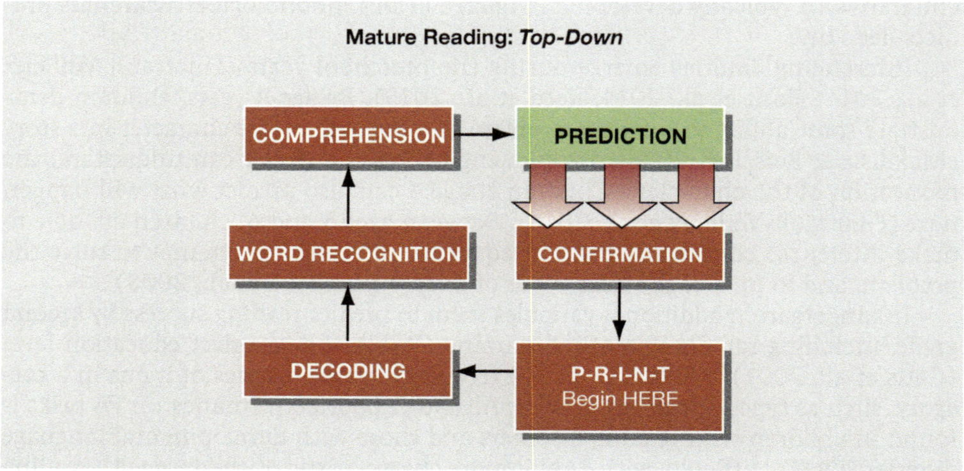

Mature readers use their language skills to predict what words or phrases will appear next in the text, then momentarily glance at the print to confirm their predictions before predicting anew what will follow.

Rapid and accurate reading is enabled by quick retrieval of orthographic and phonological information along with semantic processes. The reallocation of attention to cognitive and higher language processes is essential for comprehension (Wolf & Katzir-Cohen, 2001).

Mature readers don't simply read the text; they dialogue with it. Reading is an active process in which ideas and concepts are formed and modified, details remembered and recalled, and information checked. Much of this is the unconscious process of the brain partaking of new information.

As we mature, the types and purposes of reading change, but we can continue to enjoy the process throughout our lives. Reading skill continues to be strong through adulthood, as long as we exercise our ability and do not experience any neuropathologies, such as those in Chapter 7. Reading is one of the primary ways by which adults increase their vocabulary and knowledge.

> Establish a habit of reading now. It will serve you well as you mature.

Pearson eTextbook
Video Example 6.3

Before we begin our section on reading disorders, access this TED-Ed video of a short discussion about dyslexia.
www.youtube.com/watch?v=zafiGBrFkRM

REFLECTION QUESTION 6.2

Why might the child who has not been exposed to books or interactive reading be at a disadvantage?

Reading Disorders Through the Lifespan

Learning Objective 6.2 Characterize reading problems through the lifespan.

Language disorders that persist through preschool are associated with higher risk of poor literacy by age 8 (Jin et al., 2020). Risk of reading difficulties is greatest for children with a history of problems in both articulation and receptive and expressive language (Segebart DeThorne et al., 2006). In general, poor reading comprehenders have deficits in oral language comprehension, too, but have normal phonological abilities. In contrast, children who are poor decoders have poor phonological abilities but little or no oral language comprehension difficulties (Catts et al., 2006). The story of Liam, a young man with learning disabilities and reading difficulties, was presented at the beginning of the chapter.

One significant factor in literacy ability and in overall school success is socioeconomic status (SES). As mentioned in Chapter 3, children from low-SES environments acquire language skills more slowly than those from mid- or high-SES environments. In addition, these children have delayed letter recognition and phonological awareness and are at risk for reading disorders (Aikens & Barbarin, 2008). They experience less educational success and have the highest dropout rate, and those who do graduate from high school are 4.3 grade levels behind those of higher-SES groups (Palardy, 2008).

The ASHA website (www.asha.org) provides access to many professional articles on reading disorders. For example, select "Publications" at the top and then select "American Journal of Speech-Language Pathology." Enter "Reading" in the search box to access all the professional articles in this journal on that topic. The "Refine search" button can narrow your search to certain years.

Some children have a specific type of learning disability or disorder that is primarily manifested in reading and writing. In the past, this disorder was called *dyslexia*. The fifth edition of the *Diagnostic and Statistical Manual of Mental Disorders* (DSM-5; American Psychiatric Association, 2013), as mentioned in Chapter 4, does away with this term in favor of *specific learning disorder*. Types of specific learning disorders are not labeled but are to be described in a diagnosis. Within education, dyslexia is still used. To make this less cumbersome, this book uses the term *dyslexia* or *SLDL*, for *specific learning disorder in literacy*, interchangeably.

Pearson eTextbook
Video Example 6.4
In this video is a short, 4-minute overview of the causes of dyslexia.
www.youtube.com/
watch?v=ROPW0R54dgE

Children with SLDL or dyslexia have poor word recognition or decoding abilities, accompanied by problems with phonological processing. SLDL is a type of learning disability, is neurobiological in origin, and is characterized by difficulties with accurate and/or fluent word recognition and decoding abilities and by poor spelling (Lyon et al., 2003).

When we compare children with dyslexia to typically developing readers, we find:

- Comparable verbal IQ and/or listening comprehension
- Below-average word reading
- Well-below-average word attack or decoding skills
- Well-below-average phonological processing scores (Sawyer, 2006)

Interestingly, spelling is closely associated with word reading difficulties and often results from deficits in similar underlying skills

Three distinct types of dyslexia have been described, including a language-based disorder that may affect comprehension and/or speech sound discrimination, a speech/motor disorder that may affect speech sound blending and motor coordination, and a visual-spatial disorder that may affect letter form discrimination. The language-based disorder is the most common.

> **CASE STUDY** **Liam** *(continued)*
>
> Liam had difficulty with comprehension of both speech and reading. Recall that he was seeing a reading specialist and a speech-language pathologist several times each week. His SLP focused on Liam's language and listening skills and on his oral and reading comprehension.

Estimates of the number of children with dyslexia may go as high as 20% of all children. It's important to understand that dyslexia is not related to intelligence. In fact, across children higher intelligence results in an increased gap between reading achievement and intelligence.

The brains of children with dyslexia differ from those of the majority of children. In general, these children and adults see the world differently, leading to more creative approaches and solutions.

Several websites discuss dyslexia. The Learning Disabilities Association of America website (www.ldaamerica.org) has a brief checklist of symptoms for parents. On the home page, scroll down to and select "Parents." Under "Specific Learning Disabilities," select "Dyslexia" to learn more. Alternatively, you can go directly to www.ldaamerica.org/disabilities/dyslexia/.

Much more detailed information is available on the MedicineNet website (www.medicinenet.com). In the menu at the top, go to "Health A-Z," which will give you the "Diseases and Conditions Index." Select the letter "D," followed by "Dr-Dz," and scroll down to "Dyslexia." Alternatively, you can go directly to www.medicinenet.com/dyslexia/article.htm.

Finally, the website of public service station WETA, LD Online (www.ldonline.org), has a thorough discussion of dyslexia. In the menu at the top, go to "Getting Started" and select "Glossary." Once there, select "D," scroll down to "Dyslexia," and select "Dyslexia Basics." Alternatively, you can go directly to www.ldonline.org/ld-topics/reading-dyslexia/dyslexia-basics.

Children with DLD may be similar to those with LD, exhibiting grapheme–phoneme (letter–sound) errors and syntactic, semantic, and pragmatic errors or misinterpretations when reading (Spanoudis et al., 2019). Comprehension also may be impaired and may be related to a child's poor vocabulary.

Children with **hyperlexia** have poor comprehension but typical or above-average word recognition abilities. Hyperlexia is a near-obsessive interest in letters and words found in some children with autism spectrum disorder (ASD). Although these children appear very precocious in their reading ability, they often have poor social skills and extremely limited reading comprehension (Treffert, 2009). Many individuals with ASD have word reading skills that are more advanced than their overall reading comprehension (Church et al., 2000; Diehl et al., 2005; Smith-Myles et al., 2002; Wahlberg & Magliano, 2004).

Reading difficulties result from the interaction of a combination of risk factors that vary across individuals, including:

- Reading difficulties are heritable (Catts, 2017; Pennington & Lefly, 2001; Snowling et al., 2003). Many children at high risk for reading disability have at least one parent with a significantly slower speaking rate than children at low risk for reading disability.

- Poor oral language skills (Colenbrander et al., 2018; Murphy et al., 2016; Snowling et al., 2016; Thompson et al., 2015).

- Hearing difficulties and speech sound disorders (Carroll & Breadmore, 2018).

- Poor environmental exposure to print early in life.

- Difficulties with cognitive skills underlying language, plus other factors associated with reading abilities, such as rapid automatic naming, short-term memory, working memory, and executive functions (Alloway & Alloway, 2010; Gathercole et al., 2006; St. Clair-Thompson & Gathercole, 2006). Differences have been found in the temporal-parietal region (interior to the ear), in both the left and right linguistic processing areas of the brain, and in the cerebellum (near the brainstem) (Deutsch et al., 2005).

- Noncognitive factors.

As might be expected given their language learning difficulties, many children with ASD have accompanying literacy disorders and uneven development of skills that are predictive of reading. In general, preschool children with ASD are severely delayed in their vocabulary relative to their nonverbal mental ages (Charman et al., 2003). In addition, oral narratives are challenging for these children (Losh & Capps, 2003). As a result, children with ASD and accompanying limited verbal skills often are excluded from standard literacy curricula, under the misguided assumption that they are incapable of learning to read (Koppenhaver & Erickson, 2003).

Young children with ASD demonstrate wide variability in their emergent literacy ability (Davidson & Ellis Weismer, 2014; Westerveld et al., 2020). In general, reading comprehension is poor among many school-age children with ASD and may be affected by one or more factors, including the communication deficits mentioned previously, cognitive factors such as working memory, and active processes such as comprehension monitoring and inferencing (Davidson, 2021).

Similar to what we see in typically developing readers, children with LD acquire reading skills more rapidly in the initial stages and then gradually slow (Skibbe et al., 2008). Even so, these children are substantially below more typical readers by fifth grade.

Phonological awareness is a beginning phase for most readers. Speech perception seems to be particularly important for the development of PA (Rvachew & Grawburg, 2006). For example, 6-year-old Juan, a recent immigrant from Colombia, initially had difficulty with both English speech and English reading. As he quickly learned to speak and comprehend English, his reading ability also improved.

Most initial reading problems are related to deficiencies in both phonological awareness and processing (Catts & Kamhi, 2005). Those with phonological disorders, especially perceptual deficits, will find PA challenging. PA difficulties seem to be related to failure to analyze words into syllables and these, in turn, into smaller phonological units.

In attempting to read, some children with language disorders, especially those with poor phonological skills but average or above-average intelligence, may use memorized word shapes, letter names, or guessing rather than relying on decoding skills. As a result, they are unable to decode unfamiliar words. Without these word attack or decoding skills, by second grade, when formal decoding instruction ends, these children begin to fail.

Pearson eTextbook
Video Example 6.5

If you are not a person with dyslexia, it may be difficult to understand the disorder and how the world seems to a person with dyslexia. This video, titled "Dyslexia: Cracking the Code," may help.

www.youtube.com/
watch?v=lpO3o9U-2_s

If a beginning reader has good phonological ability and appears to decode words well, reading comprehension problems may go unnoticed (Nation et al., 2004). Although phonics-based decoding problems often decrease by third grade, comprehension problems may persist (Foster & Miller, 2007).

Poor reading comprehension is associated not with PA or phonics (letter-sound matching), but with poor oral language (Nation & Norbury, 2005). Some children have difficulty interpreting written narratives because they have poor oral narrative abilities (Naremore, 2001). Like the boy in the vignette at the beginning of the chapter, they may lack the story framework or linguistic skills for telling narratives. The majority of individuals with ASD do not become skilled readers because of their difficulties interpreting both oral and written words (Lanter & Watson, 2008).

Reading comprehension difficulties appear to be dependent on a range of oral language comprehension skills, including vocabulary knowledge and grammatical, morphological, and pragmatic skills (Hulme & Snowling, 2014). Pragmatic skills relevant to reading comprehension include overall communication ability, especially conversational skills such as social inferencing and interpersonal reasoning (Donahue & Foster, 2004). Given the low social competence of some children with language disorders, it's easy to see why this aspect of reading might be difficult (Brinton & Fujiki, 2004).

Children with DLD find reading comprehension especially challenging. This can be seen in the difficulty these children experience in answering inferential questions in comparison to literal questions. An association exists between inferencing ability and vocabulary knowledge, single word reading accuracy, grammatical skill, and verbal working memory (Gough Kenyon et al., 2018). Over 50% of children with language disorders demonstrated inferencing deficits (Lucas & Frazier Norbury, 2015).

Good readers like you actively guide and control their reading. In contrast, poor readers lack such strategies, reflecting possible deficits in executive function. They may approach reading as a random, unfathomable process. You'll recall that executive function deficit is most evident in children with traumatic brain injury. In addition, children with attention-deficit/hyperactivity disorder and LD have been described as inattentive and impulsive, disorganized, unable to inhibit behavior, and ineffective learners, which are characteristics of those with impaired executive function.

As children experience repeated reading failure, they may become frustrated or passive. Lacking persistence and with low self-esteem, they may become apathetic and resigned to failure. In contrast, some poor readers may become aggressive or display acting-out behaviors in the classroom. All these behaviors interfere with further learning and development.

Many children with language disorders are at risk for reading disorder (Hambly & Riddle, 2002; Miller et al., 2001; Potocki & Laval, 2019). In general, they:

- Begin with less language and may have difficulty catching up
- Have poor comprehension skills because they lack language knowledge that would enable them to integrate what they read
- Have poor metalinguistic skills
- Possess linguistic processing difficulties

When something goes wrong in the reading process, the result is reading that is less automatic and less fluent. Word decoding or text understanding may be impaired.

As mentioned, reading difficulties do not disappear. They are often related to other language problems. As adolescents, poor readers exhibit vocabulary, grammar, and verbal memory deficits compared to typical readers (Rescorla, 2005).

Competent readers and writers approach the task with a purpose that guides their behavior.

Remember that *metalinguistics* includes the ability to consider language out of context, to make judgments about its correctness, and to understand to some extent the process of using language.

In general, the more features of a nonmainstream American English (NMAE) dialect, such as African American English, that a child uses, the slower the growth in reading and overall literacy are likely to be (Charity et al., 2004; Craig & Washington, 2004; Gatlin & Wanzek, 2015; Terry, 2012; Washington et al., 2018). Using something other than the majority dialect used in instruction means that a child must learn to shift dialect. NMAE use is a more important factor in reading outcome than socioeconomic background and grade level. Although speaking some dialects may make reading more difficult for a child, it's important to recall that use of a NMAE dialect is not a disorder.

Assessment and Intervention for Reading Disorder

Learning Objective 6.3 Detail assessment and intervention for reading disorder.

As with the speech and language disorders discussed previously, reading disorders require an SLP to thoroughly describe a child's strengths and weaknesses and to determine the appropriate intervention methods. This requires an in-depth understanding of literacy and assessment and intervention techniques.

Given the multidimensional nature of reading, we often find low correlation across standardized reading tests used to assess reading comprehension (Keenan & Meenan, 2014). Variability in student performance on reading assessments is a function of the interaction of these factors and should be interpreted in relation to the specific reading demands of the assessment.

The focus of an assessment will vary with the child and grade level. In kindergarten, assessments of phonological awareness, letter naming, and/or letter–sound correspondence knowledge and vocabulary are appropriate. In first and second grades, the SLP may focus on the ability to read simple nonwords and frequent regular and irregular words and passage reading fluency (Gersten et al., 2009).

Assessment of Developmental Reading

In this section we discuss overall assessment, with a more detailed discussion of assessment of phonological awareness, word recognition, comprehension, and executive function. Information from multiple assessments tends to be more sensitive than information from only one assessment (Gersten et al., 2009).

Although SLPs working in preschools do not assess children for emerging reading skills, they may do so if a child fails their prekindergarten screening. More likely is a scenario in which an SLP assesses an elementary school child for emergent reading skills based on a referral from a classroom teacher or reading specialist. Identification of children likely to have reading difficulties is important because intervention can be most effective during emergent literacy and in the early school years (Catts et al., 2015; Tymms et al., 2018).

As mentioned in Chapter 4, assessments begin with an initial data-gathering step that

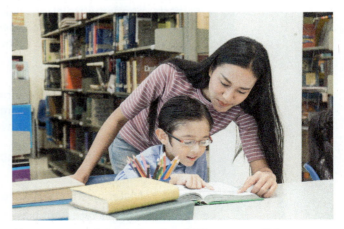

Classroom teachers may refer children to an SLP.
© Ultramansk/Shutterstock

may include use of questionnaires, interviews, referrals, and screening. Early literacy questionnaires often ask about the frequency of book reading behaviors, responses to print, language awareness, interest in letters, and early writing. Parental reports of early literacy skills of preschool children with language disorders compare favorably with professional assessments (Boudreau, 2005). Figure 6.3 presents a checklist designed to identify kindergarten and first-grade children at risk for language-based reading difficulties. No one item on its own indicates a reading problem. Children can be accurately identified at the end of first grade using a screening battery containing measures of letter-naming fluency, phonological awareness, rapid naming, or nonword repetition (Catts et al., 2015).

Additional information can be gathered from interviews with teachers, parents, and the child and by observation within the classroom. Interview questions should include the child's perceptions of the importance of reading and difficulty with different types of reading, along with the child's self-perceptions. Observation can confirm the child, teacher, and parent responses.

Collaborative reading assessment should include standardized measures, oral language samples including analysis of miscues or mistakes, and written story retelling (Gillam & Gorman, 2004). Formal testing might be accomplished by a school's reading specialist, but an SLP may also wish to give selected tests and to probe specific skills. In a more informal task, a child might be asked to read previously unread curricular materials in an attempt to assess their ability to function within the classroom (Nelson & Van Meter, 2002). The child's aloud reading can be recorded for later analysis of the child's miscues and comparison with speech. For example, children with DLD often omit morphological endings in both their speech and in oral reading (Werfel et al., 2017).

Comprehension can be assessed by using questions, retelling, or paraphrasing. Questions may range from factual to inference types.

Phonological Awareness

Phonological awareness assessment is multifaceted and should be accomplished within an overall assessment of reading, spelling, phonological awareness, verbal working memory, and RAN. In addition to formal testing, an SLP can use informal assessment of rhyming, syllabication, segmentation or breaking words into parts, phoneme isolation, deletion, substitution, and blending or putting word parts together. With school-age children, it is especially important to assess both segmenting of words and blending of sounds.

Word Recognition

Decoding skills, especially knowledge of sound–letter correspondence, is the basis for word recognition. Of interest to an SLP will be decoding of consonant blends, long (*day*) and short (*can*) vowels, different syllable structures, and morphological affixes (*un-*, *dis-*, *-ly*, *-ed*).

Word recognition assessment should adhere to the following guidelines (Roth, 2004):

- Materials appropriate to the student's age and developmental level
- Various types of tasks to assess different levels of processing
- Use of several measures
- Consideration of a child's cultural and linguistic background

FIGURE 6.3 Checklist for early identification of language-based reading disabilities.

The child . . .

_____ Has difficulty remembering words or names

_____ Has problems with verbal sequences (i.e., alphabet, days of the week)

_____ Has difficulty following instructions and directions and may respond to a part rather than the whole

_____ Has difficulty remembering the words to songs and poems

_____ Requests multiple repetitions of instructions/directions, with little improvement in comprehension

_____ Relies too much on context to understand what's said

_____ Has problems understanding questions

_____ Has difficulty understanding age-appropriate stories and making inferences, predicting outcomes, and drawing conclusions

_____ Frequently mispronounces words and names

_____ Has problems saying common words with difficult sound patterns (i.e., *spaghetti*, *cinnamon*)

_____ Confuses similar-sounding words (i.e., the *Specific Ocean*)

_____ Combines sound patterns of similar words (i.e., *nucular* for *nuclear*)

_____ Has speech that is hesitant, contains fillers (i.e., *you know*), or contains words lacking specificity (i.e., *that, stuff, thing, one*)

_____ Has expressive language difficulties, such as short sentences and errors in grammar

_____ Lacks variety in vocabulary and overuses words

_____ Has difficulty giving directions or explanations

_____ Relates stories or events in a disorganized or incomplete manner

_____ Provides little specific detail when relating events

_____ Has difficulty with rules of conversation, such as turn taking, staying on topic, and requesting clarification

_____ Doesn't seem to understand or enjoy rhymes

_____ Doesn't easily recognize words that begin with the same sound

_____ Has difficulty recognizing syllables

_____ Demonstrates problems learning sound–letter correspondences

_____ Doesn't engage readily in pretend play

_____ Has a history of language comprehension and/or production problems

_____ Has a family history of spoken or written language problems

_____ Has limited exposure to literacy in the home

_____ Seems to lack interest in books and shared reading activities

Source: Based on Catts (1997).

- Demonstration and training of unfamiliar tasks
- Children with emergent literacy skills are not the only ones with reading deficits
- Observation and interpretation of a child's test behaviors

Although traditional assessment procedures stress standardized testing, alternative approaches such as curriculum-based measures and dynamic assessment may be more appropriate for children with language disorders or from culturally or linguistically diverse backgrounds (Roth, 2004). You may recall from Chapter 4 that in dynamic assessment the SLP tries to determine the best way to teach a skill based on the learning characteristics of the child. Dynamic assessment often follows a test–teach–test format, in which a child is assessed for the amount of change they can make during the assessment process.

Materials for curriculum-based assessment usually come from the local curriculum and use criterion-referenced scoring, which measures a child against their own performance over time. In this way, progress is measured without reference to some abstract norm.

Word recognition is more than just the ability to decode a word in isolation. It's important, therefore, that word recognition testing be accomplished with various clues available to the child, such as pictures or different sentence forms, and with words both in isolation and within text. More important than test scores is describing a child's strengths and the strategies used.

When analyzing a child's recorded reading data, the SLP notes all discrepancies in the recorded reading samples. All attempts at word decoding, repetitions, corrections, omitted words and morphemes, extended pauses, and dialectal usages should be noted and analyzed for possible strategies used by the child. Reading errors can be analyzed at the word level by type, such as word order changes, word substitutions, additions, and deletions (Nelson & Van Meter, 2002). The percentage of incorrect but linguistically acceptable words indicates the extent of a child's use of linguistic cues to predict the correct word. In addition, an SLP can note the way in which the child sounds out words (Nelson & Van Meter, 2002).

Morphological Awareness

Textbooks for adolescents and young adults contain a variety of morphologically complex words, such as *regeneration*, *reptilian*, and *strenuous*. Given the importance of derived words for academic success, morphological awareness should be assessed in older children (Nippold & Sun, 2008). At the very least, SLPs should examine adolescent students' understanding of common morphemes such as *-able* (*acceptable*), *-ful* (*powerful*), *-less* (*speechless*), *-tion* (*prediction*), and the like. Actual words can be chosen based on frequency of word use in text and curricular materials.

Text Comprehension

Assessing text comprehension abilities of children is complicated by the many cognitive and linguistic processes involved. At the very least, as an SLP, you or other team members should assess a child's:

- Oral language, with special attention to the child's use of the more elaborate syntactic style used in literature

- Knowledge of narratives and text grammar
- Metacognition (Westby, 2005)

Narrative schemes or the events in a story might be assessed by having a child tell a narrative from pictures or by asking questions about the pictures that relate to the organization of the story. A child's text grammar, consisting of the parts of a story, can be assessed through spontaneous narratives or by retelling previously heard narratives.

Although several norm-referenced tests measure reading comprehension, tests should be supplemented by other measures of a child's ability to identify grammatical units, interpret and analyze text, make inferences, and construct meaning by combining text with personal knowledge and experience (Kamhi, 2003).

Executive Function

Whereas poor readers act as if reading is simply sounding out words rapidly and fluently, good readers expect text to make sense and to be a source for learning information. As a result, good readers read actively and with purpose, constructing mental models and organizing information as they go.

Self-regulation in reading can be assessed in many ways, including (Westby, 2004):

- Interview questions regarding strategies used with different reading tasks
- Verbalizing thoughts called *think-alouds* accompanying reading
- Error or inconsistency detection while a child reads

Errors and inconsistencies can be planted in texts specifically for the assessment.

Intervention for Developmental Reading Disorder

Once the diagnostic data are analyzed and a literacy problem(s) identified, a child and an SLP are ready to begin intervention. Ideally, intervention for developmental literacy disorders is a team effort. The SLP supports the efforts of all the other team members and the explicit instruction of the classroom teacher and reading specialist.

CASE STUDY   **Liam** (*continued*)

Liam received reading instruction in his class and from the reading specialist at the same time that the SLP was working on language-based issues with his reading.

Team members might cooperate in an embedded/explicit model of intervention in which younger children participate both in literacy-rich experiences embedded in the daily curriculum and in explicit, focused therapeutic teaching of reading (Justice & Kaderavek, 2004; Kaderavek & Justice, 2004). The literacy-rich environment might include a message board where children learn to decode an "important" message left daily by the teacher; snack activities in which sounds are embedded in snack names, recipes, music, and print; book and speech sound play; rhyming pictures; and book sharing with the teacher and others (Towey et al., 2004).

Effective instruction for reading should include sound and letter processes used in word identification, grammatical processes, and the integration of these

Literacy-rich environments are critical for children with literacy disorders.

with meaning and context (Gillam & Gorman, 2004). Training in phonological (sound) and orthographic (letter) processing together seems to offer a more effective strategy than working on PA skills in isolation (Fuchs et al., 2001; Gillon, 2000).

In preschool, the SLP can increase a child's print awareness with print-focused reading activities (Justice & Ezell, 2002). Print-focused strategies emphasize word concepts and alphabetic knowledge and include cues such as the following:

Show me how to hold the book so I can read.

Do I read this way or this way?

Where is the last word on the page?

How many words do you see?

Find the letter C. Whose name starts with C?

Such print-focused prompts are easy to teach, and parents have used them successfully at home with only minimal training. Print knowledge gained in this way has both short-term and long-term benefits (Justice et al., 2017).

According to the Common Core State Standards adopted by the National Governors Association and Council of Chief State School Officers in 2010, by kindergarten a child should recognize and name alphabet letters, associate sounds with letters, and be proficient in phonological awareness tasks, such as identifying phonemes in simple words and substituting phonemes in single words to create new words. Not all preschool classrooms are providing learning opportunities necessary to foster emergent literacy skills (Mihai et al., 2017).

Language-based reading intervention focuses on language that underpins and is essential for reading development, such as oral language development, listening, and reading comprehension. Oral language intervention can target language disorder as it relates to reading and writing difficulties. Language-focused intervention has a positive impact on curriculum-aligned measures of vocabulary, comprehension monitoring, and understanding narrative and expository text and on reading comprehension measures (Hui & Logan, 2019). For Spanish-speaking English learners, structured language-based English intervention in speech and reading can lead to significant gains in the production of morphosyntax in conversation and narration (Bedore et al., 2020).

Most integrated approaches to emergent literacy consider the two semi-independent sets of skills presented in Figure 6.4 (van Kleeck & Schuele, 2010):

- *Form foundations* for decoding include learning about the alphabet and becoming aware of phonological units within spoken words

- *Meaning foundations* for reading comprehension include vocabulary and sentence-level semantic-syntactic skills

Later, reading intervention might target both linguistic and metalinguistic skills, including recognition of key words, use of all parts of the text such as the glossary and the index, and application of general learning strategies such

FIGURE 6.4 Two-stage intervention.

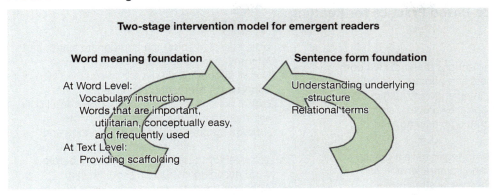

Intervention with young readers should focus on both word meaning and sentence formation.

Source: Based on van Kleeck and Schuele (2010).

as graphic organizers containing photos, drawings, and print. Now let's briefly discuss intervention for phonological awareness, word recognition, comprehension, and executive function.

Phonological Awareness

As an SLP, you'll have distinct and extensive knowledge related to PA and will play a critical role on educational teams (Cunningham et al., 2004; Moats & Foorman, 2003; Spencer et al., 2008). Many ideas for PA intervention can be found in the Terrell and Watson (2018) tutorial.

While classroom instruction focuses on children's achievement of specific curricular outcomes, SLP intervention focuses on the individual learning needs of children who have not achieved these desired classroom goals. For example, Juan, the bright elementary school child and recent immigrant from Colombia who was mentioned at the opening of this chapter, had difficulty with decoding because his phonological awareness skills were not aligned with English. Once he became more fluent in English speech, he developed PA in English and quickly caught up to his English-speaking peers.

Evidence-based practice (EBP) tells us that children who receive PA training have higher phonemic awareness, word attack, and word identification skills at the end of kindergarten than children who do not receive such training. Even short-term—as little as twice weekly for 6 weeks—high-quality, explicit phonemic instruction with small groups of children can be effective for most children (Koutsoftas et al., 2008). Other EBPs are presented in Box 6.1. In addition to working with individual students, SLPs can offer phonological awareness instruction to teachers, stressing the importance of PA and its integration into the reading curriculum (Hambly & Riddle, 2002). What seems most important is that PA intervention begin before children lag too far behind others, most likely in preschool or kindergarten (Torgesen, 2000).

Phonological awareness training alone is insufficient to increase reading comprehension (Pugh & Klecan-Aker, 2004). Whenever possible with older children, phonological awareness should be taught within meaningful text experiences, such

---

BOX 6.1   Evidence-Based Practice for Reading

General

- Code-focused interventions that included both phonemic awareness and phonics training are the most effective intervention strategies in increasing phonological awareness, alphabet knowledge, oral language, reading, and spelling skills.

- Auditory/language strategies have a greater impact on the reading comprehension of children with LD than visual strategies, demonstrating the underlying spoken–written language link.

Phonological Awareness and Metalinguistics

- We can have a moderate degree of confidence in techniques designed to improve phonological awareness in school-age children. Tasks designed to improve rhyming, sound identification, phoneme segmentation, phoneme manipulation, and grapheme–phoneme correspondence consistently yield moderately large to large effects. Similar effects can be obtained through classroom collaboration and clinician-only approaches.

- Training should be appropriate for the emergent reading or reading level of the child. In deciding whether to provide PA practice to older children, an SLP must consider both the nature of the reading deficit and the level of PA knowledge.

- Little is known about the appropriate length and intensity of intervention.
- Not all phonological skills are of equal importance. Segmenting and blending are critical skills needed for reading. Lower-level skills are important to the extent that they facilitate subsequent development of segmenting and blending. This said, we have not identified the skill level for these two that is needed before word decoding instruction should begin.
- Although the data are limited, it appears that the use of technology/computers can improve PA skills
- Some tasks are easier than others:
  - Consonants are easier to segment than vowels.
  - Initial sounds are easier to segment than final sounds.
  - Shorter words are easier to segment than longer words.
  - Initial sounds in consonant-vowel-consonant words are easier to segment than in consonant-consonant-vowel words
- Highly effective intervention is contingent on adult responses to child errors. In short, adult responses should consider the reason for the child's error and the learning level and facilitate a correct response.
- Teaching is enhanced when SLPs anticipate the types of errors that a child is likely to make and plan scaffolding or guiding strategies to elicit correct responses.

Sources: Based on Cirrin and Gillam (2008); Lee et al. (2013); Pavelko (2010); Schuele and Boudreau (2008); Sencibaugh (2007).

---

as systematic and explicit classroom instruction, so that the emergent nature of both literacy and PA can support each other.

In general, programs focusing on one or two PA skills yield better results than those that try to teach with a broader focus (National Reading Panel, 2000). It is best to work with one or two sounds at a time. An SLP should teach skills that will directly impact the child's performance of an everyday classroom task.

Intervention can begin with syllable and sound recognition and identification and can be both receptive and expressive. Next, the SLP can move to syllable segmentation and blending (*stapler → stap-ler → stapler*) and, finally, to phoneme segmentation and blending (*cat → c-a-t → cat*). In general, segmentation is easier for most children than blending.

It makes sense to target lower-level PA skills, such as rhyming, to facilitate development of more complex skills, such as segmenting and blending. Once blending and segmenting are established, an SLP can provide a link to classroom decoding and spelling instruction by providing practice that facilitates the application of phoneme awareness to spelling and decoding of words (Blachman et al., 2000).

The concept of syllables can be introduced as naturally occurring "beats" in a word. Multisensory approaches are also helpful and can make the training interesting. Clapping hands or drum beats can be used to help children recognize and identify syllables. Other examples include dropping objects into cans, stacking toys, playing hopscotch, or taking turns in any number of child games during auditory recognition training.

Phoneme intervention might progress from recognition of a target sound in isolation, through identification when paired with other sounds, to sounds in syllables, then words (Gerber & Klein, 2004). Memory can be aided by pairing sounds with real objects or pictures and finally with printed letters and words.

Morphological Awareness

Reading and spelling accuracy can be improved through instruction in morphological awareness together with other forms of linguistic awareness, including knowledge of phonology, orthography, syntax, and semantics (Kirk & Gillon, 2009). Intervention might focus on increasing awareness of the morphological structure of words and the orthographic rules that apply when suffixes, such as -*ly*, are added to a word, changing the *y* in *happy* and *crazy* to an *i* to make *happily* and *crazily*. Teaching morphology along with variations in the related English phonology and orthography results in improvement in the reading and spelling abilities for children in the mid-elementary grades (Murphy & Diehm, 2020). Apel and Werfel (2014) offer a wonderful tutorial filled with ideas for teaching morphological awareness to students with literacy deficits.

Word Recognition

The goals of intervention for word recognition are:

- To teach decoding skills
- To develop a vocabulary of written words
- To improve reading comprehension (Torgesen et al., 2005)

Success in the last two depends on achievement of the first. Teaching decoding skills can result in increases in reading accuracy, fluency, and comprehension (Torgesen, 2005). Support for learning can be provided through encouragement and positive feedback and by breaking tasks into smaller steps or by giving a child as much direction as necessary to complete the task successfully.

Context can be used to help children predict words in text. Intervention might begin with obvious words, such as *I took my umbrella because it looked like ____*. Training can then move to more ambiguous choices and the use of other strategies that include morphological and orthographic cues, such as *Let's have ___ for lunch* followed by *Let's have p___ for lunch* or *Let's have p___s for lunch*.

In this way, children can be taught to consider a word in its context and not as a single entity independent of other words. Although this may seem like encouraging guessing, it's actually helping a child use context as a tool. Recall that predicting based on what has come before is a strategy used by mature readers to increase the pace of their reading.

Text Comprehension

Comprehension relies on many different aspects of processing. As mentioned, when we read our knowledge and experience blend with the information on the page to form a mental representation of the meaning. An active reader makes inferences from the text, past knowledge, and experience. The SLP will need to identify educationally relevant reading comprehension activities and directly address the component skills and knowledge bases involved in these activities (Catts & Kamhi, 2017).

Children who lack internalized story frameworks necessary for interpreting narratives might begin intervention with telling stories (Naremore, 2001). Intervention can progress to oral and then written narrative interpretation (Boudreau & Larson, 2004). Storybook reading can be divided into before, during, and after reading activities to aid comprehension. Postreading might include creating story organizers, retelling, and creating variations of the narrative. Narratives can also be divided into story parts and then recombined.

Similarly, comprehension by children who read with difficulty can be improved by also focusing on before, during, and after reading strategies (Vaughn & Klingner, 2004). Through emergent reading techniques such as establishing the content and setting the scene or context, establishing relationships, and discussing unfamiliar vocabulary and concepts, an SLP or a teacher can assist students in constructing meaning from what they read. Activation of prior knowledge ("What do we know about farms?") can improve comprehension, especially for children with LD.

Comprehension may also be enhanced by teaching children the more explicit and precise language style found in written communication (Westby, 2005). This style can be taught through tasks in which children must follow very explicit oral instructions to be successful or tasks in which contextual cues, such as objects or pictures, are present. Literate vocabularies can be enhanced through emergent reading activities that focus on the words to be encountered and through use of visual or verbal memory aids. Complex grammar may be taught through books with familiar stories or books in which the grammar becomes increasingly complex.

Intervention strategies differ according to when they are used in the reading process. For example, prior to reading, semantic strategies, such as giving definitions or synonyms for key words, reduce reading miscues or errors. Graphophonemic strategies are more effective during reading (Kouri et al., 2006). Graphophonemic strategies include encouraging a child to "sound out" a word, calling a child's attention to phonetic regularities, and asking a child to identify initial or final sounds or consonant blends.

During reading, SLPs can facilitate comprehension through instruction, questions, visual and verbal cues, explanations, and comments (Crowe, 2003). Using a conversational style, the SLP provides cues and feedback as oral group reading occurs. It's important that questions reflect the level of comprehension targeted for each child. This semantic strategy should be accompanied by direct vocabulary instruction (Ehren, 2006).

> **CASE STUDY**   **Liam** *(continued)*
>
> Liam's SLP began with discussions and summaries of each sentence and gradually enlarged to the units. This helped him focus on the important information and to pull it together into a summary.

Ideally, students will internalize comprehension strategies and use them as they read actively. Active strategies might include the following:

- Using context to analyze word meaning
- Activating prior knowledge
- Rereading difficult passages
- Self-questioning to help frame key ideas
- Analyzing text structures to determine type of reading
- Visualizing content
- Paraphrasing in one's own words
- Summarizing (Ehren, 2005, 2006; Pressley & Hilden, 2004)

These strategies can be used along with monitoring in which a reader actively decides whether a reading passage makes sense and what to do about it if it does not. Good readers recognize when they have not comprehended a written passage, and they therefore reread it.

When we analyze eye movements of typical readers, we find that their eyes are bounding ahead and back, trying to check the accuracy of words within the surrounding meaning. Children with reading disorders can be taught to use this information to determine individual word meaning (Owens & Kim, 2007).

At another level, comprehension includes a social dialogue with the authors and characters. Comprehension training should also include discussion of the author's goals and the feelings and motivations of characters (Donahue & Foster, 2004). Knowledge of the text can be used to predict a character's behavior within a narrative.

Instruction in multistrategy approaches to inferencing seems to have a positive effect on the comprehension of struggling middle school readers (Barth & Elleman, 2017). Strategies might include such varied approaches as clarification using text clues, activating and using prior knowledge, understanding character perspectives and author's purpose, and answering inferential questions. Poor reading comprehension in adolescence can be approached by intervention targeting common deficits in word reading ability, lexical development, and syntactic development (Nippold, 2017).

Pearson eTextbook
Video Example 6.6

In this video is a TEDx Talk that discusses the dyslexic brain and its workings.

www.youtube.com/
watch?v=_dPyzFFcG7A

Executive Function

Specific areas of executive function that might be targeted in intervention include working memory, self-directed speech (*How can I figure out the meaning of this word?*), and problem solving (Westby, 2004). Just teaching these strategies is not enough. The approaches need to be embedded within reading activities. An SLP and a classroom teacher must help each child achieve independent and appropriate use of these strategies.

Of importance for more advanced readers is *distancing*, or moving away from strict dependence on the text and toward independent thinking about the text. This can be accomplished by questions that move from factual answers explicitly stated in the text (*What did she do next?*) to ones in which the question is generated by something in the text but the answer is generated from the student's knowledge (*Could she have solved the problem differently?*).

Hopefully, you're motivated to learn more. Several resources are available online. The Mayo Clinic website (www.mayoclinic.com) covers signs, symptoms, causes, and treatment of reading disability. Enter "dyslexia" in the search box at the top, then select "Symptoms and causes" or "Diagnosis and treatment." Alternatively, go directly to www.mayoclinic.org/diseases-conditions/dyslexia/symptoms-causes/syc-20353552.

Several commercial sites are available. Please be aware that with these sites, materials that are mentioned do not necessarily represent what we authors would recommend. Just browse the possibilities. For example, the Bright Solutions for Dyslexia website (www.dys-add.com) has several definitions and offers useful teaching tips.

Writing

Learning Objective 6.4 Explain important aspects of writing and their development.

In the United States, a majority of students in grades 4, 8, and 12 do not demonstrate grade-level writing skills (NCES, 2022; Persky et al., 2003). Only 28% of fourth-graders and 27% of eighth- and twelfth-graders met grade-level writing expectations. Among children with disorders, only 7% of fourth-graders and 5% of eighth- and twelfth-grade students perform at or above grade level.

Like all other modes of communication, writing is a social act. Just like a speaker, a writer must consider the audience, but because the audience is not present when the writing occurs, writing demands more cognitive resources for planning and execution than does speaking.

In short, writing is using knowledge and new ideas combined with language knowledge to create text. It's a complex process that includes generating ideas, organizing, and planning, along with acting on the plan, revising, and monitoring based on self-feedback. It includes motor, cognitive, linguistic, affective, and executive processes.

Writing is more abstract and **decontextualized** than conversation and requires internal knowledge of different writing forms, such as narratives and expository (explain, compare, contrast, convince) writing. *Decontextualized* means "outside of a conversational context."

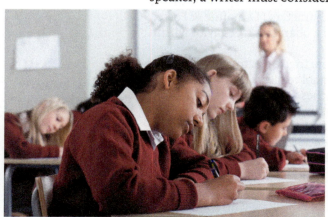

Only 27% of eighth- and twelfth-graders meet grade-level writing expectations.

© Juice Verve/Shutterstock

When you write, the entire context is contained in the writing. You create the context with your language rather than having the context created by your conversational partners.

Several aspects of the writing process are of concern for an SLP. These include (Berninger, 2000):

- Spelling
- Executive function
- Text construction, or going from ideas to writing
- Memory

As mentioned previously, executive function is self-regulation and includes attending, goal setting, planning, and the like. Memory provides ideas for content, language symbols, and rules to guide the formation of that content and is used for word recognition and storage of ideas as they are worked and reworked. As you can see, writing is a very complicated process. Let's look more closely at spelling and then writing development and disorder, followed by assessment and intervention.

Spelling

Spelling is a complex process with multiple components including letter-to-sound relationships, letter and syllable spelling patterns, and meaning based on word roots and affixes (Bear et al., 2016; Williams et al., 2017). Spelling of most words is self-taught using a trial-and-error approach. It is estimated that only 4,000 words are explicitly taught in elementary school. Rather, classroom teachers focus on strategies and regularities that children can use to determine word spelling.

Good spellers use a variety of strategies and actively search words for patterns and consistency. More specifically, mature spellers like you rely on memory; on spelling and reading experience; phonological, semantic, and morphological knowledge; orthographic or letter knowledge and mental grapheme representations; and analogy (Apel & Masterson, 2001). Semantic knowledge is concerned with the interrelationship of spelling and meaning, as in *there* and *their*, whereas morphological knowledge is knowing the internal structure of words, affixes (*un-*, *dis-*, *-ly*, *-ment*), and the derivation of words (*happy*, *unhappily*). Mental grapheme representations are best exhibited when you ask yourself, "Does that word look right?" Your representations are formed through repeated exposure to words in print. Finally, through analogy a speller tries to spell an unfamiliar word using prior knowledge of words that sound the same.

Spelling competes with other aspects of writing for our limited cognitive energy. Excessive energy expended at this level comes at the cost of higher language functions. As a result, poor spellers generally produce poorer, shorter texts. The more effective a speller becomes, the more automatic the writing process, freeing up a student's working memory to enable greater focus on other writing processes.

Your brain doesn't store words letter-by-letter; rather, it stores them by more useful units. For example, *stand* is probably stored as *st-and*, which enables you to spell *land*, *band*, *hand*, *bland*, *strand*, and so on.

Writing Development through the Lifespan

Writing and speaking development are interdependent and parallel, and many aspects of language overlap both modes. In turn, writing development includes expansion of several previously mentioned interdependent processes. For example, typically developing children and those with Down syndrome (DS) matched for reading level both exhibit oral narratives that are longer and more complex than written narratives. Among the children with DS, vocabulary comprehension is the best predictor of narrative skills (Kay-Raining Bird et al., 2008).

Emerging Literacy

Initially, children treat writing and speaking as two separate systems. Three-year-olds, for example, will "write" in their own way—usually scribbling—and don't yet realize that writing represents sounds. The story may be contained in an accompanying drawing. By age 4, some real letters of the parent language may be included.

As with reading, in early writing children expend a great deal of cognitive energy on the mechanics, such as sound–letter associations and letter formation. Gradually, spelling, like reading, becomes more accurate and fluent or automatic.

For a few years, the spoken and written systems converge, and children write in the same manner as they speak, although speech is more complex. Around age 9 or 10, talking and speaking become differentiated as children become increasingly literate. Slowly, writing overtakes speech as written sentences become longer and more complex than speaking. Children display increasing awareness of the audience through their use of syntax, vocabulary, textual themes, and attitude. Some language forms are used almost exclusively in either speech or writing, such as using *and* to begin many sentences in speech but only rarely in writing.

Mature Literacy

In a phase not achieved by all writers, speaking and writing become consciously separate. The syntax and semantics are consciously recognized as somewhat different, and the writer has greater flexibility of style. You may or may not have achieved this phase yet. If you find yourself using an enlarged vocabulary when writing or pondering how sentences flow from one to the next, then you are probably there. As with reading, practice results in improvement that should continue throughout the lifespan. In general, the writing of adults as compared to adolescents contains longer, more complex sentences and uses more abstract nouns, such as *longevity* and *kindness*, and more metacognitive and metalinguistic words, such as *reflect* and *disagree*, respectively (Nippold et al., 2005).

Writing includes, among other things, spelling; executive function; and text generation, or going from ideas to written text. Let's discuss, in that order, the aspects of particular interest to SLPs.

Spelling

Spelling development is a long, slow process. As mentioned, initial attempts at spelling consist mostly of scribbling and drawing, with an occasional letter thrown in. Later, children use some phoneme–grapheme knowledge along with letter names. For example, *bee* might be spelled as *B*. Gradually, children become aware of conventional spelling and are able to analyze a word into sounds and letters, although vowels, especially in English, will be difficult for some time.

As knowledge of the alphabetic system emerges, a child slowly connects letters and sounds and devises a system called "invented spelling" in which the names of letters may be used in spelling, as in *SKP* for *escape* or *LFT* for *elephant*. One letter may represent a sound grouping, as in **set** for **street** (*s* for *str*). Because young children lack full knowledge of the phoneme–grapheme system, they have difficulty separating words into phonemes.

As spelling becomes more sophisticated, children learn about spacing, sequencing, various ways to represent phonemes, and the morpheme–grapheme relationship. The parallel development of reading aids this process.

Children who possess full knowledge of the alphabetic system of letters and sounds can segment words into phonemes and know the conventional phoneme–grapheme correspondences. As children begin to recognize more regularities and consolidate their alphabetic system, they become more efficient spellers (Ehri, 2000). Increased memory capacity for these regularities is at the heart of spelling ability.

Many vowel representations, phonological variations (such as *later–latter*), and morphophonemic variations (such as *sign–signal*) will take several years to acquire. Gradually, children learn about consonant doubling (la*dd*er), stressed and unstressed syllables (**report–re*port***), and root words and derivations (*add–addition*).

Most spellers shift from a purely phonological strategy to a mixed one between second grade and fifth grade. As words and strategies are stored in long-term memory and access becomes fluent, the load on cognitive capacity is lessened and can be focused on other writing tasks.

Adults spell in several ways: letter-by-letter, by syllable, and by subsyllable unit, such as *ck*, used for *back*, *stick*, and *rock* but never in *ckar* (car). The method used seems to vary with the task. Next time you're typing words, notice whether your spelling is conscious letter-by-letter or more automatic.

Executive Function

It is not until early adulthood that writers develop the cognitive processes and executive functions needed for mature writing (Berninger, 2000; Ylvisaker & DeBonis, 2000). It takes this long because of the protracted period of anatomical and physiological development of your brain's frontal lobe, where executive function is housed.

Until adolescence, young writers need adult guidance in planning and revising their writing. By junior high school, teens are capable of revising all aspects of writing. Improved long-term memory results in improved overall compositional quality.

Text Generation

Once children begin to produce true spelling, they begin to generate text. In first grade, text may consist of only a single sentence, as in *My dog is old*. Early compositions often lack cohesion and use structures repeatedly, as in the following:

> *I like school. I like gym. I like recess. I like art.*

In contrast, mature writers use sentence variety for dramatic effect. The facts and events characteristic of early writing evolve into use of judgments and opinions, parenthetical expressions, qualifications, contrasts, and generalizations (Berninger, 2000).

Initially, compositions lack coherence and organization. Later, ideas may relate to a central idea or consist of a list of sequential events.

Written narratives or stories emerge first, followed by expository texts. Expository writing, the writing of the classroom, is of several genres: procedural, as in explaining how to do something; descriptive; opinion; cause-and-effect; and compare-and-contrast.

REFLECTION QUESTION 6.4

We have mentioned a few times that literacy is more than speech in print and that reading and writing are not opposite processes. How do the processes of reading and writing differ?

By adolescence, expository writing has greatly increased in overall length, mean length of utterance, multiclause production, and use of literate words that transition between thoughts, abstract nouns, and metalinguistic/metacognitive verbs (Nippold et al., 2005). Literate words include *however, finally,* and *personally;* abstract nouns are words such as *kindness, loyalty,* and *peace;* and metalinguistic and metacognitive verbs include *think, reflect,* and *persuade.*

Writing Problems Through the Lifespan

Learning Objective 6.5 Characterize writing problems through the lifespan.

Children with language disorders often have writing deficits. Unfortunately, their writing difficulties may remain through the lifespan, and the gap between their writing abilities and that of children developing typically widens.

In general, children with language disorders exhibit reduced written productivity, as measured by total number of words, total number of utterances, or total number of ideas (Puranik et al., 2007; Scott & Windsor, 2000). Similarly, these same children exhibit deficits in writing *complexity* (Fey et al., 2004; Mackie & Dockrell, 2004; Nelson & Van Meter, 2003; Puranik et al., 2007; Scott & Windsor, 2000). Finally, children with language disorders exhibit reduced *accuracy,* as measured by number of errors (Altmann et al., 2008; Mackie & Dockrell, 2004; Nelson & Van Meter, 2003; Puranik et al., 2007).

CASE STUDY   **Liam** *(continued)*

Remember that Liam, when he was evaluated at the end of first grade, wrote only one sentence to respond to reasons for liking dogs: "I lik my dods play."

Children with LD may have difficulties with all aspects of the writing process (Wong, 2000). A sample of the writing of a child with LD is presented in Figure 6.5. Because they have little knowledge of the writing process, these children fail to plan and to make substantive revisions. They are easily discouraged and may devote very little time to a given writing task. Clarity and organization are forsaken for spelling, handwriting, and punctuation, leaving little cognitive capacity for text generation. In the process, meaning suffers.

Deficits in Spelling

Poor spellers view spelling as arbitrary, random, and seemingly unlearnable. Misspellings are characterized by omission of syllables, morphological markers such as plural *s,* and letters; letter substitutions; and confusion of homonyms such as

FIGURE 6.5 Sample writing of an 11-year-old child with SLDL.

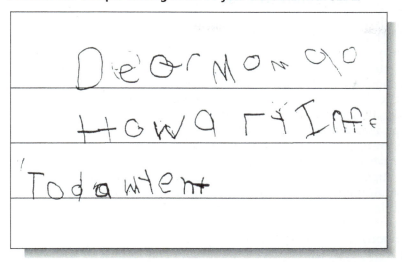

Dear mom and dad, How are you? I am fine. Today we went . . .

to/too/two. Even adults, especially those with LD, often cite spelling as their primary area of concern. Although children with DLD acquire the general knowledge of a written language's orthography, they have less well-represented word-specific knowledge than their peers with TDL (Williams et al., 2021).

Usually, deficits in spelling represent poor phonological processing and poor knowledge and use of phoneme–grapheme information. Although most spellers shift to greater use of analogy between second grade and fifth grade, poor spellers tend to rely on visual matching skills and phoneme position rules to compensate for their limited knowledge of sound–letter correspondences (Kamhi & Hinton, 2000).

Deficits in Executive Function

When you write, you begin with ideas. You convert your ideas into language. At this point, executive function becomes especially important.

When executive function or self-regulation is impaired, communication and even problem-solving abilities are diminished, especially in complex linguistic tasks such as writing. Lacking self-regulation, some children with LD follow a writing strategy of putting on paper whatever comes to mind, with little thought to planning. They produce and elaborate little, revise ineffectively and with seeming indifference to their intended audience, detect errors poorly, and experience difficulty executing intended changes. Planning is difficult because of language formulation difficulties.

One adult professional with LD uses different templates for his reports in which he fills in the blanks. Otherwise, the task of planning, writing, and revising a report would overwhelm his executive abilities. Until he and his spouse devised the templates, he would call from work at the end of each day to have his spouse talk him through the report-writing process.

Just as a poor reader expends all their energy in decoding, a poor writer becomes bogged down in the mechanics of the writing and spelling process. Both leave the poor reader or writer with little energy for higher cognitive functions such as comprehension or text generation, respectively.

Pearson eTextbook
Video Example 6.7

How does it feel to have dyslexia when notetaking in class? Try this video test from Bell House UK to see for yourself.

www.youtube.com/
watch?v=xAeaN2zCphc

Deficits in Text Generation

In narrative writing, as in storytelling, children with language disorders may lack mature internalized story models or may be unable to visualize the words even from their own spoken narratives. When compared to the narratives of chronological age-matched peers with typical language, the narratives of children with LD contained shorter, less complex sentences (Scott & Windsor, 2000). As a result, both the oral and written narratives often are shorter and have fewer episodes, contain fewer details, and fail to consider the needs of the listener.

Typical expository writing tasks follow a format, such as statement of a problem, examination of several factors, and conclusion. Children with language disorders have difficulty with these writing tasks and approach them with seemingly little thought or planning. The results are often extremely short, poorly organized, and containing numerous errors of grammar, punctuation, and spelling. There is often little revision. In addition, children with LD have substantial difficulty with morphological endings, such as regular past tense and regular plurals, even when they demonstrate accuracy with these units in their speech (Windsor et al., 2000). For example, even with assistance, a junior camp counselor with LD was unable to write a sentence or two on each child's participation in a camp activity even though he could tell others what each child did.

Assessment and Intervention for Writing Disorder

Learning Objective 6.6 Detail assessment and intervention for writing disorder.

As with the speech and language disorders discussed previously, writing disorders require an SLP to thoroughly describe a child's strengths and weaknesses and to determine the appropriate intervention methods for various aspects of writing. This requires an in-depth understanding of literacy and assessment and intervention techniques.

Assessment of Developmental Writing

One method of assessing writing in the classroom is through the use of portfolios of children's writing (Paratore, 1995). A portfolio is a collection of meaningful writing selected by a child, an SLP, and a teacher that contains samples of the child's formal and informal writing over time, thus enabling the child to demonstrate progress. The wide variety helps to increase the validity of the sample. Items in a portfolio may include SLP or teacher observation notes; work samples; first drafts of writing samples, such as journal entries and projects/papers; final drafts of the same; and peer and teacher evaluations.

Narrative samples are best for young elementary-age children. Older elementary-age children or adolescents can provide expository writing samples. Written narratives can be sorted into two broad categories: personal and fictional. Narrative tasks may be in response to storybook pictures, videos, and oral prompts, such as recalling a funny event or a topic (Price & Jackson, 2015). Perspective should be for someone who is and isn't present at an event or did not view the book or video. Expository tasks such as informational or explanatory can be elicited by describing isolated pictures, describing and explaining without pictures, comparing–contrasting tasks, and retelling of expository text (Price & Jackson, 2015).

Executive function is best measured within actual writing tasks as part of an overall writing assessment rather than separate from functional communication tasks. Samples should be written in ink to allow for analysis of revisions. For children using a computer, turn on "Track changes" but not "Show markup" as these may confuse the child. The changes can be accessed later.

It's helpful to allow children to plan and to write drafts. All notes and plans should be collected, along with the finished product, and added to the child's portfolio. Price and Jackson (2015) offer a wonderful tutorial based on the professional literature for the collection of writing samples, variables that are useful to assess, and manual and computer-aided techniques for analyzing writing samples.

Whenever possible, an SLP, a teacher, or an instructional aide can observe the writing process for evidence of planning and organizing, drafting, writing, revising, and editing. Added information can be obtained if children read their paper aloud while being recorded. This procedure aids the SLP or teacher in interpreting garbled or poorly spelled words.

Writing can be analyzed on several levels, including textual, linguistic, and orthographic (spelling). At a textual level, an SLP can note length; any indication of the amount of effort, overall quality, and structure; or the way in which comments support the topic (Berninger, 2000). Recall Liam's tendency to write one sentence. Of interest are the total number of words, clauses, and sentences, as well as the structural complexity, as measured in words per clause and clauses per sentence. Writing conventions, such as capitalization and punctuation, plus the use of sentences and paragraphs, should be noted.

> Executive function is very difficult to assess without some task to accomplish; thus, the context is very important.

Assessment of Spelling

Spelling deficits are very complex and can be difficult to describe. Collection should be of sufficient quantity to allow for a broad-based analysis. Spelling deficits should be assessed through both dictation and connected writing such as that in a child's portfolio (Masterson & Apel, 2000). Standardized tests should also be included and can be administered by a classroom teacher, writing specialist, or school psychologist. Informal assessments should include several phoneme–grapheme variations, such as single consonants in various positions in words, consonant blends (*str-*), morphological inflections (*-est*, *dis-*), diphthongs, digraphs (two letters for one sound, as in *ch* and *sh*), and complex morphological derivations.

Single-word spelling does not measure a child's ability in a real communicative context. Connected writing, such as that found in a portfolio, can offer samples closer to actual practice.

Descriptive analysis should focus on patterns in the child's spelling (Bear et al., 2000). Of interest are the most frequent and the lowest-level patterns. Figure 6.6 presents a possible analysis system that suggests several possible intervention strategies.

Assessment of Text Generation

SLPs and teachers can assess a child's writing using the papers assembled in their portfolio, including both narrative and expository examples.

Analysis may include the total number of words and the number of different words. This is an overall measure of a child's vocabulary and flexibility in its use. Other measures might include the maturity of the words used, clause and sentence length, and coherence. Narratives and expository writing can be analyzed for the presence or absence of elements of both forms. For example, does a narrative include a setting statement of *who*, *what*, *when*, and *where*?

FIGURE 6.6 Examples of language-based spelling analysis.

Phonological: Segmenting, blending, and phonemic awareness

Omission of internal and unstressed phonemes and cluster reduction

     Stop → SOP   Sand → SAD

Syllable deletion

     Elephant → ELFANT

Letter reversal (most common with liquids and nasals)

     Sing → SIGN

Orthographic: Sound–symbol relationship (/k/ = k, c, ck, cc, ch, q, x), letter combinations, letter and positional patterns, and grapheme representations

Letter-sound confusion

     Cash → CAS

Nonallowable letter sequences

     Dry → JRIE   Queen → KWEN

Possible spellings that violate location-pattern rules

     Chip → TCHIP Corn → CKORN

Different spellings on repeated attempts (no cognitive representation or graphemic representation of word)

Morphological: Inflectional (-ed, -ing, -s) and derivational (un-, dis-, -er, -ist, -ment) morphemes, relationship of root word, and inflected or derived form

More difficult if a form has more than one meaning (fast**er**, teach**er**), multiple pronunciations (walk**ed**, jogg**ed**, collid**ed**), and both phonological and orthographic properties are changed when inflected or derived (*ascend* and *ascension*).

Semantic: Effect of spelling on meaning

Homophone confusions

     Won → ONE   They're → THER   Which → WITCH

Intervention for Developmental Writing Disorder

Intervention for writing may involve both general training and more specific and explicit techniques for both narrative and expository forms. To learn to write, you must write, so intervention needs to focus on the actual writing process. Ideally, writing instruction would be explicit and systematic, promote practice, and provide ongoing structuring and feedback prior to students practicing on their own (Graham, 2006; McMaster et al., 2017). See Box 6.2 for best practices.

BOX 6.2 **Evidence-Based Practice for Writing**

English Learners

- Although there is limited evidence on using writing strategies to improve writing, self-regulation strategies, including explicit instruction, self-review, and peer modeling, show promise.
- Literacy instruction in Spanish while children continue to learn English supports English learners' literacy development in English.

General

- Data are inconclusive on the beneficial effects of the teaching of phonics on spelling.
- Direct and systematic instruction in letter–sound correspondences.
- Monitoring and self-correcting spelling errors, which provide immediate corrective feedback.
- Teaching studying strategies for spelling words and for self-monitoring, including word sorting, word hunts, flashcards, and peer practice with spelling words.
- Application of newly learned spelling skills in sentence writing and in written compositions.
- Multisensory activities, such as tracing three-dimensional letters with their fingers while saying the letters aloud to spell a given word.
- Self-regulated strategy instruction, or teaching students a strategy for approaching a writing task, works well with adolescents.
- Using writing process strategies (e.g., planning, writing, and revising); awareness of text structures (e.g., expository vs. narrative text); and guided feedback about the overall quality of writing, missing elements, and strengths.
- Questioning strategies involving self-instruction (executive function), paragraph restatements, and strategies that focus on the text structure work well in combination.

Sources: Based on Berninger et al. (2000); Brea-Spahn and Dunn Davison (2012); Brooks et al. (2008); Gersten and Baker (2001); Jacobson and Reid (2007); McLaughlin et al. (2013); McMaster et al. (2017); Suggate (2014); Thomason et al. (2007); Williams et al. (2017).

Emergent literacy/writing tasks should be considered in late preschool language assessment and intervention. PA, alphabet knowledge, and letter printing are all important factors in name writing, suggesting that in intervention, all three areas of literacy can be taught simultaneously (Pavelko et al., 2018). These skills are not singular entities to be treated in isolation but rather should all be taught in an integrated approach within developmentally appropriate activities.

A creative writing website called Druidawn (www.druidawn.org) has some practical guidelines for teaching writing. Under the "Parents and Teachers" tab, select "Learning Disabilities Articles." Then scroll down to "Writing with Dyslexia/ Dysgraphia." Other websites, such as ReadSource (www.readsource.com), offer blogs and other resources for sharing ideas. Several states and universities, such as the University of Michigan (www.dyslexiahelp.umich.edu/), also offer resources.

Spelling

Spelling intervention should be integrated into real writing and reading within the classroom. Words are the vehicles for teaching spelling principles. Ideally, intervention can occur when a child is actually writing and can be reminded of alphabetic and orthographic principles (Scott, 2000). Spelling can be taught within teaching of general executive function in which the child is taught to proofread, correct, and edit.

The way children spell is indicative of the way they read (Templeton, 2004). This would suggest that spelling intervention should also be integrated with reading to enable a child to learn and to use word knowledge.

Words selected for intervention should be individualized for each child and should reflect the curriculum, the child's desires, words attempted but in error, and error patterns (Bear et al., 2004). Spelling strategies can be discussed with a child, using the data from an SLP's analysis. The goal is to learn strategies of spelling and rules rather than specific words. For example, if a child's errors are primarily morphologic (see Figure 6.6), the SLP can target root words and the influence of various morphemes through morpheme-finding and word-building tasks. Intervention focusing on increasing awareness of the morphological structure of words, with particular attention to the orthographic rules that apply when suffixes are added, can significantly increase both spelling and reading accuracy and can generalize to new words (Kirk & Gillon, 2008). In contrast, if a child's errors are orthographic, the SLP can teach rules through key words, demonstrating alternative spellings, and acceptable and unacceptable sound–letter combinations.

> An SLP should not be teaching the class's spelling words for the week. An SLP should target spelling strategies, not individual words.

Children with LD benefit from multisensory input such as pictures, objects, or actions. Several multisensory techniques have been proposed in which the child may complete any of several steps, including listening to the SLP say and spell the word, saying the word aloud while looking at it or touching it, writing it while saying it, checking spelling, saying the letters in sequence, tracing the word while saying it, closing their eyes and visualizing the word, and rewriting the word and checking or comparing the spelling.

Word analysis and sorting tasks in which words are placed into groups can be used (Scott, 2000). Sorting tasks will differ based on the targeted error patterns found in the child's misspellings. Pairs of words that differ on the bases of these patterns, such as *pint-pit*, *meant-meat*, and *bunt-but*, can be used to demonstrate the consequences of misspelling. For example, word meaning could be used to help a child note the difference between *head* and *hid*. Other contrasting words might include *dead-did*, *read-rid*, and *lead-lid*. An SLP should begin with known, frequently used words and gradually introduce less frequently used and unknown words to facilitate generalization. Different spelling/meaning patterns might provide clues to the meaning and spelling of unfamiliar ones (Templeton, 2003). For example, a child might be helped to see the relationship between *evaluate* and *evaluation*. Some principles for word study and spelling intervention are included in Figure 6.7.

FIGURE 6.7 Principles for guiding spelling intervention.

Focus on what students are "using but confusing" in their spelling rather than beginning with focusing on what a child doesn't know.

Step back and consolidate learning before moving forward.

Use words students know and can read so that one literacy aspect influences another.

Compare words that do have the spelling feature, such as silent *e*, with words that don't, as in *dime-dim*, *tone-ton*, and *cube-cub*.

Help a child look at words in many ways through sorting tasks that include sound, sight, and meaning.

Begin with obvious contrasts first—ones that are easy to hear or clearly demonstrate a rule.

Don't hide exceptions; rather, deal with them because they will enhance generalization.

Avoid rules until a child has learned enough examples to see a rule clearly.

Work for sorting and spelling fluency.

Glean words from a child's writing and reading and then return to meaningful tasks and texts.

Source: Based on Bear et al. (2004).

Use of computers aids spelling somewhat. Although use of word processing can encourage editing in children, spell checkers, as you know, are not foolproof, and a child may learn little in the process. In general, spell checkers miss words in which the misspelling has inadvertently produced another word. Suggested spelling may also confuse the child with poor word attack skills. In addition, suggested spellings may be far afield if the original word is seriously misspelled. Spell checkers help less for children with LD than for children developing typically.

If children with literacy disorders are taught to spell phonetically when unsure of the correct spelling, spell checkers generate more correct suggestions, but a child must still select the correct one from the choices offered. Proofing and editing on a hard copy also seems to increase the number of correctly spelled words.

Word prediction programs reduce spelling errors of children with language disorders by over half, although the user must get the initial letters correct for the program to work effectively. It's important that a word prediction program's vocabulary matches the writing task. Several commercial programs incorporate word frequency or various topics.

REFLECTION QUESTION 6.5

Have you gained a new impression of how you spell and learned to spell? If so, what has changed?

Executive Function

Executive function can be targeted within the writing process by using a *goal-plan-do-review* format. An SLP can provide external support to enable children to experience some level of success (Ylvisaker & DeBonis, 2000).

When children are allowed to select their own topics, it increases motivation and shifts the focus to ideas. In the planning phase, an SLP and a child can brainstorm ideas for inclusion in the writing. Drawings and ideational maps, or "spider diagrams," can help. It is also helpful for a child to focus on the potential audience. The SLP can ask questions such as the following:

Why are you writing?

Who will read this paper?

What does the reader know?

What does the reader need to know?

The SLP and child may prefer to use computers as an assistive technology for writing (MacArthur, 2000). Software, such as Inspiration (Inspiration Software, 2017), can aid text generation, and a child or teacher can easily modify the result. Children with LD who receive training in executive function along with word processing make greater gains in the quality of their writing than children instructed only in executive function or word processing alone.

Grammar checkers miss many errors, especially if there are multiple misspellings. In addition, a child may be unable to figure out just what the error is. Speech recognition software allows a child to compose by dictation. The software cannot overcome oral language difficulties, although these can be moderated with the additional use of grammar checkers.

Narrative Text Generation

For some children, narrative writing intervention may need to begin at the oral narrative level as in the vignette at the start of the chapter (Naremore, 2001). They may need to learn to tell common event sequences, such as getting ready for school, and they may need help including all the elements of a narrative. Collectively called a story grammar, the elements, such as a "setting statement," are common in all Western literate narratives.

Children with language and writing disorders may not realize that they know a narrative or how to get it started. Story swapping with peers, spin-off stories from reading or real life, draw–tell–write methods, or topic selection from a prepared list can all be used to facilitate this process (Tattershall, 2004). Once a topic is selected, an SLP can encourage a child to write one statement, then another and another ("And then what happened?"). An SLP or a classroom teacher can guide a child by using narrative-enhancing questions and pictures that outline the story events.

During the writing process, an SLP or a classroom teacher can guide a child's writing through the use of brainstorming of ideas, story guides, prompts, and acronyms. Story guides are questions that help a student construct a narrative, and prompts are story beginning and ending phrases. Acronyms—such as SPACE for *setting, problem, action,* and *consequent events*—can also act as prompts for guiding writing (Harris & Graham, 1996). As mentioned, an SLP or a teacher can also encourage a child to write more with verbal prompts such as "Tell me more." The SLP or teacher can encourage feelings and motivations with pictures and questions such as "How do you think she felt?" (Roth, 2000).

Written narration may require explicit instruction in story grammar or structure. Story maps using pictures that highlight a narrative's main events or story frames may be initially necessary. Story frames are written starters for each main story element. The child completes the sentence and continues with that portion of the narrative. Cards or checklists can also be used to remind the child of story grammar elements.

For some children, reading and writing seem to be arbitrary, unfathomable processes.

Expository Text Generation

Procedures for intervention with expository writing may include collaborative planning and guidance by SLP/teacher and peer input; individual, independent writing; conferencing with the SLP/teacher and peers; individual, independent revising; and final editing (Van Meter et al., 2004; Wong, 2000). Collaborative planning is important. Children can think aloud and solicit opinions. Such brainstorming often provides a child with alternative views.

One promising method of teaching expository text writing is called Em-POWER, which treats writing as a problem-solving task involving six steps: Evaluate, Make a Plan, Organize, Work, Evaluate, and Rework (Englert et al., 1988). In addition, research has indicated that certain strategies, presented in Figure 6.8, are especially effective with children with LD.

Once a topic is selected and discussed in small groups, with a peer and/or with an SLP, the SLP can give the child a planning sheet to help organize their thoughts. After the child has completed the sheet, the SLP can help the child organize the information. This is a great time to challenge and help a child clarify views and prepare for independent writing.

Writing, even independent writing, can be fostered through the use of a prompt card containing key words for each major section of the paper. Figure 6.9 presents some sample prompts.

FIGURE 6.8 **Strategies for teaching expository writing.**

Include other students in a supportive environment.
Place training within a literacy-rich environment.
Provide extensive modeling.

Teach:
  Writing explicitly and systematically
  Various types of writing
  Planning and organizing strategies

Use:
  Verbal prompts to support self-regulation
  A variety of strategies to address different needs
  Graphics for display and as a means of storing test-relevant information such as words, grammar, and ideas

Move from oral to written forms by integrating the two.
Provide ample opportunity for communication and language to develop.
Collaborate with teachers in mentoring students to write.
Ensure the seamless integration of language intervention and classroom instruction and learning.

Source: Based on Singer and Bashir (2004).

FIGURE 6.9 **Sample prompts for opinion writing.**

Section of Paper	*Examples*
Introduction	*In my opinion . . .* *I believe . . .* *From my point of view, . . .* *I disagree with . . .* *Supporting words: first, second, finally, for example,* *most important is . . . , consider, think about, remember*
Counter opinion	*Although . . .* *However, . . .* *On the other hand, . . .* *To the contrary, . . .* *Even though . . .*
Conclusion	*In conclusion, . . .* *After considering both sides, . . .* *To summarize, . . .*

Sources: Based on Wong (2000); Wong et al. (1996).

After a child has completed the paper, they can conference with peers for feedback while the SLP mediates. The child then revises the paper, based on this feedback.

At each stage in the process, a child can record progress on a checklist that provides a model for the writing process. The checklist can also motivate a child as they note progress.

Summary

Although many aspects of literacy disorder clearly are the domain of the classroom teacher and reading specialist, some justifiably belong in the SLP's realm. Speech sound recognition and production are the domain of the SLP, so phonological awareness and its relationship to reading are areas in which the SLP can help emergent readers and spellers. Language intervention occurs in all forms of communication, including written text. Children with speech and language difficulties often have difficulty moving from spoken to written forms of expression.

Working with a team, including the teachers and reading specialist, an SLP helps a child obtain language-based skills on which literacy is based. This is a natural extension of the SLP's concern for language in all modes of communication.

Epilogue   Case Study: Liam

When Liam entered junior high school, he stopped seeing both the reading specialist and the SLP. Instead, his team, including both him and his parents in consultation with the reading team, decided that other measures would be attempted to compensate for his deficits. These methods included use of a word processor, recording of class lessons, and pre-preparation of lecture notes by his teachers. All through junior and senior high school, Liam met with different teachers after school for extra instruction.

When he graduated, Liam had few plans. He drifted from job to job for nearly a year before his sisters convinced him to apply to community college. Going part time, he was able to do well in his courses, and he has just been accepted into the physical therapy assistant program. Reading and writing are still difficult, but Liam is determined to do well, and his family members, especially his sisters, are extremely supportive.

As a young adult, Liam is personable and friendly, works part time, and is continuing to attend the local community college. His sisters, especially the next oldest, help him with his homework when possible.

Reflections from a School-Based Speech-Language Pathologist

Who would have guessed I'd be working with reading and writing? I mean, it's a logical extension of oral language but as an older SLP—I'm close to retirement—it wasn't an area in which I had much training. Luckily, a professor-friend let me sit in on her class and I also attended several continuing education activities.

At first everyone in the school—me included—wondered what I was going to do. There was a reading specialist and at first I think she felt threatened. But we explored my role together and she remained "the reading teacher." My job was in the "emerging reading" area, if you will. And like I said, it was a natural extension of what I was doing with speech sound awareness and narratives. Once I found my niche, working with reading and writing just became something I do. I like it.

You know, as this field expands into new areas, we sometimes need to justify what we do, what our role is. I still get teachers who say, "You teach reading?"

I say "No, I'm giving children with communication disorders what they need so they can learn to read." And write too. That's an accurate description.

Suggested Readings/Sources

Catts, H. W., & Kamhi, A. G. (2012). *Language and reading disabilities* (3rd ed.). Pearson.

Nelson, N. W. (2010). *Language and literacy disorders: Infancy through adolescence.* Pearson.

The Understood Team. (2017). *Understanding dyslexia.* www.understood.org/en/learning-attention-issues/child-learning-disabilities/dyslexia/understanding-dyslexia

7 Acquired Adult Language Disorders

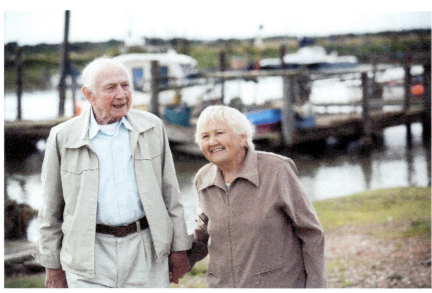

© Lord and Leverett/Pearson Education Ltd

Learning Objectives

When you have finished this chapter, you should be able to:

7.1 Outline language development beyond childhood.

7.2 Describe the main parts of the nervous system that are related to speech and language.

7.3 Discuss the different types of aphasia, concomitant or accompanying deficits, and assessment and intervention considerations.

7.4 Describe right-hemisphere damage and assessment and intervention considerations.

7.5 Describe traumatic brain injury and assessment and intervention considerations.

7.6 Describe cognitive impairment and assessment and intervention considerations.

> " The husband of my best friend had Parkinson disease for over 20 years. In the later stages of the disease, he experienced the accompanying cognitive impairment. I witnessed him go from brilliant professor to someone only able to express one-word thoughts. Sentences were impossible. I felt privileged that, according to my friend, I was one of only two men, the other being his son, whom he trusted enough to allow to help him.
>
> The disease affected not only my friend's husband but the entire family. My friend had to quit her job and provide care at home. If she went out, she was never more than a cell phone call away.
>
> At one point, my friend's husband said to me, "Don't ever tell students a disorder is interesting. From the point of view of someone like me, it's anything but. I live with the realities."
>
> So, I will not tell you that the disorders in this chapter are "interesting," but as we explore each disorder, we will try to keep in mind that we're talking about real people in difficult and challenging situations. Their entire lives have been changed, sometimes in an instant.
>
> —Robert Owens

CASE STUDY   Marsha

A single mom, Marsha has been the sole bread-winner in her family for several years. Two of her three children are grown, and her youngest is in high school. With no high school diploma, Marsha has had to work in sales or housekeeping jobs to make ends meet. Most recently, she has been a sales associate in the women's fashion section of a large department store.

Nearly a year ago, Marsha awoke one morning with a very strong headache. Although she felt somewhat unsteady on her feet, she determined that she should go to work anyway. Her right leg became weak as she walked to the bus stop, and she collapsed before she had reached her destination. Marsha had experienced an ischemic stroke caused by a blood clot.

Marsha awoke in the ambulance on the way to the hospital, confused and disoriented. Although she tried to talk with the hospital staff and with her family, she seemed unable to comprehend their speech and to form replies. She had aphasia and had lost access to language.

Marsha's medical team, consisting of her physician, a neurologist, a speech-language pathologist (SLP), a physical therapist, and an occupational therapist, went to work immediately. Her progress was rapid, although walking remained difficult. The team recommended that Marsha be released from the hospital after 1 week and that she receive services at a rehabilitation center on an outpatient basis. Both of her older children were eager to help.

As you read the chapter, think about:

- Possible interventions by the SLP while Marsha is still in the hospital
- Possible ways in which the team could coordinate services and work together
- Possible problems Marsha might still experience at work

Many future SLPs, maybe you, think they only want to work with children. That preference may change with time and experience. In this chapter, we discuss adults with language disorders.

Language disorders found in childhood often continue into the adult years. The characteristics of the disorder may evolve or alter with age. Deficits that persist may entitle these individuals to academic support services or workplace accommodations. These individuals are not our focus in this chapter.

Instead, this chapter focuses on language disorders that occur or develop during adulthood (see the Case Study). Thus, these language disorders are not developmental but acquired. In most cases, the individuals we'll meet have been functioning typically until something happened.

Specifically, in this chapter, we introduce the central nervous system related to language and explore four neurological disorders that affect adult language: aphasia, right-hemisphere brain damage, traumatic brain injury, and degenerative neurological conditions. In short, we describe language disorders related to blood supply to the brain, direct destruction of neural tissue, or a pathological process. For each disorder, we discuss characteristics, causes, lifespan issues, and assessment and intervention for language deficits.

Space precludes examining all possible neurological disorders. For example, we do not discuss disorders such as chronic schizophrenia, which typically affects pragmatic aspects of language, such as turn-taking, topic selection, and intentions (Meilijson et al., 2004). Nor do we discuss deafness (Chapter 12), which can also lead to communication challenges related to language use.

Although as an SLP you'll be concerned primarily with communication, the disorders described in this chapter also require an understanding of the medical conditions from which they originate. That means learning many new medical terms, some of which are included here. Check with your professor on what they consider to be essential for your course. As a practicing SLP, you'll be expected to know all this information and much more.

As you might suspect, the American Speech-Language-Hearing Association (ASHA) has plenty of good information on adult disorders. The ASHA website (www.asha.org) describes the role of SLPs in these disorders. Go to the website and search for "aphasia" or any of the disorders we discuss. The information the site returns will give additional information to what you'll find in this chapter.

Language Development Through the Lifespan

Learning Objective 7.1 Outline language development beyond childhood.

By adulthood, speech and language have matured, and adults are able to communicate in a variety of modes, using not only speech and language but paralinguistic and nonlinguistic signals effectively. A subtle pause or shift in word emphasis can signal important differences of meaning to a mature speaker. Reading and writing are also essential communication tools.

Unless debilitated in some way through accident, disease, or disorder, adults continue to refine their communication abilities throughout their lives. Writing and speaking abilities continue to improve with use, new words are added to vocabularies, and new styles of talking are acquired.

Language development proceeds slowly throughout adulthood. Even individuals with delayed development, such as those with intellectual developmental disorder or late-emerging language, experience continued but slowed language growth.

> Language and communication should continue to develop throughout one's life.

Use

Through the use of various communication techniques, competent adults can influence others, impart information, and make their needs known. Some adults are even capable of oratory on par with that of Martin Luther King Jr., which can call up the heroic and the selflessness in others.

Compared to children, adults are very effective communicators and skilled conversationalists who have a variety of styles of talking, from formal to casual, on a myriad of topics. Styles require modification not only in the manner of talking but also in the topics introduced and the vocabulary used. As *The Little Prince* noted when talking with adults (Saint-Exupéry, 1968):

> I would talk . . . about bridge, and golf, and politics, and neckties. And the grown-up would be greatly pleased to have met such a sensible man.

Competent adult communicators quickly sense their role in an interaction and adjust their language and speech accordingly. For example, some people are addressed as *sir* and some as *honey*, and you would do well not to confuse the two. Communication may vary from direct, as in "Turn up the heat," to indirect, as in "Do you feel a chill?". These two communications share the same goal, but their linguistic methodologies are very different.

The number of communicative intentions increases gradually, so that adults are able to hypothesize, to cajole, to inspire, to entice, to pun, and so on. A skilled speaker knows how to fulfill these intentions and when to use them.

Although adults who can read continue to refine both their writing and reading ability, these changes are not dramatic. In general, the writing of adults as compared to adolescents uses more complex, lengthy sentences (Nippold et al., 2005b).

Adult narratives improve steadily into middle age and the early senior years (Marini et al., 2005). Abilities decrease some after the late 70s. Those over age 75 have less flexibility and ease with word retrieval and make more language form errors.

> Adult language use is extremely flexible because of the variety of language forms, the large size of the vocabulary, and the breadth of language uses.

Content

Adults continue to add to their personal vocabularies, and most use between 30,000 and 60,000 words expressively. Receptive vocabularies are even larger. Specialized vocabularies develop for work, religion, hobbies, and social and interest groups. Some words fade from the language and are used less frequently, such as *dial* a phone number, while new words are added, such as *texting*. Multiple definitions and figurative meanings are also expanded.

Typical older adults experience some deficits in the accuracy and speed of word retrieval and naming. When compared to younger adults, older adults use more indefinite words, such as *thing* and *one*, in place of specific names. These deficits reflect accompanying deficits in working memory and, in turn, they affect ability to produce grammatically complex sentences (Kemper et al., 2001).

Form

Within language form, adults continue to acquire prefixes (*un-*, *pre-*, *dis-*), morphophonemic contrasts (*real*, *reality*), and infrequently used irregular verbs. Conversations become more cohesive through more effective use of linguistic devices, such as pronouns, articles, verb tenses, and aspect (which, for example, allows us to talk about the past from the vantage point of the future, as in "Tomorrow, I'll look back and say, 'That was a great picnic'"). In general, the form of written language is more complex than the form of spoken language.

The length and syntactic complexity of oral sentences increases into early adulthood and stabilizes in middle age (Nippold et al., 2005a). As mentioned previously, older seniors experience a decline in complex sentence production that seems related to word retrieval problems. There is also a decline in oral and written language comprehension, understanding of syntactically complex sentences, and inferencing.

> **REFLECTION QUESTION 7.1**
>
> *Where do you see the emphasis in adult language development? Does it differ from earlier child development? If so, how?*

The Nervous System

Learning Objective 7.2 Describe the main parts of the nervous system that are related to speech and language.

It's difficult to discuss language disorders with neurological causes, as we do in this chapter, without first understanding your nervous system as it relates to language. In this section, we briefly describe the major elements of this system, beginning with nerve cells (or neurons) and progressing through the central nervous systems as it relates to language processing. Brain involvement in movement is discussed in Chapter 10.

Your nervous system consists of your brain, spinal cord, and all associated nerves and sense organs. The **neuron** or nerve cell is the basic unit of your nervous system. Each neuron has three parts: the *cell body* where the work of the cell is accomplished, a single long *axon* that transmits impulses away from the cell body to the next neuron, and several branching *dendrites* that receive impulses from other cells and transmit them toward the cell body. A nerve is a collection of neurons. Neurons do not actually touch but are close enough so that electrochemical impulses can "jump" the tiny space, or **synapse**, between the axon of one neuron and the dendrites of the next.

Central Nervous System

Your brain and spinal cord comprise your **central nervous system (CNS)**. The CNS communicates with the rest of your body through the nerves. All incoming stimuli and outgoing signals are processed through the CNS.

The Brain

Your brain consists of the cerebrum (or upper brain), cerebellum, and brainstem. The cerebrum, depicted in Figure 7.1, is divided into right and left hemispheres. Each hemisphere consists of white fibrous connective tracts running below the surface and covered by a gray cortex of cell bodies approximately 0.25-inch thick. Each of your hemispheres is divided into four lobes: *frontal, parietal, occipital,* and *temporal*.

Hemi means "half," as in "hemisphere."

It is not entirely accurate to conceptualize your brain as having specific, localized areas with unique functions. There is a great deal of redundancy and diffuse organization of function, such that damage to a specific brain region may not completely eliminate the ability to perform that particular function. That said, there are generalized areas that are responsible for particular operations.

Although your cerebral hemispheres are roughly symmetrical, for specialized functions such as language and speech they are asymmetrical. In 98% of individuals, the left hemisphere is dominant for most aspects of receptive and expressive language processing. In general, all right-handers and 60% of left-handers are left-dominant for language, and the remainder of left-handers are right-dominant. A very small percentage of people have no apparent hemispheric dominance of language function.

The primary anatomical asymmetry in your brain is found in the left temporal lobe, where much language processing occurs. Studies using functional magnetic

FIGURE 7.1 Schematic diagram of the human brain.

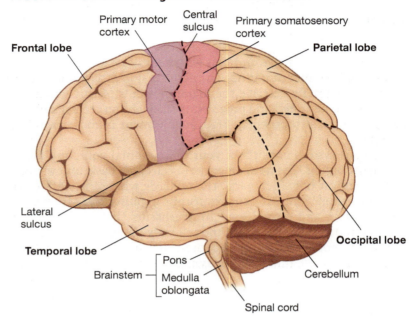

resonance imaging (fMRI) have shown a strong left-hemispheric language dominance of auditory comprehension abilities in children as young as 7 years of age (Balsamo et al., 2002). Other studies have found predominantly bilateral activation of auditory comprehension in younger children.

Language is a complex process performed by many different areas. Brain-imaging techniques have identified several regions of the brain that are active during speech sound processing. The number and location of activated regions differ across individuals and with the task, the type of input and output, the amount and kind of memory required, the relative difficulty, the attention level, and other simultaneous tasks.

Although there is little evidence of a unitary language processing area, some areas do seem to be more important than others, especially the frontal and temporal regions of the left hemisphere. These areas are more active than other regions in both perception and production.

In very succinct terms, the **frontal lobe** is important in decision making and motor control. It's the home of **executive function**, which tones and directs the brain, and **working memory**, where we hold information while we process it. The **parietal lobe** is primarily for storage and is important for memory and language processing. In the posterior region is the **occipital lobe**, important in visual processing. Finally, approximately where your ears are located is the **temporal lobe**, important in incoming and outgoing language processing.

At the base of the brain is your **cerebellum**. Although the cerebellum was historically thought to be for motor signals only, increasing evidence suggests its involvement in language as well. Neuroimaging studies indicate that the cerebellum also has considerable influence on higher-level cognitive and affective or emotional functions (Highnam & Bleile, 2011). In addition, the cerebellum contributes to executive function, working memory and attention, mentioned previously.

Information flows from the cortex to the cerebellum and back again in the form of feedback on the progress of the communication process. This said, the precise role of the cerebellum is somewhat unknown.

Language Processing

Let's discuss language processing very briefly so you will have some idea of how various disorders affect this endeavor. In most individuals, linguistic information is processed in the left hemisphere (see Figure 7.1). Nonlinguistic and paralinguistic information are primarily processed on the right. Studies of split-brain patients reveal that the right hemisphere also has a role in language processing, perhaps in storage of multiple meanings and language use. More subtle inferencing and body language may also be influenced by the right hemisphere. In addition, regions on the right are activated during speech production (Shuster, 2009; Shuster & Lemieux, 2005).

Your brain is a complex, interconnected organ, so these are gross overgeneralizations at best. Although several areas have been identified specific to language processing, it's very important to remember that brain functions are often broadly distributed. There are multiple interconnected aspects of language processing. In general, the key regions for language processing are the inferior frontal lobe, the temporal lobe, and occipito-temporal areas, presented in Figure 7.2. With neuro-imaging, researchers are able to map areas of the cerebral cortex important for language processing. Using fMRI, they measure changes in blood flow throughout the brain while people listen to or produce language.

Incoming auditory information is held in working memory in **Broca's area** in the frontal lobe while it is processed. Broca's area is relatively diffuse. Although it exists on both sides, higher cell density exists in the left hemisphere, indicating increased workings on this side of the brain.

FIGURE 7.2 **Schematic diagram of left-hemisphere language processing.**

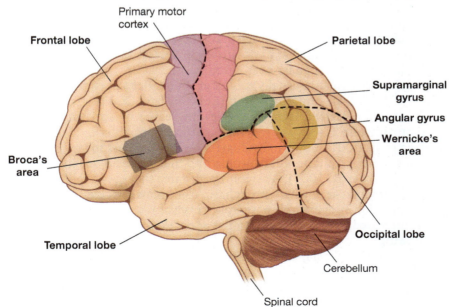

Most incoming linguistic processing occurs in **Wernicke's area** in the left temporal lobe, assisted by the angular gyrus for words and the supramarginal gyrus for grammar, although information is coming from storage areas throughout the brain. For outgoing information, the process occurs somewhat in reverse. Concepts are formed, and the **angular gyrus** and **supramarginal gyrus** contribute to the overall message formation that occurs in Wernicke's area while held in working memory in Broca's area. In addition, Broca's area sends programming information to the **motor cortex** (see Figure 7.2), which, in turn, sends signals to the motor neurons for speech.

Although the process is much more complex than we have space to discuss, you have enough understanding to comprehend why, for example, Wernicke's aphasia can be so devastating for an individual. Wernicke's area is an interface between the motor cortex for speech and temporal cortex and is important in sensory integration (Hickok et al., 2008; Wise et al., 2001).

REFLECTION QUESTION 7.2

Pick one of the areas of the brain important for language processing. What might happen if that area was damaged in some way?

With our basic understanding of language processing, let's begin. As mentioned, brain injury can occur in many places with varying results for the individual.

Aphasia

Learning Objective 7.3 Discuss the different types of aphasia, concomitant or accompanying deficits, and assessment and intervention considerations.

Aphasia means literally "without language," a feature that describes the most severe varieties of this disorder. The population with aphasia is extremely diverse. Although aphasia results from localized brain damage, the exact locations and the resultant severity and type of aphasia are not a perfect match. Individuals with mild aphasia may have language that is similar to that of typical elderly persons, but individuals with aphasia usually exhibit greater deficits in expressive language and overall efficiency of communication (Ross & Wertz, 2003).

Stroke—to be described later—is the leading cause of aphasia. Following a stroke, approximately 21–38% of individuals suffer from aphasia (Engelter et al., 2006; Laska et al., 2001). Some individuals will recover access to language, but for 40–60% of survivors, aphasia will continue into the chronic or extended stages of recovery (Pedderson et al., 2004). A recent report stated that over 2 million individuals in North America are living with aphasia (Simmons-Mackie, 2018). Because the U.S. population is aging and poststroke survival rates are increasing, we can expect an increased need for rehabilitation services, including speech, language, and swallowing.

For those with aphasia, such as Marsha, language has suddenly become a jumble of strange and seemingly unfamiliar words that may be difficult to comprehend and/or produce. Many of you are likely to have had some experience with aphasia through a relative, friend, neighbor, or possibly firsthand.

CASE STUDY   Marsha *(continued)*

Marsha's SLP began intervention as soon as her condition had stabilized some. Her SLP worked on recall of the names of family members and common objects and actions. Marsha improved rapidly, especially her comprehension, and was working on sentence production within a few days. Her speech was rapid but with frequent word substitutions and misarticulation of words. Intervention sessions were lively and contained much give-and-take between her and her SLP, who used Marsha's improved comprehension as the avenue for improving her production.

Many severities and varieties of aphasia exist and individuals differ greatly. Problems in two areas, auditory comprehension and word retrieval, seem to be common to varying degrees in all. Word retrieval difficulties suggest that memory may also be impaired in some way.

Aphasia may affect listening, speaking, reading, and/or writing as well as specific language functions, such as naming. In general, individuals with aphasia experience more difficulty with reading than with listening, especially for infrequently used words (DeDe, 2012). Related language functions such as doing arithmetic, gesturing, telling time, counting money, or interpreting environmental noises such as a dog's bark may also be difficult. The relationship between deficits in gesturing and in verbal

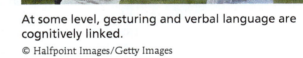

At some level, gesturing and verbal language are cognitively linked.
© Halfpoint Images/Getty Images

language suggest that at some level, though separate, the two are cognitively linked (Mol et al., 2013). Given the great variation seen in individuals with aphasia, it may be better to think of it as a general term that represents several syndromes.

Expressive deficits may include reduced vocabulary, either omission or addition of words, stereotypic utterances, either delayed and reduced output of speech or hyperfluent speech, and word substitutions. Each of these characteristics is a symptom of a deeper language-processing problem. **Hyperfluent speech**, very rapid speech with few pauses, may also be incoherent, inefficient, and pragmatically inappropriate.

Language comprehension deficits, whether spoken or written, involve the impaired interpretation of incoming linguistic information. Although individuals with aphasia may have typical hearing and vision, difficulty comes in the interpretation or the ability to make sense of the incoming signal. In general, those with aphasia and typical older adults demonstrate similar processing of complex sentences in reading, less so in speech (DeDe, 2013). In either case, more complex sentences are more difficult.

Even among those with very mild aphasia who may not evidence a disorder on standardized testing, reduction in processing speed can compromise sentence production in conversation and other contexts. These individuals have difficulty simultaneously maintaining multiple linguistic demands and other cognitive demands associated with planning and monitoring of utterances. The result may be longer

It is rare that brain injury is so precise as to affect only language. Other related areas of cognitive function and motor behaviors may also suffer damage.

pauses between and within utterances than seen in non-aphasic peers (Salis & DeDe, 2022). In general, lower language processing speed is related to more severe aphasia and to less cognitive control, which is the brain's allocation of resources and maintenance of communication intent (Faroqi-Shah & Gehman, 2021).

Severity may range from individuals with a few intelligible words and little comprehension to those with very high-level subtle linguistic deficits that are barely discernible in normal conversation. It's important to recognize that even very mild aphasia can result in language difficulties that can have an adverse effect on multiple areas of life (Cavanaugh & Haley, 2020). In addition to communication difficulties, a client may experience reduced social participation, difficulties returning to work, and a continual need to concentrate when engaging in language tasks. Clients report being keenly aware of their persisting impairments.

Although the severity of aphasia in chronic stroke survivors is typically thought to be stable by 6 months post-onset, changes are still evident years later. Approximately half improve, a quarter lose language ability, and a quarter remain stable. Factors that influence language recovery significantly during chronic aphasia include age at the time of the stroke and receipt of aphasia treatment. The age at the time of the stroke is associated with long-term outcomes and a greater number of aphasia treatment hours predict language improvement (Johnson et al., 2019).

Patterns of recovery differ across different aspects of language. In general, there are usually consistent improvements in word finding, grammatical construction, repetition, and reading (Wilson et al., 2019). Less consistent improvements are seen in word and sentence comprehension. Individuals vary greatly.

Severity is related to several variables, including the cause of the disorder, the location and extent of the brain injury, the age of the injury, and the age and general health of the individual. Differences in individual brains may account for different aphasic characteristics and for the lack of similar characteristics when similar areas of the brain are injured.

Although those with aphasia differ from one another, several patterns of behavior exist that enable us to categorize the disorder into numerous types, or *syndromes*. Although categories of the disorder describe certain similarities among individuals with aphasia, they do not adequately characterize any one individual. SLPs and other professionals, such as neurologists and psychiatrists, must thoroughly assess each individual and describe individual strengths and weaknesses.

Not all brain damage results in aphasia. Damage to the brain may result in loss of motor or sensory function, impaired memory, and poor judgment while leaving language intact. Aphasia is not the result of a motor speech disorder, cognitive impairment or dementia, or deterioration of intelligence.

Other neurogenic disorders—those that affect the CNS—such as apraxia or dysarthria, often exist along with aphasia, and these complicate classifications. Apraxia and dysarthria are discussed in Chapter 10. Individuals with aphasia may also experience seizures and depression. Depression is common in neurological disorders. Most individuals with aphasia also have a variety of attention and other cognitive deficits, indicating an association between attention, language, and other cognitive domains (Murray, 2012; Roche Chapman & Hallowell, 2021).

The complexity of our brains is reflected in the multiple areas of functioning affected by brain injury.

Concomitant or Accompanying Deficits

Physical and psychosocial problems may accompany aphasia and may be traced to the same cause. Physical impairments may include hemiparesis, hemiplegia, and hemisensory impairment. **Hemiparesis** is a weakness on one side of the body in which strength and control are greatly reduced. In contrast, **hemiplegia** is paralysis on one side. Finally, **hemisensory impairment** may accompany either and is a loss of the ability to perceive sensory information. The client may complain of cold, numbness, or tingling on the affected side and may be unable to sense or touch.

Visual processing deficits may affect communication. Individuals with deep lesions or injuries in the left hemisphere interior to the ear and across the top of the brain may experience blindness in the right visual field of each eye. This condition will affect the individual's ability to read.

When paresis, paralysis, and/or sensory impairment involve the neck and face, the client may have difficulty chewing or swallowing. There may be accompanying drooling or gagging. This condition, known as **dysphagia**, is also a concern of SLPs and is addressed in Chapter 11.

In addition, brain damage may result in seizure disorder, seen in approximately 20% of adults with aphasia. Seizures may be of the tonic-clonic type, which result in periods of unconsciousness, or the *petit mal* and psychomotor types, in which the client may lose motor control but remain conscious.

The discussion of aphasia is complicated and uses terminology that might be unfamiliar to you. As we discuss each characteristic related to aphasia, try to think of it as an advanced form of some behaviors that you already manifest. For example, occasionally we all have difficulty recalling a name or remembering a word. In its extreme form, we call this *anomia*. Some of the most common terms follow, with brief descriptions.

- *Agnosia:* A sensory deficit accompanying some aphasias that makes it difficult for the client to understand incoming sensory information. The disorder may be specific to auditory or visual information.

- *Agrammatism:* Omission of grammatical elements. Individuals with aphasia may omit short, unstressed words, such as articles or prepositions. They may also omit morphological endings, such as the plural *-s* or past-tense *-ed*.

- *Anomia:* Difficulty naming entities. Clients may struggle greatly. Individuals who have recovered from aphasia report that they knew what they wanted to say but could not locate the appropriate word. An incorrect response may continue to be produced even when the client recognizes that it is incorrect.

- *Jargon:* Meaningless or irrelevant speech with typical intonational patterns. Responses are often long and syntactically correct, although containing nonsense. Jargon may contain neologisms.

- *Neologism:* A novel word. Some individuals with aphasia may create novel words that do not exist in their language, using those words quite confidently.

- *Paraphasia:* Word substitutions in clients who may talk fluently and grammatically. Associations to the intended word may be based on meaning, such as saying *truck* for *car*; on similar sound, such as *tar* for *car*; or on some other relationship.

Pearson eTextbook
Video Example 7.1
In this video from the Australian Aphasia Association, Wendy, a nurse, talks about her aphasia and the frustrations of living with the disorder.
www.youtube.com/watch?v=Gq12cMUZPg4

This is an appropriate place to stress again that it is extremely difficult to identify the exact spot where language and speech reside in the brain. As best as we can, we try to identify the areas of the brain affected by the disorders being discussed. Some of these are presented in Figure 7.3. You'll want to refer back to this figure as we proceed. This might also be a good time for you to review the areas of the brain important in language processing before we go into different syndromes related to injury in those areas.

FIGURE 7.3 Brain schematic showing probable locations of selected aphasias.

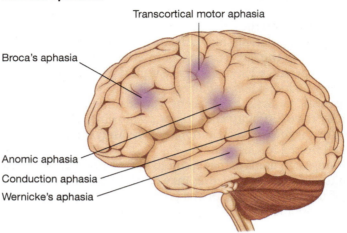

Transcortical motor aphasia

Broca's aphasia

Anomic aphasia

Conduction aphasia

Wernicke's aphasia

Types of Aphasia

Aphasias can be classified into two large categories based on the ease of producing speech: **fluent aphasia** and **nonfluent aphasia**. Not all aphasias can be so neatly classified. Other aphasias may affect primarily one communication modality, such as writing. Aphasia classification and its relationship to the location of lesions or injuries are controversial issues and areas of continued study. The most common types of aphasia and their characteristics are presented in Table 7.1.

Fluent Aphasias

The fluent aphasias are characterized by word substitutions, neologisms, and often verbose verbal output. Lesions in fluent aphasia tend to be found in the posterior portions of the left hemisphere of the brain. Let's briefly mention the most common fluent aphasias.

Before we do, it's important not to equate fluent aphasia with mild aphasia. Fluent refers to rate, not content or meaning. One way that speakers convey meaning in a conversation is by maintaining a topic. Nonspecific language and off-topic comments contribute most frequently to lower overall coherence of communication (Leaman & Edmonds, 2021b).

As a fluent aphasia, **Wernicke's aphasia** is characterized by rapid-fire strings of sentences with little pause for acknowledgment or turn taking. Individuals are often unaware of their difficulties. Content may seem to be a jumble and may be incoherent or incomprehensible, although fluent and well articulated. Notice the "stream of consciousness" quality in the following example of the speech of a client with Wernicke's aphasia:

I love to go for rides in the car. Cars are expensive these days. Everything's expensive. Even groceries. When I was a child you could spend five dollars and get a whole wagon full. I had a little red wagon. My brother and I would ride down the hill by our house. My brother served in World War II. He moved away after the war. There was so little housing available. My house is a split-level.

Adults with fluent aphasia have typical rate, intonation, pauses, and stress patterns.

Pearson eTextbook
Video Example 7.2

This video shows an example of Wernicke's fluent aphasia.

www.youtube.com/
watch?v=3oef68YabD0

TABLE 7.1

Characteristics of Fluent and Nonfluent Aphasias

Aphasia Type	Speech Production	Speech Comprehension	Speech Characteristics	Reading Comprehension	Naming	Speech Repetition
Wernicke's	Fluent or hyperfluent	Impaired to poor	Verbal paraphasia, jargon	Impaired	Impaired to poor	Impaired to poor
Anomic	Fluent	Mild to moderately impaired	Word retrieval and misnaming, good syntax, and articulation	Good	Severely impaired in both speech and writing	Good
Conduction	Fluent	Mildly impaired to good	Paraphasia and incorrect ordering with frequent self-correction attempts, good articulation, and syntax	Good	Usually impaired	Poor
Transcortical sensory	Fluent	Poor	Paraphasia, possible perseveration	Impaired to poor	Severely impaired	Unimpaired
Broca's	Nonfluent	Relatively good	Short sentences, agrammatism; slow, labored, with articulation and phonological errors	Unimpaired to poor	Poor	Poor
Transcortical	Nonfluent	Mildly impaired	Impaired, labored, difficulty initiating, syntactic errors	Unimpaired to poor	Impaired	Good
Global	Nonfluent	Poor, limited to single words or short phrases	Limited spontaneous ability of a few words or stereotypes	Poor	Poor	Poor, limited to single words or short phrases

As the name suggests, **anomic aphasia** is characterized by naming difficulties. Most aspects of speech are normal, with the exception of word retrieval. The following is an example of the speech of a client with anomic aphasia:

It was very good. We had a bird . . . a big thing with feathers and . . . a bird . . . a turkey stuffed . . . turkey with stuffing and that stuff . . . you know . . . and that stuff, that berry stuff . . . that stuff . . . berries, berries . . . cranberry stuffing . . . stuffing and cranberries . . . and gravy on things . . . smashed things . . . oh, darn, smashed potatoes.

Like the other fluent aphasias, **conduction aphasia** is characterized by conversation that is abundant and quick, although filled with paraphasia, which may be severe enough to make the speech of an individual with conduction aphasia incomprehensible. Our patient Marsha from the beginning of the chapter had conduction aphasia. The following is an example of the speech of a client with conduction aphasia:

We went to me girl, my girl . . . oh, a little girl's palace . . . no, daughter's palace, not a castle, but a pal . . . place . . . home for a sivit . . . and he . . . visit and she made a cook, cook a made . . . a cake.

The rarest of the fluent aphasias, **transcortical sensory aphasia**, is characterized by conversation and spontaneous speech as fluent as in Wernicke's aphasia but filled with word errors.

Nonfluent Aphasias

Nonfluent aphasia is characterized by slow, labored speech and struggle to retrieve words and form sentences. In general, the site of the lesion is in or near the frontal lobe.

Broca's aphasia is associated with damage to the anterior or forward parts of the frontal lobe of the left cerebral hemisphere, which is responsible for both motor planning and working memory. The most common traits are short sentences with agrammatism; slow, labored speech and writing; and articulation and phonological errors. The following is an example of the speech of a client with Broca's aphasia:

Foam, foam, phone, damn, phone . . . not ude . . . phone not ude . . . ude . . . ude . . . use . . . can't ude . . . no foam can ude.

A nonfluent counterpart of transcortical sensory aphasia, **transcortical motor aphasia**, is characterized by difficulty initiating speech or writing. Severely impaired speech is characteristic of damage to the motor cortex, although the areas that are affected may go well below the surface of the brain.

As the name implies, **global,** or **mixed, aphasia** is characterized by profound language disorder in all modalities. It is considered the most severely debilitating form of aphasia. Global aphasia has both the auditory comprehension problems found in some fluent aphasias and the labored speech of nonfluent aphasias. These symptoms are associated with a large, deep lesion in an area below the brain's surface.

Before we move on, we should mention **latent aphasia**, which is characterized by the presence of subtle impairments of linguistic abilities without clinical evidence of aphasia. In connected speech, those with latent aphasia produce fewer words and have longer silent pauses and a slower speech rate

---

Adults with nonfluent aphasia have slow rate, less intonation, inappropriately placed and abnormally long pauses, and less varied stress patterns than typical speakers.

Pearson eTextbook
Video Example 7.3

You can sense the frustrating difficulty in the speaker with Broca's aphasia in this video.

www.youtube.com/watch?v=JWC-cVQmEmY&t=142s

Pearson eTextbook
Video Example 7.4

Here is a video example of global aphasia from the Aphasia Center in St. Petersburg, Florida.

www.youtube.com/watch?v=1XIu0TUPaQI

FIGURE 7.4 Differential diagnosis of aphasia.

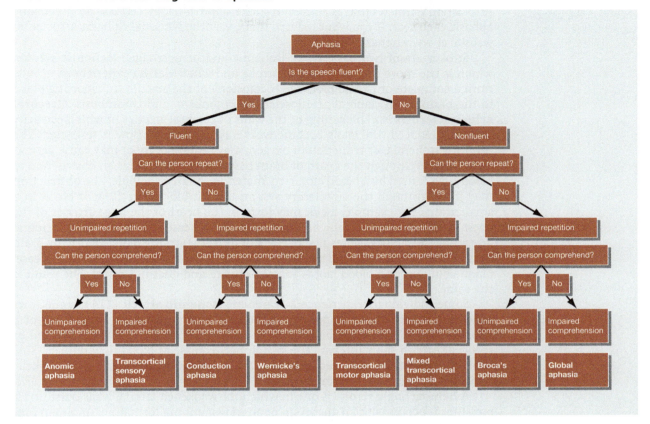

compared with neurotypical peers (DeDe & Salis, 2020). These differences indicate an impaired ability to process information from multiple cognitive domains simultaneously.

You may be thinking that these types of aphasia are all beginning to seem similar. When an SLP assesses a person with aphasia, differential diagnosis is helpful. A differential diagnosis is a step-by-step procedure, answering specific questions as you go. Figure 7.4 presents a possible differential diagnosis and the outcomes. It's another way for you to think about the types of aphasia in Table 7.1. Keep in mind that these are generalizations and no substitute for a thorough description of each individual.

Causes of Aphasia

The onset of aphasia is rapid. Usually, it occurs in people who have no former history of speech and language difficulties. The lesion or injury leaves an area of the brain unable to function as it had functioned just moments before.

The most common cause of aphasia is a **stroke**, or **cerebrovascular accident (CVA)**, one of the top five leading causes of death in the United States. Strokes affect half a million Americans annually. Seventy percent of these are over 65 years of age (Internet Stroke Center, 2005). Although strokes are rare in children, infants suffer strokes at a rate similar to older adults (Lee et al., 2005). For example,

Stroke is caused by a change in the blood supply to the brain.

the grandson of one of the authors experienced a stroke. The National Aphasia Association estimates that as a result of stroke, approximately 180,000 people acquire aphasia each year. If you want to learn more, visit the National Aphasia Association website at www.aphasia.org.

Strokes are of two basic types: ischemic and hemorrhagic. **Ischemic stroke**, which is the more common type of stroke and what Marsha experienced, results from a complete or partial blockage (occlusion) of the arteries transporting blood to the brain, as in cerebral arteriosclerosis, embolism, and thrombosis. **Cerebral arteriosclerosis** is a thickening of the walls of cerebral arteries in which elasticity is lost or reduced, the walls become weakened, and blood flow is restricted. The resulting ischemia, or reduction of oxygen, may be temporary or may cause permanent damage through the death of brain tissue. An **embolism** is an obstruction to blood flow caused by a blood clot, fatty materials, or an air bubble. The obstruction may travel through the circulatory system until it blocks the flow of blood in a small artery. For example, a clot may form in the heart or the large arteries of the chest, break off, and become an embolus as in the case of Marsha. As in cerebral arteriosclerosis, blockage results in a lack of oxygen-carrying blood, depriving brain cells of needed oxygen. Similarly, a **thrombosis** also blocks blood flow. In this case, plaque buildup or a blood clot is formed on-site and does not travel. The result is the same.

Some individuals experience a **transient ischemic attack (TIA)**, sometimes called a mini-stroke, a temporary condition whose symptoms mirror those of a stroke. A TIA occurs when blood flow to some portion of the brain is blocked or reduced. After a short interval, the symptoms decrease as blood flow returns. TIAs should be taken seriously because they can be a warning sign of increased likelihood of a stroke occurring in the future.

A **hemorrhagic stroke** is one in which the weakened arterial walls burst under pressure, as occurs with an aneurysm or arteriovenous malformation. An **aneurysm** is a saclike bulging in a weakened artery wall. The thin wall may rupture, causing a cerebral hemorrhage. Most aneurysms occur in the meninges, the layered membranes surrounding the brain, and blood flowing into this space can damage the brain or, in serious cases, cause death.

Arteriovenous malformation is rare and consists of a poorly formed tangle of arteries and veins that may occur in a highly viscous organ such as the brain. Malformed arterial walls may be weak and give way under pressure.

Patterns of recovery differ with the type of stroke. Often, with ischemic stroke there is a noticeable improvement within the first weeks after the injury. Recovery slows after 3 months. In contrast, the results of hemorrhagic stroke are usually more severe after injury. The period of most rapid recovery is at the end of the first month and into the second, as swelling lessens and injured neurons regain functioning.

The results of a stroke are further complicated by the prestroke storage patterns for language.

Damage from stroke may occur in any part of your brain. Aphasia-like symptoms also may be noted with other neurological injuries or disorders, but because other cortical areas are also affected, these result in clinically different disorders. It's also important to keep in mind that aphasia does not affect intelligence.

The human brain is extremely complex. Categorizing the types of aphasias as we have may bring some understanding to the subject but may have little practical clinical value. Each client presents unique characteristics. It is all the more important, therefore, that SLPs describe each client's abilities and disabilities carefully and clearly

Lifespan Issues

Although children and adolescents can experience aphasia, especially accompanying brain tumors, most victims are adults in middle age and beyond who previously lived healthy, productive lives. The risk of stroke is increased in an individual who has a history of smoking, alcohol use, poor diet, lack of exercise, high blood pressure, high cholesterol, diabetes, obesity, and TIAs or previous strokes. Usually, the onset of symptoms is rapid when the cause is vascular, but it can take months or years to become evident with a tumor or degenerative disease. These patterns are presented in Figure 7.5.

In the most common situation, an individual, such as Marsha in the Case Study, suffers an ischemic stroke, depriving the brain of a needed supply of oxygenated blood. First indications may be loss of consciousness, headache, weak or immobile limbs, and/or slurred speech. This condition *may* be either temporary, in which case function returns quickly, or more permanent. Some individuals may experience a series of TIAs spaced over a period of years before they become alarmed. Some TIAs go undetected by the individual.

Usually, at the onset of aphasia, regardless of the cause, the person is rushed to the hospital. Approximately a third of individuals die from the stroke or shortly thereafter. For those who survive, there may be a period of unconsciousness, followed by disorientation. Deep, long-lasting periods of unconsciousness or coma are associated with poorer eventual recovery.

For an individual who has experienced a stroke, language is probably not their immediate or central concern. Initial reaction may be fear or anxiety. The patient and the family are focused on survival and may be fearful of another stroke. For most individuals this is a novel situation, and they are unaware of how possible limitations will affect their future. As chronic effects settle in, an individual begins to focus on the physical and language complications. This can lead to frustration and depression; indeed, the mother of one of the authors refused to participate in physical therapy in this stage and thus was recommended for a nursing home.

FIGURE 7.5 Severity of symptoms by neurological condition. Individuals differ in severity and path of the disorder.

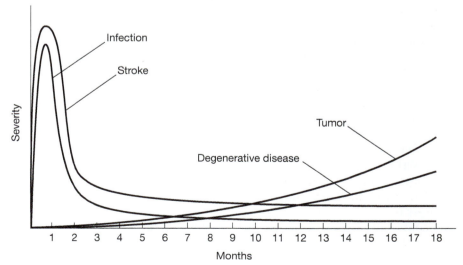

A newly aphasic patient may not be ready to receive factual information about their condition or structured intervention.

Likewise, families of individuals with aphasia are often frightened and confused. Because no one prepares in advance for stroke, families are usually ill informed. In other words, the patient and family are in crisis.

Most individuals remain in acute care for only a few days until their condition stabilizes. Following this, an individual may receive a variety of types of care, depending on the severity of the stroke. These include rehabilitative hospitalization; outpatient rehabilitation, which was recommended for Marsha; or nursing home care. Most return home but with some impairment and need for support.

CASE STUDY   **Marsha** *(continued)*

After her week in the hospital was up, Marsha was released and received outpatient services three times a week. She had improved quickly but had some continuing right-side muscle weakness. Her new rehabilitation center SLP trained her sister and two children in instructive tasks to use at home to help her retrieve her language further. Much of what family members used was instructive feedback after a language error. As Marsha continued to improve, her intervention sessions became less frequent.

Aphasia often occurs with other neurologically related disorders mentioned earlier, such as dysphagia and dysarthria (described in Chapters 10 and 11). The high incidence and co-occurrence of these disorders mean that SLPs need to be involved in every phase of stroke rehabilitation (Stipancic et al., 2019).

Although intervention services can continue for years, most individuals receive services for at least the first several months. In addition to neuromuscular deficits and seizures, an individual with aphasia may exhibit behavior changes, including perseveration, disinhibition, and emotional problems, depending on the site of the lesion. *Perseveration* is the repetition of inappropriate responses in which the client may become fixed on a single task or behavior and repeat it. *Disinhibition* is a seeming inability to inhibit certain asocial or inappropriate behaviors, such as touching others. Finally, brain damage may contribute to exaggerated swings in emotion.

Emotional behavior must be considered in light of the extreme frustration experienced by some individuals with aphasia. Depression is also common. As an SLP, you'll need to understand the compounding effects of both on intervention services and provide counseling in dealing with the effects of both on communication. Laures-Gore and colleagues (2020) have provided an excellent tutorial on poststroke depression that you are encouraged to explore.

Immediately after an incident, neurological functioning is most severely affected. Within days, the body's natural recovery process begins. As brain swelling is reduced, injured cells may recover and begin to function normally. Adjacent areas of the brain that share brain functions with the injured area may begin to play a larger role.

The course and extent of the recovery process are difficult to predict, but the rate is fastest during the first few weeks and months after the stroke, and then it slows, usually ceasing after 6 months. During this process, the entire syndrome

Speech and language services are part of a team approach to intervention for individuals who have experienced a stroke.

that the client presents may change and most certainly will lessen in severity. As with Marsha, the most frequent linguistic gains are in auditory comprehension. In general, less severely affected individuals and those who are younger, in general good health, and left-handed recover from aphasia better and faster than those who are more severely affected, older, in poor health, and right-handed.

Some individuals may be prone to repeated strokes. These may not affect overall language unless substantial volumes of additional brain tissue are affected (Goldberg et al., 2021).

Most individuals experience some type of **spontaneous recovery**, a natural restorative process. In general, individuals who experience ischemic stroke begin spontaneous recovery earlier but improve less rapidly than those who experience intracerebral hemorrhage. This recovery curve was seen in Marsha's case. Although the anatomical and physiological basis for the spontaneous recovery of language is not well understood, maximum improvement is seen in the first 3 months. This immediate physiological restitution may be complemented by reorganization of brain function in the later stages of recovery. Neuroimaging studies show use of left-hemisphere structures that were previously involved in language function and use of similar regions in the right hemisphere with a corresponding shift in some language functioning to the right (Pataraia et al., 2004; Thompson, 2004).

With or without spontaneous recovery, assessment and intervention begin as soon as an individual's condition permits. Clients who are most responsive, such as Marsha, are probably the best candidates for intervention services. A general rule is that the earlier the treatment, the better the rate of recovery, but clients do not all recover similarly. An SLP's first goal is to determine the feasibility of clinical intervention. Although it is not possible to predict accurately how much gain will result from spontaneous recovery and how much will result from intervention, an SLP attempts to determine which clients will benefit most from clinical intervention.

Communication is so entwined in our social interactions and in our very definition of who we are that the effects of aphasia reach well beyond speech and language.

CASE STUDY   Marsha *(continued)*

After Marsha's release from the hospital, she was seen for several months as an outpatient. An SLP worked with Marsha and her family to strengthen her comprehension and production of language and to improve her speech. Her intervention services were comprehensive and involved both physical and occupational therapy as well. Marsha is taking a blood thinner as a precaution against further blood clots. For similar reasons, she has also lost some excess weight.

Loss of the ability to use language efficiently changes the social role of each individual with aphasia and can result in social isolation. This situation is complicated by the often-incorrect assumption that cognitive abilities are also damaged. In addition, inability to communicate may cause an affected individual to become dependent on others for the simplest of daily tasks.

Family roles and responsibilities may also change. Partners and children may have to take on new responsibilities. If an individual supported their family prior to the incident that caused aphasia, there may be economic problems in addition to medical ones. The National Aphasia Association website (www.aphasia.org) contains stories from those who are experiencing aphasia and from family members.

Pearson eTextbook
Video Example 7.5
In this video, Mary struggles to tell her own narrative.
www.constanttherapyhealth.com/oneword/

Pearson eTextbook
Video Example 7.6
As has been mentioned, aphasia can have an effect on the entire family. In this Aphasia Center video, a wife/caregiver discusses her husband's aphasia.
www.youtube.com/watch?v=ICVjTm6U7ol

REFLECTION QUESTION 7.3

How is recovery influenced by the type of stroke? Why do you think the patterns of recovery differ?

Assessment for Aphasia

Assessment and intervention may begin in the hospital and continue as an outpatient service. Successful intervention is a team effort. A person who has had a stroke will most likely receive services from a team of professionals. Team members may include a neurologist, a physical therapist, an occupational therapist, a nutritionist, a speech-language pathologist, and an audiologist. Life changes and family concerns may necessitate the services of a counseling social worker, psychologist, psychiatrist, and/or pastoral counselor. The relative importance of each specialist will change as the client recovers. In addition, a spouse, another family member, or a close friend may be a critical participant in the recuperative process.

Counseling with the family by team members will be ongoing. The family and client may need professional counseling to cope with the enormous changes that have occurred in their lives.

Before beginning any intervention, it is necessary to complete a thorough assessment of each client's abilities and deficits. This process may continue in several stages as the client stabilizes and experiences spontaneous recovery.

Especially important are the person's medical history, the interview with the client and family, examination of the oral peripheral mechanism, hearing testing, and direct speech and language testing. The medical history can reveal information about general health and previous cerebrovascular accidents. In addition, current neurological reports and medical progress notes provide valuable information on present and changing status.

In addition to collecting data during the interview, it will be necessary for an SLP to provide information. The client may be disoriented and need reassurance. Family members will have many questions regarding recovery, family dynamics, income, medical expenses, and the like. Often a social worker will address these issues also. It is important for families to know the extent of the injuries and to have a realistic appraisal of recovery with and without professional assistance.

Comprehensive testing of clients with aphasia should include at least the two input modalities of vision and audition and the three output modalities of speech, writing, and gestures.

As an SLP, you'll find that careful observation is essential, especially shortly after the incident when more formal testing is not possible. It is important to observe the individual's general speech and language behavior and to listen to and observe what is communicated and how. Observing spontaneous language use and a client's level of engagement can give an SLP important information on the nature and extent of the disorder (Riley & Owora, 2020).

A thorough examination of the oral peripheral mechanism is important because of the potential for either neuromuscular paralysis or weakness. Speech disorders such as apraxia and dysarthria are frequently associated with aphasia and should be described or ruled out. See Chapter 10 for a fuller discussion.

Possible hearing loss must also be ascertained, especially given the older age of most individuals with aphasia. It is important in an assessment to distinguish hearing loss from comprehension deficits.

As with Marsha, initial speech and language testing often occurs at the patient's bedside. This intervention can be confounded by spontaneous recovery that decreases the need for extensive formal testing at this stage. Therefore, an SLP administers informal probes of the patient's language strengths and weaknesses. More formal testing is usually postponed until the patient has maintained a stable level on simple language tasks for at least several days. Simple tasks are administered at least once daily in a short 15-minute time frame (Holland & Fridriksson, 2001). The SLP notes subtle changes in the patient's behavior. It's important not to tire the patient because fatigue can have a negative effect on communicative ability.

Later, more formal speech and language testing and sampling should assess overall communication skills as well as receptive and expressive language in all modalities (reading, writing, auditory comprehension, expressive language, and gestures and nonlinguistic communication) and across all five aspects of language (pragmatics, semantics, syntax, morphology, and phonology). Remember that as with all of us, language and gestural use will be defined and constrained by the communication environment (de Beer et al., 2019). With higher-functioning clients, an SLP will want to assess higher language skills such as verbal reasoning and analogies, figurative language, categorization, and explanations of complex tasks. Examples of written expressive deficits of adults with two types of aphasia are presented in Figure 7.6.

Table 7.2 is an overview of some areas that ASHA recommends being evaluated in a functional assessment of communication abilities. In addition to language, data suggest that working memory (WM) should be a portion of any aphasia diagnostic. With increased WM demands, such as increased number of items, categorical naming performance decreases (Obermeyer et al., 2022). In addition, WM may affect the ability of an individual to comprehend sentences in situations with background noise (Fitzhugh et al., 2021).

FIGURE 7.6 Examples of the expressive language deficits in the writing of adults with aphasia.

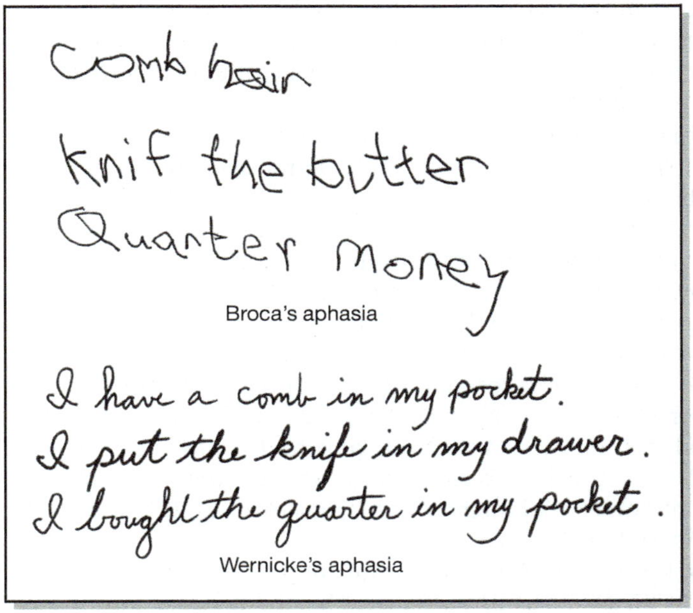

TABLE 7.2

Selected Examples from *Functional Assessment of Communicative Skills for Adults (FACS)*

Assessment Domain	Behaviors
Social communication	Use names of familiar people Request information Exchange information on the telephone Follow directions Understand facial expressions and tone of voice Participate in conversations
Communication of basic needs	Express feelings Request help Make needs and wants known Respond in an emergency
Reading, writing, and number concepts	Understand simple signs Follow written directions Understand printed material Print, write, and type name Complete forms Write messages
Daily planning	Tell time Use a phone Keep scheduled appointments

Source: Data from American Speech-Language-Hearing Association (2017).

One measure of functional language for individuals with aphasia is discourse analysis, or analysis of language used in different contexts. Data indicate that client language varies across three discourse types, expositional, narrative, and procedural, highlighting the importance of using several discourse tasks (Stark, 2019). Similarly, although single-word reading abilities underlie connected text reading accuracy, additional cognitive mechanisms are involved in text-level comprehension (Smith & Ryan, 2020). Thus, it's vital that SLPs assess both individual word-reading and connected text comprehension.

Several standardized tests are available for assessing specific language skills. Formal tests must be selected carefully. Most tests include picture or object naming, pointing to pictures named, automatic language, repeating sentences, describing pictures and answering questions, reading and answering questions and/or drawing conclusions, and writing. It is important for an SLP to remain flexible and to continue to probe a client's behavior for the duration of intervention, especially as behaviors change. In this way, assessment is an important part of intervention.

Because most individuals with aphasia have some residual communication disorder, the goal of intervention is to maximize communication effectiveness in the face of this disorder.

It's also important to consider not just the clients' performance but their subjective experience. One study found that clients had a strong awareness of their aphasia and its implications and were able to describe their language breakdown, identify relevant strategies to compensate and/or cope, and explain the impact on their emotions and social interactions (Fama et al., 2022). These factors can affect intervention and prognosis.

Interpretation of client behavior during testing is critical. For example, as an SLP, you'll want to determine whether the client failed to respond because they could not retrieve the answer or because they did not comprehend the verbal cue. Most test tasks involve decision making or problem solving, the endpoints of several cognitive and linguistic processes. Subcomponents of the process are not assessed individually, yet these points within the process may be more sensitive to individual strengths and weaknesses. This type of evaluation may require the SLP to break the task into components and evaluate the client at each step.

Intervention

The overall goal of intervention is to aid in the recovery of language and to provide strategies to compensate for persistent language deficits. Individual intervention goals are determined by the results of the assessment and by the desires of both the client and family. Goals will be individualized according to the type and severity of the aphasia and the individual needs of each client. Intervention that is effective for one person may be less so for another who differs in the type of aphasia and the severity (Edmonds & Babb, 2011).

There is very little data on the effects of treatment during the early phases of recovery. Although the focus of early aphasia management often consists of providing support, prevention, and education rather than structured language therapy, many individuals benefit from less directive, more counseling-oriented treatment (Holland & Fridriksson, 2001).

At the heart of person-centered rehabilitation is collaborative goal setting involving the SLP, the client, and the family. This model can be challenging when a client has limited communication abilities. Haley et al. (2019) offers a step-by-step model for forming a collaborative partnership with clients to develop an intervention plan. Clients with communication impairments report loss of autonomy in health care decision making. Collaborative intervention has the potential to strengthen motivation and improved real-life communication. All members of the intervention team coordinate their efforts to strengthen treatment.

Intervention approaches reflect an SLP's theoretical position on aphasia plus a strong dose of practical knowledge regarding the most effective techniques. Each clinician must decide whether to work on underlying skills, such as memory and auditory comprehension, or to begin with specific skill deficits, such as naming. Some guidelines for working with individuals with aphasia are presented in Figure 7.7.

In the discussion that follows we highlight a few areas of intervention. These include semantic feature analysis with word retrieval, cognitive skills, use of the environment, a conversational approach, consideration of augmentative and alternative communication, and concern for client and family well-being.

Semantic Feature Analysis

You may recall from the chapter on child language disorders that we discussed linking new words semantically. As adults, when we learn a word, we also connect it to related information, such as placing it in a category and connecting it to synonyms. Words are stored by association with other words. These then form interconnected webs of words that facilitate word memory and word retrieval. For example, word associations might include synonyms (e.g., *rich–wealthy*), antonyms (e.g., *short–tall*), function (e.g., *bike–ride*), themes (e.g., *kitchen–sink*), category membership (e.g., *horse–cow*), category name (e.g., *dog–pet*), rhyming, and alliteration. This semantic storage helps us remember the word.

FIGURE 7.7 Guidelines for intervention with individuals with aphasia.

Treat the client in an age-appropriate manner.

Keep your own language simple, clear, and unambiguous and control for length and complexity.

Adjust your language and the speed of production for the processing capabilities of the client.

Use everyday items and tasks and involve the family. Recall that Marsha's family was intertwined with that of the SLP.

Use repetition and familiar routines, situations, and responses to facilitate learning.

Structure tasks to improve performance and adjust the amount of structure just enough to support the client's efforts but not foster dependency.

Provide a context to support the client's language processing.

Gradually increase the demands made on the client based on the client's abilities. Teach the client to use strengths to compensate for weaknesses. Marsha's comprehension strength was used to enhance her production.

Use of semantic association or semantic feature analysis (SFA) increases naming accuracy in patients with anomic aphasia (Hashimoto, 2016). Intervention for anomia using production of sounds and sound sequences relative to word retrieval also shows promise (Kendall et al., 2015). In addition, SFA and phonological sequences generalize to word retrieval of similar but untrained words (Kendall et al., 2019).

Cognitive Skills

For some clients, it's beneficial to access the language in the left hemisphere by "bridging" from the right. This might be attempted by teaching the client to gesture or sign and simultaneously attempt to say the names of familiar objects. It is reasoned that gestures or signs, being visual-spatial in nature, are processed in the right hemisphere. Reportedly, the use of both gestures and pantomime has a positive effect on noun retrieval, although more data is needed on generalization and long-term effects (Ferguson et al., 2012). Other methods use the client's usually intact right-hemisphere ability to produce intonational patterns or rhythms. The signs or intonational patterns are gradually faded as the client begins spontaneously to produce the targeted words and phrases without their aid.

As in many other areas of language intervention, unanimity on cross-hemispheric treatment methods does not exist. Many SLPs prefer to remediate language deficits by more direct multimodality stimulation of the affected cognitive processes (Peach, 2001). The goal is reactivation of speech areas in the dominant hemisphere.

In cross-modality generalization, skills trained in one modality generalize to another. For example, some individuals with agrammatism benefit from comprehension training more than production training (Jacobs & Thompson, 2000). Comprehension training seems to generalize to comprehension and production. Similarly, generalization occurs across linguistically related structures and from more complex structures to less complex ones (Thompson et al., 2003). Another example of cross-modality intervention is reading aloud while tracing the letters with one's finger.

Intervention might also focus on cognitive abilities, such as memory and attention, in addition to more linguistic targets. Clinician-assisted intervention may also be supplemented by more minimally assisted training, such as computer-provided reading tasks, including visual matching and reading comprehension. Commercially available technology can be used as a compensatory tool to assist reading comprehension (Caute et al., 2019).

The adaptive capacity of the CNS, called *plasticity*, holds that neurons and other brain cells have the ability to alter their structure and function in response to a variety of pressures, including teaching. Plasticity may be the key to helping damaged brains either access or relearn lost behavior through intervention, although continued research is needed to translate this research to practice (Kleim & Jones, 2008).

Environmental Input

If a client's family is amenable, as was Marsha's, it is usually beneficial to involve them in the communication teaching program under the SLP's guidance. The familiar atmosphere of the home and the objects, actions, and people in it can provide a context that can facilitate a client's recovery and strengthen their relearned communicative behaviors.

CASE STUDY   Marsha *(continued)*

Marsha's sister and her children were and are valuable assets in her intervention. Her SLP taught them ways to respond to her language errors and to exercise her speech mechanism. They learned to be patient, to expect slow change, and ways to elicit her behavior. Several times each day, she engaged in family-based intervention.

Knowing what to expect poststroke is important for both clients and significant others. Despite the importance for significant others, especially within an environmental approach to intervention, these individuals may not know or understand prognostic-related information (Cheng et al., 2022). The lack of information can, in turn, affect the person with aphasia. Medical staff, including SLPs, need to consider significant others as providers of care and as those who may require help themselves.

Most SLPs in a recent survey created home programs for clients with aphasia (Donoso Brown et al., 2021). Common elements of home intervention were functional practice and spoken expression with instructional techniques such as skill building within daily routines and guided practice.

Communication partner responsiveness affects quantitative measures of spoken language and subjective reactions of clients. Although communication partners may not greatly affect a client's spoken language, they can affect the communication experience (Harmon et al., 2020). For example, ignoring a client can elicit strong emotional reactions, including increased psychological stress. This is one of many reasons why communication partner training is essential.

REFLECTION QUESTION 7.4

Why might it be better to work on language processes in a communication framework rather than separately or individually?

It is important for professionals to remember that the beneficial involvement of the family must not be at their emotional expense. Family members must not be made to feel guilty if the client shows little progress.

Medical personnel, including medical students, can also be trained to support the conversational attempts of individuals with aphasia (Baylor et al., 2019). These individuals need to acknowledge and respond to a client's interactive behaviors. Recall how Marsha's family was trained to provide conversational feedback. This feedback can affect motivation and performance, and it is an essential part of intervention.

Conversational Approaches

Inclusion of the environment can occur in two ways. First, the family can be taught to continue the intervention methods used in the clinical setting. Second, the way family members communicate within conversations in the home can also have a beneficial effect.

In both initial and follow-up intervention, conversational techniques can provide language therapy and therapeutic support, especially in the early stages of intervention (Holland & Fridriksson, 2001). Within a therapeutic conversation, the client carries as much of the "communication burden" as possible. Mindful of small improvements by the client, the SLP revises the demands made of the client. In short sessions using conversation, the SLP reassures, explains what's happening to the client, and points out positive changes. As an individual progresses, the SLP provides less support and provides a variety of communication contexts and experiences. Much of Marsha's intervention occurred within conversational give-and-take.

Increasingly, social approaches to intervention are being employed in aphasia intervention. These methods attempt to address the functional communication barriers of individuals. For example, clients might participate in conversation-based treatment with the SLP or another person or in small groups. Following conversation-based intervention, conversational skills can become more efficient with fewer difficulties and shorter repair times (Thompson Tetnowski et al., 2021). Conversational approaches may affect overall amount of communication more than correcting a client's linguistic errors (Hoover et al., 2021).

CASE STUDY Marsha *(continued)*

Marsha also attended a small-group session weekly. These sessions served a social as well as an intervention purpose and gave her a chance to use her speech and language skills in actual conversations.

By empowering agency and identity, an SLP helps a client move to greater independence. Conversation-level aphasia intervention often focuses on supportive techniques that favor progressivity of the conversation over self-repair. The SLP fixes the client's error in order to keep the conversation going. By gradually shifting the emphasis to self-repair, the SLP can maintain a supportive and engaged stance that allows clients time to repair word or sentence errors or miscomprehension.

As a result, individuals with mild to moderate aphasia reportedly contribute meaningful personal information and self-expression that directs the conversation (Leaman & Archer, 2022).

Augmentative and Alternative Communication

Sign, gesture, or some other form of augmentative and alternative communication (AAC) may become the primary communicative modality for clients who possess profoundly impaired language and/or speech disorders. Communication boards or electronic forms of communication, such as use of an iPad, may be appropriate for those who also have neuromuscular impairments. American Indian or Native American signs may also be useful because many require only one hand, important for those with hemiparalysis, and are easily guessable by others (see Chapter 13).

Although technology, such as tablet-based communication, is increasingly being used in rehabilitation, exposure and comfort with technology varies across older adults. SLPs must evaluate a client's technology ability and their ability to learn technology before considering prescribing tablet-based intervention (Sitren & Vallila-Rohter, 2019).

A collaborative rehabilitation team is essential for a continuum of care. Unfortunately, team members, such as nurses and social workers, often lack knowledge and experience in working with AAC (Gormley & Light, 2019). Collaboration may be hampered by limited funding, time, and training opportunities.

Augmentative/alternative communication may become the primary mode of communication or may be used as a facilitative tool to access verbal language.

Well-Being

Increasingly, best practices address the whole person. These approaches attempt to reduce both the disorder and the impact of aphasia on participation and quality of life. Although clinical practices vary, language and cognitive skills are addressed equally across all clinical settings; functional communication, participation, and quality of life domains are prioritized more in settings providing care to clients within the community. Unfortunately, psychological well-being is still rarely assessed or addressed in depth (Tierney-Hendricks et al., 2022).

In general, the mental health needs of people with aphasia are not being met (Santo Pietro et al., 2019) and, although SLPs are not trained mental health counselors, you will find yourself discussing psychological well-being with your clients. We are "clinician-counselors" who are concerned with thoughts and feelings as they influence a client's clinical process and with obtaining access to appropriate mental health services when needed.

Unfortunately, aphasia is frequently misunderstood among mental health care providers who may lack sufficient training in this area. Some clients with aphasia may not have access to mental health services or may resist because of the stigma often attached to need for such services (Strong & Randolph, 2021). These findings highlight the need for interdisciplinary collaboration between SLPs with their knowledge of aphasia and mental health professionals with their expertise in counseling.

It's important to recognize that people with aphasia have experienced a life-changing event that has altered their world for the foreseeable future. They may have lost their income and independence. Naturally, they will experience the grief that accompanies loss. They may be anxious and depressed. The SLP may be one of the few professionals who really communicates with them. Sandberg et al. (2021) offer an excellent tutorial with counseling strategies that you are encouraged to read.

Evidence-Based Practice

Although we can conclude from the myriad studies on intervention with individuals with aphasia that intervention promotes recovery, we cannot definitively say which intervention methods are best for the various forms of aphasia (Raymer et al., 2008). What we can say is that failure to participate in intervention has an adverse effect on recovery. Other evidence-based practice (EBP) findings are presented in Box 7.1.

Although EBP is desirable, an SLP may find it challenging to translate research findings into daily practice. A gap exists between the findings from research and the ability to implement these findings in rehabilitation settings (Cavanaugh et al., 2021). For example, hospital settings may not permit optimal service delivery

---

BOX 7.1   **Evidence-Based Practice for Individuals with Aphasia**

Overall Methods of Intervention

- Individuals with aphasia significantly benefit from the services of SLPs over those who receive no intervention. At least 80% make measurable progress affecting both the quantity and quality of language.
- Behavioral intervention promotes language recovery. In general, aphasia treatment is more effective than spontaneous recovery alone.
- The most effective forms of intervention for different forms of aphasia and different language behaviors have not been thoroughly evaluated. Most evaluative studies use test performance rather than investigate the effect of aphasia treatment for functional use of communication. More research is needed on how stroke recovery factors, such as lesion size and location, age, and type of language deficit, influence treatment, especially neural reorganization.
- Low-frequency repetitive transcranial magnetic stimulation (LF-rTMS) plus speech and language intervention is an effective and safe method for improving language performance (Yao et al., 2020).

Specific Techniques

- Although timing of intervention after an injury is critical, the optimal interval before beginning intense intervention is unknown. In general, we can say that treatment within the first 3 months is maximally beneficial but that later treatment can also improve language ability and use.
- Repetition is important for maintaining changes in brain function and physiology.
- Although more intense intervention (9 or more hours/week) yields better results, the optimal amount is unknown. In chronic aphasia, there is modest evidence for more intensive treatment. Of particular interest is *constraint-induced language therapy* (CILT; Pulvermuller et al., 2001). CILT involves (1) requiring the patient to use verbal language while limiting or constraining all other use channels and (2) massed practice or a high-intensity treatment schedule of 3 to 4 hours daily for 2 weeks. The effects are similar to those of other intensive treatments that do not employ the use of constraint (Cherny et al., 2008).
- Simultaneous auditory and written input can help clients comprehend several forms of written communication, including narratives and expository texts, such as newspapers (Knollman-Porter et al., 2019; Wallace et al., 2019). Clients with severe aphasia benefit more than those with milder forms of the disorder (Brown et al., 2019).
- Training complex language results in improvements in less complex, untrained language when the trained and untrained material are linguistically related. Training simple language has little effect on learning of more complex material.
- The results on the use of AAC (see Chapter 13) are inconclusive.
- Meta-analysis indicates that clients with aphasia have improved naming and word recall with semantic feature analysis, such as relating a word to others with similar or opposite meaning and placing words in categories (Quique et al., 2019).
- Computer-based cognitive rehabilitation interventions can have significant positive effects on the cognitive function of stroke patients in both the acute and chronic phases.

Generalization

- Research results on the generalization of treatment effects to untrained language behaviors are mixed.

- Generalization is most likely to occur to a language feature that is similar to one that is trained, such as generalization to untrained sentences that are syntactically related to trained sentences.

Sources: Based on Cha and Kim (2013); DeRuyter et al. (2008); Koul and Corwin (2010); Raymer et al. (2008); Wisenburn and Mahoney (2009).

because of scheduling and patient dismissal. As an SLP, you'll need to advocate for clients to ensure that EBP is being translated into effective intervention.

Less than 30% of recent aphasia treatment studies report race/ethnicity of participants (Nguy et al., 2022). If many studies are not demographically representative of stroke survivors living in the United States, it affects the ecological validity of aphasia research. Nonetheless, SLPs are moving forward. For example, an interactive Spanish-English online naming intervention is currently available that promises to be a useful tool with culturally and linguistically diverse clients (Sandberg et al., 2020; http://bilingualnamingtherapy.psu.edu).

Primary Progressive Aphasia

Before we move to those with right-hemisphere brain damage, we need to address on more topic. So far, we've focused on clinical improvement of the person with aphasia, but one form of aphasia, termed **primary progressive aphasia (PPA)**, is different. PPA is a neurodegenerative disorder characterized by a progressive decline of language ability and use with initial preservation of both other mental functions and activities of daily living (ADLs). The disorder takes at least 2 years to develop and over its course progresses from primarily a motor speech disorder to a near-total inability to speak. In later stages, the individual has memory and life skills loss (Insalaco, 2022). PPA is considered a subtype of frontotemporal dementia, the second most common type of cognitive impairment after Alzheimer disease.

The affected parts of speech can differentiate types of PPA. Of particular importance are the effects of PPA on content (nouns, verbs) words that carry the meaning of a sentence versus functional words that are often elaborative in nature (articles, adjectives, and adverbs) (Themistocleous et al., 2021).

The three subtypes of PPA are as follows:

- *Semantic PPA.* Impairments in object recognition and identification; understanding the content of information in spoken and written language, sometimes accompanied by agnosia; and loss of inhibition and empathy (Marshall et al., 2018). The semantic network is damaged, so items must be relearned from scratch (Suárez-González et al., 2021).

- *Nonfluent PPA.* Characterized by agrammatism with possible executive function disorder and oral and limb apraxia. Nonfluent PPA may be associated with Parkinson disease, amyotrophic lateral sclerosis, and other cortical degenerative diseases (Marshall et al., 2018).

- *Logopenic PPA.* Characterized by long word-finding pauses, phonological errors, and impaired comprehension of complex sentences. Logopenic PPA may be associated with impaired phonological memory, limb apraxia, object agnosia, and myoclonus or sudden, brief involuntary twitching of a muscle or muscle group.

Effective intervention for PPA includes conversational treatments, support groups for both the client and family, and AAC (Croot et al., 2009). Treatment attempts to use those cognitive skills that remain relatively intact (Henry et al., 2019).

As a client's vocabulary retracts in later stages, an SLP in collaboration with the client and family can select a core vocabulary for retention (Flurie et al., 2020). Consistent retrieval and semantic-based activities can help the client retain these words as others fade.

Conclusion

Aphasia is a complex disorder that varies in scope and extent across individuals. In addition, clients may have other impairments, such as paralysis, as a result of their injury. Only a careful description of individual abilities and deficits in each specific modality of communication will enable an SLP to plan and carry out effective intervention. The individual variation in symptoms and severity, the team approach to intervention, and the possibility of spontaneous recovery complicate our efforts to measure intervention effectiveness and offer opportunities for those interested in research.

The linguistic bases of aphasia can be seen in decision making. There is little difference between nonlinguistic decision making, such as matching patterns, of those with aphasia and those without. In contrast, the two groups differ greatly in linguistic decision making, especially in verbalizing a rationale for making a decision (Kim et al., 2020).

As an SLP, you'll be entering a field that is changing and adapting. For example, technological advances may change the face of intervention. Transcranial direct current stimulation (tDCS), a noninvasive, painless brain stimulation treatment, may offer some promise, although additional research is needed on the benefits of using tDCS in conjunction with more traditional intervention techniques (Keator et al., 2020). In one study, researchers concluded that electrophysiology may be useful in identifying types and severities of aphasia (Stalpaert et al., 2020).

Right-Hemisphere Damage

Learning Objective 7.4 Describe right-hemisphere damage and assessment and intervention considerations.

SLPs in health care settings are increasingly involved in the assessment and management of cognitive-communication disorders in individuals with **right-hemisphere damage (RHD)**. The term RHD refers to a group of deficits that result from injury to the right hemisphere of the brain, the nondominant hemisphere for nearly all language functions. RHD has been found to result in disorders as varied as visual-spatial neglect and other attention deficits; difficulties with memory and components of executive function, such as problem solving, reasoning, organization, planning, and self-awareness; and a wide range of communication disorders (ASHA, n.d; Blake, 2006; Lehman & Tompkins, 2000; Myers, 2001; Tompkins et al., 2013). Although it is estimated that 50 to 78% of individuals with RHD exhibit one or more communication disorders, many do not receive treatment for these difficulties (Blake et al., 2002; Côté et al., 2007; Ferré et al., 2009).

Less information exists on RHD than on damage to the left hemisphere, although approximately half the individuals who have suffered stroke have right-hemisphere involvement. The communication disorders that individuals with RHD experience do not seem to be strictly language based. Rather, a combination of cognitive deficits results in the communication problem. As a result, the efficiency, effectiveness, and accuracy of communication are affected.

Although there is greater activation in the left hemisphere during both reception and production, some right-hemisphere involvement also occurs (Fridriksson et al., 2009). The role of the right hemisphere in language processing has not been explored as much as that of the left. Linguistic information is processed on the left, and nonlinguistic and paralinguistic information are processed on the right. In general, the right plays a role in some aspects of pragmatics, including the perception and expression of emotion; understanding of jokes, irony, and figurative language; and production and comprehension of coherent discourse. The right hemisphere also plays a greater role in processing emotion in nonverbal contexts.

The right hemisphere is involved in semantic processing. Let's take a look at sentence processing for a moment. In the sentence "Ann bumped into Kathy, and she fell over," the person who fell is in doubt. We don't know who fell. If we measure brain activity using event-related potentials, a measure of the electrical activity generated by the brain, we find that the right hemisphere is much more involved in processing sentences such as this as the brain attempts to clarify the meaning (Streb et al., 2004).

There are many misperceptions about RHD. The website Right Hemisphere Brain Damage has a "Myths & Facts" page that you might want to read. You'll find it at www.righthemisphere.org/about.

Characteristics

Deficits in RHD are not as obvious as those that result from left-hemisphere brain damage. Deficits may be very subtle but can have a great effect on everyday life. Although these deficits may seem nonlinguistic in nature, they can have a great effect on communication. The most common characteristics of RHD include the following:

- Neglect of all information from the left side
- Unrealistic denial of illness or limb involvement
- Impaired judgment and self-monitoring
- Lack of motivation
- Inattention

Disturbances can be grouped into attentional, visual-spatial, and communicative. Attentional disturbances are characterized by a client's lack of response to information coming from the left side of the body. This phenomenon is exhibited in the drawings of individuals with mild RHD who may omit all or provide few left-side details. Figure 7.8 shows an example of left-side neglect in a drawing. More severely impaired individuals may even refuse to look to the left of themselves.

Visual-spatial deficits may include poor visual discrimination and poor scanning and tracking. The client may have difficulty recognizing familiar faces, remembering familiar routes, and reading maps. Some clients fail to recognize family members.

About half of the individuals with RHD have communication disorders.

FIGURE 7.8 Drawings of an individual with mild RHD that demonstrate left-side neglect.

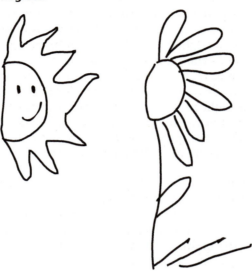

Data from ASHA's National Outcomes Measurement System (NOMS; 2008) reveal that individuals with RHD resulting from stroke are treated for difficulties in swallowing (52%), memory (41%), and problem solving (40%). Intervention for disorders of expression (22%), comprehension (23%), and pragmatics (5%) occurs far less frequently. These low percentages of treatment may be due, in part, to the difficulty in identifying right-hemisphere communication disorders, to the few available assessment tools available, and to lack of clarity regarding the types of communication intervention available (Lehman Blake et al., 2013). For more information, check the ASHA website at www.asha.org/practice-portal/clinical-topics/right-hemisphere-damage/.

The communication deficits associated with RHD affect the exchange of communicative intent through nonlinguistic and paralinguistic as well as linguistic means. Facial expression, body language, and *prosody* (intonation) are all nonverbal means of conveying intent. Intent can also be conveyed by words, sentences, and *discourse*, which is two or more sentences organized to convey information.

Individuals with RHD may exhibit poor auditory and visual comprehension of complex information and limited word discrimination and visual word recognition. When we interpret a word or sentence, we activate a web of meanings and categories, some closely related to the word and others more distant. The word *banana* might activate closely related terms such as *tropical fruit*, but less closely relates to ones such as *slippery*. The right hemisphere is important for activation of distant word and sentence meanings. It is believed that those with RHD have reduced activation that affects their conversation (Tompkins et al., 2008, 2013). The use and frequency of various question types may reflection the cognitive limitations of those with RHD (Minga et al., 2020).

Many words have multiple meanings. It's believed that all the multiple meanings of a word are activated when that word is heard or read but that the brain quickly inhibits meanings that do not fit the context (Blake, 2009; Blake & Lesniewicz,

2005; Tompkins et al., 2000, 2001, 2004). A listener's failure to suppress irrelevant or inappropriate information affects comprehension (Tompkins et al., 2000). When we hear about a *bride's train*, we suppress meanings related to railroads. An individual with RHD is slower in suppressing those meanings, making them less inefficient in interpreting conversations (Tompkins et al., 2000, 2013).

Of the various aspects of language, pragmatics, or the functional use of language in context, seems to be the most impaired (Myers, 2001). For example, topic maintenance, appreciation of the communication situation, and determination of listener needs are affected. In general, the expressive language of individuals with RHD is characterized as tangential to the topic and more egocentric. There are also extremes of either verbosity or paucity of speech (Lehman Blake, 2006). Contextual cues such as familiarity with the communication partner, social status of speaker and partner, or use of a specific speaking style may be missed or ignored (Blake, 2007; Ferré et al., 2011).

Sentence and discourse deficits can affect efficiency and effectiveness of both comprehension and production (Myers, 2001). Discourse is frequently described as disorganized, tangential, and overpersonalized (Blake, 2006; Myers, 2001). The narratives of individuals with aphasia and those with RHD differ and demonstrate differences related to areas of the brain that have been damaged (Schneider et al., 2021).

Comprehension deficits include misinterpretation of intended meaning, which is related to difficulties using contextual cues and generation of inferences or links between sentences. This can also include deficits in comprehension of nonliteral language, including metaphors, idioms such as *hit the roof*, humor, sarcasm, and indirect requests such as "Is it chilly in here?". It is unclear whether such a difficulty is due to an underlying deficit in nonliteral language processing or a deficit in the use of nonlinguistic and contextual cues.

Individuals with RHD exhibit poor judgment in determining which incoming information is important and which is not. A similar pattern of difficulty with selectivity is noted in expressive use of language. Clients may include unnecessary, irrelevant, repetitious, and unrelated information, seemingly unable to organize their language in meaningful ways or to present it efficiently. Other problem areas include naming, repetition, and writing, especially letter substitutions and omissions.

Paralinguistic deficits include difficulty comprehending and producing emotional language. The speech of individuals with RHD may lack normal rhythm or prosody and the emphasis used to express joy or sadness, anger or delight. Called *aprosodia*, it is the reduced ability or inability to produce or comprehend affective aspects of language (Baum & Dwivedi, 2003; Pell, 2006). Speech production may sound "flat," or monotone.

People with a right-hemisphere stroke are vulnerable to interpersonal relationship change. Sources of difficulty include altered communication style, impairments in social cognition, and reduced insight and/or motivation (Hewetson et al., 2021). Spouses often facilitate social engagement.

Pearson eTextbook
Video Example 7.7
You'll find an interview with a client with RHD and an explanation of associated behaviors in this video.

www.youtube.com/
watch?v=YgfSgn0Brmc&
list=PLX_PzwBeQwbKDX5T0
XeKnW-RqfBqHcREP

REFLECTION QUESTION 7.5

Why are the symptoms of RHD different from those for aphasia?

Assessment

As with aphasia, the assessment of individuals with RHD is a team effort involving many of the same professionals and diagnostic tasks described with aphasia. An SLP is interested in visual scanning and tracking, auditory and visual comprehension of words and sentences, direction following, response to emotion, naming and describing pictures, and writing. For example, an SLP may ask a client to re-create patterns with blocks or to find two objects or pictures that are the same; to recall words or sentences heard, seen in print, or both; and to describe a picture accurately enough for the SLP to re-create it.

Because of the diffuse effects on behavior seen in RHD, we know less about the treatment of these patients.

Limited guidance exists for assessment and intervention of cognitive-communication disorders associated with right-hemisphere stroke. Although SLPs routinely assess cognitive disorders using standardized tests, communication disorders are less likely to be formally assessed. Nonstandard procedures include interviewing, observation, and ratings of the client's behavior, along with testing of communication. Sampling and observational data are essential in assessing pragmatic abilities in conversational contexts. Free or low-cost resources for evaluating pragmatics, prosody, and awareness are readily available (Ramsey & Lehman Blake, 2020).

Intervention

Intervention often begins with visual and auditory recognition. These skills are essential before progressing to more complex tasks such as naming, describing, reading, and writing. Self-monitoring and paralinguistics are introduced, and the complexity of the content is gradually increased. Despite increasing knowledge about the deficits of individuals with RHD, knowledge about how to treat them is limited (Lehman Blake, 2007). What we do know is presented in Box 7.2.

BOX 7.2   **Evidence-Based Practice for Individuals with Right-Hemisphere Brain Damage**

General

- Cognitive rehabilitation intervention has positive effects on attention, functional communication, memory, and problem solving.
- Approximately 70 to 80% of clients who receive SLP intervention services make significant measurable improvements in communication.
- Communication intervention services as part of a broader interdisciplinary approach including physical, emotional, vocational, and communication, plus family education and support, resulted in greater independence in daily living and return to modified work programs.
- Despite promise, treatment studies have been few and have included a relatively small number of participants.

Specific Interventions at the Sentence and Conversational Level

- In interventions for aprosodia or difficulty expressing emotion through intonation, both imitation and cognitive-linguistic treatment show promise.
- In interventions for receptive language, techniques that provide prestimulation of word meanings prior to interpretation show promise, although generalization data are still lacking.
- The use of narratives to improve organization of conversations has mixed results on very limited data.
- Pragmatic intervention, whether a social skills–based treatment using a combination of video-recorded feedback, modeling, coaching, and rehearsal strategies or an auditory stimulation approach to enhance attending and attentional control, has mixed results.

Sources: Based on Lehman Blake et al. (2013) and Lehman Blake and Tompkins (2008).

For individuals with expressive aprosodia, SLPs may use several methods. In imitative treatment, a client repeats a sentence in unison with the SLP in response to a question. Another approach, called cognitive-linguistic treatment, uses various cues to modify the client's prosody, or the rhythm, stress, and intonation of speech. These include use of an emotion label such as happy or angry, a description of the prosodic characteristics for conveying that emotion, and a facial picture depicting the emotion. When the client is successful, the cues are systematically removed.

In order to interpret nonliteral or figurative language, such as "Home is where the heart is," an individual must be able to combine the literal meaning of the words *home* and *heart* with the metaphorical sense of these words. For example, *heart* is used to signify a warm, comforting feeling, as is *home*. In a semantic intervention approach, word meanings and connotations are mapped using spider diagrams and the two words connected in this way (Lundgren et al., 2011).

Intervention for activating meanings and for suppression of noncontextual ones can be accomplished through a technique called *contextual prestimulation*. In this method, still in its infancy, a client is given sentences to activate different meanings prior to being given a word. For example, the client might hear "He slipped and fell on the floor" before being asked to connect *banana* with *slippery* (Tompkins et al., 2011).

Clients are helped to respond appropriately to common communicative initiations and to track increasingly complex information in conversations. Beginning with questions from the SLP that require precise information, the client learns to make responses that come to the point. These questions become more open-ended as the client learns to make off-topic responses less frequently. Similarly, time restraints may limit conversational turns to keep the client from rambling.

Sequencing tasks and explanations of common multistep actions, such as making coffee, will be introduced to help the client organize linguistic content and make relevant contributions. Cues such as objects or pictures may be used initially to aid organization.

Finally, within conversations, an SLP will help a client synthesize these many skills. Visual and verbal cues may aid in turn taking. Important nonlinguistic markers such as eye contact, body language, and gestures may be targeted. Topic maintenance and relevant conversational contributions are stressed.

Traumatic Brain Injury

Learning Objective 7.5 Describe traumatic brain injury and assessment and intervention considerations.

A traumatic brain injury (TBI) is a disruption of normal functioning caused by a blow or jolt to the head or a penetrating head injury, such as a firearms incident or suicide. Please be aware that different sources list varying percentages for cause. According to the National Center for Injury Prevention and Control (2009), the leading causes of TBI are falls (28%); motor vehicle/traffic crashes (20%); blows to the head, often from sports (19%); and domestic violence and assaults (11%). Falls mostly affect the very young and the very old. The two age groups at highest risk for TBI are 0- to 4-year-olds and 15- to 19-year-olds.

The increase in use of motor vehicles, motorcycles, and off-road vehicles is directly related to the increase in TBI among teens and young adults. Another disturbing increase is the rise in attempted homicides and gun-related injuries, especially in urban areas. The authors have worked with adult clients with TBI resulting from automobile, motorcycle, and bicycle collisions; falls; violent crime; and failed suicide attempts involving firearms.

Annually, approximately 1.7 million people sustain TBI in the United States (National Library of Medicine, 2022). Most are treated in emergency rooms and released, but 64,000 die and 223,000 require longer hospitalization (Centers for Disease Control and Prevention, 2022). Motor vehicle accidents result in the greatest number of hospitalizations. The number of people with TBI who do not seek medical treatment or care is unknown. It's estimated that as a result of TBI, approximately 6 million Americans—around 2% of the U.S. population—currently have a long-term or lifelong need for help performing ADLs. Males are about twice as likely as females to sustain a TBI.

The statistics tell a chilling story but do not begin to explain the pain and suffering or the long struggle to recover. For further information, you can check the National Institute of Neurological Disorders and Stroke website.

You will recall from our discussion of language disorders in children that, unlike stroke, which usually injures a specific area of the brain, TBI can include diffuse injury to the entire brain. Diffuse injury comes from the blow and counter blow resulting from the brain shifting within the skull due to acceleration forces. In general, closed head injuries that include swelling of the brain result in diffuse injury. In contrast, open head injury may accommodate swelling, resulting in less damage that is more focused. For this reason, neurosurgeons may elect to open the skull to allow for brain swelling. In either case, damage may result from:

- Bruising and laceration of the brain caused by forceful contact with the relatively rough inner surfaces of the skull
- Secondary **edema**, or swelling due to increased fluid, which can lead to increased pressure
- Infection
- Hypoxia (oxygen deprivation)
- Intracranial pressure from tissue swelling
- **Infarction**, or death of tissue deprived of blood supply
- **Hematoma**, or focal bleeding

Aphasia-like symptoms are rare, but linguistic disorders related to cognitive damage are not. In addition, an individual with TBI may have sensory, motor, behavioral, and affective disabilities. Neuromuscular disorders may include seizures, hemisensory impairment, and hemiparesis or hemiplegia. The symptoms and the life changes that result can be profound.

Characteristics

Adults with TBI are a heterogeneous group with a diverse collection of physical, cognitive, communicative, and psychosocial deficits. Usually, the most devastating aspect is an inability to resume interests and daily living tasks to the level that existed before the injury. Some clients exhibit nearly total dependence on others. Cognitive difficulties may be evident in orientation, memory, attention, reasoning and problem solving, and executive function, which is the planning, execution, and self-monitoring of goal-directed behavior.

Language is affected in three of four individuals with TBI. The two most commonly reported symptoms for TBI are anomia and impaired comprehension.

As with children, the most disturbed language area and that with the most pervasive problems is pragmatics. Most published tests target language form and content and may miss pragmatic deficits that are evident in conversation. Pragmatic disorders result from the inability to inhibit behavior and from errors of judgment. The result may be rambling speech and incoherence, as manifested by off-topic and irrelevant comments and inability to maintain a topic, as well as by poor turn-taking skills, such as frequent interruption of others. In addition, communication may be marked by poor affective or emotional language abilities and inappropriate laughter and swearing.

Disorders of discourse associated with severe TBI can affect everyday outcomes relating to work, relationships, and independence (Elbourn et al., 2019). You may recall that discourse or longer connected speech is characterized as the type of communication, such as narration or conversation.

In addition, people with TBI often struggle with complex reading, which, in turn, limits participation in work and educational settings. Global reading ability, including both comprehension and speed, is negatively impacted by brain injury, even for those with mild TBI (Pei & O'Brien, 2021).

Communication deficits are not limited to language and may include speech, voice, and swallowing difficulties. Approximately a third of all individuals with TBI exhibit dysarthria, a disorder resulting from weakness or incoordination of the muscles that control speech production (see Chapter 10). Language deficits reflect underlying disruptions in information-processing, problem-solving, and reasoning abilities. In addition, psychosocial and personality changes may include disinhibition or impulsivity, poor organization and social judgment, and either withdrawal or aggressiveness. Physical signs may include difficulty walking, poor coordination, and vision problems. A more complete list of the possible outcomes of TBI is presented in Figure 7.9.

Personality changes may complicate the essential support of family that's needed to aid recovery. Read the story of David to help you understand the sometimes devastating effects of personality change on loved ones at www .brainline.org/blog/getting-back-bike/leaning-loss-after-brain-injury.

FIGURE 7.9 Possible outcomes of TBI.

Cognition

Inattention, disorientation, poor memory, poor problem-solving abilities

Language, Speech, and Oral Mechanism

Dysphagia, dysarthria, possible mutism, pragmatic difficulties (talks better than can communicate), confused language (irrelevance, confabulation or casual unfocused chatting, circumlocution, off-topic comments, lack of logical sequencing, and misnaming)

Emotion/Personality

Aggression/withdrawal, apathy and indifference, denial, depression, disinhibition and impulsivity, impatience, phobias, socially inappropriate behavior and comments, suspiciousness and anxiety

Severity seems to be related to initial levels of consciousness and posttraumatic amnesia. Consciousness levels can be classified along a continuum from extended states of unconsciousness or coma, in which the body responds only minimally to external stimuli, to consciousness with disorientation, stupor, and lethargy. Amnesia, or memory loss, is a frequent result of TBI.

The duration of both coma and amnesia has been used successfully, but not infallibly, to predict severity and prognosis. In general, the shorter both are, the less severe the resultant deficits of TBI and the better the potential outcome.

One overall measure of brain damage in TBI, such as brain volume loss, may be predictive of general cognitive functioning but not conversational narrative ability (Lê et al , 2014). Measures of atrophy in specific regions of the brain may be more informative about specific language functions.

Before we move on, we should mention concussions. Maybe you, like many people, have experienced a concussion. Although SLPs are rarely involved in cases of concussion, it's important for SLPs to understand the multiple-factor interactions involved. Attention to the factors that increase the risk of patients developing prolonged symptoms are vitally important. Although more study is needed, signs of possible long-term risk include an inability to concentrate for extended periods of time, cognitive fatigue, retrograde amnesia or difficulty recalling memories from before the concussion, and multiple concussions (Mayo Clinic, 2022).

Lifespan Issues

Most adults with TBI are young and have experienced a motor vehicle or motorcycle accident. Imagine that you, a college student, are riding in a friend's car. The next thing you remember is waking in the hospital, dazed, disoriented, and unaware of your surroundings. You may have language or other disorders that will change your life forever, or at least for the immediate future.

Several phases of recovery exist, and clinical intervention varies with each. Most individuals will not reach full recovery, and some residual deficits will most likely remain. Unfortunately, for some individuals with moderate-to-severe TBI, magnetic resonance imaging and performance testing indicate neurodegenerative and progressive symptoms long term (Pettemeridou & Constantinidou, 2021).

Initially, the individual may be nonresponsive to stimuli and may need total assistance in a hospital setting. When the individual does begin to respond, their behavior may not reflect the varying nature of the stimuli. In other words, the patient may persist with a response, although the situation has changed. Responses may be delayed. Vocalizations may seem purposeless.

Gradually, the individual begins to respond differently to different stimuli and to recognize familiar individuals. Response to commands is still often inconsistent.

As the individual becomes more alert, they may seem confused or agitated. Short-term memory and goal-directed behaviors may be poor. Although the client is able to sit and walk, these behaviors are performed without purpose. The client may be subject to mood swings and may have incoherent, inappropriate, or emotional language. Although the individual still needs rehabilitative hospital care, they have recovered enough to move from intensive care.

As agitation fades and language continues to return, the individual can remain alert for short periods of time and hold brief conversations if strong external cues, such as pictures or objects, are used. There are still periods of nonpurposeful behavior. Short-term memory is still severely impaired. With structure, the patient can perform learned tasks but is still unable to learn new behaviors.

As the individual continues to improve, they need less assistance. Able to attend for up to 30 minutes with redirection, the individual is aware of the appropriate responses to self, family, and basic needs, which become more goal directed. Relearned tasks exhibit some carryover to other situations, although new learning does not. Language is used appropriately only in highly familiar contexts.

Gradually, the individual becomes oriented to person and place. Time is still confusing, and the individual demonstrates only superficial understanding of their condition. Usually in outpatient status, the individual is able to learn and carry over this learning to other tasks and to monitor their own behavior with minimal assistance. Still unable to recognize inappropriate social behavior, the client is often uncooperative, unrealistic in their expectations, and unaware of the needs and feelings of others.

As the individual gains more of an understanding of their condition and is able to plan and initiate routine tasks, frustration may build, and they may become depressed, argumentative, irritable, or overly dependent or independent. Living at home and possibly having returned to work, the individual may be able to concentrate for an hour even with distractions, to recall past and present events, and to learn new tasks with only minimal assistance.

Increasing abilities may not reduce the individual's low tolerance for frustration, although behavioral responses may be less. In the later stages of recovery, the individual can shift between tasks for up to 2 hours and initiate and carry out familiar tasks. Able to acknowledge their impairment, the client is able to consider the consequences of their actions and to recognize the needs and feelings of others.

Finally, the individual may be able to consistently act in a socially appropriate manner, to respond appropriately to others, and to plan, initiate, and complete both familiar and unfamiliar tasks. Periodic depression may occur, and irritability may reappear with illness, inability to perform a task, and in emotional situations.

An individual with TBI may face a long period of rehabilitation. Even those who have made a nearly full recovery will have some lingering deficits, especially in pragmatics. The authors have worked with college students with TBI who were able to gain their degrees with only minimal adaptations.

Before we move to a discussion of assessment and intervention, you might want to check out the National Institute of Neurological Disorders and Stroke website (www.ninds.nih.gov) for a description of TBI and links to several other useful sites. Enter "Traumatic brain injury" in the search box. Another informative website is the National Center for Injury Prevention and Control (www.cdc.gov/traumaticbraininjury/).

Assessment

An SLP is a member of an interdisciplinary team of rehabilitation specialists who collaborate in assessment of and intervention with persons with TBI. As such, the SLP is responsible for assessing all aspects of communication, cognitive-communicative functioning, and swallowing.

Assessment of cognition should be multifaceted and consider both the typical profile of cognitive impairment and patient-specific factors influencing cognitive abilities, such as psychological well-being. Memory and executive function deficits are common cognitive difficulties associated with acute TBI (Johnson & Hall, 2022).

Unlike individuals with aphasia, those with TBI progress through recognizable stages of recovery outlined previously. Assessment must be ongoing and varies with each stage. Neurological, psychiatric, and psychological reports will aid in the planning of both assessment and intervention. Observation can aid the SLP in deciding which areas to probe, especially in determining pragmatic deficits that may be missed in formal testing.

To date, few standardized tools exist for a comprehensive assessment of language skills in individuals with TBI. Many SLPs working with this population have compiled a series of individual tests for aspects of both language and cognition. These tests are often portions of larger test batteries that focus on daily living skills. Language testing must be comprehensive. Tests that emphasize language form and content may fail to adequately assess pragmatics, thus underestimating the extent of the language disorder.

Sampling is essential because pragmatic behavior that varies across communicative contexts cannot be adequately assessed in a testing context alone. Sampling contexts should include functional activities, such as talking on the phone or grocery shopping, in natural environments, such as the home. Sampling should occur within a discourse unit, a series of related linguistic units that convey a message.

Written expression challenges following TBI can greatly affect quality of life and the reintegration success. Although some formal assessment tools are available, multiple assessment methods reveal writing challenges not always obvious through testing. An informal procedure might describe microstructural (e.g., productivity, sentence structure, spelling accuracy) and macrostructural (e.g., topic adherence, organization, story grammar) difficulties (Dinnes & Hux, 2022a). Examination of multiple aspects of writing is essential to a comprehensive evaluation.

Intervention

As we've stressed throughout this chapter and text, as an SLP working with clients with TBI, you'll be part of a team. Many TBI clients are eager to return to work (RTW). SLPs play a vital role in identifying, managing, and collaborating with an RTW team. This requires a working knowledge of vocational rehabilitation (VR) models that can inform practice when working with clients who have work return as a goal. An article by the ANCDS TBI Writing Committee (2022) is an excellent tutorial on RTW and VR models.

Unfortunately, a majority of first-line health care providers (physicians, physician assistants, nurse practitioners, nurses, and athletic trainers) lack knowledge in the role of the SLP in the management of mild TBI (Knollman et al., 2021). This is reflected in the low referral patterns of these professionals.

Traditionally, restorative strategies are attempted first and may include rehearsal and encoding strategies and the use of memory aids. Compensatory methods are typically used when restorative attempts have failed. Slowly, professionals are recognizing that compensatory strategies aid in restorative development, and both methods are being used simultaneously. A cautionary note: Use of compensatory strategies specific to writing is unlikely as long as the client's awareness remains limited (Dinnes & Hux, 2022b). Although some adults with TBI are aware of writing challenges, others may deny any changes in writing performance.

With or without intervention, the pattern of recovery for individuals with TBI is predictable. Unlike those with focal damage such as a stroke, who progress smoothly, those with TBI usually recover in a plateau fashion characterized by periods of little or no change interspersed with periods of rapid improvement. After a period of unconsciousness, the person often responds indiscriminately and

Pearson eTextbook
Video Example 7.8

There are many variables in intervention following TBI. This video demonstrates an overview of pragmatic intervention.

www.youtube.com/watch?v=UQJ3VFvT7SA

seemingly without purpose. Attention may be fleeting, and overall level of arousal may fluctuate. The client is often hyperresponsive to stimuli and easily irritated and agitated. Clients may become very emotional and exhibit shouting, emotional language, and, in some cases, repetitive, stereotypic movements such as rocking. With recovery, a client's behavior becomes more purposeful, although restlessness and irritability may persist.

As the client becomes more oriented in place and time, they are better able to respond to simple requests, although attention span is short and distractibility high. Memory and abstract reasoning may continue to be a problem even as the client becomes better able to manage daily living and to begin to function independently.

Intervention for cognitive-communicative deficits with individuals with TBI is called **cognitive rehabilitation**, a treatment regimen designed to increase functional abilities for everyday life by improving the capacity to process incoming information. The two primary approaches are restorative and compensatory. The restorative approach attempts to rebuild neural circuitry and function through repetitive activities, while the compensatory approach concedes that some functions will not be recovered and develops alternatives. Restorative techniques might include classification tasks and word associations. In contrast, compensatory strategies to improve memory might include focused attending and rehearsal of new information.

Traditionally, intervention has focused on episodic memory tasks. Episodic memory involves recollection of personal experiences including time- and place-specific storage. Retrieval depends on semantic memory or world knowledge that provides the context for encoding and information storage. Deficits in episodic memory are common in patients with TBI.

For some clients, a combined memory therapy including both episodic and semantic memory may result in significant improvements in both (Cochran D'Angelo et al., 2021). Semantic memory tasks might include identifying meaningful connections between diverse concepts represented by sets of two or three words.

An SLP is responsible for designing and implementing treatment programs to decrease the effects of the disorder. Evidence-based practices are presented in Box 7.3. In addition to providing direct intervention, an SLP helps to identify functional supports, such as memory logs, and work adjustments that aid in successful independent living.

> Cognitive rehabilitation promotes independent functioning in daily life by focusing on specific cognitive processes such as memory and language processing.

BOX 7.3   **Evidence-Based Practice for Individuals with Traumatic Brain Injury**

General

- The most effective interventions are those that are tailored to the individual client's unique needs and situation. Those receiving communication intervention make gains in cognitive communication, activities, and social participation.
- Embedding intensive intervention in real-life situations fosters learning and generalization.
- Those receiving communication services are discharged with higher levels of cognitive functioning and in greater percentages to home versus long-term care.
- More than 80% of clients with TBI make significant measurable gains in memory, attention, and pragmatics.

Sources: Based on Coelho et al. (2008); Gilmore et al. (2022).

Although not appropriate for all clients, collaborative client–clinician models of goal setting can increase client motivation and functional outcomes for those with mild TBI and high self-awareness (Brown et al., 2021). The SLP and client work collaboratively to identify strengths and challenges, select and prioritize goals, and discuss and develop meaningful, personalized intervention activities. For example, working collaboratively on social media goals and having a supportive network of rehabilitation professionals, family, and friends can enable people with TBI to develop social media mastery (Brunner et al., 2021). In contrast, professionals' concerns regarding potential risks associated with using social media can lead to restricted social media use.

Impairments to self-regulation and social communication can strain relationships for those with TBI. Video self-modeling provides evidence of what clients do well and what they could improve. When conducted in the context of authentic exchanges with their everyday partners, this training supports positive change in social communication (Hoepner et al., 2021). For example, a voice email task can be used to work on appropriate communication within the work environment (Meulenbroek & Cherney, 2019).

Intervention programs vary depending on the stage of recovery. During the early stages, intervention focuses on orientation, sensorimotor stimulation, and recognition of familiar people and common objects and events. Early intervention results in shorter rehabilitation and higher levels of cognitive functioning.

In the middle stages, training becomes more structured and formal. The goals are to reduce confusion and improve memory and goal-directed behavior. Much of the training involves increasing the client's orientation to the everyday world. Consistency and routines are important in orientation training. An SLP may target active listening and auditory comprehension and following directions with increasingly more complex information. Word definitions, descriptions of entities and events, and classification of objects and words are also targeted. Conversational speech training is also attempted. For example, one SLP, recognizing that the act of taking a conversational turn is too difficult for some clients, begins by using an object that is passed back and forth to signal turn changes. Over time, the object is replaced with subtle nonverbal signals, such as eye contact.

During the late stages of recovery, the goal is client independence. Targets include comprehension of complex information and directions and conversational and social skills. An SLP helps a client to explore alternative strategies for word recall, memory, and problem solving. Conversational problem-solving tasks are also targeted, along with self-inhibition and self-monitoring. Real-world contexts are emphasized, especially those that are potentially confusing or emotional.

Lastly, realizing the perspective of someone with a TBI can be difficult. WETA, a public broadcasting station has a website with nine things not to say to someone with a TBI (www.brainline.org/article/9-things-not-say-someone-brain-injury). The "nine things" are important and the remarks, especially by those with a TBI, are very enlightening.

Cognitive Impairment

Learning Objective 7.6 Describe cognitive impairment and assessment and intervention considerations.

We live in a youth-oriented culture. Commercial images lead to the stereotype of elderly people with deteriorated bodies and minds. Although physical decline with age is inevitable, intellectual capacity is frequently unimpaired. Fewer than

15% of older adults experience dementia or cognitive impairment, and as many as 20% of these respond positively to treatment (Shekim, 1990). The incidence of cognitive impairment is increasing as the percentage of the U.S. population over age 65 increases. It is estimated that as many as 48% of new admissions to long-term care facilities have a diagnosis of cognitive impairment (Magaziner et al., 2000).

Cognitive impairment is an umbrella term for a group of both pathological conditions and syndromes that result in the decline of memory and at least one other cognitive ability that is significant enough to interfere with daily life activities (American Psychiatric Association, 2013). It is acquired and is characterized by intellectual decline due to neurogenic causes. Language performance deficits are often seen

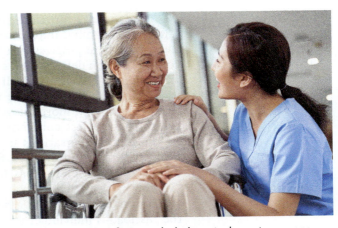

As many as 48% of new admissions to long-term care facilities have a diagnosis of cognitive impairment.
© Imtmphoto/Shutterstock

before other characteristics, which uniquely qualifies SLPs to be on the front lines in assessing mild cognitive impairment (McCullough et al., 2019).

> Cognitive impairment or dementia is an impairment of intellect and cognition.

Memory, as mentioned, is the most obvious function affected. Additional deficits include poor reasoning or judgment, impaired abstract thinking, inability to attend to relevant information, impaired communication, and personality changes. Irreversible cognitive impairment is most frequently caused by Alzheimer disease (AD), vascular cognitive impairment (VCI) in which the blood supply to the brain is restricted, or multi-infarct dementia following repeated strokes, or a combination, referred to as mixed cognitive impairment (Ritchie & Lovenstone, 2002).

Cognitive impairment can be divided into cortical and subcortical types, based on patterns of neurophysiological impairment. The characteristics of cortical cognitive impairments that affect the cortex of the brain, such as Alzheimer and Pick diseases, resemble those of aphasia and RHD. These include visual-spatial deficits, memory problems, judgment and abstract thinking disturbances, and language deficits in naming, reading and writing, and auditory comprehension. Also included in this category would be individuals in advanced stages of PPA, mentioned earlier in this chapter. Alzheimer disease accounts for 60 to 80% of all cognitive impairment cases, or 6.5 million adults, in the United States (Alzheimer's Association, 2022).

Subcortical cognitive impairments result from damage to areas of the brain below the cortex, such as the thalamus, basal ganglia, and brainstem, and may accompany disorders such as multiple sclerosis and Parkinson and Huntington diseases. A slow, progressive deterioration of cognitive functioning occurs with deficits in memory, problem solving, language, and neuromuscular control. Disorders that involve neuromuscular functioning, such as Parkinson, are discussed in Chapters 9 and 10.

Differences in the brain location of cognitive impairment affect behavior in different ways. Individuals with **Parkinson disease**, such as the friend's husband mentioned at the beginning of the chapter, produce fewer formulaic expressions than those with AD. *Formulaic language* consists of fixed, unitary expressions, such as "You betcha," "You've got to be kidding," "That's the way the cookie crumbles," and "When it rains, it pours"; it is used as a compensation strategy that enables individuals to participate in conversations. In comprehension, those with AD perform significantly worse than participants with Parkinson (Van Lancker Sidtis et al., 2015).

The language functions that most depend on memory seem to be primarily affected by cognitive impairment. Communication disorders associated with cognitive impairment progress over time and include anomia, discourse production and comprehension deficits, and, eventually, the inability to express oneself via speech and language (Bourgeois & Hickey, 2009).

A significant decline is noted in naming and word retrieval. Language form—phonology, morphology, and syntax—is generally less disordered, although syntax may be less coherent than before as the client struggles with anomia. As a result, conversations may lack coherence and may be filled with repetitions, stereotypic utterances, false starts, verbal repairs, jargon, neologisms, and the use of phrases such as *that one* and *you know*. One client would repeat "I know" several times.

For an SLP working in a health care setting, maybe you, a large proportion of the caseload is individuals with cognitive impairment. Only individuals with dysphagia and aphasia are a larger portion of the caseload (ASHA, 2008).

Alzheimer Disease

Alzheimer disease (AD) is a cortical pathology that affects approximately 13% of individuals over age 65 and possibly as many as 50% of those over age 85, or approximately 6.5 million individuals, in the United States (Alzheimer's Association, 2022). Given the aging U.S. population, the prevalence of Alzheimer disease will nearly double to 12.7 million by 2050 unless science finds a way to slow the progression of the disease or prevent it. Alzheimer is the most expensive disease in the United States, costing families and society around $305 billion annually, most of this total spent on long-term care (Wong, 2020). Individuals with AD are a heterogeneous population and may be primarily impaired in memory, language, or visual-spatial skills. AD is twice as common in women as in men, primarily because women tend to live longer.

> Alzheimer disease is characterized by microscopic changes in the neurons of the cerebral cortex.

The cause of AD is unknown but may be a combination of genetic and environmental factors. The neuropathology is characterized by the presence of twisted neurofilaments in the cytoplasm or gelatinous liquid of neurons that deteriorate cell functioning. These tangles are most pronounced in the temporal lobe and in associational areas of the brain (see Figure 7.10). Nerve fibers degenerate, resulting in brain atrophy that may decrease brain weight as much as 20%, especially in the temporal, frontal, and parietal lobes. Other physical changes include extensive damage to the hippocampus, located on the interior portion of the temporal lobes, and formation of senile plaques or protein growths within the cortex that affect nerve cell interactive functioning.

A variation of the *APOE* gene found in all humans greatly increases the likelihood of developing AD. Environmental risk factors include head trauma, heart and circulatory problems, poor overall health, and diabetes.

Both normal aging and mild cognitive impairment (MCI) may be characterized by name recall (anomia) difficulties. For those with MCI, we also find difficulty processing complex sentences (Sung et al., 2020), occasional disorientation, and memory loss. Memory problems are the most obvious changes. Retention of newly learned information is most impaired. Long-term memory is unimpaired initially but deteriorates as the disease progresses.

It's important to realize that memory affects multiple aspects of daily living. In addition, there may be accompanying challenges, such as in ADLs.

FIGURE 7.10 **Alzheimer disease.**

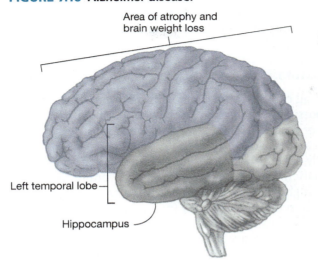

Language is not affected in all individuals initially. Early problems involve word finding, off-topic comments, and comprehension. At these early stages, deficits are mostly pragmatic and semantic-conceptual in nature, and syntax is relatively unaffected compared to that of elderly individuals not affected by AD (Kavé & Levy, 2003).

Both quantitative and qualitative findings support the notion that lexical–semantic impairments underlie word retrieval problems (Paek & Murray, 2021). When matched with healthy older adults, individuals with cognitive impairment produce fewer verbs, especially mental state verbs. Those with AD also produce verbs with shorter phoneme and syllable lengths, higher word frequency, and earlier age of acquisition.

Later characteristics include paraphasia (word substitution) and delayed responding. In more severe stages, expressive and receptive vocabulary and complex sentence production become reduced; pronoun confusion, topic digression, and inability to return to and to shift topic are more pronounced; and writing and reading errors occur. In the most severe form of AD, the language of individuals is characterized by naming errors and the use of generic words (*this, that*), syntactic errors, minimal comprehension, jargon, echolalia, or mutism. As might be expected, increased severity results in more conversational breakdowns.

All areas of communication, including writing, are affected. Writing disorders may arise at several different steps in the process, including planning, sequencing, and organization at the letter, word, sentence, and narrative levels (Neils-Strunjas et al., 2006). Deficits may include misspelling, poor narrative organization, content word errors, perseveration (or repetition of words or ideas), grammatical errors, and reduced syntactic complexity. Problems with writing reflect general language deficits as well as deficits in working memory, attention, and motor control. Both the Centers for Disease Control and Prevention (www.cdc .gov/aging/aginginfo/alzheimers.htm) and the Alzheimer's Association (www .alz.org/alzheimer_s_dementia) have helpful online guides to Alzheimer disease and dementia.

Exploration of effective cognitive-communication practices is needed. The number of SLPs who work with adults with MCI and early-stage dementia from AD is increasing and this is an expanding area of our field (Lanzi, Saylor & Cohen, 2022).

Lifespan Issues

In many if not all cases, AD is a genetic disorder that lies in hiding, although early screening is possible. Often the person who will be afflicted with the disease is unaware and/or ignores early signs. At present there are no cures, but some early drug therapies seem to lessen the effects.

In the early stages of AD, the individual experiences memory loss, especially of new information. The individual experiences word retrieval problems and some difficulty with higher language functions, such as humor and analogies. The individual may seem indifferent and may initiate little communication. Able to live at home, the individual can become an increasing burden on an elderly spouse or on adult children who may have families of their own.

As the disease progresses, memory loss increases, resulting in a decrease in vocabulary. Comprehension is reduced. There is a gradual weakening of syntax–semantics integration needed for complex sentence processing (Cohen Sherman et al., 2021). Language production may be reduced to ritualistic or high-usage phrases accompanied by poor topic maintenance and repair of errors, frequent repetition and word retrieval problems, and insensitivity to conversational partners. Irritability and restlessness may increase. The individual may be able to live at home with visiting nurse or health aide care to help with ADLs.

In the most advanced stages of the disease, all intellectual functions including memory are severely impaired, and almost all individuals reside in nursing homes. Language may be meaningless or the individual may be mute or echolalic. Most clients cannot recall the names of loved ones and may undergo radical personality changes. Motor function is also severely impaired, and the individual needs total care.

> **REFLECTION QUESTION 7.6**
>
> *Try to visualize the four cognitive disorders discussed. Begin with causes. How do they differ? Which are progressive? Which are not? How is language affected?*

Assessment

Definitive diagnosis of AD is difficult in the early stages of the disease. Use of neuroimaging techniques may help in early identification, especially for protein buildup in the brain (DeKosky, 2008). Pupil dilation tests may also indicate the presence of the disease in the early stages. Finally, computer-based assessments, such as the Computerized Assessment of Mild Cognitive Impairment, a self-administered test, have good sensitivity and specificity (Saxton et al., 2009). Such measures usually test attention, recognition, and recall of both words and pictures. It's important that SLPs not neglect comprehension and production of longer, more complex units of communication.

Working as a member of a diagnostic team, an SLP usually helps identify changes in language performance that may signal intellectual deterioration and aspects of behavior amenable to change (Hopper, 2005). The results of this assessment may help differentiate AD from other neuropathologies.

Genetic history and general and neurological health data are important elements in the assessment process. Observation of the individual in different communication environments is also important. In the early stages, cognitive impairment may be confused with other disorders such as depression. The progressive nature of the disorder makes it imperative that the SLP remain current on the changing condition and learning ability of a client.

Although SLPs are often responsible for assessing cognitive disorders that affect communication for individuals with diagnosed or suspected acute or degenerative neurological conditions, there is little consensus on appropriate assessment tools for various neurological disorders. Few definitive language tests for this population exist.

SLPs collect a considerable amount of clinical evaluative data supported by informal observation and/or the completion of select subtests of standardized assessment tools (Roitsch et al., 2021). Of importance are assessment of retrieval, perceptual, and linguistic deficits and the client's ability to participate in the give-and-take of daily communication in a number of areas. Language samples should consist of both structured tasks, such as narration, and unstructured tasks to provide a comprehensive description of an individual's language (Leaman & Edmonds, 2021a).

Writing assessment is important because decline in written language may precede other cognitive and spoken language deficits (Kavrie & Neils-Strunjas, 2002). Functional writing tasks, such as writing a letter, are one of the earliest affected areas of linguistic performance.

Several scales exist for rating the severity of a client's loss. Of particular importance are memory deficits. In addition, many assessment batteries that are used with individuals with aphasia can be helpful in evaluating the communication skills of persons with cognitive impairment. Detailed understanding of a client's strengths and weaknesses is essential for helping family members choose the most effective communicative strategies.

> With cognitive impairment, language is affected by deficits in memory.

Intervention

Intervention with those with progressive disorders can sometimes feel like trying to hold back the tide. Decline is inevitable, given the present state of our knowledge. However, this does not mean that we do nothing. Quite the contrary: Clinical intervention by an SLP can help maintain the client at their highest level of performance and help others maximize the client's participation in conversational interactions. It is imperative, therefore, that an SLP emphasize the use of intact cognitive abilities to compensate for deficient ones (Hopper, 2005). ASHA defines the role of the SLP with clients with cognitive impairment (go to ASHA's website and enter "cognitive impairment" into the search box).

Both healthy older adults and those with mild-to-moderate AD have the ability to learn new content. Involvement of family is crucial. When describing familiar images, healthy older adults modify their expressions depending on the current partner's knowledge, but individuals with AD are less likely to do so, increasing the importance of a range of conversational partners (Paek & Yoon, 2021).

Professionals use three general approaches with individuals with cognitive impairment. In *cognitive rehabilitation*, the client, health professionals, and families develop individualized goals and implement strategies based on those goals. Goals may be very basic, such as appropriately recalling a family member's name, or, in less impaired clients, reading a book to grandchildren.

A second approach, *cognitive training*, is used to denote structured practice to improve specific cognitive functions, such as attention, memory, and executive functions. Tasks might include memorizing a grocery list or attending to a prerecorded conversation for a short period.

Finally, a third intervention method, called *cognitive stimulation*, is less direct. Usually conducted in groups, cognitive stimulation is concerned with general enhancement of cognitive and social functioning and might involve relaxation exercises or music therapy.

With no cure for cognitive impairment on the immediate horizon, much research and intervention has focused on nonpharmacological therapies to lessen the symptoms of cognitive impairment and to improve the quality of life for individuals with cognitive impairment and for their caregivers. A wide range of nonpharmacological therapies are used to treat cognitive impairment or MCI. These include direct interventions focused on the person with cognitive impairment, such as computer-assisted cognitive interventions, reminiscence or recall therapy, errorless learning, simulated presence therapy, spaced retrieval, and vanishing cues, as well as indirect interventions for use with caregivers, such as caregiver-administered cognitive stimulation and caregiver education in communication strategies (Olazarán et al., 2010). While it isn't possible to discuss all these methods in detail, we try to give you a taste of many of them. Today's best evidence on effectiveness is presented in Box 7.4.

Many communication intervention methods involve the use of cues or prompts to elicit the correct behavior, such as a request for a desired item or for assistance,

Pearson eTextbook
Video Example 7.11

Even with our best efforts, until some medical breakthrough occurs, we are faced with the inevitable decline of the patient. It isn't fair to you to not show the effect of this on family and loved ones. Be forewarned that this healthline video is very sad.

www.youtube.com/watch?v=0T6UbR-pR6U

BOX 7.4 **Evidence-Based Practice for Individuals with Cognitive impairment**

Guidelines

- Although evidence is limited for individuals with moderately severe and severe cognitive impairment, those with mild and mildly moderate to moderate cognitive decline may be able to learn and relearn facts and procedures using specific cognitive intervention strategies.
- Spaced retrieval, errorless learning, vanishing cues, and specific cueing are promising techniques, although more research is needed.
- Intervention tasks should be as functional as possible and should include ecologically valid facts and procedures.
- Although improvement on trained items may be expected, carryover and long-term maintenance of facts and procedures may be limited unless there is additional intervention.

- Improvement in general cognitive functioning should not be expected from intervention on specific cognitive tasks and information.
- SLPs should consider ethnic, cultural, linguistic, and educational factors when making prognostic statements about learning outcomes.
- Patients with AD have more positive outcomes in individual treatment than in group therapy.
- Restorative strategies are most effective at improving cognitive and functional abilities. These include general cognitive stimulation, such as practicing conversation skills, prompting recall of remote memories, reading, problem solving and participating in creative activities; computerized visual-spatial drills; and memory drills that emphasize repetition.

Sources: Data from Hopper et al. (2013); Sitzer, Twamley, et al. (2006).

names, and events. In errorless learning, a memory intervention technique, SLPs use cues or instructions to prevent or reduce the likelihood of individuals making mistakes (Clare & Jones, 2008). In this way, desired information is accessed and, presumably, the neural pathway to that information is enhanced. As a client progresses, the SLP may use vanishing cues (VC), a technique in which cues or prompts are gradually decreased one at a time, following each successful recall trial. In a variation of VC, cues may be withheld and then added one at a time following an incorrect response. When a correct response is achieved, the cues are decreased (Sohlberg et al., 2005). Finally, with spaced retrieval, the prompted recall of a response occurs at spaced or delayed intervals.

An SLP may target memory or word retrieval by working on word associations and categories; auditory attending and comprehension in conversational contexts; coherent verbal responses; and formation of longer, more complex utterances with the help of memory aids. Interactive strategies that result in the least communication breakdown include eliminating distractions, speaking in simple sentences, and using yes/no questions. Relatively intact reading and visual memory can be used to facilitate verbal memory (Hopper, 2005).

With treatment, individuals with mild memory impairments can learn to use external memory aids (EMAs), such as pictures, to enhance participation in functional activities (Lanzi & Bourgeois, 2020). Similarly, individuals with cognitive deficits from Parkinson disease can also improve cognitive functioning and social interaction (Spencer et al., 2020). If applied carefully and systematically within individualized client-specific intervention, such compensatory strategies can be used in everyday tasks.

EMAs are not limited to mild impairment. Within skilled nursing facilities, it's important that everyone on the intervention staff be involved in providing services. For example, certified nursing assistants (CNAs) can be trained by the SLP to use EMAs to enhance the communication and independence of residents with more severe dementia (Douglas & Affoo, 2019).

Intervention is not undertaken in isolation. As in the other disorders discussed in this chapter, an SLP is a member of a team. Professionals consult with one another and with the client and family on the best course of action. In addition, SLPs include families in the intervention process. Unfortunately, these practices tend to be inconsistent. As such, these efforts may be insufficient. Family members need assistance enhancing their own daily lives as well as those of the client (Mach et al., 2021).

Family members can help to keep conversations focused on the present, to validate the client's comments, to reduce distractions and limit the number of participants, and to foster comprehension and participation by slowing the rate and decreasing the complexity of their utterances, using nonlinguistic cues and yes/no response questions (Small & Perry, 2005). In skilled nursing facilities, CNAs can be trained to implement positive communication behaviors when communicating with clients (Douglas & MacPherson, 2021). In turn, negative responsive behaviors of people with AD also decrease.

Appropriate and effective intervention requires that the SLP understand what the family of the client is experiencing.

New drug and gene therapies and bioengineering techniques hold the promise that many of the diseases that cause cognitive impairment may one day be controllable. At present, intervention that stimulates cognitive processes combined with pharmacological approaches that increase certain neural chemicals important for memory is best.

Summary

Aphasia, right-hemisphere damage (RHD), traumatic brain injury (TBI), and cognitive impairment describe very different types of language disorders. Aphasia, which results from a focal brain injury, most likely a stroke, may result in a wide variety of deficits that may affect one or more modalities of communication; comprehension, speech, and naming are usually impaired. Stroke is also the primary cause of RHD. Comprehension and production of paralinguistics and complex linguistic structures are affected. Pragmatics is the most affected aspect of language. This is also true for TBI, which, in contrast to aphasia and RHD, is a diffuse injury rather than a focal injury. Finally, cognitive impairment, particularly Alzheimer disease, is a degenerative disease. Word-finding difficulties, off-topic comments, and comprehension deficits are the most common characteristics.

In the adult language disorders discussed, an SLP functions as a member of a multidisciplinary collaborative team. The role of the SLP includes assessment of communicative abilities and the implications of other cognitive deficits, swallowing, and associated neurological disorders. SLP responsibilities include treatment planning and programming, direct intervention services, interdisciplinary consultation, and family training and counseling. Intervention usually focuses on retrieval of language skills and on compensatory strategies.

Even though there is great diversity in the brain injuries presented here, a few themes emerge. In addition to considering individual client differences, the SLP should:

- Use descriptive methods during assessment
- Focus on cognition as it affects communication
- Collaboratively plan with the client, family, and medical team
- Include the client's communication environment in intervention by enlisting the aid of family and other professionals
- Link cognitive abilities via a multimodality approach
- Use real-life teaching situations as much as possible, including conversation
- Underpin word learning with semantic organization
- Consider client and family well-being
- Be flexible and able to change as your clients change

Epilogue

Case Study: Marsha

Marsha is now 6 months poststroke. To date, she has recovered much of her speech and language. Some speech sounds are slightly slurred, especially when she talks quickly, and she still has some lingering word-retrieval difficulties that affect sentence production.

Fortunately, Marsha was able to return to her job, where she is able to communicate with only limited lingering symptoms. She expressed genuine happiness upon returning to work, which also reduced some of her financial concerns.

The intervention plan is for Marsha to still meet with her SLP and attend evening group sessions on a weekly basis. At this point, her SLP has recommended dismissal but is letting her ease out of the group sessions, which provide some emotional support.

Reflections from a Rehabilitation Hospital Speech-Language Pathologist

If you had told me in graduate school that I would be working with adults, I would have questioned your sanity. My focus was completely on working with children. The younger the better. That was before my adult practicum.

I was placed in a group program with adults with brain injury, some from strokes but most were from TBIs. I had no idea how rewarding it could be, and here I am. I wouldn't change it for the world.

Because I work in a rehabilitation setting, most patients have recovered some communication and swallowing skills, basic stuff such as word finding. I'm not belittling those accomplishments but it's not a major focus of what I do. In general, I consult with the medical staff and families and the client and we sort of collaboratively decide on intervention goals. Much of what I do is working with small groups on social goals, pragmatics. I don't neglect more basic skills but it's not a major focus. Word-finding challenges don't disappear but I try to work on them in service to larger communication goals. If we're going to be discussing travel or cooking, we decide collectively on the words we'll need and I use pictures as reminders.

For example, one young man has difficulty determining when enough is enough, when he has provided enough information and it's time to stop and let someone else talk. That's the beauty of being in a small group. We started with very specific questions to the group and, at first, I had to thank him and move on even though he was revving up for a long-winded explanation. Afterward, we would discuss what was asked and what was needed. And thankfully he is improving. This may sound trivial—talking too much—but it's not if you're in a conversation. Turns move quickly and no one wants to listen to a 10-minute lecture. The question is, "When have I given enough of the relevant information?"

That gives you some idea. We often focus on conversational skills because that is often the culmination of how we use language but we also work on comprehension of both speech and reading. Often, we work on skills needed for the patient to return to work.

I truly enjoy my job. And, like I said, I wouldn't trade it for the world.

Suggested Readings/Sources

Brookshire, R. H., & McNeil, M. R. (2014). *Introduction to neurogenic communication disorders* (8th ed.). Elsevier.

Davis, G. B. (2007). *Aphasiology: Disorders and clinical practice* (2nd ed.). Pearson.

Martin, N., Thompson, C., & Worrall, L. (2007). *Aphasia rehabilitation: The impairment and its consequences.* Plural.

8 Fluency Disorders

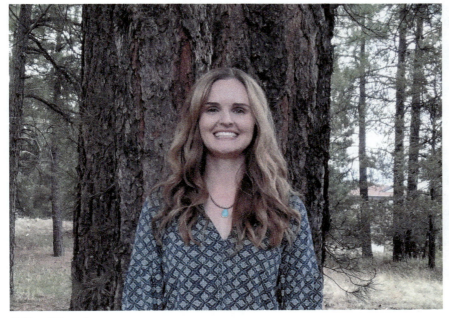

© Myra Crimmel

Several exceptional SLPs believed in me and gave me the tools to speak freely. My experience as a PWS [person who stutters] gave me insight into the frustration caused by the inability to communicate to my fullest potential. My experiences have helped me immensely in my work with children with communication disorders. I hope others with personal knowledge of communication disorders consider joining this field!

—Myra Crimmel

Learning Objectives

When you have finished this chapter, you should be able to:

8.1 Describe the differences between fluent speech and stuttering.

8.2 Outline and describe the onset and development of stuttering through the lifespan.

8.3 Describe the major etiological theories and conceptual models of stuttering.

8.4 List and briefly describe the components of a comprehensive stuttering evaluation.

8.5 Describe efficacious treatment approaches for children and adults who stutter.

> " While not my original plan, I completed my dissertation in pediatric stuttering with a fantastic mentor who now teaches at the University of Georgia. It was interesting to learn the similarities between models and theories about motor-based speech sound disorders in children (i.e., childhood apraxia of speech), my true passion, and stuttering. My treatment-focused dissertation provided me the clinical experience to deliver direct interventions to young children who stutter. I never thought my knowledge/experience in this area might come to the forefront of my own life.

My son is now 6 years old and has exhibited borderline stuttering for about a year. He is left-handed (more about this in the chapter) and has mild fine motor delays that continually improve with practice, experience, and occupational therapy services. Because he is not anxious or fearful about speaking, and he has no awareness of disfluencies, I haven't intervened all that much. There also is no family history of stuttering.

(continued)

Periodically I interject and have my son repeat his "bumpy" phrase after I provide a "smooth" model (more on this treatment later, too). I continue to monitor him for any negative feelings, fear, or embarrassment he may have about speaking. I recognize I have the skills to intervene directly and on a more consistent basis. However, my goal as a mom is to help my son become a warm, kind, empathetic human being. If he is also someone who stutters, we will manage it together with the help of an SLP

as needed. I try to focus on my son as a person and enjoy the time we spend together rather than always operating as an SLP focused on his speech and disfluencies.

Still, I'm grateful for my background, and my research and clinical experience in this area. There is always so much to learn, though, and my son keeps me on my toes in all aspects of life.

—*Kimberly Allyn Farinella*

CASE STUDY   ## Dylan

Dylan was 29 years old when he decided to go back to college to get his master's degree in education. For the previous 7 years, he had worked as a grant writer for an environmental consulting firm in his hometown. Dylan always wanted to be a science teacher working with high school students but, as a person who stuttered, he feared he would be perceived as inadequate and unintelligent. He believed it wasn't possible for him to achieve his career goal. Dylan became a grant writer after he graduated with his bachelor's degree because it required minimal communicative interactions with others. He didn't need to worry about what people thought about his stuttering. After enrolling in the master's degree program, he sought treatment for

his stuttering at the university's speech-language-hearing clinic. A comprehensive evaluation revealed Dylan's stuttering was severe. Secondary behaviors included head nodding and slapping of his leg. Dylan often avoided certain words, including his name. He also had a difficult time starting conversations with people because of his stuttering.

As you read this chapter, think about:

• The social-emotional challenges associated with stuttering
• Key areas to assess when evaluating a person who stutters
• The role of the speech-language pathologist (SLP) in counseling persons who stutter

---

Fluent speech is the consistent ability to move the speech production apparatus in an effortless, smooth, and rapid manner, resulting in a continuous, uninterrupted forward flow of speech. Several conditions that adversely affect speech and language production can also disrupt the fluency of speech. Dysarthria, apraxia, and some forms of aphasia affect the fluency of speech. These disorders and their effects on speech and language production are discussed in Chapters 7 and 10 of this book. The focus of this chapter is on a disorder of speech called *developmental stuttering*. Developmental stuttering, or simply *stuttering*, primarily influences the speaker's ability to produce fluent speech. Stuttered speech is characterized by involuntary repetitions of sounds and syllables (e.g., *b-b-b-ball*), sound prolongations (e.g., *mmmmm-mommy*), and blocks (e.g., *b—oy*). All three of these interruptions are considered to be stuttering behaviors, and they have a negative impact on a speaker's ability to produce fluent speech. The Case Study provides an example of an adult who stutters and is revisited throughout this chapter to highlight the key points in the learning objectives.

In this chapter, we define stuttering and discuss how stuttering begins and develops as a disorder, paying particular attention to how stuttered speech differs from fluent speech. Consideration is given to some of the major theories regarding stuttering, the clinical diagnosis of stuttering, and evidence-based treatment practices.

The cause of stuttering remains elusive, and our understanding of stuttering is incomplete despite its long and diverse history. Stuttering has been part of the human condition for all recorded time. Clay tablets found in Mesopotamia dating from centuries before the birth of Christ record the disorder, hieroglyphics from the 20th century B.C. depict stuttering, and poems written in China more than 2,500 years ago allude to stuttering (Van Riper, 1992). Stuttering occurs all over the world and affects people regardless of age, sex, race/ethnicity, or intellectual level.

The *incidence* of stuttering or number of people who have stuttered at some point in their lives is between 5% and 8% (Felsenfeld et al., 2000; Yairi & Ambrose, 2013). How stuttering is defined and differences in data collection procedures among researchers seem to contribute to discrepancies in incidence rates for stuttering (Guitar, 2019). The fact that a high percentage of children who begin to stutter will recover without treatment also contributes to difficulties in accurately determining stuttering incidence. Yairi and Ambrose (1999) reported a natural recovery rate of 74% after a minimum of 4 years postonset of stuttering in 84 children. In 51 preschool children, Mansson (2000) reported that 71% naturally recovered within 2 years after starting to stutter, and 85% recovered over the next few years, at around 8 or 9 years of age.

It is not well understood why most children naturally recover from stuttering whereas some do not. However, certain factors seem to contribute to the persistence of stuttering in some children. For example, females appear to recover from stuttering more frequently and more quickly than males. A family history of stuttering increases the risk that it will persist. A child with a later onset of stuttering (after 3.5 years of age), or a child who continues to stutter more than a year postonset, is also at greater risk for persistent stuttering (Singer et al., 2020).

The prevalence of stuttering is determined by ascertaining the number of cases in a population (usually school-age children) who currently stutter. Research findings of many studies conducted around the world suggest an average prevalence rate of 1% for school-age children (Andrews et al., 1983; Bloodstein & Ratner, 2008). Prevalence data are higher for preschool-age children (over 2% according to some estimates). This makes sense given that natural recovery with or without treatment will occur between kindergarten and the upper grades (Guitar, 2019; Yairi & Ambrose, 2013).

Stuttering affects more males than females; however, reported sex ratio differences are age dependent. In very young children (age 3 and under), there is no statistically significant difference between boys and girls who stutter (Yairi & Ambrose, 2013). By first grade, however, the sex ratio difference has been found to be about 3 to 1 (Bloodstein & Ratner, 2008). This difference has been attributed to differences in the physical maturation rates of boys and girls and to differences in speech and language development. However, genetic factors are more likely responsible for the sex difference (Ambrose et al., 1997).

Stuttering has a high degree of familial incidence; approximately 30–60% of people who stutter report that they have a relative who stuttered at some time in their life (Yairi et al., 1996). Persistent stuttering also runs in families; children who do not naturally recover from stuttering are likely to have a relative whose stuttering persisted. On the other hand, children who do recover tend to come from a family where a relative who stuttered eventually recovered (Ambrose et al., 1997). In addition, if one twin stutters, there is a high probability that the other twin will stutter, and the rate of concordance (both twins exhibiting the disorder) is higher for genetically identical (monozygotic) twins than for fraternal (dizygotic) twins. Because there isn't a 100% concordance of stuttering in twins, environmental factors must also play a role in the onset and persistence or recovery of stuttering, in addition to genetic factors (Ambrose et al., 1997).

Differences between Fluent Speech and Stuttering

Learning Objective 8.1 Describe the differences between fluent speech and stuttering.

Anyone who has listened carefully to a young child speak can attest to the fact that the flow of most children's speech is not continuously forward and uninterrupted. Children exhibit many hesitations, revisions, and interruptions in their utterances. Children are not born as fluent speakers. Fluency requires some degree of physical maturation and language experience, but it does not develop linearly as the child matures. Longitudinal research indicates that children around 25 months of age are more fluent than they will be at 29 months and at 37 months of age (Yairi, 1981, 1982). There is a gradual increase in disfluent speech behaviors beginning around 2 years of age that peaks around the third birthday. Fluency then improves after age 3, and the types of disfluency change.

Typical Disfluencies

The type of disfluency exhibited by a typically developing child changes between the ages of 25 and 37 months. At approximately 2 years of age, typical disfluencies are whole-word repetitions ("I-I-I want a cookie"), interjections ("Can we, uhm, go now?"), and syllable repetitions ("I like ba-baseball"). Revisions such as "He can't, he won't play baseball" are the dominant disfluency type when the child is approximately 3 years old (Yairi, 1982). Typical disfluencies persist throughout the course of one's life, but they do not tend to adversely affect the continuous forward flow of speech. Typically, fluent speakers frequently interrupt the forward flow of speech by repeating whole multisyllabic words ("I really-really like hockey"), interjecting a word or phrase ("He will, uhhhhh, you know, not like that idea"), repeating a phrase ("Will you, will you please stop that"), or revising a sentence ("She can't—she didn't do that").

Children who exhibit typical disfluencies are rarely aware of them and are not bothered or negatively affected during times when they are aware of them. Repetitions are the more common type of typical disfluency in children between 2 and 3 years of age, whereas revisions are more common in older children (Guitar, 2019).

Stuttering

What is stuttering? How is it different from fluent and typically disfluent speech? These are not simple questions, and there are no simple answers. The issue of what stuttering is and how to define it lies at the center of some unresolved issues (e.g., Ingham & Cordes, 1997). Can clinicians determine reliably whether and when stuttering has occurred? Do typical disfluencies and moments of stuttering lie along the same continuum, or are they entirely different behavioral events? There are no absolute answers to these questions. At present, no universally accepted definition of stuttering exists. However, a reasonable framework from which one can begin to distinguish between typical disfluencies and those that are likely to be regarded as stuttering has been proposed.

Stuttering, or stuttered speech, involves certain core behaviors, including repetitions of sounds, syllables, or one-syllable words, prolongations of sounds, or blocks, where an inappropriate stop in the flow of air or voice occurs during speech production (Guitar, 2019). Part-word repetitions and single-syllable word repetitions are the most frequently observed stuttering behaviors reported by parents when their child is just beginning to stutter. In addition, children who stutter exhibit more repeats of a word or syllable (more than two), and repetitions are three times faster than the repetitions produced by typically disfluent children (Guitar, 2019; Yairi & Ambrose, 2013). Children who stutter generally do not exhibit repetitions of multisyllabic words. Repetitions, revisions, and pauses that frequently occur in children with typical speech and language development are not considered to be stuttering behaviors (Guitar, 2019).

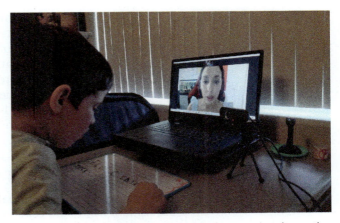

Here a 6-year-old child receives speech therapy via telepractice with speech-language pathology assistant Karina Kadhi.

© Kimberly Allyn Farinella

Pearson eTextbook
Video Example 8.1
Stuttering: For Kids, By Kids (Clip 1)
Watch this video from the Stuttering Foundation to meet a few children who stutter.
www.youtube.com/watch?v=rw04lXYpQgQ

CASE STUDY **Dylan** (*continued*)

When Dylan was 3 years old his parents noticed he would often repeat the first sound in words when beginning to speak (e.g., "C-c-c-c-can I have cookie?", "I-I-I-I need help!"). They also noticed occasional sound prolongations (e.g., "Mmmmmy toy!"). He sometimes became frustrated and stopped talking right in the middle of a sentence without finishing.

In young children, there continues to be debate about when speech disfluencies constitute stuttering behaviors. Some studies have shown that children who stutter produce many more within-word disfluencies, including part-word repetitions and prolongations, than do children who are exhibiting typical disfluencies. Other studies have found that the amount of disfluency is important when differentiating stuttering from typical disfluencies, regardless of the type of disfluency produced. Young preschool children who are typically disfluent tend to produce fewer than 10 disfluencies per 100 words, with an average of 6 disfluencies per 100 words. These disfluencies may be within-word (e.g., syllable repetitions) or between-word disfluencies (e.g., whole-word repetitions). However, stuttering frequency by itself is not a definitive clinical measure for stuttering because some typically disfluent children may exhibit more than 10 disfluencies per 100 words on occasion (Guitar, 2019).

Stuttering behaviors are also differentiated from typical disfluencies by the number of repetition units. As previously stated, more than two repetitions of a sound or word is considered stuttering, but only one extra repetition (e.g., "I-I want more juice"; "I li-like ice cream") is believed to be a typical disfluency (Guitar, 2019). Similarly, one or two repetitions of an interjection (e.g., "um") is generally considered a typical disfluency, but more than two repeats of an interjection represents stuttering. Table 8.1 provides specific examples of stuttering behaviors and typical disfluencies.

> **REFLECTION QUESTION 8.1**
>
> *Considering what you have learned so far about speech and language acquisition, why might children exhibit typical disfluencies during development?*

You can visit the Stuttering Foundation website (www.stutteringhelp.org) to listen to the personal stories of children and adolescents who stutter; enter "videos" into the search bar at the bottom of the webpage to check out some "Must-See" videos. You can also enter the following titles into the same search bar: "Stuttering: Straight Talk for Teens" and "Stuttering: For Kids, by Kids." You'll find firsthand examples of the core stuttering behaviors discussed in this section (i.e., repetitions, prolongations, and blocks) in each video clip.

More than one type of within-word disfluency may be present in a disruption that interferes with the forward flow of speech. Consider the following disfluent production of the word *mommy* that contains elements of both sound repetition and a prolongation: *m-m-m-mmmommy* (Yaruss, 1997). Such productions, called "clustered disfluencies," are quite common in the speech of young children who

TABLE 8.1

Examples of Stuttering Behaviors and Typical Disfluencies

Type of Disfluency	Stuttering Behavior	Typical Disfluency	Examples
Sound/syllable repetitions (more than two repeats)	X		*He's a b-b-b-boy.* *G-g-g-g-go away.* *Yes, puh-puh-puh please.*
Sound prolongation	X		*Ssssssee me swing!* *My name is Tiiiiiiiiimmy.*
Block	X		*Base-(pause)-ball.*
Monosyllabic whole-word repetitions	X		*I-I-I hit the ball.* *It's my-my-my turn.*
Multisyllabic whole-word repetitions		X	*I'm going-going home.*
Phrase repetition/interjection		X	*She hit—she hit me.* *I like, uh, ya know, big boats.*
Revisions		X	*He went, he came back.*

Sources: Based on Guitar (2019); Yairi and Ambrose (2013).

stutter. Some researchers have suggested that the presence of clustered disfluencies may also indicate stuttering that is just beginning.

Other behaviors may accompany instances of speech disfluency. Such behaviors that occur concomitantly with stuttered disfluencies are called *secondary behaviors* or *accessory characteristics* and are widely varied and idiosyncratic. Some common secondary behaviors include blinking of the eyes, facial grimacing, facial tension, and exaggerated movements of the head, shoulders, and arms. Children who are typically disfluent generally do not exhibit secondary behaviors, although occasionally tense pauses may be observed (Guitar, 2019). In older individuals, interjected speech fragments that are superfluous to the utterance are also considered to be secondary behaviors, particularly when they occur in conjunction with a stuttered disfluency. An example of an interjected speech fragment is the superfluous phrase *that is to say* in the utterance "I met her in M-M-M-M, that is to say, I met her in Mexico."

Secondary behaviors are adopted to reduce instances of stuttering (Bloodstein, 1995). The person who stutters discovers through trial and error that some action (e.g., bodily movements) momentarily distracts from the act of speaking and that action appears to help terminate or avoid an instance of stuttering. Behaviors such as eye blinking, however, soon lose their apparent power to reduce stuttering, and the individual is forced to replace the ineffective behavior with a new behavior, such as shrugging the shoulders, to reduce stuttering. Unfortunately, the eye-blinking behavior may have become so strongly habituated that it will remain permanently associated with a person's stuttering. How do these cardinal stuttering behaviors and secondary behaviors develop, and how do they change over the course of an individual's life?

The Onset and Development of Stuttering Through the Lifespan

Learning Objective 8.2 Outline and describe the onset and development of stuttering through the lifespan.

Although stuttering can develop at any age, the most common form of stuttering begins in the preschool years and is called *developmental stuttering*. Developmental stuttering is contrasted with another form of stuttering, called **neurogenic stuttering**, which is typically associated with neurological disease or trauma and is acquired after childhood. Neurogenic stuttering is discussed in Chapter 10.

It is generally accepted that the onset of developmental stuttering occurs between the ages of 2 and 5 and that 75% of the risk of developing stuttering occurs before the child is 3½ years old (Yairi, 1983, 2004; Yairi & Ambrose, 1992a, 1992b, 2004). The onset of stuttering is gradual for most children who develop the condition, with stuttering severity increasing as the child grows older. When stuttering develops in a gradual manner, some general trends regarding stuttering behaviors, reactions to stuttering, and conditions that seem to promote stuttering can be observed. We outline some of these developmental trends in the following sections (Bloodstein, 1995; Guitar, 2019).

Not all children follow this developmental framework of stuttering exactly, but it generally does capture the onset and progression of the disorder. This developmental framework is divided into four specific age groups that are sequentially

Pearson eTextbook
Video Example 8.2
Stuttering: For Kids, By Kids (Clip 2)
Watch this video from the Stuttering Foundation to hear what stuttering is from the perspective of kids who stutter.
www.youtube.com/watch?v=rw04IXYpQgQ

Some parenthetical interjections or asides that are common interruptions in adult speech are devices that help to maintain listener interest. An example of a parenthetical interjection is "When John slipped on the stairs—like Mary slipped in the same spot last week—he broke his ankle."

related: younger preschool, older preschool, school age, and adolescents and adults (Guitar, 2019). The development and progression of stuttering by age group are summarized in Table 8.2.

In the younger preschool years, roughly between 2 and 3½ years of age, stuttering may resemble typical disfluency but with increased frequency (i.e., more than 6–10 disfluencies per 100 words), raising parental concern (Tumanova et al., 2014). Children may go back and forth between stuttering behaviors (e.g., part-word repetitions; prolongations) and typical disfluencies (e.g., interjections; revisions) and may have periods of fluency followed by an increase in stuttering

TABLE 8.2

Summary of the Development and Progression of Stuttering

Developmental Age Group/ Level of Stuttering	Approximate Age	Highlights
Younger preschool/ Borderline stuttering	2–3½ years	Stuttering is highly variable. More than 6–10 disfluencies per 100 words. More than one or two units in repetitions.
		Higher proportion of part-word and monosyllabic whole-word repetitions and prolongations. Child seems unaware of stuttering; rarely expresses frustration. Few, if any, secondary behaviors.
Older preschool/ Beginning stuttering	4–6 years	Stuttering is still variable, but the child is aware of stuttering and may become frustrated when speaking.
		Stuttering repetitions begin to sound rapid and irregular; blocks and muscular tension begin to appear. Increases in pitch may accompany prolongations and repetitions. Secondary behaviors such as eye blinking may appear.
School-age/ Intermediate stuttering	6–13 years	Fear of stuttering and attempts to avoid certain speaking situations are common. Certain words are regarded as more difficult than others.
		Circumlocutions and word substitutions are frequent. Blocks with increased muscular tension become more frequent, although repetitions and prolongations with increased pitch are still common. Secondary behaviors to avoid or escape stuttering become more complex.
Adolescence and adulthood/ Advanced stuttering	14+ years	Stuttering is at its apex of development.
		There is fearful anticipation of stuttering. Longer, more tense blocks accompanied by lip, tongue, or jaw tremors mixed with repetitions and prolongations are frequent. Certain sounds, words, and speaking situations are carefully avoided. Circumlocutions, word substitutions, and interjections are used extensively as avoidance strategies.

Sources: Based on Bloodstein (1995); Guitar (2019).

behaviors (Bloodstein, 1995; Guitar, 2019). This period is called "borderline stuttering" since children exhibit disfluencies characteristic of both typical disfluency and stuttering (Guitar, 2019). Stuttering moments are characterized mainly by initial sound and syllable repetitions, along with monosyllabic whole-word repetitions, compared to multisyllabic word and phrase repetitions (Yairi & Ambrose, 2013). Repetitions with more than one or two units occurs more frequently with borderline stuttering (Yairi & Lewis, 1984; Zebrowski, 1991). Most children at this age are unaware of the interruptions in their speech or are not bothered by them. They generally do not exhibit secondary behaviors, although there may at times be a slight degree of tension during stuttering moments (Guitar, 2019).

In older preschoolers between about 4 and 6 years of age, a progression of the disorder occurs, or in some cases, stuttering appears suddenly during stress or excitement. Stuttering repetitions may begin to sound rapid and irregular. Blocks, or the inappropriate stoppage of the flow of air or voice, may begin to appear and increased tension of the speech mechanism may be observed (Guitar, 2019). Previously repeated sounds may now be prolongations, and stuttering moments may occur on initial and middle sounds accompanied by a rise in pitch. Secondary behaviors such as eye blinking or head nodding may begin to appear. The child has a conscious awareness of stuttering and may become frustrated or embarrassed. At this point, the child is exhibiting beginning stuttering onset (Guitar, 2019).

By school age, fear and avoidance of stuttering begin to emerge. Stuttering seems to be in response to specific situations such as speaking to strangers or speaking in front of groups. The individual who stutters will approach these situations with dread and will later try to avoid these situations at all costs (Guitar, 2019). In addition, certain words are regarded as more difficult than others, and the person who stutters attempts to avoid such words by using word substitutions and circumlocutions. An example of a word substitution is "I want a ni-ni-ni-five cents"; the individual substitutes *five cents* for the originally intended word *nickel*. Circumlocutions are roundabout or indirect ways of speaking. A circumlocution used to avoid the term *fire truck* in a child's request for a toy might take on the following form "I want a—ya know—red thing—sirens and ladders—truck for my birthday."

More complex secondary behaviors used to escape or avoid stuttering also emerge and might include a combination of head nodding, eye blinking, and slapping of the leg. Blocks are more common and characterized by excessive muscular tension; the increased tension is believed to result from negative feelings of fear, embarrassment, and helplessness about the anticipation of stuttering. Repetitions and prolongations are still common, and many will occur with increased pitch due to the increase in muscular tension that accompanies these moments of stuttering (Guitar, 2019).

Pearson eTextbook
Video Example 8.3
Stuttering: For Kids,
By Kids (Clip 3)
Watch this video from the Stuttering Foundation to hear how some kids feel about their stuttering.
www.youtube.com/
watch?v=rw04IXYpQgQ

CASE STUDY Dylan *(continued)*

Dylan was bullied by peers throughout his school-age years because of his stuttering. He feared introducing himself to new people because he often stuttered when saying his name; this was usually accompanied by head nodding and slapping his leg. As Dylan got older, he began avoiding peers at school, and would not initiate conversation with new people to avoid the embarrassment and shame he felt about his stuttering.

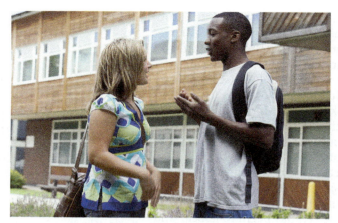

In older teens and adults, the individual has developed a self-concept as a person who stutters and will often refer to themselves in this way.

© Mark Bowden/123RF

Pearson eTextbook
Video Example 8.4

Watch this video of an adult explaining their feelings about their stuttering.

www.youtube.com/
watch?v=Iz7LC4Qog1k

In older teens and adults, stuttering is in its most advanced form; the individual has developed a self-concept as a person who stutters and will often refer to themselves in this way. A primary characteristic of this age group is vivid and fearful anticipation of stuttering. The person who stutters tries to control the environment so that situations in which stuttering might occur are avoided (Guitar, 2019). Certain sounds and words are carefully avoided also; the person with advanced stuttering may plan the verbal message ahead of time to ensure they avoid sounds and/or words believed to be more difficult. Longer, tense blocks are the most frequent core stuttering behavior and may be accompanied by visible tremors. Repetitions still occur but they are more rapid and irregular and may co-occur with tense blocks (Guitar, 2019). Secondary behaviors such as word substitutions, interjections (e.g., "um"), and circumlocutions continue to be frequent avoidance strategies.

Adults who stutter have reported a sensation of being stuck or losing control. Some also report a negative impact on self-esteem and quality of life (Tichenor & Yaruss, 2019). Feelings of embarrassment, helplessness, fear, shame, and hopelessness are common in individuals with advanced stuttering (Guitar, 2019).

REFLECTION QUESTION 8.2

What kinds of jobs require a great deal of speaking? Do you think people who stutter avoid such jobs?

Stuttering does not always develop gradually. For some individuals, when stuttering is first diagnosed in young children, the symptoms appear to be very advanced, and secondary characteristics may be present (e.g., Van Riper, 1982; Yairi, 2004). The onset may be a distinct and sudden event for as many as 36% of children, and the stuttering behaviors may be considered moderate to severe (Yairi & Ambrose, 1992a). More research is needed about the onset and development of stuttering and the factors that underlie persistence and natural recovery.

Theories and Conceptual Models of Stuttering

Learning Objective 8.3 Describe the major etiological theories and conceptual models of stuttering.

Let's look now at past and present theoretical perspectives that consider genetic and/or environmental factors associated with onset and persistence of stuttering. Etiological theories and models are classified into the following categories: organic, behavioral, psycholinguistic, or a combination thereof. Several of these are described next.

Organic Theory

Organic theories propose an actual physical cause for stuttering. Speculations about a physical cause for stuttering date back to the writings of Aristotle, who suggested that stuttering is a disconnection between the mind and the body and that the muscles of the tongue cannot follow the commands of the brain (Rieber & Wollock, 1977). Many organic theories have been proposed since Aristotle's writings, but they have all failed in one manner or another to explain stuttering satisfactorily.

For example, the *theory of cerebral dominance* or the "handedness theory," proposed by Samuel Orton and Lee Travis in the 1920s and 1930s, suggested that people who stutter do not exhibit left cerebral hemisphere dominance for speech and language the way fluent individuals do. They speculated individuals who stutter were born left-handed, but then were forced to learn to use their right hand as children. This ultimately resulted in neither cerebral hemisphere becoming dominant, thereby causing the right and left hemispheres of the brain to send competing neural impulses to their respective muscles of speech. This resulted in a discoordination between the right and left halves of the speech musculature causing stuttering (Boberg & Kully, 1989; Orton & Travis, 1929).

While there is no strong empirical support to date, renewed interest in this theory has come about due to more recent findings from brain imaging studies that revealed structural and functional differences in the brains of adults with persistent developmental stuttering. Specifically, evidence from limb motor control studies suggests individuals who stutter may have right-hemisphere interference on left-hemisphere motor planning structures. This is believed to disrupt the function of left-hemisphere motor structures responsible for planning, initiating, and sequencing speech motor output (Guitar, 2019; Webster, 1993a).

Current brain imaging research may facilitate the development of a comprehensive neurophysiological model for both fluent and stuttered speech that could lead to new stuttering prevention and treatment methods (e.g., Butler et al., 2020).

Behavioral Theory

Behavioral theories assert that stuttering is a learned response to conditions external to the individual. Wendell Johnson developed a prominent behavioral theory, the *diagnosogenic* theory, during the 1940s and 1950s. According to this theory, stuttering began in the parent's ear, not in the child's mouth. Overly concerned parents would react to the child's typical speech hesitations and repetitions with negative statements, admonishing the child to speak more slowly and not to stutter. Such parental behaviors made the child anxious about speaking, and the child's anxiety fostered further hesitations and repetitions.

Not only is there no evidence to support this theory, there is evidence to the contrary. Studies have shown that the process of natural recovery may be due in part to parents explicitly telling

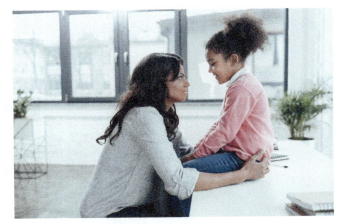

The process of natural recovery may be due in part to parents telling their child to slow down, stop, and start again.

© LightField Studios/Shutterstock

their child to slow down, stop, and start again, or think before speaking when their child is stuttering (e.g., Ambrose & Yairi, 2002; Langford & Cooper, 1974; Martin & Lindamood, 1986).

Language and Stuttering

The *covert repair hypothesis*, based on a language production model, assumes that stuttering is a reaction to some flaw in the speech production plan (Postma & Kolk, 1993). Speakers have the capability of monitoring their speech as it is being formulated and detecting errors in the speech plan. People who stutter have poorly developed phonological encoding skills that cause them to introduce errors (repetitions, prolongations, and blocks) into their speech plan. If there are more errors in the speech plan, there will be more occasions for error correction. Stuttering is not the error; rather, stuttering is a "normal" repair reaction to an atypical phonetic plan.

Another conceptualization of stuttering is the *demands and capacities model* (DCM; Starkweather, 1987, 1997). This model asserts that stuttering develops when the environmental demands placed on a child to produce fluent speech exceed the child's physical and learned capacities. The child's capacity for fluent speech depends on a balance of motor skills, language production skills, emotional maturity, and cognitive development. Children who stutter presumably lack one or more of these capacities for fluent speech. Parents of a child who lacks the required motor skills for fluency might talk rapidly; rapid rates of speech may put time pressure on the child that exceeds their motoric ability to respond. Other parents might insist on the use of advanced language structures that exceed the child's language development. In every case of stuttering within the DCM, there is an imbalance between the environmental demands that are placed on the child and the child's capacity for fluent speech.

The DCM is not a theory of stuttering, and it does not suggest a cause for stuttering. Rather, the DCM is a useful tool that helps clinicians understand the dynamics of forces that contribute to the development of stuttering. Therapeutically, the DCM provides useful guidelines for understanding what capacities a child may lack for fluent speech production and the elements of the child's environment that may be challenging those capacities.

Current Conceptual Models of Stuttering

A model of stuttering that takes the DCM theory a step further, referred to as the Packman and Attanasio model (or P&A model), suggests that there are three factors that cause moments of stuttering: (1) a deficit in the neural processing of language and inherent instability of the speech production system; (2) triggers, or certain features of spoken language that are associated with greater speech motor demands that negatively affect an already unstable speech production system; and (3) modulating factors, such as physiological arousal in an individual that can alter the threshold at which a stuttering moment occurs (Packman, 2012).

In other words, in individuals who stutter, there exists an impairment in brain function that affects speech motor stability, such that attempts to produce longer or more linguistically complex utterances result in an increased probability for stuttering moments to occur. Fear and anxiety about speaking, influenced by an individual's past experiences (e.g., bullying in childhood), contributes to the variability of stuttering in the individual in different speaking situations (Packman, 2012; Smith et al., 2010). The P&A model of stuttering is an attempt to address the complex, multifactorial nature of stuttering, including an individual's perceptions and/or reactions to stuttering, which must be addressed in treatment, discussed later in this chapter.

A similar perspective proposed by Anne Smith and colleagues also views stuttering as a multifactorial disorder, where motor, linguistic, and emotional factors interact in complex ways, contributing to the development of stuttering. In addition, the researchers consider the "dynamic" aspects of these neurobehavioral systems during development—or the rapid, nonlinear changes that occur in the speech motor control, language, and emotional regulatory systems when stuttering emerges in young children. This *multifactorial dynamic pathways theory* attempts to describe the critical factors (e.g., genes, experience, environmental influences) contributing to the diagnosis of stuttering in children. It focuses on the interactions of these factors with developing systems over time that lead to recovery from stuttering for most children, but not all. An important goal of the theory, as stated by the researchers, is to motivate research and clinical efforts to better understand how to lead all children toward a path to recovery from stuttering (e.g., Smith & Weber, 2017).

Evaluation of Stuttering

Learning Objective 8.4 List and briefly describe the components of a comprehensive stuttering evaluation.

When parents are concerned that a child is stuttering, the SLP must determine whether there is cause for concern and, if so, to plan an appropriate course of action. Two important components of the evaluation of a child suspected of stuttering are observations of the child speaking and a detailed case history with relevant individuals in the speaker's life, including parents, teachers, other caregivers, and the speakers themselves (Brundage et al., 2021). See Figure 8.1 for some common questions for parents with a disfluent child.

An important component of a stuttering evaluation is a detailed analysis of the child's speech behaviors. The SLP determines the average number of each type of disfluency the child produces (e.g., within-word repetitions, sound prolongations, interjections). More than 10 disfluencies per 100 words spoken may indicate that the child has a fluency problem (Guitar, 2019). The presence of interjections, revisions, and whole-word repetitions tend to be more common in nonstutterers, whereas sound prolongations and part-word repetitions may be more indicative of stuttering. The SLP will also measure the number of units that occur in each repetition or interjection. Recall that more than two repetitions likely represents stuttering versus typical disfluency.

Standardized tests such as the *Stuttering Severity Instrument—Fourth Edition* (SSI-4; Riley, 2009) may also be used in a stuttering evaluation. The SSI-4 may be used with children or adults. This test determines frequency of stuttering measured in percent of syllables stuttered, duration of stuttering moments, and secondary behaviors. An SLP will also record the types of secondary behaviors. A wide variety of secondary behaviors may indicate a progression of the disorder.

CASE STUDY   Dylan *(continued)*

The SSI-4 (Riley, 2009) was administered to Dylan by the graduate student clinician in speech-language pathology at the university clinic. Using this standardized assessment, Dylan's percentage of syllables stuttering on both a reading task and a speaking task were determined. Duration of stuttering was assessed by measuring the length of the three longest stuttering moments and calculating a mean duration. Finally, physical tension and secondary behaviors were observed and counted to derive a "Physical Concomitants" score. In addition to the standardized evaluation, the percentages of syllables stuttered were calculated for speaking tasks that Dylan determined were either low stress or high stress and for speaking situations outside the clinical setting. This enabled the graduate student clinician to obtain a comprehensive picture of Dylan's core stuttering behaviors. The SSI-4 total overall score, as well as disfluent calculations on all other speaking tasks, indicated Dylan had a severe stuttering impairment.

FIGURE 8.1 **Common questions for parents of a disfluent child.**

Introduction

Why are you here today?

Tell us (me) about your child and any concerns you may have.

Medical/Health History

Were there any problems with your pregnancy or with the birth of your child?

Does your child have any medical or health concerns?

Does your child take any medications?

Was your child ever hospitalized?

Family History

Do any other family members have speech, language, or hearing problems?

Did they receive speech therapy?

Does anyone in the family currently stutter or previously stuttered at some point in their life?

Speech/Language and Motor Development

When did your child say their first words?

When did your child say their first phrases and sentences?

Describe your child's motor development.

How does your child's speech-language and motor development compare with their siblings or peers?

History/Description of the Problem

Describe your child's speaking problems.

When did the problem start?

Can you describe your child's disfluencies when they were first noticed?

Have they changed over time?

Is your child aware of their disfluencies?

Do they avoid certain words or avoid talking in certain situations?

Does your child have any excessive body movements when talking?

Have you done anything about your child's disfluency problem?

Have you seen a doctor or other specialist for your child's disfluency problem?

Family Interactions

How does your child get along with siblings or other children?

What is a typical day like for you and your child?

What kinds of things do you do as a family?

Sources: Based on Guitar (2019); Shipley and McAfee (2016).

Determining the child's or adult's feelings and attitudes about stuttering is an essential component of the stuttering evaluation. Informal assessment tools are available for young children through to adulthood for this intended purpose. One such tool for children is the *KiddyCAT Communication Attitude Test for Preschool and Kindergarten Children Who Stutter* (Vanryckeghem & Brutten, 2006), which consists of 12 yes/no questions that the SLP asks the child. An example of a question is "Is talking hard for you?" Research has shown that this questionnaire effectively taps into children's awareness and attitudes about stuttering and can help differentiate children who stutter from their typically fluent peers (e.g., Vanryckeghem et al., 2005).

Similar qualitative assessment questionnaires are available for adolescents and adults also. One such questionnaire is the *Overall Assessment of the Speaker's Experience of Stuttering* (OASES; Yaruss & Quesal, 2006). This assessment tool is for individuals who are 18 years and older and includes four sections: I. General Information, II. Reactions to Stuttering, III. Communication in Daily Situations, and IV. Quality of Life. Its purpose is to determine the overall impact the stuttering impairment has on an individual's life, as well as document changes in more functional communication outcome measures, such as the speaker's difficulties communicating in daily situations, before and after treatment (Yaruss & Quesal, 2006).

CASE STUDY   Dylan *(continued)*

Dylan completed the OASES (Yaruss & Quesal, 2006) so the graduate student clinician could determine his thoughts and feelings about stuttering and how stuttering impacted his daily life. Based on his responses, Dylan views his speech as highly disfluent in most speaking situations and has significant difficulty communicating what he wants to say. He is very concerned about how others will react to his speech and avoids social interactions whenever possible. Stuttering is a factor when making decisions about day-to-day activities, as well as major life decisions (e.g., career). He reports feelings of shame, hopelessness, and depression because of his stuttering. Dylan's responses and overall scores on the OASES indicate a highly negative impact of stuttering on his quality of life.

An SLP's decision to recommend treatment is not based on any single behavior or test result. Certain risk factors associated with persistent stuttering (e.g., family history of persistent stuttering) will play a role in determining the need for immediate treatment. Children exhibiting borderline stuttering (i.e., more than 10 disfluencies per 100 words with no tension or hurry during the first 12 months after onset), with no significant family history, may not need immediate treatment. Rather, following these children and monitoring their disfluencies to ensure stuttering behaviors decrease during that first year may be all that is needed. The following are some risk factors for persistent stuttering in children:

- A family history of one or more relatives who required treatment to recover from persistent stuttering or continues to exhibit persistent stuttering (Ambrose et al., 1997).

- The child is male (Ambrose et al., 1997; Singer et al., 2020).
- Receptive and expressive language, phonological skills, or overall intellectual abilities are below average (Yairi et al., 1996).
- Stress brought on by high expectations for academic, athletic, and social or verbal performance (Guitar, 2019).
- Possibly having a more sensitive temperament, along with greater emotional reactivity to stuttering (Guitar, 2019; Richels & Conture, 2010).

Treatment for Stuttering

Learning Objective 8.5 Describe efficacious treatment approaches for children and adults who stutter.

If the SLP determines that a child has a stuttering problem or a high probability of developing stuttering, therapeutic intervention is indicated. In general, two broad intervention strategies can be used with young children who stutter: indirect treatment and direct treatment. Indirect approaches are considered viable for children who are just beginning to stutter and whose stuttering is mild. Direct approaches are typically reserved for children who have been stuttering for at least a year and who exhibit moderate to severe stuttering.

For older children and adults, treatment focuses on the core stuttering behaviors as well as the affective and cognitive components of stuttering that impact daily life (Yaruss et al., 2012). Treatment also involves education about stuttering to improve the individual's knowledge of the disorder. This allows them to become an effective self-advocate and educate others, including peers, about stuttering, which serves to empower the person who stutters (Coleman et al., 2015; Reardon-Reeves & Yaruss, 2013).

Indirect Treatment

An indirect approach does not explicitly try to modify or change a child's speech fluency; it focuses instead on the child, the child's caregivers and family, and the child's environment. Important aspects of indirect treatment are sharing information and teaching parents to provide a slow, relaxed speech model for the child. Play-oriented activities that encourage slow and relaxed speech are the central component of such intervention. Working with family to decrease anxiety about their child's disfluencies, understand their feelings, modify family–child communicative interactions, and reduce general stresses felt by the child is also central to this approach. There is no explicit discussion about the child's fluent or stuttering speaking behaviors.

The goal of indirect treatment is to facilitate fluency through environmental manipulation. This approach is often effective for younger preschool children over a period of 1–2 months. If stuttering does not decrease within 6 weeks, more direct treatment approaches may be recommended (Guitar, 2019).

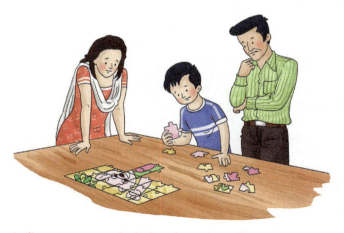

Indirect treatment includes play-oriented activities that encourage slow and relaxed speech.

© Pradip Kumar Bhowal/Pearson India Education Services Pvt. Ltd

Direct Treatment

Direct approaches involve explicit and direct attempts to modify the child's speech and speech-related behaviors. It may also involve teaching the child to stutter more easily (Guitar, 2019).

In direct treatment, concepts such as "hard" and "easy" speech may be introduced. Hard speech is rapid and relatively tense (such as a tense sound prolongation of /s/ in *sssssssss-snake*), whereas easy speech is slow and relaxed. The terms "hard" and "easy" are simple and carry little negative connotation for the child. Children are taught to identify both types of speech, indirectly at first, while the clinician models "hard" and "easy" speech during play interactions and comments about it to the child. Later, the clinician has the child identify these types of speech in their own ongoing productions. Once the child can identify hard and easy speech segments accurately and reliably, the SLP teaches the child strategies that will help increase easy speech and change from hard speech to easy speech when required.

The therapeutic sequence of identification followed by identification/modification forms the core elements of many strategies for children and adults. Other examples of direct evidence-based treatment approaches are provided in Box 8.1 later in this section.

CASE STUDY **Dylan** *(continued)*

When Dylan was 4 years old, he was evaluated by an SLP for parental concerns about his disfluencies. Because he was already showing some negative feelings about his disfluencies, the SLP initiated home-based treatment services with Dylan and his family. The SLP engaged in play activities with Dylan at his home and provided models of "easy stuttering" (Guitar, 2019), in which slow, relaxed repetitions were modeled following his rapid, tense repetitions. In addition, parents were encouraged and shown how to provide empathetic, calming statements to Dylan when he became frustrated about his stuttering. Within a few months, he was making steady progress in treatment.

Soon after, Dylan and his family moved out of state and did not seek further treatment at that time for his stuttering. He continued to show improvement in his speech; however, at the start of second grade, his stuttering suddenly seemed to become worse. He was reevaluated and began treatment with the SLP at his school. Direct treatment focused on reducing physical tension and secondary behaviors (e.g., leg slapping) associated with stuttering and improving negative feelings and reactions to stuttering.

REFLECTION QUESTION 8.3

If a person who stutters no longer exhibited overt stuttering (e.g., sound prolongations, blocks, repetitions), but reported feeling fearful of certain speaking situations or avoiding certain words, would treatment by an SLP still be warranted? Why or why not?

Direct Therapeutic Techniques

Therapeutic techniques designed to modify stuttering behaviors are classified generally into two broad categories: *fluency-shaping techniques* and *stuttering modification techniques*. When used properly, both techniques have a powerful effect in reducing stuttering.

Fluency-shaping techniques involve changing overall speech timing patterns to reduce or eliminate stuttering. This is typically accomplished by lengthening the duration of sounds and words and greatly slowing down overall rate of speech. Stuttering modification techniques involve changing only the stuttering behaviors. This is done by lengthening the duration of or in some way modifying only the speech segment on which the stuttering is occurring. Treatment programs for stuttering often combine these two approaches (Guitar, 2019).

Addressing negative feelings and thoughts related to stuttering and effectively managing negative reactions from others are integral to the direct therapeutic treatment process. This may involve counseling with an SLP trained in cognitive-behavioral therapy techniques (Menzies et al., 2009) and desensitization activities like practicing newly learned fluency-enhancing strategies in feared speaking situations or role-playing to explore potential reactions to bullying or teasing (Coleman et al., 2015).

Fluency-Shaping Techniques

Reducing speech rate, known as **prolonged speech**, is one of the most powerful ways to reduce or eliminate stuttering. Prolonged speech may be a specific therapeutic goal or it may involve use of various techniques that serve to reduce speaking rate and increase fluency. The term *prolonged speech* arose from research conducted in the 1960s regarding the effects of delayed auditory feedback (DAF) on speech production. DAF is a condition in which a speaker hears their own speech after an instrumental delay of some finite period of time, such as 250 or 500 milliseconds. When a person speaks under DAF, their speech is slowed involuntarily because the duration of syllables is prolonged. For example, when people who stutter speak under conditions of DAF, speaking rates decrease dramatically. The longer the delay, the slower the speech. This slowing of speech rate under DAF conditions is accompanied by a substantial decrease in stuttering.

When DAF is used clinically to prolong speech, the feedback delay is set to promote speaking rates of about 30 to 60 syllables per minute. During this initial phase, the person who stutters is taught to prolong the duration of each syllable but not to increase the duration of pauses between syllables (Boburg & Kully, 1995; Max & Caruso, 1997). This prolonged speech pattern is systematically altered over the course of intervention by adjusting the DAF times to reduce the magnitude of syllable prolongation while maintaining fluent speech. Speech rates ranging from 120 to 200 syllables per minute are typical targets for the termination of treatment.

Behavioral techniques that serve not only to reduce speech rate but also reduce physical tension in the speech musculature before and during occurrences of stuttering, promoting smooth speech, are *light articulatory contacts* and *gentle voicing onsets*. The therapeutic use of light articulatory contacts involves instructing the speaker to use less tension in the articulators, particularly during production of stop consonants (/p/, /b/, /t/, /d/, /k/, and /g/) that involve a complete constriction of the vocal tract (Max & Caruso, 1997).

Delayed auditory feedback systems use a microphone and earphones. A person wearing the earphones speaks into the microphone, which transmits the speech to a device that electronically delays sending the speech to the earphones. If the delay were set at 250 milliseconds (or ¼ second), the speaker would hear their utterance ¼ of a second after it was produced. Delaying the auditory feedback causes the speaker to reduce the rate of speaking.

People who stutter frequently use excessive articulator pressure when producing sounds. They may, for example, press the tongue very hard on the roof of the mouth during the production of /t/ and /d/ sounds. Teaching the individual to reduce such pressure, or make light articulatory contacts, promotes fluency.

Reducing articulatory tension is believed to prevent occurrence of prolonged articulatory postures that interfere with smooth articulatory transitions from sound to sound. Light touches promote continuity and ease of articulation by preventing excessive pressure and tension in the articulators (Boburg & Kully, 1995).

Gentle voicing onsets (GVOs) are a cardinal feature of many treatment programs, and they are known by many different names, such as Fluency Initiation of Gestures (FIGS; Cooper, 1984). The basic characteristic of GVOs is a tension-free onset of voicing that gradually builds in intensity. You can appreciate the dynamics of this technique by initiating production of the vowel /a/ in a whisper, gradually engaging the vocal folds such that the vowel is produced with a breathy voice quality, and finally increasing the vowel's intensity. GVOs are typically learned in a hierarchical fashion beginning with vowel production, followed by syllable production, and then word production.

Another powerful fluency-shaping therapeutic intervention consistently found to reduce or eliminate stuttering is response-contingent stimulation (RCS). RCS procedures have their origins in learning theory and are based on B. F. Skinner's behavioral (operant) conditioning paradigm. Operant conditioning results in the association between a behavior (response) and the stimulus that follows (consequence), and thus determines the future occurrence of that behavior.

Response-contingent procedures form the basis of the *Lidcombe Program*, which involves parent-administered verbal contingencies for stutter-free speech (e.g., "That was nice and smooth") and stuttering (e.g., "Oops, that was bumpy"), as well as requests for self-correction (e.g., "Can you say that more smoothly?"). The Lidcombe Program is highly successful in eliminating stuttering in young children, although it remains uncertain which aspects of the program are responsible for its positive effects. It is important that parents are taught to administer the program in the way it is described in the treatment manual; search online for the Lidcombe Program Treatment Guide to find the newest manual available (free) from Mark Onslow and colleagues.

> Effective treatment for stuttering involves addressing both the overt stuttering behaviors (e.g., prolongations, blocks, repetitions), as well as the covert, or more hidden, behaviors associated with stuttering (e.g., shame, hopelessness, fear).

Stuttering Modification Techniques

Unlike the fluency-shaping approach that seeks to reduce or eliminate stuttering by teaching the individual who stutters to speak in a way that prevents stuttering, the stuttering modification approach teaches the person who stutters to react to their stuttering calmly, without unnecessary effort or struggle (Prins & Ingham, 2009). Stuttering modification procedures are based on Charles Van Riper's conceptualization of stuttering as a disruption in speech timing, causing fluency breakdowns and the triggering of negative reactions to such breakdowns.

Three techniques developed by Van Riper work to not only modify speech timing but also modify atypical reactions to stuttering (Prins & Ingham, 2009). They are known as *cancellations*, *pull-outs*, and *preparatory sets*.

These three techniques are introduced therapeutically in sequential order, beginning with stuttering cancellation. During the cancellation phase of treatment, an individual is required to complete the word that was stuttered and pause deliberately following the production of that stuttered word. The individual pauses for a minimum of 3 seconds and then reproduces the stuttered word in slow motion. Stuttering cancellation provides practice with the motoric integration and speech timing movements that are required for a fluent production of that word. When a criterion level of cancellation proficiency is reached, the individual will move to the second technique, known as pull-outs.

> Dr. Charles Van Riper was a distinguished professor of SLP for many years at Western Michigan University. Dr. Van Riper learned to control his stuttering and spent most of his life searching for the cause and cure of stuttering. Intervention techniques that he developed are still in use today.

During the pull-out phase of treatment, the individual does not wait until after the stuttered word is completed to correct the behavior. Rather, the stuttered word is modified during the actual occurrence of the stuttering. This modification involves slowing down the sequential movements of the syllable or word when stuttering occurs, similarly to the slowed and exaggerated movements used in the cancellation phase of treatment. In this way, the individual is modifying the stuttering online, "pulling out" of the stuttering behavior and completing it with a more fluent production of the intended word. Once again, when the individual reaches a criterion level of proficiency, they will move to the last stage, known as preparatory sets.

The preparatory sets stage involves using the slow-motion speech strategies that were learned during the first two phases of treatment, not as a response to an occurrence of stuttering but in anticipation of stuttering. A person who stutters typically knows when and on what word a stuttering moment will occur. When an individual anticipates stuttering, they start preparing to use the newly learned fluency-producing strategies before the word is attempted. The goal of this phase of treatment is to initiate the word in a more fluent manner, even though the individual is producing consecutive speech movements and transitions in a slowed manner.

CASE STUDY Dylan *(continued)*

Halfway through fifth grade, Dylan decided he didn't want to attend speech therapy sessions at school anymore. Bullying and teasing became worse, especially when it came to his stuttering. When he met anyone new for the first time, they would often ask him why he talks the way he does. Although Dylan had learned many different fluency-shaping techniques from the SLP that effectively reduced or eliminated his stuttering, he didn't like how unnatural he sounded when his speech was slower than usual or when he used equal stress on each syllable of every word.

After Dylan was reevaluated at the university clinic as an adult and treatment was recommended, he explained to the graduate student clinician and clinical faculty educator that he wanted to learn to be more accepting of who he was and reduce his shame and embarrassment about his stuttering. Dylan also wanted to stutter in a more open, "acceptable" fashion and not shy away from social interactions or careers that might expose his stuttering.

Cognitive-Behavioral Therapy Techniques

Counseling individuals who stutter is an important part of the therapy process to address negative thoughts, feelings, and reactions to stuttering. While not readily apparent to the communication partner, physical tension, anxiety, and fear are all part of the overall experience of the moment of stuttering (Tichenor & Yaruss, 2019). Cognitive-behavioral therapy, a psychotherapy approach, can help restructure negative thought patterns by eliminating atypical behaviors and replacing them with more positive patterns of behavior (Mustofa, 2010; Palasik & Hannan, 2013).

Techniques such as attitude modification with effective self-talk to support fluency skills, increasing awareness and confrontation of cognitive-emotional concerns, and practicing communication in social skills training have been found to be effective with adolescents and adults who stutter (Kully et al., 2003). Recent research on an automated Internet cognitive-behavioral treatment program that requires no clinician contact shows promise in addressing social anxiety in adults who stutter (Menzies et al., 2019).

Selecting Intervention Techniques

An SLP's selection of a specific management technique depends on many factors, including the individual's age, severity of the stuttering problem, the motivation and specific needs of the person who stutters including psychosocial variables, and the SLP's knowledge of the specific techniques available. Careful and detailed observation of an individual's stuttering behaviors before initiating treatment and during the treatment process is essential to successful clinical management of stuttering.

> **CASE STUDY**   **Dylan** (*continued*)
>
> Dylan's treatment program at the university clinic included practice with stuttering modification strategies (e.g., cancellations) to enable him to stutter less severely, along with the strategy of "self-disclosure." This strategy involved having him tell new communication partners in certain speaking situations that he is a person who stutters. Self-disclosure has been shown to positively influence listeners' perceptions of individuals who stutter (e.g., Byrd et al., 2017).
>
> During the student-teaching experience, Dylan self-disclosed his stuttering to school personnel and his high school students by stating, "Hi, my name is Mr. Madden, and I am a person who stutters. You might hear me repeat words or prolong sounds when I speak, but if at any time you don't understand me, please let me know and I'll be happy to say it again." This strategy eased his anxiety about speaking in front of his class and eliminated his avoidance behaviors. Dylan also participated in a self-directed e-therapy cognitive-behavioral treatment program. The online program was individualized using pretreatment assessments about his negative thoughts, feelings, and reactions toward stuttering, as well as specific feared situations (Menzies et al., 2019). Dylan was provided access to the treatment website and completed all modules of the program at home over the course of 6 months.

Effectiveness of Stuttering Intervention through the Lifespan

Determining the effectiveness of stuttering treatment depends largely on how *effectiveness* is defined. This is a complex issue. Treatment for stuttering might be considered *effective* if it resulted in the person being able to speak with disfluencies within typical limits whenever and to whomever they chose, without undue concern or anxiety about speaking (Conture, 1996). The treatment of stuttering differs across an individual's lifespan in terms of frequency, nature, and rates of recovery. Therefore, the review of treatment efficacy is best considered relative to age group: preschool, school-age children, teenagers, and adults. Several treatment approaches and/or techniques are briefly reviewed in Box 8.1.

> ## BOX 8.1 Evidence-Based Practices for Individuals with Stuttering
>
> **Specific Behavioral Treatment Approaches or Techniques**
>
> - Indirect treatment approaches that teach parents to reduce their conversational speaking rate have been shown to facilitate fluent speech in preschool children.
> - The long-term effectiveness of the parent-administered behavioral intervention, the *Lidcombe Program*, is well established, particularly for preschool children. Parents are taught to provide positive praise for their child's fluent speech by saying, "Good job, that was nice and smooth" and to acknowledge or correct stuttered speech by saying, "Oops, that was bumpy, can you say _____ again." The program recommends more verbal contingencies for stutter-free speech than stuttered speech.
> - Syllable-timed-speech (STS) is a promising treatment approach for school-age children who stutter. With STS, the child is taught to place equal stress on each syllable in a sentence (e.g., "My-cat's-name-is-Ti-a") while using their typical speech rate and intonation. This technique is practiced during daily conversations with the parent or caregiver.
> - A program of gradual increase in length and complexity of utterances, called GILCO, in which a child progresses from one-word stutter-free responses to 5 minutes of stutter-free speech during reading, monologue speaking, and conversation has been found to be highly effective with older children.
> - Prolonged speech techniques (e.g., prolonging syllable durations; use of light articulatory contacts or GVOs) have been found to be highly effective with older children and adults, particularly when taught in the context of a
> structured program with opportunities for daily practice. No one technique has been found to be effective on its own, however.
> - Smooth speech, a derivative of prolonged speech, uses multiple strategies (i.e., pausing/phrasing, GVOs, light articulatory contacts) to first slow speech rate and prolong syllables and then increase speech rate to typical levels. This approach has been shown to be effective with older children and adolescents who stutter and tends to result in more natural-sounding speech and so may be preferred over other prolonged speech treatments.
> - Response Contingent Time-Out (RCTO) from speaking is based on behavioral (operant) conditioning and involves the individual pausing briefly from speaking immediately after a stuttering event. RCTO is highly effective in reducing stuttering in adolescents and adults. Usually, the SLP tells the individual to stop speaking after an instance of stuttering; however, individuals can be taught to self-deliver a time-out from speaking following a self-identified stuttering moment.
> - Cognitive-behavioral therapy strategies, widely used in clinical psychology, can be learned and applied by SLPs. These strategies have been shown to effectively decrease social anxiety and reduce avoidance in adults who stutter.
> - A program on stuttering education and bullying awareness and prevention for third- through sixth-grade children delivered by classroom teachers was successful in improving students' knowledge and attitudes about children who stutter. More research is needed to determine the overall effectiveness and long-term benefits of this program for school-age children who stutter.

Sources: Based on Andrews et al. (2012); Bothe et al. (2006); Conture and Yaruss (2009); Craig et al. (1996); Ellis and Beltyukova (2012); Guitar (2019); Hewat et al. (2006); Iverach et al. (2017); Langevin and Narashimha Prasad (2012); Menzies et al. (2009); Nippold and Packman (2012); Nye et al. (2013); Packman et al. (2015); Ryan (1974); Ryan and Van Kirk Ryan (1995); Sawyer et al. (2017).

Efficacy of Intervention with Preschool-Age Children

In general, the findings of most recent studies are quite encouraging and indicate the potential benefits of early diagnosis and treatment of stuttering. Indirect and direct treatment approaches for preschool children have both been found to be effective (Franken et al., 2005) and may be even more effective when combined

(Gottwald, 2010). Among preschool-age children enrolled in a parent-conducted intervention program, all maintained their fluent speech in long-term clinical follow-up studies after dismissal from treatment (e.g., Jones et al., 2008; Lincoln & Onslow, 1997).

Efficacy of Intervention with School-Age Children

Research has shown that the various treatment approaches and techniques available for school-age children who stutter are effective in establishing fluent speech; however, the child's ability to use these techniques in different settings and maintain improvements in fluent speech over time appears to be problematic (Yaruss & Pelczarski, 2007). With school-age children, it is important to address the psychosocial aspects of stuttering—namely, the fear, anxiety, avoidance, and other negative reactions commonly associated with stuttering—for treatment to be effective in the long term (Yaruss et al., 2012).

Efficacy of Intervention with Adolescents and Adults

Teenagers who stutter can be difficult to manage clinically; establishing a collaborative relationship based in trust and mutual respect is essential to success with this population (Zebrowski & Wolf, 2011). Similarly, a positive client–clinician relationship has also been shown to contribute to successful treatment outcomes in adults who stutter (e.g., Plexico et al., 2010). In addition, a wide variety of adult stuttering treatment techniques have been investigated, ranging from behavioral conditioning techniques to participation in self-help support groups. Collectively, these studies suggest a 60–80% improvement rate, regardless of the therapeutic technique used. Treatment that addresses negative feelings and attitudes, in addition to establishing fluency, is more effective than treatment that just focuses on speech alone.

In summary, stuttering intervention across all age groups results in an average improvement for about 70% of all cases, with preschool-age children improving more quickly and easily than people who have a longer history with stuttering. The clinical research that we have considered indicates that effective treatment of stuttering involves a comprehensive approach that considers the broader consequences of stuttering, in addition to the observable stuttering behaviors.

The Effects of Stuttering through the Lifespan

Evidence suggests that stuttering affects the ability to communicate and participate in life situations from an early age (Millard & Davis, 2016). More than 50% of disfluent preschool children are aware of their stuttering and develop negative feelings about their speech. As a result, they may use more gestures to communicate or withdraw from play interactions with peers (Boey et al., 2009; Langevin et al., 2009). School-age children who stutter are more likely to be bullied, teased, viewed negatively by peers, and less likely to be nominated as leaders (Davis et al., 2002). Reduced classroom participation and poorer academic achievement are also more common in children who stutter compared to their nonstuttering peers (e.g., Daniels et al., 2012).

The educational and personal disadvantages stuttering may impose on a young person do not end when the child leaves school. Stuttering can also have a negative impact in the workplace and is a vocationally disabling condition because employers view it as a disorder that decreases employability and opportunities for promotion (Hurst & Cooper, 1983; Palasik et al., 2012). However, employers' perceptions of adults who stutter improved for those who sought treatment for their stuttering compared with those who did not. This enhanced perception is further reflected by increased numbers of job promotions among employees who sought treatment and were successful in maintaining fluency following treatment (Craig & Calvert, 1991).

Stuttering has a potentially negative effect on an individual's emotional well-being and overall quality of life (Boyle, 2015). Individuals who stutter tend to withdraw from people and social situations due to their fear and embarrassment about their stuttering, thereby causing social isolation and reduced social support networks. There is also a high rate of social anxiety among individuals who stutter (Iverach & Rapee, 2014). Consequently, individuals who stutter are more prone to anxiety, depression, and negative affect. Encouraging individuals who stutter to engage in social activity, and helping them accept who they are, is integral to the treatment process.

Summary

Stuttering is a disabling condition primarily characterized by sound and syllable repetitions and sound prolongations that interrupt the smooth forward flow of speech. Stuttering is a universal problem that affects males more than females. In most cases, stuttering appears between the ages of 2 to 4 years, and as the disorder progresses it increases in severity. Stuttering can adversely affect an individual's school performance, employment, and social interactions. The treatment of stuttering is most effective when it is initiated in early childhood, although treatment at any age can reduce stuttering. Successful treatment approaches, particularly for older children and adults, address both the overt (e.g., prolongations; blocks) and covert (e.g., fear, shame, anxiety) behaviors associated with stuttering.

Various theories and integrative frameworks have been proposed to explain the onset and development of stuttering. The exact cause of stuttering, and our understanding of why most children recover from stuttering while some persist, is still largely unknown. Pinpointing the exact cause of stuttering will undoubtedly require expertise from many specialists, including speech-language pathologists, neurolinguists, geneticists, and medical specialists.

Epilogue   Case Study: Dylan

Dylan completed his student-teaching experience successfully and was hired by the school as an environmental science teacher. His dream of becoming a high school teacher came to fruition, something Dylan never thought possible.

Reflections | from an Expert Speech Researcher in the Area of Stuttering: Dr. Ehud Yairi

1. *Why/how did you become a speech-language pathologist?*

   Actually, my interest in becoming a professional speech pathologist was inspired relatively late in life. During high school, living in a farm community and milking cows in the afternoons, I was interested in agriculture and veterinary medicine. During my military service, I also entertained the idea of extending my expertise in explosives and mines to civilian usage.

   When these early aspirations could not be materialized, my interests shifted to very different fields and options, ending up majoring in psychology and African studies at Tel Aviv University in Israel. In 1964, when I was a senior in the Department of Psychology, one important assignment was writing a serious term paper on a topic of our choice. Being afflicted with rather severe stuttering since early childhood (others in my expanded family also stuttered), I chose stuttering as my topic. An intensive literature search at several universities as well as other libraries revealed very few resources. Among them was Wendell Johnson et al.'s (1948) book, *Speech Handicapped School Children*. Johnson's chapter on stuttering, especially his diagnosogenic theory, as well as learning that such a famous leader in the field was a stutterer, left an overwhelming impression on me. Thus, the idea of becoming a speech clinician despite my stuttering was born.

   I immediately wrote to Johnson at the University of Iowa and was happy to receive his lengthy, very kind reply. In September 1965, just a few months later, I arrived at the world-renowned University of Iowa Department of Speech Pathology and Audiology and began graduate studies. Unfortunately, Johnson had died a short three weeks earlier, depriving me of the opportunity of meeting him.

2. *What advice might you give to students interested in pursuing a clinical expertise in this area someday in the future?*

   Choosing a professional career as a clinician in the field of speech-language pathology should involve an honest, thoughtful process. First, be highly informed of what you might be getting into. Hence, obtain a good general knowledge of the wide scope of practice involving speech and language disorders. You will discover, for example, that these range from delayed language problems to severe speech disorders resulting from medical conditions such as cleft palate and laryngectomy [the surgical removal of the larynx]. These affect people across a very wide age range. Perhaps you have never encountered individuals who exhibit some of these conditions, or even heard of them.

   Next, educate yourself about the different types of jobs settings available in the field where services to people with such diverse disorders are provided, demands for clinicians, workloads, salary ranges, etc. Ask yourself, are you prepared to spend your working years in the school setting? In hospital settings? Other types of clinics? With preschool-age children? With the geriatric population? etc.

Now, if you are still inclined to enter this profession because of a desire to be a clinician who "helps people," be advised from the outset that the profession involves much more than providing therapy. Good clinicians must also understand why they do what they do. What is the theory or rationale behind a specific clinical approach? What are the relevant scientific findings? Then, be able to clearly communicate this knowledge to clients and their families, as well as to other professionals. You also must tailor what you know and what you do in assessment and treatment to the real-life communication needs of your clients.

Furthermore, clients and their families confront clinicians with questions about what they believe or have heard about the disorder of concern. For example, "Is it true that stuttering is caused by brain damage?" "Is it true that stuttering is psychological?" "Is it true that stuttering is genetic?" Therefore, once they obtain a degree in speech and language disorders, clinicians must keep up with updated scientific literature to be able to respond intelligently and professionally to such questions and to adjust their treatment accordingly.

Finally, there are several assets of good clinicians you should strive to nurture (and these can be developed if you are not naturally endowed with them). Among these is the constant self-reminder to *respect* the clients who seek your help, as well as their perspectives about their expressed problems, regardless of what you may not like, or with which you disagree, when you meet them. Of course, *empathy* for your clients is another essential asset. That is, the ability to put yourself in your client's place, imagining what that person is feeling and their beliefs about the nature of the problem. This is only possible when you take the time to listen to and endeavor to understand, to the best of your ability, their individual perspectives. Personally, with the passage of time, as I have encountered many clients who stuttered and/or their concerned parents, I noticed a decrease in my sensitivity to their plight and had to constantly remind myself to stay on guard. My point: Be honest with yourself with all these issues when considering the field of speech-language pathology as your potential professional career.

Suggested Readings/Sources

Bothe, A., Davidow, J., Bramlett, R., & Ingham, R. (2006). Stuttering treatment research 1970–2005: I. Systematic review incorporating trial quality assessment of behavioral, cognitive, and related approaches. *American Journal of Speech-Language Pathology, 15*, 321–341.

Guitar, B. (2019). *Stuttering: An integrated approach to its nature and treatment* (5th ed). Wolters Kluwer.

Menzies, R., Packman, A., Onslow, M., O'Brian, S., Jones, M., & Dögg Helgadóttir, F. (2019). In-clinic and standalone internet cognitive behavior therapy treatment for social anxiety in stuttering: A randomized trial of iGlebe. *Journal of Speech, Language, and Hearing Research, 62*, 1614–1624.

Prins, D., & Ingham, R. (2009). Evidence-based treatment and stuttering—Historical perspective. *Journal of Speech, Language, and Hearing Research, 52*, 254–263.

Tichenor, S., & Yaruss, S. (2019). Stuttering as defined by adults who stutter. *Journal of Speech, Language, and Hearing Research, 62*, 4356–4369.

9 Voice and Resonance Disorders

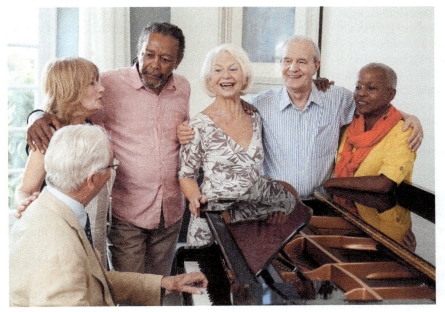

© Shutterstock

Learning Objectives

When you have finished this chapter, you should be able to:

9.1 Explain the normal processes of phonation and resonance.

9.2 Briefly describe voice and resonance disorders and describe the classification system for voice disorders.

9.3 Describe the primary components of a voice and resonance evaluation.

9.4 Describe the major goals of voice and resonance treatment and effective voice and resonance treatment approaches and techniques.

> " Perhaps the reason I studied speech-language pathology is because at age 14, I was diagnosed with bilateral vocal nodules. At that time in my life, I was the wannabe cheerleader yelling at every school sporting event. Many times, I was mistaken for a male on the phone or told I had a "sexy froglike voice." I didn't pursue treatment when I was younger. I only received treatment when my esteemed professor in graduate school told me it was important that I receive voice therapy for the health and safety of my voice, especially since I would be using my voice daily in my chosen career.
>
> At age 14, I never would have imagined myself working with clients with similar voice issues. It's interesting how my early circumstances turned into helping others manage and understand their voice disorder. Having a voice disorder allows me greater empathy for my clients and has led me and many of my clients on a journey of self-discovery. I wouldn't have it any other way.
>
> *–Sherril Howard, an SLP expert in voice disorders*

Voice is our primary means of emotional and linguistic expression and is an essential feature of the uniquely human attribute known as speech (Boone et al., 2010; Titze, 1994). Your voice reflects gender, personality, personal habits, age, and the general condition of your health. Research has shown that certain characteristics of the voice help listeners infer

CASE STUDY   Blake

Blake is 15 years old and currently a sophomore in high school. He was born with 22q11.2 deletion syndrome (22q11.2 DS), also known as velocardiofacial syndrome (VCFS). 22q11.2 DS is the most common microscopic (or submicroscopic) chromosomal deletion syndrome where a tiny piece of genetic material on chromosome 22 is missing. 22q11.2 DS is also the most common genetic cause of cleft palate (Robin & Shprintzen, 2005). In addition to velopharyngeal insufficiency, laryngeal abnormalities are also common (e.g., vocal fold paralysis secondary to cardiac surgery). Blake had a complex medical history that included multiple heart surgeries between 1 and 3 years of age to correct severe cardiac malformations

and surgical repair of a submucous cleft palate (i.e., levator veli palatini muscle is separated but overlying mucosa is intact) at 6 years of age.

As you read the chapter, think about:

- The impact of Blake's complex medical history on his communication development
- The collaborative team approach to assessing and treating clients with complex medical needs like Blake
- The importance of having a strong foundation in anatomy and physiology of the voice and speech mechanism to accurately diagnose and effectively treat clients like Blake

psychosocial traits about the speaker such as friendliness and trustworthiness (e.g., McAleer et al., 2014). Your voice is an emotional outlet that mirrors your moods, attitudes, and general feelings. You can express anger by shouting and express affection by speaking softly. These types of vocal expression have great potential to evoke emotional responses from a listener.

Resonance refers to the quality of the voice that is produced from sound vibrations in the pharyngeal, oral, and nasal cavities. Recall from Chapter 3 that sound energy produced by the vibrating vocal folds travels through the vocal tract, an acoustic resonator that serves to enhance or reduce certain frequencies of that sound. Thus, the size and shape of the pharynx, oral cavity, and nasal cavity will directly affect the perceived sound, or quality of your voice.

In addition, the velopharyngeal mechanism, responsible for coupling and decoupling the oral and nasal cavities during speech and swallowing, regulates sound energy and air pressure in the oral and nasal cavities (Kummer, 2011a; Kummer & Lee, 1996). Recall that the production of most speech sounds requires the velum to be elevated to prevent air from escaping through the nose. Velopharyngeal closure also ensures adequate air pressure buildup in the oral cavity to produce high-pressure consonants (e.g., /p/, b/, /s/). Failure of the velopharyngeal mechanism to separate the oral and nasal cavities during speech production and swallowing is called **velopharyngeal dysfunction (VPD)**. VPD is a frequent result of malformations of the hard and soft palate early in embryonic development.

In this chapter, we extend some of the basic concepts related to normal voice and resonance, as well as discuss disorders of voice associated with structural pathologies, neurological disorders, and psychological and stress conditions. We also discuss disorders of resonance related to *craniofacial anomalies*, or congenital malformations involving the head and face (i.e., cleft palate). Finally, we discuss assessment, treatment, treatment efficacy issues, and evidence-based practices as they pertain to voice and resonance.

Normal Voice and Resonance Production

Learning Objective 9.1 Explain the normal processes of phonation and resonance.

As discussed in Chapter 3, production of normal voice depends on the integrity of the phonatory system (e.g., larynx), while normal resonance depends on the opening and closing of the velopharyngeal port. The physiologic and perceptual correlates of normal voice and resonance are discussed in the following section.

Vocal Pitch

Recall from Chapter 3 that speech production begins with phonation, or sound produced by vocal fold vibration. Fundamental frequency is associated with the speed of vocal fold vibration and is measured in **hertz (Hz)**, or the number of complete vibrations per second.

The perceptual correlate of fundamental frequency is *pitch*. For example, on average, adult men have fundamental frequencies of around 125 Hz (the vocal folds open and close 125 times per second), whereas adult women have fundamental frequencies around 250 Hz. On average, male voices are perceived as lower in pitch compared to female voices. The fundamental frequency of young children's voices can be as high as 500 Hz, resulting in a very high-pitched voice. The difference in vocal fundamental frequency (and resulting vocal pitch) among men, women, and children is due largely to the structure of the vocal folds themselves. The structural changes of the vocal folds and the relationship to vocal fundamental frequency through the lifespan are summarized in Table 9.1.

During one complete vibratory cycle of vocal fold vibration, the vocal folds move from a closed or adducted position to an open or abducted position and back to the closed position. Figure 9.1 depicts the normal vocal folds in the abducted position during endotracheal intubation.

FIGURE 9.1 Normal, healthy vocal folds in abducted (open) position during endotracheal intubation.

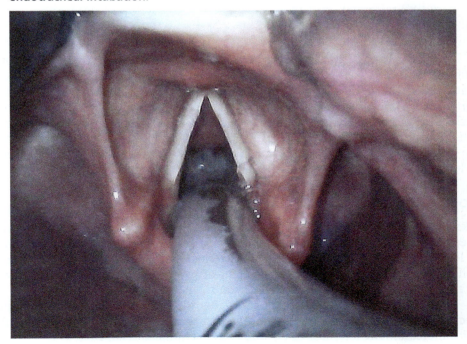

(Photograph courtesy of Steven R. Knight)

TABLE 9.1

Summary of Laryngeal Development and Fundamental Frequency Characteristics through the Lifespan

Time	Structural Development	Fundamental Frequency
Birth	Larynx positioned high in the neck close to the hyoid bone; vocal fold length is 4–6 mm. Laryngeal framework is soft and pliable. Vocal fold composition is homogenous and undifferentiated in the newborn.	Average is about 500 Hz with high variability
Childhood	Vocal folds double in length to about 8–9 mm in both sexes. Interior of the larynx becomes less pliable.	About 200 to 300 Hz in both males and females
Puberty	Increases to about 12–17 mm in girls and 15–25 mm in boys. Structural makeup of the vocal folds becomes adult-like beginning around 16 years of age.	Large, downward change in males to about 130 Hz; much less downward change in females
Adulthood	Vocal fold length is about 17–29 mm in men, and 12.5–21 mm in women.	Males' average is 125 Hz; females' average is 250 Hz

Sources: Based on Hixon, Weismer, & Hoit (2014); Kent (1997).

Although individuals have a habitual speaking frequency (average pitch), the frequency of the voice constantly varies during speech production. A monotonous or **monopitch** voice is the result of not varying the habitual speaking frequency during speech production. People who use a monotone voice may not be interesting to listen to, and listeners may quickly lose interest.. Varying the pitch of the voice also has linguistic significance. Consider these two sentences:

Macy is an artist.

Macy is an artist?

The words in these two sentences are identical, but the sentences' meanings are quite different. "Macy is an artist" is a statement of fact (a declarative), whereas "Macy is an artist?" is a question (an interrogative). Say those two sentences out loud, paying particular attention to what happens to your pitch at the end of each sentence. For the declarative, the pitch of your voice will decrease or fall off as you are saying the word *artist*. In contrast, for the interrogative, the pitch of your voice will increase when you are saying the word *artist*. How do you change the pitch of the voice? Modifications in length and tension of the vocal folds are necessary to produce pitch changes.

Vocal Loudness

Like changing the pitch of the voice, changing vocal loudness is also necessary for adequate communication. **Monoloudness**, or a voice that lacks normal variations of loudness that occur during speech, may reflect an inability to change loudness voluntarily due to neurological impairment or psychological disability, or it may be merely a habit associated with the person's personality.

Vocal loudness is the perceptual correlate of intensity, which is measured in **decibels (dB)**. In general, as vocal intensity increases, the perceived loudness of the voice increases. The loudness of normal conversational speech, such as conversations at the dinner table, averages around 60 dB. Changes in vocal intensity require the vocal folds to stay together longer during the closed phase of vibration, but alveolar pressure is the major determinant of vocal intensity (Hixon et al., 2020; Zemlin, 1998). As discussed in Chapter 3, alveolar pressure is the pressure placed on the vocal folds by the lungs. Every time alveolar pressure doubles, there is an 8 to 12 dB increase in vocal intensity.

The *Guinness Book of World Records* reports that the loudest scream ever recorded was produced at 123.2 dB, and a man named Anthony Fieldhouse won the World Shouting Contest with a yell that was registered at 112.4 dB (Kent, 1997). Unless you are a record seeker, this kind of behavior is not recommended, as we see later in this chapter.

Voice Quality

Voice quality is a perceptual attribute related to the sound of the voice that is difficult to quantify like fundamental frequency or vocal intensity (Behrman, 2007; Titze, 1994). The unique traits of an individual's voice quality are derived from the anatomy of the larynx, the shape of the vocal tract, and its resonant characteristics. Suprasegmental aspects of speech such as rate and rhythm can also alter the way the vocal folds vibrate. Therefore, voice quality is based on genetics (e.g., laryngeal anatomy is partially determined at birth) and learned behaviors (e.g., how fast or slow you talk) (Titze, 1994).

Lifespan Issues

After the structure and function of the larynx reach full maturity in early adulthood, it continues to change with age, causing functional changes in the voice. For instance, beginning in the third decade for men and the fourth decade for women, some of the laryngeal cartilages and joints begin to ossify, or turn to bone, while others calcify, or turn to salt, causing the larynx to become stiff and brittle (Hixon et al., 2020). Changes in pulmonary function, neuromuscular properties of intrinsic muscles, and vocal fold tissue also occur with advancing age. These changes can result in reduced movement of laryngeal structures in older individuals and interfere with the ability of the vocal folds to fully come together during phonation (Kahane, 1988). Age-related changes to the larynx can lead to **presbyphonia**, a voice disorder characterized by perceptual changes in pitch, pitch range, loudness, and voice quality in the voice of older individuals. The voice of someone with presbyphonia may sound weak, hoarse, breathy, and unsteady (e.g., Sauder et al., 2010).

Hormonal changes with age are associated with vocal changes for both women and men (Kirgezen et al., 2017). As mentioned in Chapter 3, fundamental frequency gets lower in women and higher in men with advancing age. After menopause, vocal folds thicken, and they have increased *edema* or swelling due to an accumulation of fluid. Age-related declines in testosterone in men contribute to thinning of the vocal fold tissue. Thickening and thinning of the vocal folds are believed to contribute to fundamental frequency changes in women and men with age (Abitbol et al., 1999; Pontes et al., 2005). Age effects on the larynx tend to be more pronounced in men due to laryngeal muscle **atrophy**, or loss of tissue. This results in a decrease in the overall mass of the vocal folds that increases fundamental frequency. We perceive this as a higher-pitched voice commonly heard in elderly men (Hixon et al., 2014; Hirano et al., 1989; Kahane, 1987).

Check out the National Center for Voice & Speech website at www.ncvs.org and go to "Education" to access some interesting videos on normal voice production, voice simulation, and the importance of taking care of the voice.

Because hormones differentially affect men and women's voices throughout the lifespan, voice therapy programs developed for typical or disordered voice in older individuals should consider sex differences in their design (Lenell et al., 2019).

> **REFLECTION QUESTION 9.1**
>
> *How might vocal training with a speech-language pathologist improve voice function in individuals with age-related voice changes or disorders?*

Resonance

The sound produced by the vibrating vocal folds would not result in a rich, full, or loud enough voice without the additional component of resonance (Boone et al., 2010). Normal resonance is largely determined by the velopharyngeal structures and the adequacy of their function. Structures of the velopharyngeal mechanism include the velum (soft palate), the lateral pharyngeal walls, and the posterior pharyngeal wall. Velopharyngeal closure is achieved by the combined action of velar elevation in a flaplike fashion and movement of the lateral pharyngeal walls and posterior pharyngeal wall in a sphincter-like fashion. The velopharyngeal port remains open most of the time to allow for nasal breathing. It is also open for production of the nasal consonants (i.e., *m*, *n*, *ng*) but must achieve complete or nearly complete closure for production of oral speech sounds (Hixon et al., 2020).

Lifespan Issues

Velopharyngeal closure patterns vary among individuals and can change over time with age. For instance, young children with enlarged adenoids may achieve velopharyngeal closure via elevation of the velum against the adenoid mass. If an adenoidectomy is performed, the child may experience hypernasal-sounding speech, or speech that sounds like it is resonating through the nasal cavity, following the surgery. Luckily, most children undergo a natural reorganization of their systems during development such that velopharyngeal closure patterns slowly begin to involve movement of the pharyngeal walls to accommodate for the lack of adenoid tissue (Hixon et al., 2020). From young adulthood through to advanced age, velopharyngeal function during speech production remains intact and unchanged (Hoit et al., 1994).

CASE STUDY **Blake** *(continued)*

Blake received speech-language therapy from infancy through middle school for receptive and expressive language disorders, speech sound production deficits (including childhood apraxia of speech), and hypernasality. When he started high school, he had accommodations for residual learning difficulties (e.g., small-group instruction; visual aids; repetition of information) and strategies to ensure others understood his overall message (e.g., use of gestures when speaking; talking louder; indicating a change in conversational topic).

As Blake began 10th grade, some of his teachers noticed that he seemed anxious and withdrawn.

When they talked to him, he said there seemed to be more group presentation projects expected this year. He was worried about how his peers might feel about presenting with him in a group. Blake still had residual voice and resonance disorders and was concerned about what others might think.

Blake's teachers asked if he might want to see the speech-language pathologist (SLP) at his high school to address concerns about his voice and hypernasality. He agreed to meet with her at the end of the school day to discuss possible options to improve his voice quality and reduce his hypernasal resonance.

Disorders of Voice and Resonance

Learning Objective 9.2 Briefly describe voice and resonance disorders and describe the classification system for voice disorders.

Voice disorders are characterized by deviations in voice quality, pitch, and/or loudness resulting from disordered laryngeal, respiratory, and/or vocal tract functioning. Approximately 1 in 13 adults in the United States will experience a voice disorder each year, but only a small percentage (10%) will seek treatment (Bhattacharyya, 2014).

In children 3–10 years of age, the prevalence of voice disorders is about 6%, with boys affected more often than girls (Black et al., 2015; Carding et al., 2006). It is believed that children with voice disorders may be underidentified or underserved despite data suggesting a relatively high prevalence of pediatric voice disorders. Most standardized speech-language screenings and evaluations do not provide enough opportunities to correctly identify vocal abnormalities. Additionally, many school-based SLPs report a lack of confidence in treating voice disorders in children (Childes et al., 2017).

Specific vocal behaviors such as loud talking, coughing, or throat clearing may predispose some individuals to voice disorders (Titze, 1994). Certain occupational groups like teachers and singers, who regularly engage in vocally intense activities, are also more prone to voice disorders. Teachers are two to three times more likely to develop a voice disorder compared to the general population (Martins et al., 2014). Risk factors for teachers include working more than 40 hours per week, high student numbers per class, environmental noise, inappropriate classroom facilities (e.g., classroom dryness; echo), and teaching fourth grade or below (e.g., Byeon, 2019). Similarly, singers are likely to report voice disorders regardless of singing style or skills (Pestana et al., 2017). While singers represent less than 1% of the workforce in the United States, it is estimated that 11.5–29% of those who seek voice treatment are singers (Kridgen, 2019; Titze et al., 1997).

Pediatric and adult voice disorders are quite varied and can be associated with vocal misuse or abuse behaviors, neurological disorders, psychological conditions, or some combination of these factors. Perceptual signs of a voice disorder are related to specific characteristics of a person's voice and are evaluated by the SLP.

Clinically, perceptual signs in conjunction with a person's case history serve as the initial benchmarks in the differential diagnosis of a voice disorder. When one or more perceptual aspects of voice such as pitch, loudness, or voice quality are outside the typical range for an individual's age, sex, cultural background, or geographic location, we say a voice disorder exists (Boone et al., 2010).

Individuals who access voice treatment services for gender-affirming or transgender care do not exhibit a voice disorder but a voice difference. Voice and communication therapy are critical in supporting individuals to develop voice and communication that best reflect their gender identity and expression (Russell & Abrams, 2019). The role of the SLP in gender-affirming care is discussed throughout this chapter.

Classification of Voice Disorders

Several different classification schemes exist to characterize voice disorders (cf. Stemple, 2007; Verdolini et al., 2006). Here we classify voice disorders into two distinct categories: *organic*, which have an underlying physical or neurological basis, and *functional*, which manifest as the result of vocal misuse or abuse and/or psychological factors (e.g., stress) but do not result in changes in structure. Voice disorders can overlap, however. For instance, vocal misuse or abuse (functional etiology) can lead to structural abnormalities such as vocal fold lesions (organic consequence). For our purposes here, we discuss structural abnormalities at the level of the larynx as "organic" disorders and voice disturbances that do not alter laryngeal structure as "functional" disorders.

Organic Voice Disorders

Two types of organic voice disorders can occur: those associated with structural changes or abnormalities of the laryngeal mechanism and those associated with neurological disorders. As mentioned previously, physical changes to the larynx can result from aging (e.g., laryngeal muscle atrophy; cartilage ossification) or structural abnormalities (e.g., vocal fold lesions), both of which negatively impact voice. Neurological disorders, on the other hand, interfere with normal vocal fold vibration as the result of damage to central or peripheral nervous system substrates that control laryngeal functioning. The following sections describe some of the more common structural abnormalities of the larynx, along with neurological disorders that result in deviations in voice quality, pitch, and loudness.

Structural Abnormalities Resulting in Voice Disorders

As stated, structural abnormalities of the laryngeal mechanism result in disordered voice, or **dysphonia**. In the following sections, we discuss etiologies and primary voice symptoms of common structural abnormalities of the phonatory system, including:

- Vocal nodules
- Vocal polyps
- Contact ulcers and granulomas
- Laryngitis
- Papillomas
- Webs
- Cancer

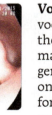

Pearson eTextbook
Video Example 9.1
This video is of a child with bilateral vocal fold nodules.

Vocal Nodules. Vocal nodules are a common vocal fold pathology secondary to vocal misuse or abuse. Nodules are localized growths on the medial edge between the anterior one-third and posterior two-thirds of the vocal folds, the point of maximal contact during vocal fold vibration (Stemple et al., 2018). They are generally bilateral (appearing on both vocal folds), although they can appear on only one vocal fold (see Figure 9.2). Nodules are soft and pliable early in their formation. Over time they become hard and fibrous, interfering significantly with vocal fold vibration.

Nodules occur frequently in male and female children who engage in vocally abusive behaviors such as excessive loud talking or screaming (Stemple et al., 2018). They are the most frequent cause of pediatric dysphonia (Martins et al., 2016). Nodules occur more frequently in adult women than men, possibly due to susceptibility of the female larynx to hormonal effects (Chagnon & Stone, 1996).

The primary perceptual voice symptoms of vocal nodules are *hoarseness*, or a rough-sounding voice, and **breathiness**, or the perception of audible air escaping

FIGURE 9.2 Unilateral vocal fold nodule.

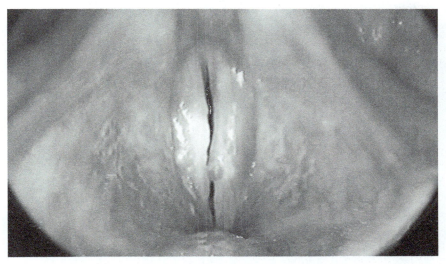

Photograph courtesy of Robert Orlikoff, East Carolina University, Greenville, NC.

through the glottis during phonation due to inadequate glottal closure during vocal fold vibration. People who have vocal nodules may complain of soreness in the throat and an inability to use the upper third of their pitch range.

Vocal Polyps. Vocal polyps, like vocal nodules, are caused by trauma to the vocal folds associated with vocal misuse or abuse. Polyps develop when blood vessels in the vocal folds rupture and swell, developing fluid-filled lesions. Polyps tend to be unilateral, larger than nodules, vascular, and prone to hemorrhage. Unlike vocal nodules, polyps can result from a single traumatic incident such as yelling at a sporting event (Colton et al., 2011).

Two general types of polyps have been identified: sessile and pedunculated. A **sessile polyp**, closely adhering or attaching to vocal fold tissue (see Figures 9.3 and 9.4), can cover up to two-thirds of the vocal fold. A **pedunculated polyp**

FIGURE 9.3 Sessile polyp.

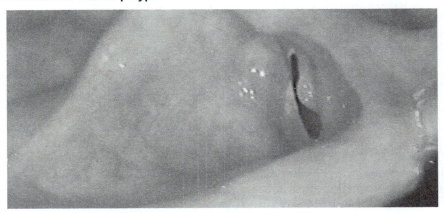

Photograph courtesy of Robert Orlikoff, East Carolina University, Greenville, NC.

FIGURE 9.4 Two sessile polyps stacked on top of each other on the right vocal fold.

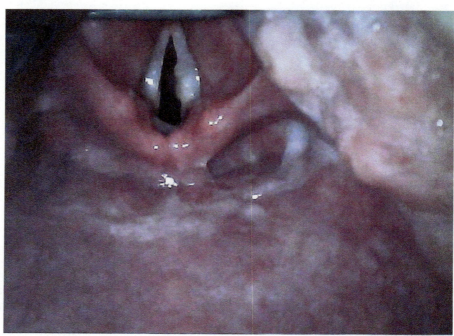

(Photograph courtesy of Steven R. Knight)

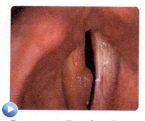

Pearson eTextbook
Video Example 9.2

This video shows a patient with a sessile polyp.

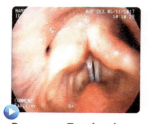

Pearson eTextbook
Video Example 9.3

This video is of an individual with a granuloma.

appears to be attached to the vocal fold by means of a stalk; it is usually found on the free margins of the vocal folds and the upper and lower surfaces of the folds.

Hoarseness, breathiness, sudden voice breaks, and **diplophonia**, or the perception of two different pitches during phonation, are the primary voice symptoms. Diplophonia occurs because of the increase in mass due to the polyp on one vocal fold. Individuals who have a vocal polyp may also report the sensation of something in the throat. Airway obstruction can also occur if the polyp is significantly enlarged (Deem & Miller, 2000).

Contact Ulcers and Granulomas. Contact ulcers are small, reddened ulcerations that develop on the posterior surface of the vocal folds in the region of the arytenoid cartilages. Contact ulcers, like vocal nodules, are usually bilateral but, unlike nodules they can be painful. Pain is either unilateral or bilateral, and it may radiate into the ear. As contact ulcers heal, they are replaced by granulated tissue, referred to as a **granuloma** (see Figure 9.5).

It was once believed that contact ulcers, which occur predominantly in older men, resulted primarily from forceful and aggressive speaking behaviors (Colton et al., 2011). Contemporary thought, however, suggests that gastroesophageal reflux disease (GERD) is a significant contributing factor. Stomach acids irritate vocal fold tissue and promote excessive throat clearing, which is also abusive to tissue, thereby causing the ulcerations (Colton et al., 2011). The condition is complicated by regurgitation of stomach acids into the esophagus and throat during sleep, causing further irritation of the ulcer (Deem & Miller, 2000).

In rare cases, contact ulcers and granulomas can develop as the result of trauma induced during surgical intubation of the larynx (respiratory tube placed

FIGURE 9.5 Granuloma.

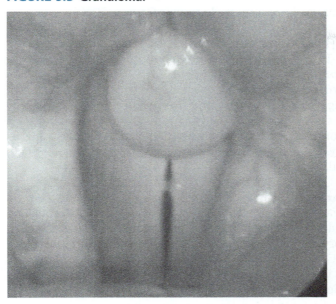

Photograph courtesy of Robert Orlikoff, East Carolina University, Greenville, NC.

between the vocal folds). The risk is greater in women and children who have smaller airways (Boone et al., 2010).

The primary voice symptoms of contact ulcers are vocal hoarseness and breathiness. Throat clearing and vocal fatigue accompany the disorder.

Laryngitis. Acute laryngitis and **chronic laryngitis** are inflammation of the vocal folds that can result from exposure to noxious agents (tobacco smoke, alcohol, etc.), allergies, GERD, or vocal abuse (Colton et al., 2011). Acute laryngitis is a temporary swelling of the vocal folds that can result in vocal hoarseness, lowered pitch, and intermittent voice breaks (Stemple et al., 2018).

Chronic laryngitis is a result of vocal abuse during periods of acute laryngitis, and it can lead to serious deterioration of vocal fold tissue. The vocal folds appear thickened, swollen, and reddened because of excessive fluid retention and dilated blood vessels in the vocal folds. If chronic laryngitis persists, a marked atrophy (wasting-away of tissue) of the vocal folds will occur. The vocal folds become dry and sticky, resulting in persistent cough and complaints of sore throat (Stemple et al., 2018). The voice symptoms of chronic laryngitis range from mild hoarseness to near-aphonia, lowered pitch, effortful speaking, and complaints of vocal fatigue (Jetté, 2016; Stemple et al., 2018).

Papillomas. Laryngeal papillomas are small wartlike growths that cover the vocal folds and the interior aspects of the larynx. These lesions are caused by the human papillomavirus (HPV) and are the most common abnormal laryngeal pathology in children younger than 6 years (Boone et al., 2010), although an adult-onset form also exists (Rivera & Morrell, 2021). Papillomas are noncancerous, but they can obstruct the airway, hindering breathing. Children with the disorder exhibit inspiratory **stridor**, or noisy breathing during inhalation. This indicates a narrowing in the airway (Stemple et al., 2018). Papillomas are the second most

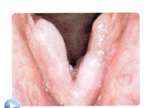

Pearson eTextbook
Video Example 9.4
This video shows an individual with papillomas.

common benign laryngeal abnormality in children and the second most frequent cause of childhood hoarseness (Larson & Derkay, 2010).

Webs. Laryngeal webs are the result of connective tissue growing between the vocal folds. They can be congenital (present at birth) or acquired as the result of trauma or prolonged infection (Boone et al., 2010). Congenital laryngeal webs typically form on the anterior aspects of the vocal folds and can obstruct the airway, causing inspiratory stridor and shortness of breath. Laryngeal webbing must be removed surgically. Voice quality can range from normal to severely dysphonic, depending on the severity of the web. Webs may produce a high-pitched, hoarse voice quality, and/or **aphonia**, the complete absence of voice (Boone et al., 2010; Deem & Miller, 2000).

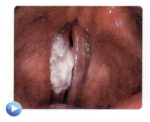

Pearson eTextbook
Video Example 9.5

This video shows an individual with laryngeal cancer.

Cancer. Laryngeal cancer is the most serious organic disorder of the voice. It is linked to cigarette smoking and excessive use of alcohol, although other risk factors have been identified, including HPV infection, obesity, poor nutrition, age, race, family history, GERD, workplace chemical exposure, and inherited gene mutations (American Cancer Society, 2021). Figure 9.6 is a photo of laryngeal cancer that is obstructing view of the vocal folds in a chronic smoker and heavy alcohol user. Figure 9.7 depicts the thickened and precancerous vocal folds of a heavy smoker.

Laryngeal cancer is the second most common head and neck cancer in the United States, with over 13,000 new cases diagnosed annually. It is estimated that 99,000 people in the United States are currently living with laryngeal cancer (e.g., Regan & Joshi, 2019). One of its early signs is persistent hoarseness or difficulty

FIGURE 9.6 Laryngeal cancer.

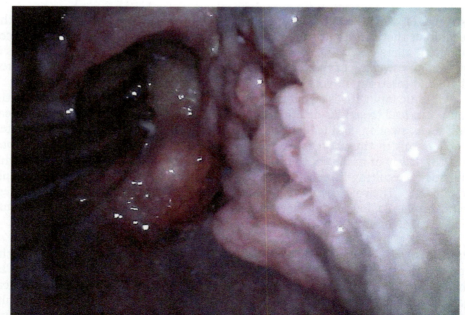

(Photograph courtesy of Steven R. Knight)

FIGURE 9.7 **Hypertrophic (thickened) and precancerous vocal folds of a heavy smoker.**

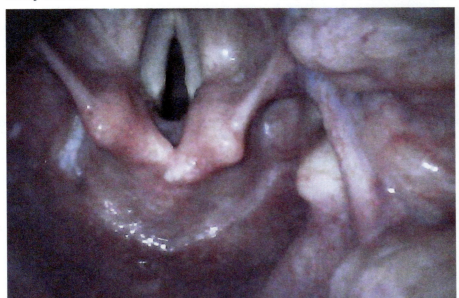

(Photograph courtesy of Steven R. Knight)

breathing in the absence of colds or allergies (Stemple et al., 2018). Once cancer is diagnosed, it is frequently necessary to remove the entire larynx to prevent the spread of the cancer to other parts of the body. When the larynx is removed surgically, the trachea is repositioned to form a stoma (mouthlike opening) on the anterior aspect of the throat for breathing purposes.

Table 9.2 summarizes the voice characteristics frequently associated with each structural abnormality just described.

Neurologic Voice Disorders

The second major group of organic voice disorders is that caused by damage to the central nervous system (CNS) or peripheral nervous system (PNS). Recall from previous chapters that the CNS comprises the brain and spinal cord, and areas of the brain such as the primary motor cortex in the frontal lobe control activation of muscles that initiate speech and voice production via connections with the PNS. The PNS consists of the 12 cranial nerves that activate the muscles responsible for speech and voice after receiving signals from the CNS. Cranial nerve X (vagus) innervates the muscles of the larynx and is primarily responsible for voice production.

Disorders of the CNS or PNS can result in speech and voice disorders that are characterized by muscle weakness, paralysis, discoordination, or involuntary movements. Most of these disorders, generally called *dysarthrias* (discussed further in Chapter 10), involve generalized neurological damage resulting in complex patterns of speech and voice symptoms. Table 9.3 describes the voice characteristics associated with several types of neurological damage or disease.

Pearson eTextbook
Video Example 9.6
This video shows a patient with unilateral vocal fold paralysis.
https://youtu.be/Dfqj69Gxvuw

Pearson eTextbook
Video Example 9.7
This video shows a patient with bilateral vocal fold paralysis.
https://youtu.be/uCjU0B16bNM

Because the left recurrent laryngeal nerve leaves the brainstem, travels down into the chest cavity, loops around the heart's aorta, and then courses upward inserting into the larynx from below, it was frequently severed in the early days of open-heart surgery. This resulted in postoperative aphonia. Improved surgical procedures have minimized this problem, although the risk still exists.

TABLE 9.2

Dysphonic Voice Characteristics Associated with Structural Abnormalities

Structural Abnormality	Voice Characteristics of Dysphonia
Vocal nodules	Hoarseness and breathiness
Vocal polyps	Hoarseness, breathiness, sudden voice breaks, and diplophonia (i.e., perception of two different pitches during phonation)
Contact ulcers and granulomas	Hoarseness and breathiness
Acute and chronic laryngitis	Acute: hoarseness; lowered pitch; intermittent pitch and voice breaks Chronic: narrowing of the airway; inspiratory stridor (i.e., noisy inhalation); sharp cough; hoarseness
Papillomas	Hoarseness; inspiratory stridor
Webs	High-pitched hoarseness; possible airway obstruction and inspiratory stridor
Cancer	Persistent hoarseness

TABLE 9.3

Voice Characteristics Associated with Neurological Damage or Disease

Neurological Damage or Disease	Description	Voice Characteristics
Damage to cranial nerve X (vagus)	Damage to the cranial nerve that controls the laryngeal muscles for phonation. Specifically, the **recurrent laryngeal nerve (RLN)** of the vagus is the nerve supply for most of the laryngeal muscles associated with voice production. Damage results in unilateral and bilateral **vocal fold paralysis**.	*Unilateral damage:* Hoarse, breathy voice quality; reduced loudness and monoloudness; **pitch breaks**, or sudden uncontrolled upward or downward changes in pitch; diplophonia (i.e., vibration of folds at two different frequencies). *Bilateral damage:* Severe breathiness; possible aphonia. Potentially life-threatening if folds are paralyzed in adducted position obstructing the airway.
Parkinson disease (PD)	Degenerative disease that results in depletion of dopamine, interfering with *basal ganglia* circuitry functioning. Rigidity of intrinsic laryngeal muscles and vocal fold bowing are common.	Reduced loudness; monopitch; monoloudness; hoarseness; harshness; breathiness; **voice tremor**.
Amyotrophic lateral sclerosis (ALS)	Motor neuron disease characterized by degeneration of upper and lower motor neurons. Results in flaccid and spastic weakness and, ultimately, paralysis.	Reduced loudness; monoloudness; inspiratory stridor; harshness; strain; strained/strangled; wet-gurgly.
Spasmodic dysphonia (SD)	Neurological voice disorder reflecting damage to basal ganglia and cerebellar control circuits. Involves abnormal, involuntary movements of the larynx, with adductor-type SD occurring in most cases. Average age of onset is 45 to 50 years of age, with more women affected than men.	Strained, effortful tight voice and intermittent voice stoppages.

Visit the LSVT Global website at www.lsvtglobal.com and watch the pre-/post-treatment video of Shirly, a woman with Parkinson disease. Note her complaints about her voice before treatment.

Functional Voice Disorders

As mentioned previously, functional voice disorders can result from misuse, abuse, or overuse of the voice or psychological or stress factors, without causing physical changes to the larynx. Several functional voice disorders you may encounter as an SLP are described in Table 9.4.

Pearson eTextbook
Video Example 9.8
This is a video of a patient with muscle tension dysphonia.
https://youtu.be/c1HExyNPeY8

TABLE 9.4
Common Functional Voice Disorders

Functional Voice Disorders	Description	Voice Characteristics
Muscle tension dysphonia (MTD)	Generally associated with hyperfunction of laryngeal muscles, including excessive or abnormal muscle activity in the absence of structural or neurological abnormalities. The underlying cause of abnormal muscle activation is not well understood, but certain factors may contribute to development of abnormal laryngeal tension, including significant emotional stress, excessive use or misuse of the voice, GERD, or learned compensatory behaviors. Women are more affected than men.	Hoarseness; strain; harshness; aphonia; intermittent pitch breaks; pain and discomfort when the laryngeal area is palpated.
Conversion (functional) dysphonia or aphonia	Functional or **psychogenic voice disorders** believed to result from psychological suppression of emotion. The term **conversion disorder** is used when an individual is converting stress, anxiety, depression, or emotional conflict into physical symptoms. The vocal folds are structurally normal during nonspeech behaviors like coughing or throat clearing, indicating the capacity for normal glottal closure. Individuals with conversion dysphonia or aphonia believe they have a physical condition that prevents them from using their typical voice.	**Conversion dysphonia**: Hoarseness with or without a strained component; pitch breaks; breathiness; intermittent whispering, or other abnormal voice characteristics. **Conversion aphonia**: Loss of voice; involuntary whispering. Whisper may be pure, harsh, or sharp, and sometimes accompanied by high-pitched, squeaky traces of phonation, or even normal traces of phonation.
Functional mutism	May occur in schizophrenia, severe depression, or other psychiatric conditions. May also be a sign of conversion disorder.	May make no attempt to speak or may mouth words without voice or whispering. Vocal fold adduction is normal based on ability to produce a normal cough.

Sources: Based on Desjardins et al. (2022); Duffy (2020).

Resonance Disorders

Resonance disorders can accompany voice disorders, particularly in cases when the CNS or PNS are damaged or disordered; they result when there is any disruption to the normal balance of oral and nasal resonance. They can also be caused by structural abnormalities, including clefts of the palate. A cleft is an abnormal opening in an anatomical structure (Shprintzen, 1995) caused by failure of structures to fuse or merge correctly early in embryonic development. Alternatively, a resonance disorder may develop when there is a blockage in the nasopharynx that impedes sound energy from traveling through the nose for production of nasal sounds (Kummer & Lee, 1996).

REFLECTION QUESTION 9.2

What impact might a cleft palate have on family–infant bonding?

When the velopharyngeal mechanism fails to decouple the oral and nasal cavities, **hypernasality** secondary to VPD occurs. VPD is a frequent result of palatal clefts and is associated with velar soft tissue and muscle tissue deficiencies. VPD also occurs in neurodegenerative diseases like ALS that result in damage to the motor neurons that control the velopharyngeal mechanism. People with VPD are said to have a hypernasal voice quality; however, hypernasality is not a problem associated with phonation. Rather, it is a result of not partitioning the oral and nasal cavities by actions of the velopharyngeal mechanism. Hypernasality is a resonance problem created by the nasal cavity acting inappropriately as a second "filter," coupled to the oral cavity. Addition of this second filter alters the vocal tract's output in such a way that it sounds as though the individual is talking through the nose.

VPD can also result in **audible nasal emission**, particularly during production of high-pressure consonants (e.g., /p/, /b/, /s/, *sh*, *ch*, *j*). When an individual with VPD attempts to build up the necessary air pressure in the oral cavity for production of high-pressure sounds, the air pressure subsequently escapes through the nasal cavity. This may be heard as a very loud, turbulent sound called a *nasal rustle*, or *nasal turbulence*, believed to be a friction noise caused by a large amount of air moving through a small velopharyngeal opening (Kummer & Lee, 1996; Peterson-Falzone et al., 2006). When there is an insufficient amount of nasal resonance as is needed during production of the nasal sounds /m/, /n/, and *ng*, speech may sound hyponasal. Your voice may have a hyponasal quality when you experience

---

CASE STUDY   **Blake** *(continued)*

Blake met with the school-based SLP. While he mentioned concerns and feelings of self-consciousness about his voice and nasal-sounding quality, the SLP could hear a mild breathy-hoarse voice quality and inconsistent hypernasality and nasal emission, especially in words containing /s/, *sh*, and *ch*, and in multisyllable words. The SLP discussed possible treatment options for voice and resonance but stressed the importance of first seeing an ear, nose, and throat doctor to visualize the structures of Blake's larynx and velopharyngeal mechanism using special instrumentation. This was necessary to ensure there were no structural abnormalities present and that voice and resonance therapy would not exacerbate any possible underlying medical condition.

a bad head cold. **Hyponasality** occurs when there is a partial blockage somewhere in the nasopharynx or nasal cavity. When there is a complete blockage, denasality occurs, resulting in a more severe resonance disorder where nasal sounds are imperceptible from oral consonants produced with the same place of articulation (Peterson-Falzone et al., 2017).

Evaluation of Voice and Resonance Disorders

Learning Objective 9.3 Describe the primary components of a voice and resonance evaluation.

Evaluation of voice and resonance disorders requires a multidisciplinary team approach. The specific nature and cause of a disorder determines the precise composition of the team. At a minimum, a voice evaluation requires an otolaryngologist (or ear, nose, and throat doctor) and an SLP. For evaluation of resonance disorders, particularly of VPD secondary to cleft palate, a cleft palate or craniofacial team comprising but not limited to surgeons, SLPs, dental specialists, audiologists, and social workers is necessary for effective clinical management of this population.

The Voice Evaluation

The primary objectives of the clinical voice evaluation are to determine the (1) presence or absence of a voice disorder, (2) nature of the voice disorder, and (3) severity of the voice disorder (Barkmeier-Kramer, 2016). It is necessary for the individual presenting with a suspected voice disorder to have an examination performed by an otolaryngologist. The otolaryngologic examination provides information about vocal fold tissue damage and presence of nodules, polyps, or other abnormal growths, including more serious conditions like laryngeal cancer. A direct examination of the vocal folds and other laryngeal structures is essential to determine whether the voice disorder has an organic basis.

Direct observation of laryngeal structures can be achieved with an **endoscope**, which is a camera lens coupled to a light source. The light source illuminates the larynx, and laryngeal structures are viewed through the lens. The endoscope may be rigid or flexible. Rigid endoscopy involves placing the camera into the oropharynx while the tongue tip is held out of the mouth by the clinician. This allows a closer view of the larynx and vocal folds and a higher-quality image. Vocal fold vibration is viewed while the patient prolongs a vowel (usually /i/). Some individuals cannot tolerate rigid endoscopy due to having a hypersensitive gag reflex but most can be coached through the procedure successfully.

Flexible endoscopy involves insertion of a flexible scope (Figure 9.8) through the nasal passage and advanced over the velum into the pharynx. An advantage of this method over rigid endoscopy is that the vocal folds can be viewed during a variety of connected speech tasks, not just vowel prolongation. Image quality is poorer with the flexible endoscope due to the smaller diameter of the light source compared to the rigid endoscope (Stemple et al., 2018).

Endoscopy provides a constant light source that permits imaging of laryngeal structures while stationary or moving slowing. Imaging the rapid movements of the vocal folds during vocalization requires use of a flashing strobe light that creates

Pearson eTextbook
Video Example 9.9

In this video of a rigid laryngeal stroboscopy examination, there is an optical illusion created by the strobe light. It looks as if the vocal folds are vibrating in slow motion and can be viewed quite easily.
www.youtube.com/watch?v=9Tlpkdq8a8c

FIGURE 9.8 An endoscope.

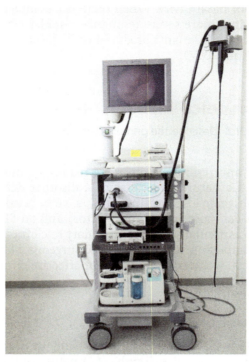

(© KPG Payless/Shutterstock)

the illusion of the vocal folds vibrating in slow motion. Thus, **videostroboscopy** gives us a detailed view of vibratory characteristics of vocal fold movement during phonation that we can see with the naked eye (Hixon et al., 2020).

CASE STUDY **Blake** (*continued*)

The SLP and school nurse helped Blake's family coordinate the appointments to first see his primary care physician and obtain a referral for an otolaryngologist. School personnel worked to ensure appointments were scheduled so Blake didn't miss any academic coursework. Collaboration with family ensured appointments were convenient for them also.

Videostroboscopy and fiberoptic nasoendoscopy were performed by the ENT to visualize laryngeal and velopharyngeal structures, respectively. A flexible endoscope was used in both cases to permit visualization of structures during connected speech tasks. Blake tolerated the endoscopic procedures without difficulty.

Videostroboscopic results indicated the left vocal fold appearing shorter and fixed in the paramedian (near the midline) position. The left vocal fold was also reduced in tone and fluttered during phonation, contributing to asymmetrical vocal fold vibration. A small posterior opening during phonation was also observed. The right vocal fold was normal in mobility. Dynamic assessment revealed that, with increased vocal effort, Blake could achieve increased glottal closure and glottal closure duration. In other words, when he put forth high effort using a louder voice, he could achieve adequate vocal fold closure during phonation despite having a weakened left vocal fold.

The SLP involved in the voice evaluation begins by obtaining a thorough case history. Gathering of a case history will help determine the following information:

- Description of the voice problem
- When the voice problem started
- Duration of the problem
- What the client believes may be causing the problem
- How the voice problem affects daily life activities
- Current social and vocational use of their voice
- Overall physical and psychological condition

For individuals seeking gender-affirming care, case history gathering will involve listening to what the client wants in terms of gender expression. Some transgender clients are binary and may identify as the opposite gender as that assigned at birth. Others may be nonbinary and identify as genders in between male and female or they may be agender, or not having a gender. Sometimes clients are unsure, and their gender expression evolves during the therapy process. SLPs should expect to adapt treatment goals and targets to help the client find the voice that matches their gender expression (Smith, 2020).

The SLP also conducts an auditory-perceptual evaluation to describe the pitch, loudness, and voice quality characteristics. The *Consensus Auditory-Perceptual Evaluation of Voice (CAPE-V)* is a tool developed to help SLPs standardize the way these parameters of voice are evaluated and judged (Kempster et al., 2009). The CAPE-V uses continuous visual analog scales for judgments of the following parameters of voice: overall severity, roughness, breathiness, strain, pitch, and loudness. The SLP places a tick mark on a 100 mm horizontal line to indicate perceived severity of the disorder, with higher scores indicating greater severity (Zraick et al., 2011). Hoarseness was excluded from the protocol because many consider "hoarseness" a combination of "roughness" and "breathiness" (Fairbanks, 1960; Kempster et al., 2009).

Speech tasks to perceptually judge voice include sustained vowel prolongation of /a/ and /i/, sentence repetition, and elicitation of a 20-second spontaneous speech sample. A copy of this assessment tool can be requested for noncommercial purposes at www.asha.org/Form/CAPE-V/. In addition to auditory-perceptual assessment, the clinical voice evaluation may also involve detailed acoustic and aerodynamic measurements regarding vocal function that can be compared to normative data. Quantitative acoustic measurements of voice are easily made by using specially designed computer hardware and software. Kay Elemetrics, for example, manufactures a computer-based instrument called the Visi-Pitch (see Figure 9.9), a user-friendly instrument that permits numerous objective assessments of the physical correlates of voice, such as average fundamental frequency, frequency variability, and average vocal intensity.

Similar measures can be made using a free software program called PRAAT, which you can download to your computer from www.fon.hum.uva.nl/praat/.

Spectrograms, or graphic representations of frequency and intensity of sound as a function of time, can also be generated with the Visi-Pitch or PRAAT software. These graphs can also provide useful visual feedback during voice treatment. Quantitative measurements of voice are not necessary to accurately diagnose a voice disorder but are used to supplement the auditory-perceptual evaluation.

Pearson eTextbook
Video Example 9.10

This video provides an overview of how to use an online version of *CAPE-V* using the Visi-Pitch to record and rate voice samples.

www.youtube.com/
watch?v=uXcwJ6qcOBc

FIGURE 9.9 Kay Elemetrics Visi-Pitch.

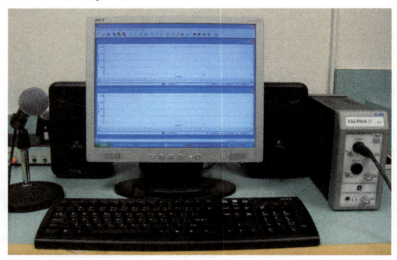

(Photograph courtesy of Kim Farinella)

Aerodynamic voice measures provide information about airflow and air pressure during vocal fold vibration. A **pneumotachometer** measures airflow through the larynx and indicates the average openness of the larynx and degree to which air passes between the trachea and pharynx (Isshiki & von Leden, 1964). Additionally, pressure inside the oral cavity can be measured and used to estimate pressure below the vocal folds (Boone et al., 2010; Patel et al., 2018). Aerodynamic data provide information about the physiology of voice production including voice use and breathing patterns (Schneider, 2019).

After auditory-perceptual and instrumental assessment of voice, obtaining information about how the disorder may be impacting quality of life is also important. The *Voice Handicap Index* (VHI; Jacobson et al., 1997) is a 30-item questionnaire that can help determine the psychosocial handicapping effects of a voice disorder. Patients respond to questions such as "My voice makes me feel incompetent" and "I use a great deal of effort to speak" using a 5-point scale from 0 ("never") to 5 ("always"). Similar instruments include the *Voice-Related Quality of Life* (V-RQOL; Hogikyan & Sethuraman, 1999) and the *Voice Outcome Survey* (VOS; Gliklich et al., 1999). Each instrument can be accessed online. These instruments can also be used as patient-reported outcome measures pre- and post-treatment to determine the patient's perspective on treatment effectiveness (Francis et al., 2017).

The voice evaluation would not be complete without perceptual judgments of resonance since abnormalities of resonance can affect the perception of voice quality or can lead to hyperfunction of the voice as a compensatory response. Behavioral and instrumental techniques for assessing resonance are discussed in the next section.

The Resonance Evaluation

Before making clinical judgments about resonance, it's important to obtain case history information about velopharyngeal function. Interviewing the client or client's caregiver about the history of the presenting problem is essential to the

FIGURE 9.10 Two examples of scales used to rate the degree of resonance disorders: (a) a 7-point scale emphasizing hypernasality and (b) an 8-point scale for rating nasal resonance.

(a)

			Hypernasality			
Normal		Mild		Moderate		Severe
1	2	3	4	5	6	7

(b)

		Hypernasality					
Hyponasality	Normal	Mild		Moderate		Severe	
−1	0	1	2	3	4	5	6

Source: Based on Peterson-Falzone, s., Hardin-Jones, M., & Karnell, M. (2010). Cleft palate speech (4th ed.). st. Louis, Mo: Mosby.

evaluation process. If the client has a cleft, obtaining information about medical and surgical history is necessary for appropriate treatment planning.

Auditory-perceptual evaluation of resonance is still the "gold standard" when determining whether or not a resonance disorder is present. There are several standardized rating scales for assessing resonance. Rating scales permit the assignment of numbers to express increasing severity of the disorder. In general, such rating scales are reliable and valid. Two such rating scales are presented in Figure 9.10.

To determine the presence or absence of hypernasality and rate its severity during speech production, you might ask the client to repeat sentences containing voiced, oral sounds with few high-pressure consonants (i.e., "How are you?"); if you were rating hyponasality, you might ask the client to repeat sentences that contain mostly nasal sounds (e.g., "Mom made lemonade") (Kummer, 2011b, 2014a, 2014b). The presence of *audible nasal emission*, or air escaping from the nose during production of oral sounds, can best be determined by having the client repeat sentences loaded with high-pressure consonants (e.g., "Sissy sees the sun in the sky") (Kummer, 2011b, 2014c). Additional speech tasks for assessing resonance include counting, syllable repetition (e.g., "pa, pa, pa, pa"), and connected speech (Kummer, 2014a). You can listen and judge severity of abnormal resonance in connected speech samples at the following sites: www.acpa-cpf.org/speech-samples/ and www.rit.edu/ntid/slpros/assessment/speechvoice/training/10.

Specially designed instruments are also available to assess resonance disorders. Direct and indirect instrumental assessments are sometimes necessary to confirm what the SLP is hearing during the auditory-perceptual evaluation. Instrumental procedures are not used as substitutes for clinical judgments of resonance, however (Peterson-Falzone et al., 2010).

An indirect technique to quantitatively evaluate resonance requires use of an instrument called a **nasometer**. A nasometer measures simultaneously the relative amplitude of acoustic energy being emitted through the nose and mouth during speech production. A numerical value, the **nasalance score**, is computed to reflect the magnitude of hypernasality. Nasalance scores have been determined to correlate well with perceptual ratings of hypernasality in some studies, but other studies have observed a poor correlation with clinical judgments of hypernasality (cf. Dalston et al., 1991; Keuning et al., 2002). Nasometry can also be used as an effective therapeutic feedback technique, especially with young children, since it includes virtual games and animated graphics (Perry & Schenck, 2013).

A cost-effective direct imaging technique to directly visualize velopharyngeal function during speech production discussed previously is endoscopy. **Videonasendoscopy**, or fiberoptic endoscopy, involves insertion of a flexible endoscope through the nose providing an image of the nasal airway as it travels back and is positioned in the nasopharynx above the velum. From here, structures of the nasopharynx and velopharyngeal function can be examined (Hixon et al., 2020).

CASE STUDY **Blake** *(continued)*

Nasoendoscopic images revealed evidence of previous surgical repair of the soft palate. Recall that Blake received surgical intervention for management of a submucous cleft at 6 years of age. Inconsistent closure of the velopharyngeal port was observed (manifesting as an intermittent hypernasal-sounding resonance) during pressure-loaded sentence repetition tasks (e.g., "Buy Bobby a puppy"). When repetition and modeling were provided, Blake was able to achieve complete closure of the VP port for all pressure sounds in words during sentence tasks, thereby achieving typical resonance without hypernasality or nasal emission.

ENT diagnoses included left unilateral vocal fold paralysis and normal structure for VP closure with inconsistent, impaired function during connected speech.

X-ray imaging using a technique called **multiview videofluoroscopy** provides for dynamic assessment of velopharyngeal structures from three different perspectives: the front (frontal), the side (lateral), and from beneath (base). These images provide a complete picture of the velopharyngeal mechanism and may be useful when trying to determine or rule out **apraxia of speech** as velar movements can be viewed during production of complex speech tasks (Perry & Schenck, 2013). Videofluoroscopy (discussed again in Chapter 11 for evaluation of swallowing) is costly and involves radiation exposure. Unless you work in a hospital setting, you probably won't have immediate access to this imaging technique.

Magnetic resonance imaging (MRI) provides a safe and effective way to visualize the velopharyngeal mechanism in real time during speech production (Hixon et al., 2020). MRI data can even be obtained in young children with velopharyngeal insufficiency and assist in determining the nature and extent of defects in the primary muscle of velar elevation, the palatal levator, in those with craniofacial anomalies (Kollara et al., 2017).

Management of Voice and Resonance Disorders

Learning Objective 9.4 Describe the major goals of voice and resonance treatment and effective voice and resonance treatment approaches and techniques.

Treatment for voice and resonance disorders and differences may involve behavioral, medical, surgical, and/or prosthetic interventions by the multidisciplinary

Pearson eTextbook
Video Example 9.11

This is video of an MRI of the velum (and other articulators) moving during speech (inaudible).

www.youtube.com/watch?v=uTOhDqhCKQs

Blake (*continued*)

After receiving results of Blake's instrumental evaluation, the SLP obtained permission from his parents to conduct an auditory-perceptual assessment of voice and resonance. The CAPE-V (Kempster et al., 2009) was administered. Results indicated a mild to moderate dysphonia characterized by mild breathiness and mild to moderate roughness. Loudness was moderately reduced with slightly high pitch during connected speech tasks. Sustained vowel prolongation was reduced in duration, with intermittent pitch breaks and diplophonia.

Blake completed the VHI (Jacobson et al., 1997). Responses revealed Blake's avoidance of social situations because of his voice, along with vocal fatigue even after brief, communicative interactions at school. He also reported feeling "shame" about his voice and resonance difficulties, and again stated he was concerned about required group presentations in his academic classes.

Ratings for hypernasality during pressure-loaded sentences (e.g., "The blue spot is on the key") indicated mild but inconsistent hypernasality. Occasional nasal emission was heard in words containing /s/, *sh*, and *ch* sounds. Blake could correctly produce words with high-pressure sounds (e.g., /s/) with repeated practice of the target word following clinician modeling. Repetition and backward chaining of words in sentences (e.g., "key"; "the key"; "on the key"; "is on the key"; "spot is on the key") helped significantly reduce hypernasality.

In addition, 20 multisyllabic words from the Single Word Test of Polysyllables (Gozzard et al., 2004) were administered to informally assess sound sequencing in multisyllabic words, hypernasality and nasal emission in words with high-pressure sounds (e.g., octopus, washing machine), and prosody. Recall from Chapter 5 that multisyllabic words are used to assess motor planning/programming skills. Initially, Blake demonstrated difficulty sequencing sounds in the correct order and presented with inconsistent hypernasality and nasal emission. His performance improved, however, when numerous models were provided by the SLP. On occasion, multisyllabic words were segmented (choppy). Improvement was noted when models and practice were provided.

The following speech diagnoses were determined by the SLP based on assessment results:

- Mild to moderate flaccid dysphonia secondary to unilateral vocal fold paralysis
- Mild, inconsistent hypernasality, likely secondary to residual motor planning/programming deficits (i.e., childhood apraxia of speech)
- Mild residual childhood apraxia of speech characterized by difficulties with sound sequencing and sound segmentation in multisyllabic words (abnormal prosody)

Dynamic assessment (i.e., trial therapy) results indicated Blake was a good candidate for behavioral voice and resonance intervention, and further medical/surgical procedures were not necessary to achieve successful clinical outcomes. Blake expressed interest in participating in treatment to address his voice, resonance, and speech production difficulties.

team depending on the specific needs of the client. SLPs treat voice and resonance disorders and differences using evidence-based behavioral interventions tailored to the individual. Treatment aims to restore or modify voice and resonance for purposes of effective communication and improved quality of life.

In the next sections, we describe behavioral, medical, surgical, and prosthetic management of voice and resonance associated with structural abnormalities, neurological diseases, functional disorders, and gender-affirming care. Specific therapeutic approaches and techniques for voice and resonance are described in Box 9.1.

BOX 9.1 **Evidence-Based Practices for Individuals with Voice and Resonance Disorders**

General Intervention for Voice Disorders

- SLP-administered voice intervention is effective when medical intervention, such as surgery, is not warranted.
- For some types of laryngeal pathology, SLP voice intervention may be as or more effective than medical intervention.
- In general, voice treatment before and after surgery results in better outcomes than surgery alone.

Direct Physiologic Voice Treatment Approaches

- Vocal function exercises, which include sustained vowels, pitch glides, and sustained low and high pitches practiced twice per day, are effective in treating functional voice disorders, as well as voice disorders associated with vocal hyperfunction, by strengthening and balancing the laryngeal mechanism and facilitating production of a more relaxed voice.
- Resonant voice therapy focuses on production of voice through the hearing and feeling of vibratory sensations produced with a "forward focus" in the oral cavity, particularly in the palate, tongue, and lips. It is based on techniques that improve voice production in actors and singers. The goal is production of a strong, clear voice accomplished with minimal impact of the vocal folds. It has been shown to be effective for individuals with hyperfunctional voice disorders.
- Confidential voice therapy or use of breathy phonation is effective in reducing laryngeal hyperfunction by facilitating a continuous, relaxed voice with increased airflow. After several weeks, clients gradually increase voicing and reduce airflow while maintaining relaxed laryngeal muscles.
- The *Lee Silverman Voice Treatment* (*LSVT*) is an evidence-based treatment repeatedly shown to improve voice production in both children and adults with neurological diseases (e.g., cerebral palsy, Parkinson disease, multiple sclerosis). Treatment focuses exclusively on increasing vocal loudness during multiple high-effort productions of maximum phonation trials and functional speech tasks of increasing complexity. This intensive treatment approach is delivered four times per week for 4 weeks, with recommended "tune-up" sessions to maintain positive results.

- Case studies involving a combination of individual and group treatment focused on mindfulness/relaxation, vocal function exercises and resonant voice therapy, shared gratitude and feedback, and counseling showed positive changes for voice and improved verbal and nonverbal communication for gender-nonconforming individuals.

Direct Symptomatic Treatment Techniques

- The yawn–sigh technique, or instructing the client to simulate a real yawn completed with a sigh, effectively lowers the larynx and opens the glottis, thereby decreasing laryngeal tension and facilitating ease of phonation. This technique is suggested for individuals with laryngeal pathology associated with vocal hyperfunction (e.g., vocal nodules).
- Semi-occluded vocal tract phonation involves having the client phonate through a straw to partially close the mouth, thereby increasing air pressure above the vocal folds. The increased air pressure maintains the folds in a slightly abducted position during phonation, allowing vocal fold vibration to occur more easily and with less muscular effort. The straw is eventually eliminated. This technique is useful in achieving a more "resonant" voice.

Surgical Intervention for Cleft Palate

- Although about 90% of children with nonsyndromic clefts are expected to have good velopharyngeal function after the first surgery, speech treatment may still be needed. As structures of the head and face grow, velopharyngeal function may deteriorate.
- The type of secondary surgical procedure used in some children (i.e., secondary palatal surgery and/or pharyngeal flap surgery) depends on the severity of velopharyngeal inadequacy. Following secondary surgery, speech treatment is often needed to eliminate habituated compensatory misarticulations and nasal air emission during production of pressure consonants.

Specific Behavioral Treatment Approaches or Techniques for Resonance Disorders

- Continuous positive airway pressure (CPAP) is best suited for individuals with a small velopharyngeal gap (less than 2 mm) and a movable velum, and it has been found to be effective in some patients with mild to moderate hypernasality.

- A technique called **electropalatography (EPG)** uses an artificial palatal plate containing electrodes connected to a computer. The palatal plate is fitted in the mouth so when the tongue contacts these electrodes during speech production, the articulatory patterns can be seen on the computer screen. EPG provides visual feedback on the location and timing of tongue–palate contacts and continues to show promise for remediation of speech sound errors in children with a history of cleft palate.
- Bottom-up articulation drill procedures that focus on phonetic placement and sound shaping

are recommended for children with repaired clefts, and they may be effective for sounds that are often difficult for this population. For instance, to teach the production of /s/ without nasal emission, have a child produce /t/ with the teeth closed. Then have the child prolong this sound, which should result in the correct production of /s/. The technique can be applied to other fricative or affricate sounds.

- **Enhanced milieu teaching (EMT)** is a naturalistic method of stimulating speech and language development in young children that parents can do at home. This child-led approach involves organizing the environment such that a child must request or comment on objects to receive them.

Sources: Based on Colton et al. (2011); Fox et al. (2002, 2006); Hardin-Jones et al. (2006); Kuehn et al. (2002); Kuehn and Henne (2003); Kummer (2014a); Peterson-Falzone et al. (2017); Pickering (2015); Pindzola (1993); Ramig and Verdolini (2009); Roy et al. (2001); Stemple et al. (2018); and van der Merwe (2004).

Intervention for Structural Abnormalities Associated with Voice and Resonance

Treatment of voice and resonance disorders associated with structural abnormalities may involve behavioral, medical, surgical, or prosthetic interventions. A combination of treatments may also be recommended by the multidisciplinary team, depending on the specific needs of the individual (Colton et al., 2011).

Behavioral Treatment for Voice and Resonance

Behavioral voice therapy is often the clinical method of choice for voice disorders associated with benign structural abnormalities (e.g., vocal nodules) that are caused and maintained by vocal misuse or abuse (e.g., Colton et al., 2011). In such cases, identifying the behaviors that contributed to the laryngeal pathology (e.g., frequent yelling, throat clearing, coughing) is an important first step in the treatment process.

Once identified, clients are educated about vocally abusive behaviors and how forceful adduction of the vocal folds can result in trauma to tissue mucosa, leading to laryngeal pathology. Pictures, videos, and descriptions of voice anatomy and physiology can help increase client awareness of the negative consequences of vocal hyperfunction (Stemple et al., 2018). Clients are also educated about good vocal hygiene (see Figure 9.11). These indirect treatment techniques can be beneficial for both children and adults with voice disorders.

Clients may be taught to modify hyperfunctional behaviors more directly. Direct treatment approaches teach clients to eliminate vocally abnormal or abusive behaviors (e.g., talking too loudly or too forcefully) by producing voice that balances the speech production subsystems—respiratory, laryngeal, and upper airway—called *physiologic therapy*. Symptomatic voice treatments work to modify various aspects of the voice, such as reducing a pitch that is deemed too high (Stemple et al., 2018). Specific physiologic and symptomatic voice approaches and techniques that are effective in reducing or eliminating hyperfunctional vocal patterns are described in Box 9.1.

FIGURE 9.11 Behaviors that promote good vocal hygiene.

Drink plenty of fluids, especially water.

Limit the intake of caffeine.

Limit the intake of alcoholic beverages.

Avoid tobacco products.

Avoid yelling and screaming.

Speak at a comfortable loudness level; don't "push" your voice.

Avoid loud, dry, or smoky environments.

Do not use "unnatural" voices, such as imitating cartoon characters.

Practice vocal rest.

Avoid excessive throat clearing and coughing.

REFLECTION QUESTION 9.3

If you were prescribed a specified period of vocal rest, how would your daily life activities be affected? Could you comply with this treatment approach?

For patients with laryngeal cancer who require total removal of their larynx, an alternate method of producing voice will be needed. Some alaryngeal (without larynx) speakers learn to use **esophageal speech** by bringing air into the oral cavity and using the esophagus as a vibratory source in the form of "burps." It can be challenging and time-consuming for individuals to learn esophageal speech. For some, up to 12 months of therapy and daily practice may be necessary, whereas others may never succeed in learning this technique (Regan & Joshi, 2019).

Clefts of the lip and/or palate are the most frequent craniofacial defects in the world, with an estimated prevalence of 1 in 700 births (e.g., World Health Organization, 2006). While surgery is effective in improving the structure of the velopharyngeal mechanism in individuals with cleft palate, it does not improve function of the velopharyngeal mechanism for speech. As such, behavioral treatment by the SLP to manage VPD, resulting in varying degrees of hypernasality, following surgical repair of a cleft palate is often necessary.

Behavioral treatment programs based on exercise physiology principles like progressive resistance training, may be beneficial in treating VPD. Progressive resistance training asserts that when muscles are subjected systematically to weights greater than those to which they are accustomed, they adapt by adding muscle tissue, and strength is increased. To continue building muscle tissue, weights are increased systematically until the desired muscle strength is achieved.

One such program is called continuous positive airway pressure (CPAP). CPAP treatment is an 8-week muscle resistance home-training program designed to strengthen the muscles of the soft palate during speech production. A CPAP device, like the one used for patients with obstructive sleep apnea (see Figure 9.12), generates continuous positive air pressure that is delivered through a nose mask. The procedure attempts to strengthen the muscles of the velopharyngeal mechanism

FIGURE 9.12 **Individual using a continuous positive airway pressure (CPAP) device.**

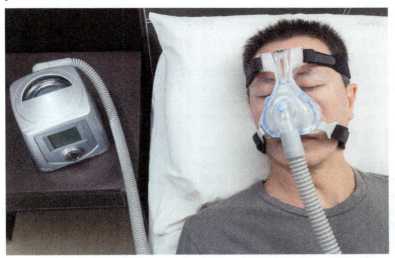

© Chalermpon Poungpeth/Shutterstock

by having velar muscles work against systematic increases of weight. Heightened air pressure in the nasal cavity is the "weight" that the velopharyngeal mechanism works against (Tomes et al., 1997). Treatment involves production of 50 specified words and six sentences while pressure is delivered through the nose. The amount of pressure delivered and the amount of practice time each week progressively increases (Peterson-Falzone et al., 2010).

Individuals with clefts are also at high risk for disordered articulation. Direct intervention for speech sound development should begin prior to the first palatal surgery and as early as 5 to 6 months of age, just before the onset of babbling (Peterson-Falzone et al., 2017). Early speech-language intervention focusing on increasing the child's consonant inventory, especially pressure consonants, and on increasing oral airflow is also recommended (Hardin-Jones et al., 2006). The behavioral treatment approaches and techniques described in Chapter 5 for children with speech sound disorders also apply to the treatment of the cleft population. The procedures and techniques used in bottom-up drill approaches may be particularly useful for treating habituated, compensatory misarticulations.

Medical/Surgical Treatment for Voice and Resonance

When behavioral therapies have been exhausted, medical and surgical management of persistent benign structural abnormalities (e.g., vocal nodules) is usually necessary. For certain types of structural abnormalities like papillomas and laryngeal webs, surgical removal is required. Papillomas have a high rate of recurrence in children and adults, requiring repeated surgical procedures and often causing scarring of the vocal folds (Colton et al., 2011).

Small unilateral polyps require surgical removal (Colton et al., 2011). Vocal polyps are effectively treated with a combination of surgical removal of the polyp and voice treatment to eliminate vocal misuse or abuse to prevent recurrence.

Contact ulcers and granulomas tend to reappear after surgical removal, so managing gastroesophageal reflux with medication in combination with behavioral treatments that address vocal hygiene prior to surgical intervention is strongly recommended (Colton et al., 2011).

Early-stage laryngeal cancers are frequently managed with radiation or, more recently, transoral microsurgery where the surgeon resects the glottal tumor using an endoscopic laser coupled to an operating microscope (Regan & Joshi, 2019). This surgical technique allows for greater preservation of laryngeal structure and function (Silver et al., 2009). Total laryngectomy (removal of the entire larynx) is still performed in more advanced cases of laryngeal cancer, however. Behavioral voice treatment with an SLP is beneficial in improving voice and quality of life following medical/surgical management of laryngeal cancer (Regan & Joshi, 2019).

Treatment of hypernasality secondary to VPD in individuals with cleft palate typically begins with surgical intervention. Normal velopharyngeal function cannot be achieved without structural integrity of the velopharyngeal mechanism. Children born with palatal clefts undergo surgical closure of the cleft, called a **primary palatoplasty**, around 12 months of age (Peterson-Falzone et al., 2010). If a child also has a cleft of the lip, surgery to repair it frequently occurs before 3 months of age (Kuehn & Henne, 2003).

Superiorly based pharyngeal flap or sphincter pharyngoplasty are secondary surgeries effective for managing continued velopharyngeal incompetence in individuals with repaired palatal clefts. Superiorly based pharyngeal flap surgery involves a U-shaped surgical incision at the midline of the oropharynx, the tissue dissected away from the pharyngeal wall, and then brought forward and inserted into an incision made on the nasal surface of the velum (Peterson-Falzone et al., 2010). Sphincter pharyngoplasty involves dissection of the posterior faucial pillars from their lower attachments and lateral pharyngeal wall and suturing them to a pharyngeal flap (Peterson-Falzone et al., 2010), narrowing the pharyngeal opening. The advantages of this surgery include creation of a dynamic portlike structure for velopharyngeal closure and the ease of surgical revision should hypernasality persist (Nam, 2018).

Prosthetic Treatment for Voice and Resonance

Following total laryngectomy, a prosthetic device can provide an alternative form of voicing for alaryngeal speakers. One such device is a battery-powered **electrolarynx**. The electrolarynx has a vibrating diaphragm that is placed on the lateral aspects of the neck. This vibration excites the air in the vocal tract, serving as an alternate form of voicing. The electrolarynx is easy to learn to use for purposes of communication. Alaryngeal patients are advised to own one even if just to use as a backup form of communication (Hutcheson, 2016), despite its undesirable electronic sound quality and cost (Regan & Joshi, 2019).

Some alaryngeal speakers may be candidates for a **tracheoesophageal puncture (TEP)**, regarded as the gold standard for alaryngeal voice restoration in the United States (Regan & Joshi, 2019). The TEP is a one-way prosthetic valve inserted through a surgical opening created between the trachea and esophagus. The speaker occludes the stoma and exhaled air is redirected via the one-way valve from the trachea into the esophagus, allowing the speaker to use respiratory air and a muscle of the esophagus, the cricopharyngeous muscle, for voice production (Regan & Joshi, 2019; Stemple et al., 2018). TEP can provide alaryngeal speakers immediate restoration of voice without a mechanical-sounding quality (Regan & Joshi, 2019).

Following surgical repair of a cleft palate, a *fistula*, or open hole between the nasal and oral cavities, may spontaneously occur (Peterson-Falzone et al., 2010).

FIGURE 9.13 **A speech bulb obturator.**

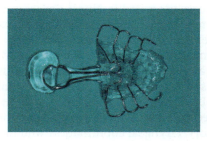

Source: Bispo, ME Whitaker, HC Aferri et al(2011), Speech therapy for compensatory articulations and velopharyngeal function: a case report, Journal of Applied Oral, Vol. 19, Issue 6, pages 679–684.

A prosthetic device called a **palatal obturator** can be used to cover the fistula until further surgery is warranted.

For a velum that is too short, a **speech bulb obturator** may be used. The bulb fills the space between the velum and pharyngeal walls, reducing perceived hyper-nasality during speech (Kummer & Lee, 1996). Obturators are made of acrylic material and are custom-built to conform to the configuration of the oral cavity. An obturator is held in place by clasps that anchor it to the teeth (Figure 9.13).

Intervention for Voice and Resonance Disorders Associated with Neurological Diseases

Treatment of voice and resonance disorders secondary to neurological disease often aims to increase overall speech intelligibility, since progressive neurological disease tends to affect all aspects of speech production.

Behavioral Treatment for Voice and Resonance

Voice and resonance abnormalities commonly associated with dysarthria second-ary to neurological disease, discussed further in Chapter 10, benefit from specific behavioral approaches or techniques to increase respiratory, laryngeal, and velo-pharyngeal function and from speech supplementation strategies such as alphabet cues (i.e., pointing to the first letter of each word on an alphabet board) or topic cues (i.e., pointing to the topic word or picture prior to sharing information with the listener) to improve understanding of the speaker's message (Figure 9.14).

An evidence-based behavioral approach directly targeting the respiratory and laryngeal systems is LSVT, discussed also in Chapter 10. LSVT is an intensive treat-ment program originally designed for patients with Parkinson disease. Its focus

FIGURE 9.14 **Topic board.**

family	friends	feelings	schedule
home	health	hobbies	money
food	medication	TV	transportation
clothing	therapy	sports	current events
weather	work	the past	the future
you	travel	communication	it's not on here

is systematic increase of phonatory effort using intensive treatment and multiple repetitions of productions. Increased loudness occurs in the context of good voice quality and a focus on sensory awareness of the increased vocal loudness and effort. LSVT has proven to be beneficial for improving voice function not only in patients with Parkinson disease (e.g., Fox et al., 2002) but also in individuals with other progressive and nonprogressive neurological diseases across the lifespan (e.g., **multiple sclerosis**, cerebral palsy) (e.g., Fox & Boliek, 2017). In addition, "spreading effects" of LSVT include increased velopharyngeal closure and reduced hypernasality, decreased speaking rate, increased range of motion of the articulators, improved respiratory/laryngeal coordination, and improved swallowing function (Peterson & Galgano, 2019).

Medical/Surgical Management for Voice and Resonance

Indirect benefits to voice and resonance may be achieved with pharmacological management of neurological diseases. Examples include dopamine replacement agents used to treat Parkinson disease and Mestinon, a medication for **myasthenia gravis**, an autoimmune disease characterized by rapid weakening of muscles due to inadequate transmission of nerve impulses to the muscles, causing sudden and significant hypernasality and articulatory imprecision with continued speaking (Duffy, 2020).

Botulinum toxin (Botox) injections into laryngeal muscles is the standard of care for treating spasmodic dysphonia to improve voice function (Boutsen et al., 2002) and may be beneficial for some patients with voice tremor. Patients receiving Botox injections may also benefit from behavioral voice interventions (Barkmeier-Kraemer, 2012).

Medialization laryngoplasty, or *type I thyroplasty*, is a surgical procedure that may be used for unilateral vocal fold paresis (weak) or paralysis. It involves surgical placement of an implant into the weakened or immobile vocal fold, displacing the paralyzed fold medially to facilitate vocal fold approximation during phonation. Patients who undergo this surgical procedure demonstrate improved pitch, loudness, and prosody, although breathiness, harshness, and vocal fatigue may persist (Franco & Andrus, 2009). The procedure is reversible so it can be undone if the vocal fold paralysis heals on its own and returns to normal functioning (Duffy, 2020).

For resonance abnormalities, injection **pharyngoplasty** is a less invasive surgical technique that involves injection of a gel material into the posterior and lateral pharyngeal walls in individuals with small to medium-sized gaps in velopharyngeal closure secondary to acquired velopharyngeal insufficiency. Improved perceived resonance and nasalance scores were achieved following the procedure in adults with neurological etiology (e.g., brainstem stroke) (Duffy, 2020).

Prosthetic Management for Voice and Resonance

For those with progressive deterioration of muscles due to motor neuron disease (e.g., amyotrophic lateral sclerosis), and who are poor candidates for behavioral treatments focused on high-effort exercise (e.g., LSVT), a portable voice amplifier may be used to improve vocal loudness levels.

A simple and cost-effective way to manage significant hypernasality and nasal emission in those with motor neuron diseases involves plugging the nares with a swimmer's nose clip. For some patients, the swimmer's clip quickly improves speech intelligibility in connected speech, and patients who talk extensively on the phone for work prefer this treatment option to manage hypernasality when possible during the course of the disease.

Botulinum toxin (Botox) is one of the most poisonous substances known. It is produced by bacteria found in contaminated meat products. When ingested, it causes paralysis of muscles in the body, including the respiratory muscles that regulate breathing, and can lead to death. In small doses injected into localized areas, Botox has been found to be a safe and effective way to weaken or paralyze selected muscles temporarily for medical and cosmetic reasons, including reducing abnormal muscle contractions, managing pain, and reducing the appearance of wrinkles.

FIGURE 9.15 **A palatal lift.**

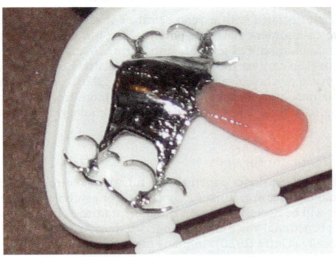

Source: https://en.wikipedia.org/w/index.php?curid=6270160

A more costly option to manage an immobile velum due to paralysis secondary to neurological disease is a **palatal lift**. A palatal lift works to either elevate the velum into full contact with the posterior pharyngeal wall or positions the velum such that pharyngeal wall movement is sufficient to achieve closure (Duffy, 2020). Many patients find the palatal lift (Figure 9.15) to be uncomfortable and some even throw it away (despite the cost) because they dislike using it so much.

CASE STUDY   Blake *(continued)*

During their first treatment session, the SLP explained that because of Blake's anxiety about group presentations, assessment of coursework competencies could be arranged in another format (e.g., individual project) and he could opt out of the group presentation assignments. Blake felt participating in the group presentations would motivate him to work hard during speech therapy sessions. As such, speech treatment stimuli included scripts that Blake was working on for his first-quarter group presentation in world history.

A daily home practice program of vocal function exercises (e.g., maximum phonation tasks; pitch glides from lowest pitch to highest on open vowels) designed to strengthen and balance the laryngeal musculature and balance airflow with muscular effort was prescribed. Additionally, Blake met with the SLP twice weekly for drill production practice of complex, multisyllabic words related to

coursework vocabulary (e.g., dynasty, theocracy, hieroglyphics). The goal was to achieve correct articulation, resonance, and prosody in each word. Repeated practice following clinician models and feedback, with progression from single words to words in sentences, and finally paragraph reading resulted in significantly reduced hypernasality and nasal emission on high-pressure sounds. Overall articulation and prosody also improved for all targeted words.

Blake participated in daily homework practice focused on correct articulation, prosody, and resonance of his targeted multisyllabic words. The SLP created videos for him on his tablet of a close-up of her mouth producing each targeted word. Blake was required to record at least one of his productions of each target word for playback during treatment sessions to ensure he was practicing correctly at home.

Intervention for Functional Voice Disorders

Voice disorders associated with psychological or stress conditions, referred to as functional voice disorders, have the potential for full recovery since structural or neurological abnormalities are not contributing. Many times, these voice disorders occur in the context of acute emotional distress or stress in individuals who are otherwise psychologically healthy (Duffy, 2020). Some research suggests depression, trauma, and adverse life events occur more frequently in these individuals compared to those with disorders of organic etiology, however (e.g., Ludwig et al., 2018).

Behavioral Treatment for Voice

It may seem intuitive to refer patients with functional voice disorders associated with emotional conflict or trauma for psychiatric or psychological treatment and, for some, this will be necessary. However, highly trained SLPs are not only experts in diagnosing functional voice disorders but often play a central role in managing them behaviorally (Duffy, 2020). In many cases, when behavioral speech therapy is successful, referral to other providers is unnecessary.

Whether the individual has muscle tension dysphonia, conversion aphonia or dysphonia, or functional mutism, in some cases, significant improvement or even a return to normal voice can be accomplished in just a few treatment sessions. Each of these disorders has been shown to respond positively to symptomatic treatment that addresses vocal hyperfunction and involves empathetic discussion about the possible link between psychological factors (i.e., the role of stress, anxiety, or conflict) and their physical voice symptoms. Such discussions can occur during symptomatic treatment or afterward following improvements in voice function (Duffy, 2020).

Behavioral treatment for functional voice disorders by the SLP, based on Duffy (2020), includes the following:

- Discussion of the diagnosis (i.e., functional voice disorder) that includes a rationale for the diagnosis, explanation for the potential for success with symptomatic treatment, and reassurance that there are no organic barriers (e.g., neurological diseases) that could interfere with treatment success.

- Identification of the behaviors that represent the disorder (e.g., mutism; intermittent whispering; tight, effortful voice).

- Symptomatic treatment strategies that provide opportunities to approximate normal voice without tension. These strategies may include initiation of voice from a grunt or sigh, gentle production of "uh-huh," or prolongation of a sound. Directing attention to how the voice sounds and feels during these simple tasks and reinforcement of all attempts that represent behaviors that are different from the abnormal patterns are provided. Once normal phonation is achieved consistently, treatment can progress to syllables, words, sentences, reading paragraphs, and spontaneous speech.

- Light-touch laryngeal manipulation or massage, which has the physical benefit of relieving hyperactivation of laryngeal muscles and the psychological benefit of building a bond with the patient.

- Debrief discussion following successful symptomatic treatment that serves to validate the patient's initial patterns of voice abnormalities and their active participation in overcoming them. The debrief helps the individual develop a plausible explanation for the initial voice disorder and the successful clinical outcome following treatment that then can be shared with others. See Utianski and Duffy (2022) for debrief explanation examples following successful clinical outcomes.

Not all patients with functional voice disorders associated with stress or psychological conditions emerge successfully from behavioral treatment. Some individuals have more complex, chronic mental health conditions or the situation causing distress or stress is still active and ongoing (e.g., physical, sexual, or emotional abuse). In such cases, referral to other healthcare providers and relevant others is warranted.

For those unwilling to accept the diagnosis of "functional" and who continue to assert an organic basis for their voice disorder, successful management is likely not a priority. Therefore, behavioral voice therapy alone is unlikely to yield positive outcomes in such cases (Utianski & Duffy, 2022).

Intervention for Gender-Affirming Voice and Communication Patterns

Gender is complex and includes gender identity (i.e., the intrinsic sense of being male, female, or an alternative) and the relationship with one's body, appearance, gender roles, gender norms, and gender stereotypes (Russell & Abrams, 2019). In contrast, sex (male/female) refers to biological identity assigned at birth. For some, gender identity may not be consistent with assigned sex. As such, characteristics associated with gender stereotypes relating to body type, hairstyle, clothing, relationships, activity preferences, and verbal and nonverbal communication may be incongruent with the gender identity they wish to express (Russell & Abrams, 2019). The SLP, as part of a multidisciplinary team, plays a critical role in providing voice, resonance, and communication therapy to individuals who wish to better reflect their authentic self.

Behavioral Treatment for Voice and Resonance

Behavioral treatments that address the unique needs of the client and focus on self-expression, self-esteem, feelings, and attitudes while emphasizing empathy and trust are most effective (Pickering, 2015; Smith, 2020). Therapy sessions and homework may involve the individual reflecting and observing their own gender-expressive strategies as well as those of others to help determine how they may want to modify their presentation (Smith, 2020). Treatment targets will develop and change throughout the therapy process as the individual explores their self-identity.

For some, altering speaking fundamental frequency to be consistent with perceived masculine, feminine, or nonbinary intonation can be achieved with behavioral voice therapy alone. Education about vocal health and good vocal hygiene is necessary when altering voice expression. Treatment focused on listening to male and female voices, vocal drill practice, and even singing with progression to speech to achieve the vocal range of intonation and resonance associated with the desired gender expression has proven successful in clinical case studies (Russell & Abrams, 2019; Smith, 2020).

Because females' vocal tracts are shorter than males', vocal tract resonances for women are typically higher. Behavioral techniques to achieve a more

Pearson eTextbook
Video Example 9.12
This video highlights gender-affirming treatment for voice and resonance.
www.youtube.com/
watch?v=Cq5bskEpdpg

The World Professional Association for Transgender Health promotes the highest standards of care for evaluation and treatment of gender-nonconforming individuals seeking to better reflect their authentic gender identity (Davies et al., 2015).

Person-centered counseling by the SLP assists the transgender client with voice and communication changes that enable them to present themselves authentically while maintaining a safe voice and preventing vocal harm (Adler, 2017).

feminine-sounding resonance include slight retraction of the lips, effectively shortening the vocal tract (Carew et al., 2007). Research has shown it is necessary to shift both voice fundamental frequency and resonant formant frequencies for an individual to be perceived as the opposite gender (Pasricha et al., 2008). Treatment may also involve practicing stereotypically female or male language and nonverbal communication behaviors (Russell & Abrams, 2019).

Counseling by the highly trained SLP in gender-affirming care is critical in helping the transgender client reach their treatment goals. Person-centered counseling involves connecting with the client and guiding them to feel independent and self-confident as their voice and communication characteristics are modified. The client–clinician relationship must first be developed before effective counseling can be provided (Quinn, 2012; Riley, 2002).

Medical/Surgical Treatment for Voice and Resonance

Hormone medications are common treatments for transgender males and females. If started early in puberty, secondary sex characteristics can be suppressed and lowering of pitch prevented in transgender females if the adolescent meets eligibility criteria for treatment (Russell & Abrams, 2019). While testosterone therapy alone can lower voice in individuals assigned female at birth, most individuals benefit from behavioral interventions to optimize voice and resonance to best match their gender expression. Hormone replacement therapy for transgender females, on the other hand, does not significantly alter pitch (Russell & Abrams, 2019).

Surgical treatments to alter length and tension of the vocal folds to change vocal pitch range are available. Average pitch elevation has been achieved through surgical creation of a laryngeal web between the anterior portion of the vocal folds using gel injection augmentation. This procedure serves to effectively shorten the vocal folds. Dramatic increases in pitch with minimal adverse effects were reported (Anderson, 2014), although additional surgeries may be necessary for patient satisfaction (Yilmaz et al., 2017).

Many barriers exist in accessing medical and surgical interventions as part of transgender health care (Smith, 2020). Discriminatory behaviors by medical professionals include exclusionary practices and blocking individuals from transitioning who they deem unready, seemingly making medical decisions for transgender individuals (Williams, 2015). Financial issues including lacking insurance or insurance not covering gender-affirming health care also interfere with service access.

More highly trained medical professionals and SLPs are needed to provide care to transgender individuals. Culturally competent training and education for SLPs to adequately serve this population must be expanded (Hancock & Haskin, 2015). As such, universities are working to develop clinical methods and techniques to address the unique needs of transgender clients in their speech-language pathology training programs (Smith, 2020).

Efficacy of Voice and Resonance Treatment

Assessing the efficacy of treatment for voice and resonance disorders is complex because of the variety of conditions that produce voice and resonance disorders, the varying severity levels of the specific types of these disorders, the variety and combinations of behavioral and medical treatments available, and the way treatment efficacy is defined. Despite these complexities, clinical and experimental data suggest general clinical effectiveness. For voice disorders, particularly those associated with vocal misuse and abuse (such as disorders with structural tissue damage), neurological conditions like Parkinson disease, and functional disorders associated with psychological or stress conditions, treatment has been shown to be reasonably effective. Similarly, individuals born with cleft palate who receive medical and behavioral treatment earlier in their life generally speak normally by the time they are adolescents (Peterson-Falzone et al., 2010). Voice and communication therapy as part of gender-affirming care is effective when provided by SLPs with technical expertise, experience working with voice clients, and a nurturing, caring clinical approach. Box 9.1 earlier briefly summarized specific approaches and techniques that have been shown to be effective in treating voice and resonance disorders.

In addition, it's important for an SLP to help clients who have voice or resonance disorders comply with specific treatment techniques by being patient and encouraging during treatment sessions. Changing habituated behaviors that contribute to vocal misuse or abuse is hard work and takes time. As an SLP, your dedication to your clients through your hard work and your enthusiasm about even small gains in progress can be overwhelmingly motivating to clients.

SLPs specialize in *communicating*, which we often equate with *talking*, but it is sometimes more important to compassionately listen to our clients and their caregivers. This is particularly the case for parents who have children with cleft palate, which can cause significant anxiety for caregivers about their child's future. While you as an SLP will probably not have specific answers or be able to make any reliable inferences about prognoses for speech and language development, you can listen attentively, acknowledge caregivers' concerns and fears, and act in a caring and empathetic fashion. Your success as an SLP will depend on your ability to build trusting relationships with clients and caregivers, and these relationships will not only contribute to your effectiveness as a clinician but also serve to add genuine meaningfulness to your career.

Summary

The human larynx is a versatile instrument that, in addition to its primary biological function of protecting the lower airways from invasion of foreign substances, serves as the primary sound generator for spoken communication. The human voice reflects one's personality, general state of health and age, and emotional condition. The human vocal tract, made up of the pharyngeal, oral, and nasal cavities, acts as a filter, changing in size and shape to alter the sound generated by the larynx, thus contributing to the resonance, or quality, of the voice. Closure of the velopharyngeal mechanism is necessary to produce most speech sounds in the English language and inadequate closure due to structural abnormalities such as cleft palate results in the perception of hypernasality, or sound energy inappropriately resonating through the nasal cavity.

Disorders of voice and resonance affect a substantial number of people and vary in both etiology and severity. Voice and resonance disorders can range from relatively uncomplicated abnormalities such as vocal hoarseness resulting from yelling excessively at a sporting event, or hyponasal-sounding speech due to an upper respiratory infection, to cancer of the larynx or bilateral cleft of the lip and palate. The specific method of treatment is largely dictated by the etiology and severity of the disorder.

SLPs play a pivotal role in the treatment of voice and resonance disorders, but effective and ethical management requires a team approach. In many instances, surgical intervention followed by behavioral treatment is the standard protocol. In other instances, medical intervention alone, as in the case of a nasal blockage, or behavioral treatment alone, as is sometimes the case for individuals with vocal nodules, is sufficient. Effective treatment for individuals with voice and resonance disorders requires detailed and specific knowledge about normal and abnormal function of the laryngeal and velopharyngeal mechanisms. Many voice and resonance disorders and differences respond well to techniques used by SLPs and working with such cases can be a rewarding and exciting clinical endeavor.

Epilogue   Case Study: Blake

After 6 months, Blake made excellent progress with articulation, resonance, and prosody during production of his core multisyllabic vocabulary words. Progress with voice was adequate, but abnormal features of voice quality were not eliminated. Blake reported feeling that his vocal loudness had improved, and he felt more confident about his voice in general. Group presentations were going well so far, but he indicated concerns about vocal fatigue during lengthier oral presentations. The SLP recommended a portable voice amplifier to use as needed to sustain the necessary vocal loudness and optimal voice quality for extended periods. The SLP suggested they practice a few times with it before he was dismissed from services. The SLP also recommended that Blake participate in LSVT at a nearby university clinic over the summer, given the intensity of the treatment. She believed this treatment would further improve his voice quality and vocal loudness. Blake was agreeable to this plan.

Reflections   from an SLP in an Ear, Nose, and Throat Clinic in a University Hospital: Sherril Howard

My career life as a speech-language pathologist has been so rewarding both educationally and personally. I had the great pleasure of working in an ENT clinic in a university hospital setting. Aside from seeing a variety of voice disorders, transgender voice, accent reduction, and cleft lip and palate cases, the other half of my practice was head and neck cancer. We saw many complex cases such as oropharyngeal cancers involving total glossectomy (total removal of the tongue). More often I worked with laryngectomy patients and their families. This involved collaborating with other specialists including but not limited to oncologists, radiologists, otolaryngologists, internists, occupational therapists, physical therapists, dieticians, and social services.

The science involved in managing the above type of cases was stimulating and challenging and my learning never ceased. And yes, knowing normal and abnormal anatomy and physiology is important, but beyond the science were my patients who many times were my best teachers. They helped me develop a deep listening—a listening beyond and beneath their words so that I could listen for their depth of feelings.

Being able to help my laryngectomy patients find their voices again was extremely rewarding and truly beyond words. Fitting a patient with a voice prosthesis or teaching them esophageal speech or use of an electrolarynx and witnessing them say, "I love you" to their family in their "new voice" was what always made my day. I am forever grateful for the breadth of our field and all the rich experiences that I've had throughout my career.

Suggested Readings/Sources

Davies, S., Papp, V., & Antoni, C., (2015). Voice and communication change for gender nonconfirming individuals: Giving voice to the person include. *International Journal of Transgenderism, 16,* 117–159.

Patel, R., Awan, S., Barkmeier-Kraemer, J., Courey, M., Deliyski, D., Eadie, T., . . . Hillman, R. (2018). Recommended protocols for instrumental assessment of voice: American Speech-Language-Hearing Association expert panel to develop a protocol for instrumental assessment of vocal function. *American Journal of Speech-Language Pathology, 27,* 887–905.

Peterson-Falzone, S., Hardin-Jones, M., & Karnell, M. (2010). *Cleft palate speech* (4th ed.). Mosby.

Peterson-Falzone, S., Trost-Cardamone, J., Karnell, M., & Hardin-Jones, M. (2017). *The clinician's guide to treating cleft palate speech* (2nd ed.). Mosby.

Utianski, R., & Duffy, J. (2022). Understanding, recognizing, and management functional speech disorders: Current thinking illustrated with a case series. *American Journal of Speech-Language-Pathology, 31,* 1205–1220.

10 Motor Speech Disorders

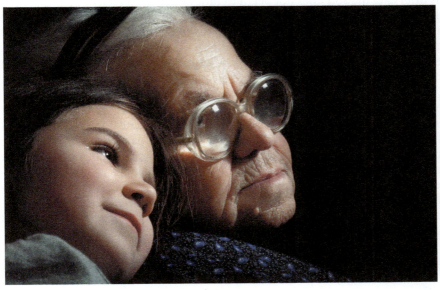
© tcsaba/Shutterstock

Learning Objectives

When you have finished this chapter, you should be able to:

10.1 Describe the structures of the brain important for motor speech control.

10.2 Define dysarthria and briefly describe each type and common etiologies.

10.3 Define apraxia of speech (AOS) and describe speech characteristics associated with AOS and common etiologies.

10.4 Describe assessment techniques for motor speech disorders.

10.5 Briefly explain evidence-based treatments for dysarthria and apraxia.

I decided to return to school to obtain a doctoral degree in the area of motor speech disorders. I had a particular interest in childhood apraxia of speech (CAS) based on my clinical experiences working in schools. My doctoral mentor, however, did not believe in CAS. He thought apraxia in children was a subtype of dysarthria (it's not), or perhaps a variant of stuttering (it's not that either). That was mostly fine with me. I knew if he trained me in speech science and speech motor control, I would have a strong foundation to eventually pursue my passion.

Finally, after 5 years as a full-time doctoral student, I was done and knew it was time to embark on a post-doctoral experience. My mentor asked me if I was still "hung up" on CAS, or if he had helped me "get over it." I told him I wasn't over it. He said, "Well, if you want to seriously pursue a career in motor speech disorders across the lifespan, including CAS, you must go to the best. You need to go to Mayo Clinic." I thought, "Great, I can live in Scottsdale, Arizona." He said, "No, you need to go to Rochester, Minnesota." While I'm not a fan of (extreme) cold, I was accepted (because of my mentor's letter of recommendation) and trained with Dr. Joseph Duffy and Edythe Strand in the Department of Neurology, an experience of a lifetime.

I am grateful my mentor pushed me in that direction and knew that while he didn't believe in CAS, he believed in me and wanted to make sure I was as passionate about my career as he had been about his in respiratory physiology. I am forever grateful to my mentor for helping me become the professional I am today.

–Kimberly Allyn Farinella

Motor speech disorders are difficulties related to problems of movement resulting from neurological disorder or injury. They are a heterogeneous group of neurological impairments that affect motor planning, programming, coordination, timing, and execution of movement patterns used for speech production in both children and adults. Any or all of the processes of respiration, phonation, resonation, and articulation described in previous chapters may be affected. Language disorders often co-occur with motor speech disorders; these are described in Chapter 7.

This brief explanation does not begin to hint at the complexity of the disorders that fall within the boundaries of motor speech disorders. So fine and precise are the movements needed for speech that more area in the brain is devoted to control of vocal folds, tongue, lips, and other articulators than to any other bodily movement, even walking. Given this complexity, it is amazing that the process of speech production becomes so automatic that we give little thought to it when speaking. In fact, we rarely consider the process unless something goes wrong.

As with language, there does not seem to be a specific area of the brain devoted to speech motor control. Even those areas of the frontal lobe that are important for speech are not solely devoted to speech-specific tasks. They also participate in nonspeech motor tasks. In this chapter, we limit our discussion to motor speech. We discuss the two main types of motor speech disorders: dysarthria and apraxia of speech. In addition, we discuss five different types of dysarthria and briefly explain how to differentiate each from one another as well as from apraxia of speech. The Case Study below is an example of a woman with motor speech and other motor control disturbances as the result of a neurodegenerative disease commonly seen in adults over the age of 65.

CASE STUDY   Genevieve

Genevieve is a 69-year-old woman diagnosed with Parkinson disease by her local neurologist 3 years ago. She presents to the university speech-language clinic with complaints about a hoarse voice and disfluencies when speaking, and a reduced pitch range while singing. Genevieve reports that others tell her that her voice sounds quieter than usual, but she has not noticed this herself. She also reports her gait (manner of walking) is getting slower, and it takes her longer to finish meals, particularly when in social situations. She states these issues have caused her to avoid gatherings with friends and family recently and to drop out of the church choir.

As you read this chapter, think about:

- The brain structures involved in Genevieve's difficulties

- The impact on quality of life that can result from changes in motor control and motor speech production

- Treatment goals to increase social and communicative participation to increase quality of life

Structures of the Brain Important for Motor Speech Control

Learning Objective 10.1 Describe the structures of the brain important for motor speech control.

Neurons, or nerve cells (Figure 10.1), are the basic unit of the nervous system responsible for generating, receiving, transmitting, and synthesizing electrical and chemical impulses. The human brain has 15 to 20 billion neurons that generate these nerve impulses to communicate within and between the nervous system and

FIGURE 10.1 A neuron.

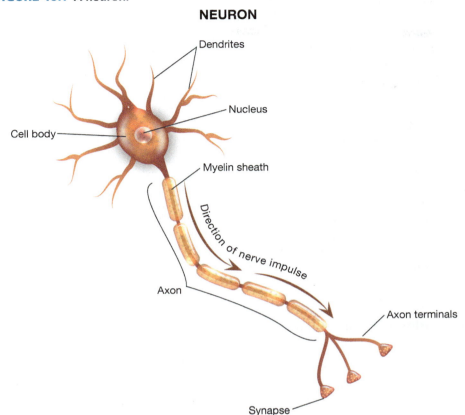

NEURON

Dendrites

Nucleus

Cell body

Myelin sheath

Direction of nerve impulse

Axon

Axon terminals

Synapse

© Tefi/Shutterstock

body structures (Bhatnagar, 2013). Voluntary movement requires the integrated activity of many neurons.

Lower motor neurons (LMNs) are responsible for muscle activation and represent the *final common pathway*, the peripheral mechanism through which all motor activity is mediated, including motor speech control. LMNs are the paired cranial and spinal nerves that travel between the central nervous system (i.e., brain and spinal cord) and the sensory and motor structures they innervate on the ipsilateral (same) side of the body (Duffy, 2020). For instance, you can smile, frown, or raise your eyebrows in surprise because of the paired facial nerves (cranial nerves) that innervate the muscles of your face. The cranial and spinal nerves important for motor speech production are discussed later in this chapter.

Damage to LMNs may result in weakness (paresis) if some of the LMNs supplying that muscle are still functioning. Damage can also result in paralysis (complete loss of ability to move) if the muscle is deprived of all input from its LMNs (Duffy, 2020). Figure 10.2 shows a LMN innervating a muscle fiber.

REFLECTION QUESTION 10.1

What types of injury or disease might lead to complete paralysis of muscles verses muscle weakness?

FIGURE 10.2 A lower motor neuron innervating a muscle fiber.

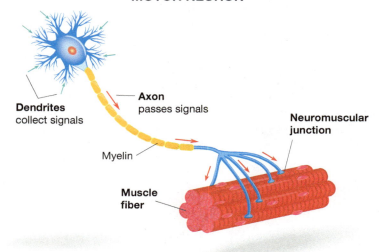

© designua/123RF

FIGURE 10.3 Schematic diagram of the human brain.

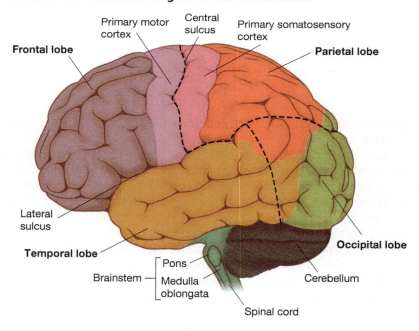

The *direct activation pathway*, also known as the **pyramidal tract**, connects directly to the final common pathway. The pyramidal tract originates mainly from the **primary motor cortex**, a 2-centimeter-wide strip located in the right and left frontal lobes responsible for initiation of voluntary movement (see Figure 10.3). The pyramidal tract is responsible for rapid, discrete voluntary movement of the limbs and of the articulators for speech production on the contralateral (opposite) side of the body.

The *indirect activation pathway*, or **extrapyramidal tract**, is important for regulating reflexes and maintaining posture and muscle tone. It provides the necessary framework to facilitate movement carried out by the direct activation system. Figure 10.4 depicts both the direct activation pathway (pyramidal tract) and the rubrospinal tract, one of the descending tracts of the extrapyramidal, or indirect activation pathway, of the upper motor neuron system.

FIGURE 10.4 **Direct and indirect activation pathways of the upper motor neuron system.**

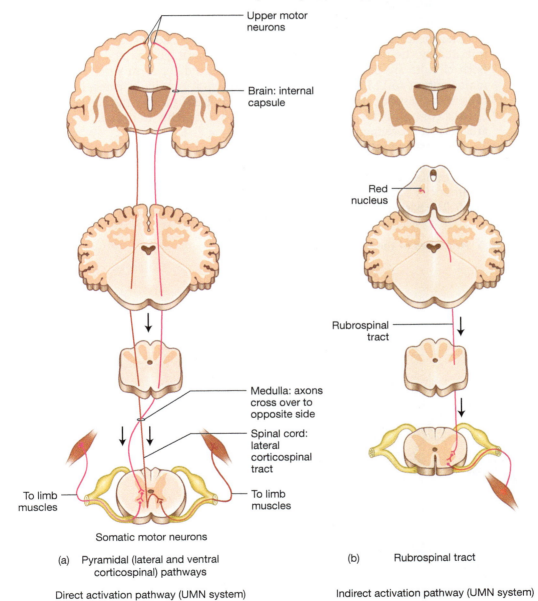

(a)   Pyramidal (lateral and ventral corticospinal) pathways

Direct activation pathway (UMN system)

(b)   Rubrospinal tract

Indirect activation pathway (UMN system)

Together, the direct and indirect activation pathways form the upper motor neuron system (Duffy, 2020). As mentioned, the *upper motor neurons (UMNs)* are primarily a crossed system, meaning damage to UMNs in one cerebral hemisphere will affect the opposite side of the body—resulting in weakness, loss or reduction of skilled movements, and **spasticity** (resistance to passive stretch in one direction).

Unlike the limbs, where generally the right UMNs originating in the primary motor cortex activate the left side of the body (via the spinal nerves), and vice versa, the speech musculature is activated bilaterally. This means UMNs in the right and left cerebral hemispheres are activated at the same time to drive the LMNs (cranial nerves) that activate the right and left sides of the jaw, tongue, face, larynx, and pharynx during speech production. As such, unilateral UMN damage has far less impact on speech production than does bilateral UMN damage (Duffy, 2020). This is discussed later in this chapter in the section on dysarthria.

The control circuits of the brain that indirectly influence or modify movement initiated by the primary motor cortex are the basal ganglia and the cerebellum. Both circuits are part of the brain's extrapyramidal system since neither has a major output to LMNs. As such, damage to basal ganglia or cerebellum will not cause weakness or paralysis of a body structure. Basal ganglia and cerebellar control circuits communicate back and forth and work together to initiate, refine, adjust, and correct movements as they are executed.

The **basal ganglia** are large subcortical nuclei (Figure 10.5) that regulate motor functioning, maintain posture and muscle tone and participate in motor planning/programming and motor learning of skilled movement sequences, as well as the automaticity of those learned movement sequences (e.g., riding a bicycle or driving a car). The basal ganglia control circuit modulates the activity of the primary motor

FIGURE 10.5 Structures of the basal ganglia.

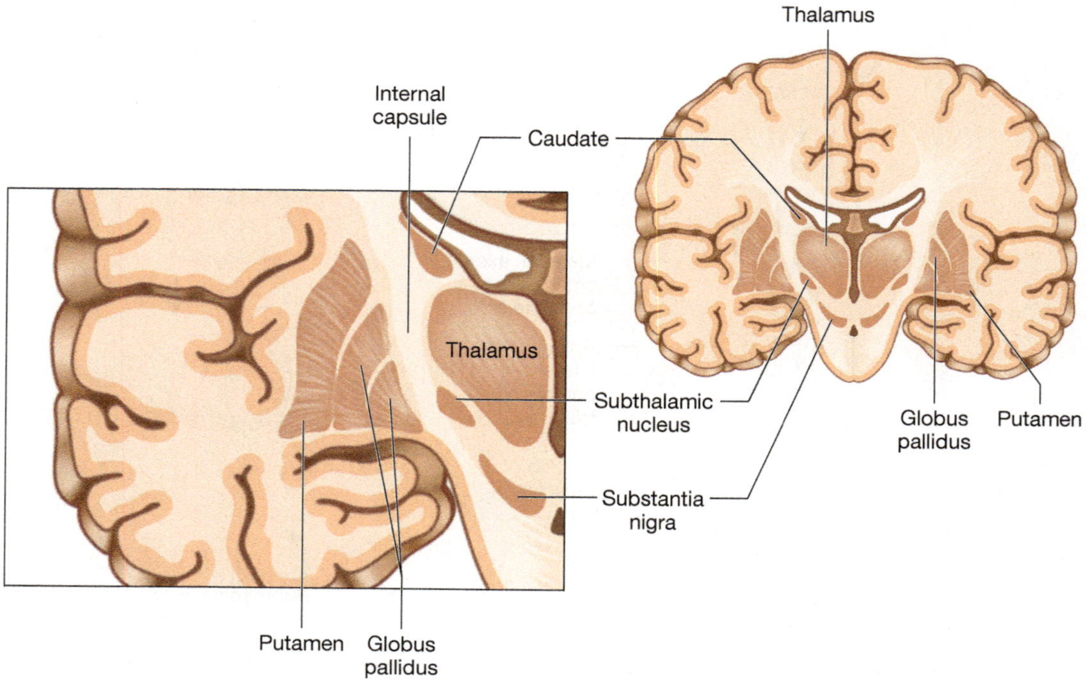

cortex through direct and indirect control loops that have opposing functions. Both are regulated by the neurotransmitter dopamine. The direct pathway serves to increase or facilitate movement, while the indirect pathway serves to decrease or inhibit movement. The balance of activity in these two pathways determines the quality of movement. Damage to the basal ganglia will either result in reduced or slowed movement, as seen in Parkinson disease, or in abnormal, involuntary movements, as seen in the chorea associated with **Huntington disease**. Chorea involves quick, continuous, and purposeless movements of the head, face, tongue, and/ or limbs, discussed later in this chapter. Figure 10.6 depicts normal basal ganglia structures compared to that of a person with Huntington disease.

The **cerebellum**, or "little brain," helps coordinate movement by constantly monitoring all input received from various parts of the brain and spinal cord, comparing motor commands with intended movements, and issuing correcting signals as needed (Bhatnagar, 2013). The cerebellum and cerebellar control circuitry coordinates the control of fine, complex motor activities like speech production; maintains muscle tone; and participates in the planning of movements and motor learning of new physical skills. Damage to the cerebellum or its circuitry results in discoordination of voluntary movements. Temporary impairment of the cerebellum can result when a person has consumed too much alcohol. For example, if during the finger-to-nose sobriety test the person demonstrates over- or undershooting of the target (the nose), this represents discoordination as reflected in impaired estimation of distance and **range of motion**. If the movements appear segmented or jerky, this represents discoordination as reflected in decomposition (lack of smoothness) of movements (Duffy, 2020).

Figure 10.7 summarizes the areas of the brain important to motor control. Search online for "2-Minute Neuroscience Videos" for more information and to review each motor control substrate discussed in this section (e.g., 2-Minute Neuroscience: Cerebellum) (Dingman, 2022).

FIGURE 10.6 Normal basal ganglia structures versus Huntington disease.

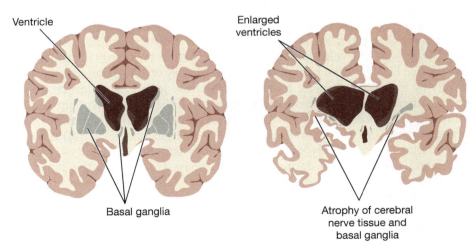

© Blamb/Shutterstock

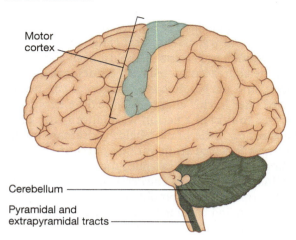

FIGURE 10.7 **Areas of the brain important for motor function.**

Motor
cortex

Cerebellum

Pyramidal and
extrapyramidal tracts

Cranial Nerves Important for Speech Production

Whereas the central nervous system (CNS) comprises the brain and spinal cord, the **peripheral nervous system (PNS)** consists of 12 pairs of cranial nerves, most of which originate in the brainstem, and 31 pairs of spinal nerves that exit the vertebral column and travel to and from muscles of the body. By transmitting messages to muscles and receiving sensory information, the PNS helps the CNS communicate with the body.

The **cranial nerves** (Figure 10.8) are especially important for speech production. Because they are arranged vertically along the brainstem, they are referred to by Roman numerals corresponding to their vertical order. Thus, number VII, the facial nerve, is seventh from the top. The **spinal nerves**—22 of the 31 pairs of these nerves—are important for activating chest wall musculature important for speech breathing. In contrast, special control centers in the brainstem govern breathing to sustain life.

In summary, the LMN system, or final common pathway, includes the paired cranial nerves that activate the muscles of speech production and paired spinal nerves that activate the voluntary muscles of respiration for speech breathing. The mostly crossed UMN system controls the LMNs directly via the pyramidal tract and indirectly by the extrapyramidal tract. A single UMN lesion has minimal impact on speech production since the speech mechanism is driven by both right and left primary motor cortices simultaneously (bilateral innervation), whereas the limbs are driven mainly by one cerebral hemisphere (e.g., right hand is activated by left primary motor cortex). UMN lesions affect a body structure on the opposite side (contralateral), while LMN damage affects a body structure on the same side (ipsilateral).

The basal ganglia and cerebellar control circuits have no direct connection to LMNs, and therefore damage to these structures or their circuitry will not cause weakness or paralysis. Rather, the control circuits influence and modulate movement initiated in the primary motor cortex to ensure movements are smooth, refined, and executed as intended.

FIGURE 10.8 Cranial nerves important in speech production.

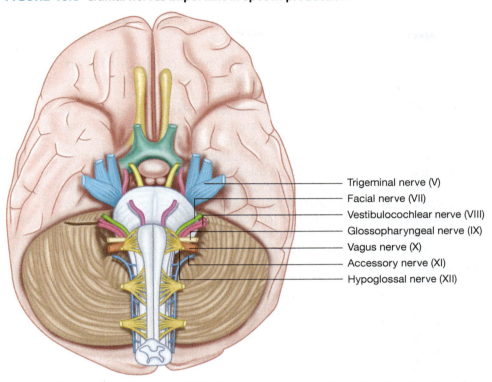

Trigeminal nerve (V)
Facial nerve (VII)
Vestibulocochlear nerve (VIII)
Glossopharyngeal nerve (IX)
Vagus nerve (X)
Accessory nerve (XI)
Hypoglossal nerve (XII)

Trigeminal (V): A mixed nerve, with both sensory and motor functions for the jaw and tongue for speech and chewing.

Facial (VII): A mixed nerve for sensation of taste and motor control of the facial muscles important in facial expression, such as smiling, tearing, and salivation.

Vestibulocochlear (VIII): A sensory nerve with two branches. The vestibular division maintains balance and head orientation in space, and the acoustic (cochlear) branch mediates hearing. While not directly involved in speech production, hearing one's own speech is important to speech motor learning in childhood and important later in life for regulating suprasegmental aspects of speech production (e.g., regulation of loudness).

Glossopharyngeal (IX): A mixed nerve, with sensory input from the tongue for taste and motor control of the pharynx for salivation and swallowing.

Vagus (X): A mixed nerve serving the heart, lungs, and digestive system. A sensory nerve to the larynx and throat. A motor nerve to the larynx for phonation, to the soft palate for lifting, and to the pharynx for swallowing.

Accessory (XI): A motor nerve controlling muscles of the pharynx, soft palate, head, and shoulders.

Hypoglossal (XII): A motor nerve controlling the muscles of tongue movement.

Damage to any structure or pathway involved in the speech production process can cause a motor speech disorder. Motor speech disorders are a heterogeneous group of neurological impairments that reflect a disturbance in the motor planning, programming, coordination, timing, and execution of movement patterns used for speech production. Motor speech disorders include the dysarthrias and apraxia of speech (Duffy, 2020).

Motor Speech Disorders: Dysarthria

Learning Objective 10.2 Define dysarthria and briefly describe each type and common etiologies.

Dysarthria is a general diagnostic term for a group of speech disorders resulting from disturbances in the central and peripheral nervous systems that control the muscles of speech production. Dysarthria can affect the speed, range, direction, strength, and timing of motor movements for respiration, phonation, resonance, and articulation. These abnormalities are the result of weakness, spasticity, discoordination, or involuntary movements (Duffy, 2020). Motor movements that were previously established may have been lost or modified in some way, though the pattern for that movement still exists.

Dysarthria is not a language disorder. An individual can present with dysarthria alone and yet exhibit good language structure and vocabulary, good reading comprehension skills, and effective participation in the give and take of conversation. An individual with profoundly severe dysarthria can convey by other means, such as a computer device, sentences that they may be unable to produce freely through speech.

The muscular disorders that cause dysarthria represent a variety of neurological diseases. Although individuals with dysarthria share some common symptoms, there are distinct clusters of neurological and speech characteristics that describe specific types of the disorder.

Different types of dysarthria result from lesions to different parts of the CNS and/or PNS. Certain commonalities exist across these types, as shown in Table 10.1, including inadequate respiratory drive; voice disturbances such as pitch and loudness problems; prosodic abnormalities such as excessive stress patterns; rate difficulties such as slow, rapid, or varying speeds; hypernasality; and imprecise articulation.

Five distinct types of dysarthria can be identified by their speech characteristics and the impaired neuromuscular processes, including **flaccid**, **spastic**, **ataxic**, **hypokinetic**, and **hyperkinetic** dysarthria (Duffy, 2020). Each type is discussed here.

Flaccid Dysarthrias

Your body's immune system is a network of cells, tissues, and organs that work to prevent foreign substances that cause infection from entering your body and destroy invading microorganisms once they have entered. Autoimmune diseases occur when the immune system mistakes healthy cells and tissues as infected and attacks and destroys them. The reason the immune system responds in this way toward healthy body tissues is unclear. Some dysarthrias are caused by an autoimmune attack on the structures of motor speech control.

Muscles that exhibit flaccid paralysis are weak and soft, exhibit low tone (i.e., hypotonia), and fatigue quickly. Flaccid dysarthria results from damage to cranial and spinal nerves (LMNs), the neuromuscular junction (the space between the neuron and the muscle), or to the muscle itself. Affected muscles may cause reduced respiratory drive for speech breathing, continuously breathy voice quality, reduced pitch and loudness, hypernasality, and imprecise articulation. Speech and voice characteristics associated with flaccid dysarthria reflect weakness and low tone in one or more of the speech production subsystems.

Search online for interviews with Bobby Rush (former U.S. Representative from Illinois), who underwent surgery and chemotherapy to treat cancer of his salivary gland in 2008. LMN (cranial nerve) damage may have occurred during cancer treatment, as evidenced by voice (dysphonia) and resonance (hypernasal-sounding) abnormalities, as well as mild articulatory imprecision, consistent with flaccid dysarthria.

TABLE 10.1

Characteristics of the Dysarthrias

Type of Dysarthria	Lesion Location	Speech Characteristics
Flaccid dysarthria: Muscles are weak and reduced in tone; decreased reflexes; flaccid paralysis; eventual atrophy of muscles	Damage to lower motor neurons (i.e., cranial and spinal nerves) or to the muscle itself	Continuous breathiness; monopitch; hypernasal; short phrases; imprecise articulation
Spastic dysarthria: Weak, spastic muscles; hyperactive reflexes; increased muscle tone	Bilateral damage to upper motor neurons (i.e., direct and indirect activation pathways)	Slow rate; strain-strangled voice quality; hypernasal; imprecise articulation; excess and equal stress
Ataxic dysarthria: Incoordination; reduced muscle tone; poor accuracy and timing of movements	Damage to the cerebellum or cerebellar control circuitry	Irregular breakdowns in articulation; imprecise consonants; vowel distortions; prosodic abnormalities (e.g., excess and equal stress; prolonged pauses)
Hypokinetic dysarthria: Reduced movement; muscle rigidity and stiffness; difficulties starting and stopping movements	Damage to basal ganglia and basal ganglia circuitry	Accelerated speech rate; imprecise articulation due to reduced range of motion of the articulators; breathy/harsh/hoarse voice quality; reduced loudness; disfluencies
Hyperkinetic dysarthria: Involuntary movements	Damage to basal ganglia and basal ganglia circuitry	Irregular breakdowns in articulation; prosodic abnormalities; variable speech rate
Mixed dysarthrias: Combination of two or more dysarthrias	Damage to multiple brain structures or circuits	Imprecise articulation; slow rate; harsh voice; monopitch; monoloudness; hypernasality; excess and equal stress

Source: Based on Duffy (2020).

Spastic Dysarthria

Spastic paralysis of muscles reflects the combined effects of weakness and loss of inhibitory motor control. As a result, reflexes become hyperactive, muscle tone is increased at rest, and individuals exhibit *spasticity* or increased resistance to passive stretch. Spasticity of the speech mechanism is the hallmark of spastic dysarthria, causing movements of the articulators to become slowed and reduced in force and range of motion. Spasticity at the level of the larynx causes the vocal folds to inappropriately adduct (close) during speech production, resulting in a strained or strain-strangled voice quality (Duffy, 2020).

Ataxic Dysarthria

Damage to the cerebellum or cerebellar control circuitry results in incoordination and reduced muscle tone, called *ataxia*. Ataxic dysarthria reflects the effects of incoordination and the improper timing of movements, causing irregular breakdowns in articulation and abnormalities of prosody. Ataxia and ataxic dysarthria are not caused by weakness. Muscles are not reduced in strength. Instead, they

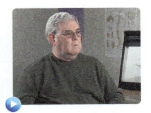

Pearson eTextbook
Video Example 10.1
Identifying Spastic Dysarthria
Go to the link for a video of a 58-year-old man with spastic dysarthria.

are poorly timed and improperly coordinated during movement. Movements are inaccurate, jerky, and lacking smoothness. Too much alcohol consumption can result in temporary ataxia. Individuals who have had a stroke in the cerebellum, or who have a neurological disease that causes degeneration of the cerebellum, often complain that they look and sound drunk.

Search online for recent interviews with Montel Williams (a former talk show host) about his cerebellar stroke. He also has a diagnosis of multiple sclerosis, also associated with cerebellar lesions that lead to ataxic dysarthria. Though his speech abnormalities are subtle, if you listen carefully, you can hear mild irregular articulatory breakdowns (i.e., drunk-sounding speech) in his connected speech.

Hypokinetic Dysarthria

Hypokinetic movements are slow and reduced in range of motion due to effects of rigidity or increased resistance to passive stretch in all directions. Individuals with *hypokinesia* (i.e., reduced movement) feel stiff and find it difficult to get movements started. Once started, they then struggle to stop. Reduced range of motion is the hallmark of hypokinetic dysarthria. The articulators appear to be barely moving during speech production. As a result, speech rate becomes very fast and loudness gradually diminishes. Disfluencies such as sound, syllable, and word repetitions, sound prolongations, and inappropriate silences are common. Disfluent speech that is the direct result of neurological disease is called **neurogenic stuttering** and differs from developmental stuttering in that fear and anxiety about speaking are not common complaints (Duffy, 2020).

Search online for interviews with actor Michael J. Fox, who has a probable genetic, early-onset variant of Parkinson disease (PD). He has been on medication for PD for a good portion of his life, as he was diagnosed with PD at age 29. As such, he not only exhibits the hypokinetic dysarthria consistent with PD (e.g., short rushes of speech; reduced range of motion of the articulators; imprecise articulation), but at times also exhibits hyperkinetic dysarthria (i.e., speech that is interrupted by abnormal involuntary movements) induced by the medications he takes for his PD.

CASE STUDY   Genevieve *(continued)*

Recall that Genevieve was diagnosed with Parkinson disease, which is the most common neurological degenerative disease in individuals over 65 years of age. It is associated with progressive loss of dopaminergic neurons. The loss of dopamine disrupts the balance of direct and indirect control loops in basal ganglia circuitry. This results in slowed, rigid movements; reduced range of motion; and hypokinetic dysarthria.

Hyperkinetic Dysarthria

Hyperkinetic dysarthria is also due to damage to the basal ganglia control circuitry; however, in this case the indirect pathway and/or structures of basal ganglia that inhibit unwanted movements are damaged. As a result, *hyperkinesia* (i.e., increased movement) occurs. Hyperkinetic dysarthria is essentially the production of motorically normal speech that is interrupted in some fashion by abnormal involuntary movements (Duffy, 2020). A number of hyperkinetic movement disorders can result in hyperkinetic dysarthria.

Tremor, the most common involuntary movement disorder, involves rhythmic movement of a body part, such as the limbs, head, or voice. The best way to determine whether an individual has voice tremor is to ask the person to sustain the vowel /a/ for as long as possible. Voice tremor may go unnoticed during conversational speech but is quite evident during vowel prolongation.

Tics are rapid, patterned movements that are not completely involuntary and can be suppressed for brief periods with effort. Vocal tics are the hallmark of hyperkinetic dysarthria in individuals with Tourette syndrome, with rapid production of noises, sounds, or words causing significant interruption to the normal flow of speech.

Dystonia is a slow hyperkinesia that may involve the entire body (i.e., generalized dystonia) or may be localized to just one body part (i.e., segmental dystonia). Involuntary movements are characterized by slow, sustained abnormal posturing, with possible twisting of body parts (e.g., arm, leg, head). Hyperkinetic dysarthria in individuals with dystonia may include excessive pitch and loudness variation, irregular breakdowns in articulation, variable rate, and inappropriate silences (Duffy, 2020).

Unlike dystonia, **chorea** is characterized by rapid and unpredictable movements of the limbs, face, and tongue. The term is derived from the Greek word meaning "dance," and patients with chorea appear to move continuously, in an unstable, dancelike fashion. Hyperkinetic dysarthria in individuals who exhibit chorea is characterized by variable speech rate, irregular articulatory breakdowns, and significant prosodic abnormalities.

The more common etiologies of each type of dysarthria are briefly described in Table 10.2.

Mixed Dysarthria

When two or more types of dysarthria are present in an individual, a speech-language pathologist (SLP) diagnoses the individual with mixed dysarthria. Mixed dysarthrias are common in neurodegenerative diseases that cause damage to multiple areas of the central nervous system, such as **amyotrophic lateral sclerosis (ALS)**, also known as Lou Gehrig's disease. Typically, a mixed spastic–flaccid dysarthria secondary to UMN and LMN degeneration is associated with ALS. Mixed dysarthria is also common after traumatic brain injury, discussed in Chapter 7. Typically, a mixed spastic–ataxic dysarthria is seen following TBI, such as a motor vehicle accident or a fall.

Lifespan Issues

Dysarthria can occur in children due to congenital impairments that were present since birth, such as cerebral palsy, discussed in Chapter 5. Most acquired dysarthrias occur in adulthood. An individual with even mild dysarthria may be reluctant to speak, perhaps leading others to assume the person is tense, shy, or unfriendly. For some, even a slight speech abnormality can be cause for embarrassment or

TABLE 10.2
Common Etiologies of Dysarthria

Etiology	Characteristics
Flaccid Dysarthria	
Bell's palsy	Sudden onset of unilateral facial paralysis. Exact cause is unknown but believed to be due to inflammation of the facial (VII) nerve. Most people recover within weeks to a year.
Progressive bulbar palsy	Degenerative motor neuron disease that primarily affects the cranial nerves that supply the muscles of speech and swallowing. Death occurs 1 to 3 years postonset of the disease.
Myasthenia gravis	Reflects an autoimmune response targeting the neuromuscular junction, the space between the neuron and the muscle. Characterized by rapid weakening of muscles due to inadequate transmission of nerve impulses to the muscles. The disease is effectively managed with medication.
Muscular dystrophies	Group of hereditary, progressive muscle diseases associated with degeneration of muscle fibers and replacement with fat and connective tissue. These disorders tend to lead to early death.
Spastic Dysarthria	
Vascular disorders	Strokes that involve the upper motor neuron (UMN) system in both the right and left cerebral hemispheres or a single brainstem stroke where right and left UMN pathways travel closely together.
Primary lateral sclerosis	Rare, degenerative motor neuron disease resulting in loss of UMNs in primary motor cortices.
Cerebral palsy	Congenital disorder with diverse causes. Frequently associated with bilateral UMN abnormalities.
Ataxic Dysarthria	
Spinocerebellar ataxias	Hereditary, degenerative diseases that affect the cerebellum.
Vascular disorders	Lesions caused by aneurysms, arteriovenous malformations (abnormal tangle of blood vessels that can rupture and interrupt normal blood flow), hemorrhage, or stroke affecting the blood supply to the cerebellum.
Multiple sclerosis	Autoimmune, demyelinating disease of the central nervous system that destroys the insulating sheath around nerves; frequent cause of cerebellar lesions.
Hypokinetic Dysarthria	
Parkinson disease	The most common neurological movement disorder; associated with degeneration of neurons that produce dopamine, the neurotransmitter important in regulating the direct and indirect control loops of the basal ganglia.
Hyperkinetic Dysarthria	
Huntington disease	Inherited progressive disease that results in degeneration of neurons in structures of the basal ganglia and cortex. Clinical features include generalized chorea, dementia, depression, and personality changes. Average survival rate is about 20 years.
Tourette syndrome	Neurodevelopmental disorder that emerges in childhood; characterized by multiple motor and vocal tics (brief, involuntary movements or sounds like eye blinking or throat clearing). Due to abnormalities in basal ganglia circuitry.

depression. In more severe cases of dysarthria, individuals may be frustrated as loved ones and acquaintances attempt to communicate for them by finishing their sentences or ordering for them in restaurants. In turn, they may communicate or socialize less. Difficulty communicating may limit opportunities to participate in social, occupational, and educational activities, leading to feelings of isolation. As an SLP, you can provide a person with dysarthria and their communication partners strategies to promote increased communicative participation and improve the quality of their lives.

Motor speech disorders are not limited to speech production and may have a negative effect on many aspects of life.

In the later stages of progressive degenerative diseases, an individual with dysarthria may be unable to live independently and may need daily living assistance or institutional care. Movement may become difficult, and the person may be unable to care for themselves. The person may eventually be unable to speak at all, and you as an SLP can continue to work to improve the quality of life for individuals with profound dysarthria with the help of augmentative and alternative communication (AAC) devices.

REFLECTION QUESTION 10.2

How might the impact of a motor speech disorder differ for an individual with a congenital impairment versus an acquired impairment?

Motor Speech Disorders: Apraxia of Speech

Learning Objective 10.3 Define apraxia of speech (AOS) and describe speech characteristics associated with AOS and common etiologies.

Apraxia of speech is a clinically distinct neurological speech disorder that impairs the ability to plan or program the sensory and motor commands needed for speech production. Unlike dysarthria, apraxia of speech is not a result of damage to speech muscles, nor does it involve muscle weakness. Rather, it is a higher-level deficiency in motor control.

The motor speech production process begins with a motor program being retrieved from memory. A motor program is an organized set of motor commands that specify all the necessary parameters of movement for speech production; they are learned and consolidated in memory over time. Apraxia of speech results in an inability to adequately retrieve these speech motor programs, which causes disordered articulation of vowels and consonants, slowed rate, and prosodic disturbances (e.g., inappropriate pausing or lengthening of speech segments; incorrect word and sentential stress patterns). It generally occurs following damage to the left cerebral hemisphere, particularly motor and premotor areas of the left frontal lobe, often due to stroke or degenerative disease.

The speech of individuals with apraxia is characterized by groping attempts to find the correct articulatory position, with great variability (inconsistency) over repeated attempts. Frequent sound substitutions, omissions, and additions of sounds occur, along with significant difficulties sequencing sounds when producing multisyllabic words. Unlike a person with dysarthria who produces predominately sound distortion errors and/or related sound substitution errors, a person with apraxia often produces unrelated substitutions, repetitions, or additions.

A person with apraxia of speech recognizes their errors and will make repeated attempts to correct them. As the person tries to produce the correct sound or word, there may be frequent pauses, lengthened sound segments, and re-initiations of words and sentences. As a result, speech production may appear like stuttering in nature. Unlike a person with dysarthria who repeats the same error, an individual with apraxia of speech often produces widely varying productions on repeated attempts. Such inconsistencies are specific to apraxia of speech, and thereby help you as an SLP correctly diagnose apraxia of speech from dysarthria. A speech sample from a person with apraxia follows:

> O-o-on . . . on . . . on our cavation, cavation, cacation . . . oh darn . . . vavation, oh, you know, to Ca-ca-caciporenia . . . no, Lacifacnia, vafacnia to Lacifacnion . . . on our vacation to Vacafornia, no darn it . . . to Ca-caliborneo . . . not bornia . . . fornia, Bornifornia . . . no, Balliforneo, Balliffornee, Balifornee, Californee, California. Phew, it was hard to say Cacaforneo. Oh darn.

Consonants and consonant clusters and blends are particularly challenging for those with apraxia, although more frequently used phonemes and words are produced with more accuracy. As you might expect, complex, long, and unfamiliar words are most difficult to produce.

Individuals with apraxia of speech may have no difficulty producing words on one occasion that they struggle to produce on another. In fact, clients may exhibit periods of error-free speech during automatic or emotional utterances. It is not uncommon to have a client struggle with volitional production of a word such as *vacation* only to hear the client easily say later, "Wow, I sure had a lot of trouble with *vacation*!"

A person with apraxia of speech is usually aware of their errors, as mentioned previously, and may even anticipate them but be unable to correct them. Monitoring of speech in anticipation of these errors tends to result in a slowed, almost cautious rate of speech, with equal stress and spacing, although prosodic abnormalities such as slow rate and equalized stress patterns are hallmark characteristics of this disorder. Clients frequently report that they know what they want to say but can't initiate the sequence or keep it going. Faced with a naming task, these individuals frequently respond, "I know it, but I can't say it."

Although apraxia and aphasia often co-occur, the two are not the same. Aphasia is a language disorder, while apraxia is a motor speech disorder. An individual with aphasia has difficulty with word recall in all modalities, whereas a person with apraxia of speech may be able to recall a word more easily when writing but be unable to say it correctly. In addition, apraxia of speech can be an individual's only diagnosis, and thus language structure may be perfectly intact.

While there appear to be overlapping characteristics between the dysarthrias and apraxia of speech, the two are distinctly different types of motor speech disturbances. Correct diagnosis of a client is essential for speech treatment to be effective. Table 10.3 presents the major differences between the disorders, although there will be many individual variations.

Lifespan Issues

The impact of acquired apraxia of speech on a person's life depends on the etiology of the disorder, as well as the severity. Most individuals who acquire apraxia of speech do so following a stroke in the left hemisphere, specifically Broca's area in the left frontal lobe. Recall that damage to Broca's area also results in aphasia.

TABLE 10.3

Differences between Dysarthria and Apraxia

Dysarthria	Apraxia of Speech
Speech-sound distortions	Speech-sound substitutions
Substitution errors related to target phoneme	Substitution errors often not related to target phoneme
Highly consistent speech-sound errors	Inconsistent speech-sound substitutions
Consonant clusters simplified	Schwa (/ə/) often inserted between consonants in a cluster
Little audible or silent groping for a target speech sound	Audible or silent groping for a target speech sound
Rapid or slow rate	Slow rate characterized by repetitions, prolongations, and additions
No periods of unaffected speech	Islands of fluency
Little difference between reactive or automatic speech and volitional speech; both affected	Often very fluent reactive or automatic speech, nonfluent volitional speech

It is not uncommon for patients with damage in this region to present with both apraxia of speech and aphasia. Depending on the severity of the stroke, individuals can make a full recovery and speech may return to normal. In other cases, speech may recover to some extent, but mild prosodic abnormalities such as slow rate and incorrect stress patterns may persist.

For an individual who has apraxia of speech secondary to a progressive neurological disease (e.g., corticobasal degeneration), an SLP might consider AAC options earlier in treatment for their patient. Such individuals are likely to lose most or even all ability to speak. It is helpful to encourage clients to continually practice speaking when they can or are able and utilize their AAC device often to increase communicative participation and maintain quality of life. Encouraging a positive attitude in clients with apraxia of speech and other types of motor speech disorders also helps to maintain a satisfactory quality of life throughout the course of a degenerative disease.

Evaluation of Motor Speech Disorders

Learning Objective 10.4 Describe assessment techniques for motor speech disorders.

To correctly identify motor speech disorders, you must first obtain a thorough case history from the client or client's caregiver, as motor speech disorders are often accompanied by predictable complaints and symptoms. In addition, it is important to have a client attempt various speech production tasks specifically designed for purposes of differential diagnosis, along with perceptual and objective measures of the speech production subsystems (i.e., respiratory, phonatory, resonatory, articulatory). Such measures will allow you to determine the most effective treatment approach for the client.

As an SLP, you will likely serve on a diagnostic team with medical professionals, particularly when your client is exhibiting generalized neurological impairments. By correctly identifying different speech patterns consistent with a particular type of motor speech disorder, you as an SLP provide valuable information to other members of the team responsible for differential diagnosis of underlying neurological conditions.

When assessing a child or adult client, the purposes of the motor speech evaluation are many and include the following:

- To determine whether a significant long-term problem exists
- To describe the nature of impaired functions, specifically the types of problems, their extent and severity, and the effect of these impairments on everyday functional communication
- To identify functions that are not impaired
- To establish appropriate goals and decide where to begin intervention
- To form a well-reasoned prognosis, based on the nature of the disorder, the client's age, the age or stage of injury or disease, the presence of other accompanying conditions, client motivation, and family support

You as an SLP will evaluate the structure and function of a client's oral mechanism, connected speech, and speech in special tasks. Although a few commercial test procedures are available, many SLPs working in hospitals or outpatient clinics have assessment protocols they use for their motor speech evaluations in pediatric and adult populations. These procedures may or may not rely on the use of instrumental approaches.

To begin, you examine the oral peripheral mechanism and note the following with particular interest:

- Symmetry, configuration, color, and general appearance of the face, jaw, lips, tongue, teeth, and hard and soft palate at rest
- Movement of the jaw, lips, tongue, and soft palate
- Range, force, speed, and direction of the jaw, lips, and tongue during movement

You will also determine either directly (using instrumental methods) or indirectly (during nonspeech tasks or perceptual speech production tasks) the following:

- Respiratory function during speech production
- Phonatory initiation, maintenance, and cessation
- Pitch and pitch variability
- Loudness and loudness variability
- Volitional pitch–loudness variations
- Velopharyngeal function

For adults who may have acquired apraxia of speech, the following speech production tasks will help in differential diagnosis:

- Imitation of single words of varying lengths
- Sentence imitation
- Reading aloud
- Spontaneous speech
- Rapid repetition of "puh," "tuh," "kuh," and "puh-tuh-kuh" (or "buttercup")

CASE STUDY   Genevieve *(continued)*

During the structural functional examination, Genevieve exhibited an expressionless face at rest. Her jaw, lips, and tongue were normal in strength but mildly reduced in range of motion. Conversational speech was characterized by moderately reduced loudness, rapid speech rate, short rushes of speech, and reduced articulatory precision. Sound and syllable repetitions were occasionally heard. Vowel prolongation was reduced in loudness and had a breathy-hoarse voice quality. Nonspeech and speech characteristics were consistent with hypokinetic dysarthria secondary to her medical diagnosis of Parkinson disease.

Genevieve completed the 10-item Communication Participation Bank questionnaire (Baylor et al., 2013). Her responses indicated that her speech and voice difficulties were significantly impacting her ability to effectively communicate with friends, family, and others in her daily life.

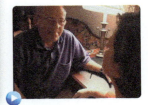

Pearson eTextbook
Video Example 10.2
Examining the Oral Peripheral Mechanism

Go to the link for a video of a speech-language pathologist examining the structures and function of the upper airway system in an older adult male client.

Speech production assessment tasks for apraxia are repetitive and imitative. Recall that performance in apraxia of speech will likely vary with repeated performance, and errors may be inconsistent. Modes of stimulus presentation are also important because the person with apraxia responds better to auditory-visual stimuli than to either auditory or visual stimuli alone. Additional assessment techniques for children suspected of having childhood apraxia of speech are discussed in Chapter 5.

Treatment of Motor Speech Disorders

Learning Objective 10.5 Briefly explain evidence-based treatments for dysarthria and apraxia.

Some basic principles underlie treatment of motor speech disorders in children and adults. These include (1) restoring lost function, (2) using compensatory strategies, and (3) adjusting for lost function (Duffy, 2020). For adults with acquired motor speech disorders like dysarthria or apraxia, a full recovery is quite possible, particularly in mild cases of stroke, for instance. Generally, residual motor speech deficits persist for long periods of time in many individuals with acquired disorders, and especially in those with congenital disorders such as cerebral palsy. Compensation for inadequate functioning of the motor speech system will be necessary. For degenerative diseases such as ALS or Parkinson disease that are progressive, ongoing adjustment to lost function will be necessary. Compensatory strategies and the use of prosthetic devices may be effective throughout the course of the disease.

Management of Dysarthria

Because dysarthria affects all aspects of speech production, management must address a client's difficulties with respiration, phonation, resonance, articulation, and prosody. Various medical, prosthetic, and behavioral interventions are available to improve all aspects of speech production for speakers with dysarthria. Several ways speakers with dysarthria can modify their respiration, phonation, resonance, articulation, and prosody to improve their overall speech intelligibility are discussed below.

A behavioral technique to improve speech breathing is reading aloud using a breath-patterning strategy. The client is trained to pause and take a breath when they see a back slash (/) while reading sentences (Tjaden & Liss, 1995). Say the following sentence aloud: *She sat quietly all through high school*. Now say it again and pause and take a breath at the slash mark: *She sat quietly/all through high school*. Helping speakers with dysarthria learn to increase pauses and breaths during speech helps improve respiratory drive and coordination, thereby increasing speech intelligibility.

If respiratory muscle weakness impedes use of such a strategy, as in the case of ALS or in some children with spastic cerebral palsy, an abdominal binder is an effective prosthetic for increasing respiratory drive, thereby improving loudness and voice quality (Figure 10.9). Patients with severe respiratory weakness and significantly reduced loudness levels may choose to use a voice amplifier (Figure 10.10).

Specific medical interventions and techniques for improving voice and voice quality are described in Chapter 9. To recap one of these, an evidence-based behavioral approach to increasing phonatory competence in adults with Parkinson disease and for treating respiratory and phonatory deficits in children with spastic cerebral palsy is the *Lee Silverman Voice Treatment (LSVT)*. LSVT is an intensive 4-week speech treatment program that has been shown to produce marked and long-term improvement in voice and speech function. LSVT trains speakers to use a louder voice with good voice quality and to self-monitor use of this new loud voice.

While voice and voice quality improve with LSVT, indirect benefits of this treatment have also been seen in velopharyngeal function, articulation, and swallowing. Visit the LSVT Global website at www.lsvtglobal.com and go to "Videos" for demonstrations of LSVT LOUD, along with the physical therapy equivalent treatment, LSVT BIG.

FIGURE 10.9 Abdominal binder.

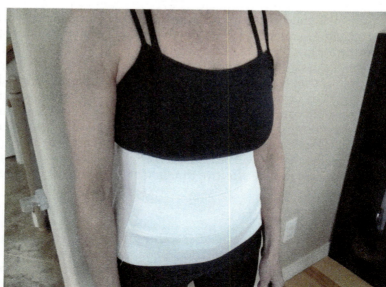

© Kimberly Allyn Farinella

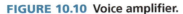

FIGURE 10.10 **Voice amplifier.**

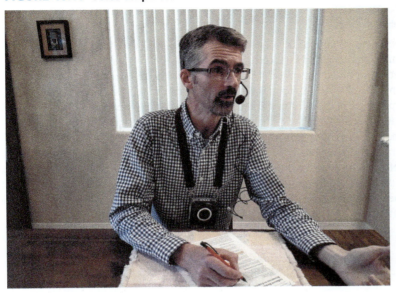

© Thomas Parker

Techniques and prosthetic devices to improve velopharyngeal function are described in detail in Chapter 9, including continuous positive airway pressure and use of a palatal lift. These same techniques may be useful in individuals with dysarthria secondary to velopharyngeal weakness. As mentioned previously, LSVT has also been shown to improve velopharyngeal function in adults and children with dysarthria of varying etiologies.

Intensive, repetitive speech production drill practice with meaningful words and phrases is an effective way to increase articulatory accuracy and improve speech intelligibility. Electropalatography (EPG), mentioned in Chapter 9, has utility in increasing articulatory precision in children with dysarthria due to cerebral palsy and in adults with acquired dysarthria. EPG provides visual feedback of tongue movement placement for articulatory accuracy. Although the device may be awkward at first, wearing an EPG palate for as little as 2 hours in a period of a day results in speech that sounds typical (McLeod & Searl, 2006). Through a combination of EPG computer display, speech monitoring, and biofeedback, some pediatric and adult clients with dysarthria learn better tongue control for improved articulation of speech sounds.

Speech supplementation strategies increase listener comprehension of speech produced by adults with dysarthria. Alphabet cues, where the speaker points to the first letter of each word on an alphabet board as they say the word, combined with topic cues, or stating the topic of conversation and indicating topic changes, help to slow speech rate, as well as allow listeners to better predict the speaker's intended message (Hustad et al., 2003; Yorkston & Beukelman, 2013) (see Figure 10.11). Such strategies may also be effective for older children with dysarthria.

For children and adults with markedly severe to profound dysarthria, the use of AAC (see Chapter 13) in conjunction with verbal forms of communication are most beneficial. Individual assessment is needed to determine the optimal system, including the client–device interface or input mode.

> **CASE STUDY** **Genevieve** (*continued*)
>
> Genevieve participated in 16 sessions of LSVT LOUD over four weeks with two graduate student clinicians certified in LSVT at the university clinic. Example functional phrases practiced each session included, "How was your day?", "Can you please take the dog for a walk?", and "Turn the television on, please." After completing LSVT LOUD treatment, Genevieve participated in LSVT BIG with physical therapy students and their clinical educators at the university. In the following semester, she participated in a combined speech therapy and physical therapy program at the university's Interprofessional Practice Clinic. Dual-task activities targeted in the combined treatment program with speech and PT student clinicians included practice using her LSVT LOUD voice in functional phrases while simulating household chores, like picking up clothes from the ground and placing them into a laundry basket or putting away dishes from the dishwasher into upper cabinets.

FIGURE 10.11 Alphabet board.

A	B	C	D		
E	F	G	H		
I	J	K	L	M	N
O	P	Q	R	S	T
U	V	W	X	Y	Z
Space					

Historically, intervention to improve articulation in individuals with dysarthria has included nonspeech oral-motor treatments (NSOMTs), including exercise, massage, blowing, positioning, icing, cheek puffing, and other nonspeech activities. Data on the value of these techniques are weak. Despite popularity of NSOMTs, evidence-based practice suggests that there is insufficient evidence to support their use, and NSOMTs are not recommended to improve articulation in adults and children with dysarthria.

Management of Apraxia of Speech

One of the most effective treatments for acquired apraxia of speech continues to be *integral stimulation*, a speech production approach developed by Rosenbek et al. (1973). This approach uses the visual-auditory cued instructions "watch me, listen to me," along with an eight-step task continuum of speech production practice (e.g., simultaneous production, immediate production, delayed production). The SLP uses these cues to help the client with apraxia re-establish their motor planning/programming abilities necessary for volitional production of functional words and phrases that are meaningful and motivating for the client.

Integral stimulation procedures incorporate the principles of motor learning (e.g., intensive practice distributed throughout the week), which is important for retraining motor skills that can no longer be accessed following brain injury (e.g., stroke). For a comprehensive discussion of the principles of motor learning, see Maas et al. (2008).

Other useful therapeutic approaches for apraxia of speech include *melodic intonation therapy (MIT)*, an approach that focuses on prosody, emphasizing the melody, rhythm, and stress patterns of spoken utterances. With this approach, the SLP models an utterance for a client by "singing" the phrase and tapping out the rhythm while the client attempts to imitate. As the client is producing the utterance, the SLP works to fade the rhythmic cues until the client imitates speech without such cues (Yorkston et al., 2010). Because acquired apraxia of speech typically involves an infarct in the left hemisphere, melodic intonation therapy is believed to facilitate motor planning/programming for speech production by accessing functions more associated with the right hemisphere (i.e., singing).

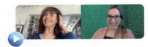

Pearson eTextbook
Video Example 10.3
Apraxia of Speech

This is a video of a woman with apraxia of speech practicing the word *family* with the graduate student clinician. The treatment approaches of backward chaining and integral stimulation (i.e., watch me, listen to me, do what I do) are used in this video to enable the client to eventually achieve correct production of the word *family*.

> **REFLECTION QUESTION 10.3**
>
> *How are treatment techniques for childhood apraxia of speech (see Chapter 5) and acquired apraxia of speech in adults similar, and how and why do they differ?*

Another treatment approach for acquired apraxia of speech that focuses on prosody is contrastive stress. In this approach, the client practices producing sentences by emphasizing stress on particular words in the sentence and thus changing the meaning of that sentence (e.g., *I* didn't say he stole the money"; "I *didn't* say he stole the money"; "I didn't say *he* stole the money"). Contrastive stress practice is most effective for clients with mild to moderate apraxia of speech who continue to exhibit prosodic abnormalities while having otherwise adequate speech articulation skills (Yorkston et al., 2010). Box 10.1 summarizes the evidence-based treatment approaches that may be beneficial for individuals with motor speech disorders.

BOX 10.1   **Evidence-Based Practice with Motor Speech Disorders**

Repetition/Practice

- Repetition is important for maintaining changes in the brain and their related functional benefits. In general, maintenance of intervention gains requires long-term consistent use of a skill.

Intensity of Intervention

- Given the need for repetitive motor speech production practice, intensive and individualized treatment is stressed for individuals with apraxia of speech, nonprogressive dysarthria, and in

some cases of slowly progressive dysarthria (e.g., Parkinson disease). There are more beneficial results from prolonged practice distributed over time to promote speech motor learning.

Dysarthria

- Electropalatograph technology offers modest gains in speech production.
- Using a breath-patterning strategy, where backslashes are strategically placed in reading passages to remind the client to pause and take

(continued)

a breath, is an effective way to improve loudness and overall speech clarity when reading aloud. It can be difficult to generalize this strategy to conversational speech, however.

- Overenunciating and maximizing prosody (i.e., stress and inflection) can improve articulation and overall speech intelligibility.

- Supplementation strategies such as specifying the topic of conversation and using an alphabet board (pointing to the first letter of every word produced) have been shown to significantly improve listeners' ability to comprehend speakers with dysarthria, particularly those with severe to profound dysarthria secondary to neurodegenerative disease (e.g., amyotrophic lateral sclerosis).

- Familiarizing listeners with dysarthric speech, even with only brief exposure, is very effective in improving listeners' ability to subsequently understand a speaker with dysarthria.

- Parkinson disease
  - LSVT produces long-term clinically meaningful improvement in voice, speech, and swallowing functions.
  - Clinical ratings of loudness, prosody, and speech intelligibility all showed improvement following SPEAK OUT!® treatment, where clients with Parkinson disease are taught to speak with intent.
  - Surgical interventions, such as deep brain stimulation, may improve limb motor function but may cause further motor speech and swallowing deficits.

Apraxia of Speech

- Integral stimulation is beneficial when addressing speech production difficulties in individuals with acquired apraxia of speech.
- Melodic intonation therapy is useful during the early stages of acquired apraxia of speech, when speech production may be very difficult.
- Contrastive stress is beneficial for mild to moderate apraxia of speech when prosodic abnormalities persist.

Sources: Based on Boutsen et al. (2018); Broadfoot et al. (2019); Duffy (2020); Tjaden and Liss (1995); Wambaugh et al. (2013); Yorkston et al. (2010),

Summary

The two main types of motor speech disorders are dysarthria and apraxia of speech. Dysarthria is a group of speech disorders that affect the speed, range, direction, strength, and timing of motor movement as a result of paralysis, weakness, or discoordination of the speech muscles. Five distinct types are flaccid, spastic, ataxic, hyperkinetic, and hypokinetic dysarthria. Disorders affecting multiple motor systems may yield a mixed dysarthria.

Dysarthria can be acquired in adulthood because of neurological disease (e.g., Parkinson disease) or traumatic brain injury (e.g., motor vehicle accident) or can be congenital as in cerebral palsy. Dysarthria is also associated with neurodevelopmental disorders like Tourette syndrome.

Apraxia is an acquired disorder in voluntary motor planning and programming of movement gestures for speech that is unrelated to muscle weakness or paralysis. Apraxia of speech often results from a lesion in the central programming area for speech in the left frontal lobe that details and plans the coordination of sequenced motor movements for speech.

Motor speech disorders, both congenital and acquired, offer a special challenge to the affected individual, family, friends, and SLP. Many clients are in the very frustrating position of being able to formulate a message but are unable to produce it intelligibly.

Intervention methods differ greatly. A child with cerebral palsy may learn to communicate using an AAC device. Meanwhile, an older adult with motor speech deficits may relearn or retrieve previously learned speech patterns. Finally, an individual with a progressive degenerative disease, such as Parkinson disease or amyotrophic lateral sclerosis, may attempt to maintain the level of effective communication that was previously possible or may explore additional methods of communication. Changing intervention techniques and promising new surgical procedures and medical management continue to offer hope to individuals with motor speech disorders of neurogenic origin.

Epilogue   Case Study: Genevieve

After completing treatment, Genevieve now reports that her voice feels stronger, she doesn't notice disfluencies as often anymore, and she feels more confident when speaking in most situations. Her steps are more typical in size when she walks, and it doesn't take her as long to complete basic, everyday activities like eating or doing household chores. Genevieve returns one time per month to the university for LSVT LOUD and BIG follow-up treatments to maintain her gains and participates in the SING OUT!® Virtual Choir online through the Parkinson Voice Project, a nonprofit organization. Her family reports also that she is more outgoing and interactive during family gatherings and seems more like herself again.

Reflections   from Kim's Uncle Joe, who has Parkinson Disease: Joseph B. D'Antoni

At long last, I am rediscovering the LOUD program which I had completed over five years ago. Now, I find myself sitting with a different speech pathologist renewing and reviewing my speech skills. Not only is this speech pathologist using the tenets of the LOUD Program, but she is also incorporating other programs to enhance my speech. Through the miracle of technology, I have an app on my phone that keeps me apprised of my loudness of speech and [has] a daily message pop up on my screen, reminding me to be loud and clear. With the help of my speech pathologist, my speech is improving gradually. My speech pathologist is patient and caring and encourages me to keep moving forward.

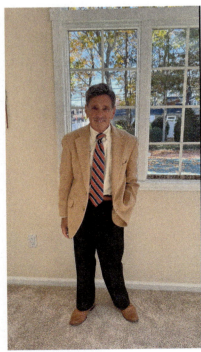

© Joseph B.D Antoni

Suggested Readings/Sources

Duffy, J. (2020). *Motor speech disorders: Substrates, differential diagnosis, and management* (4th ed.). Elsevier.

Yorkston, K., Beukelman, D., Strand, E., & Hakel, M. (2010). *Management of motor speech disorders in children and adults* (3rd ed.). PRO-ED.

Yorkston, K. M., Miller, R. M., & Strand, E. A. (2004). *Management of speech and swallowing disorders in degenerative disease* (2nd ed.). PRO-ED.

11 Disorders of Swallowing

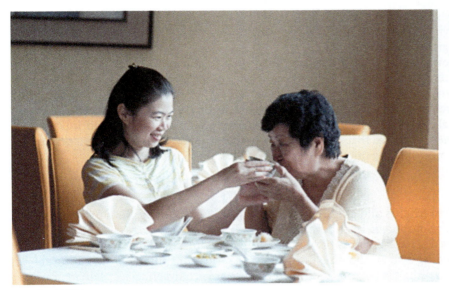

© szefei/123RF

Learning Objectives

When you have finished this chapter, you should be able to:

11.1 Describe the normal and disordered processes of swallowing.

11.2 List and describe common etiologies of pediatric and adult dysphagia.

11.3 List and describe the important components of the swallowing evaluation.

11.4 Describe evidence-based swallowing treatments for children and adults.

> " I was in graduate school when I learned that my grandpa was diagnosed with cancer. I didn't know what kind of cancer but knew he was being treated with chemotherapy and radiation. After his treatments, he ended up in the hospital with aspiration pneumonia [a respiratory infection that occurs when foreign material enters the lungs] because of difficulties swallowing. It was then that I learned he had received radiation to the pyriform sinus, a cavity located near of the back of the larynx. I watched him receive speech therapy for swallowing in the hospital. It was then that I vowed to do what I could to prevent cases like his and to help patients with swallowing disorders as the focus of my career.
>
> —*Carolyn Abraham, medical speech-language pathologist*

Speech-language pathologists (SLPs) play a major role in the evaluation and management of *dysphagia*, or swallowing disorders. The American Speech-Language-Hearing Association's (ASHA's) 2021 *Health Care Survey in Speech-Language Pathology* found that 59% of SLPs who work in adult settings said swallowing disorders were among the top five areas they treated. Swallowing ranked more often (33%) than any other area (e.g., aphasia, acquired brain injury) treated by clinical service providers who treat adults. In this same survey, 36% of SLPs working in pediatric hospital settings reported that they provide feeding and swallowing

CASE STUDY   **Steve**

Steve was 57 years old when he had a stroke. After a week in the hospital and 10 days in acute rehabilitation, his dysphagia had not resolved. He was referred to the outpatient SLP who specialized in treating patients with swallowing difficulties. The referral order read "oropharyngeal dysphagia, on thickened liquids." The SLP recognized the need to ensure Steve's safety when swallowing. Any difficulty swallowing foods or liquids can result in choking, aspiration (foreign material entering the lungs), or even **aspiration pneumonia** (respiratory infection that occurs when foreign material enters the lungs).

During their first session, the SLP learned that Steve was having difficulty swallowing his favorite

drink, Diet Coke. He was not eating his favorite foods, such as nuts or toast. If he ate a piece of toast, it would take him 2 hours to finish. Steve stated that it felt as if food was getting stuck at the level of his voice box, and he had to cough after eating.

As you read this chapter think about:

- How damage to the brain could interfere with swallowing
- Why certain textures of foods or consistencies of liquids can contribute to swallowing difficulties
- How a swallowing disorder might affect a person's quality of life

services to infants and children (ASHA, 2021). Additionally, SLPs may be required to manage dysphagia in children in their school-based setting (e.g., Homer, 2015). You, the SLP, are responsible for screening, evaluating, and treating individuals with feeding and swallowing disorders. With the continually growing number of adult and pediatric patients identified every year with dysphagia, specific knowledge about normal and disordered swallowing is essential to effectively evaluate and manage feeding and swallowing disorders. The Case Study in this chapter describes a man with disordered swallowing after having a stroke.

Swallowing and the efficient intake of food have both medical and psychosocial implications. Eating is essential to physical health. Without proper nourishment, one cannot grow, develop, or survive. Swallowing disorders increase the risk of choking and may lead to **aspiration** of food into the lungs and respiratory illnesses such as pneumonia. Problems or weakness related to the anatomy of swallowing may result in **gastroesophageal reflux (GER)**, the movement of food or acid from the stomach back into the esophagus. Eating is also one of our major social activities. Feeding difficulties in children may stress the parent–child relationship. Among older people, dysphagia may lead to isolation, depression, frustration, and diminished quality of life.

The term *dysphagia*, which comes from the Greek, literally means "difficulty with eating."

REFLECTION QUESTION 11.1

What special skills and knowledge does the SLP bring to swallowing therapy?

In this chapter, we describe the normal processes involved in feeding and swallowing. We describe the characteristics and common etiologies associated with disordered swallowing and discuss how to evaluate and manage feeding and swallowing disorders.

Normal and Disordered Swallowing

Learning Objective 11.1 Describe the normal and disordered processes of swallowing.

We generally don't think about how we swallow food or liquid. We know that we put something edible in our mouth, chew for a while, and then swallow. Sometimes, however, we have trouble that calls attention to the process. For example, we might eat and cough or feel that the food has "gone down the wrong pipe." Before we can understand disorders of swallowing, we need to examine processes involved in normal swallowing.

Normal Swallowing

Normal swallowing can be described in four stages: oral preparation, oral transport, pharyngeal, and esophageal. The following section describes each of these stages in detail.

Oral Preparation Phase

When you are ready to eat, your senses heighten. You may salivate in anticipation of food coming to your mouth. In the oral preparation for swallowing solid foods, the tongue and cheeks move the food to the teeth for chewing and mixing with saliva to form a solid **bolus**. When preparing to drink, the tongue forms a cupped position and holds the fluid in a liquid bolus. The back of the tongue raises to contact the velum and forms a back wall separating the oral and pharyngeal cavities. This ensures the prepared liquid or solid bolus doesn't spill into the pulmonary airways (Hoit et al., 2022).

Oral Transport Phase

Once the bolus is formed, the oral transport (or transit) stage begins. This stage consists of the movement of the bolus from the front to the back of the mouth. Approximately when the substance reaches the level of the anterior faucial pillars at the rear of the mouth, the pharyngeal swallow reflex is triggered. Oral transport typically takes less than 1 second (Hoit et al., 2022). Figure 11.1 depicts the oral transport phase of swallowing, which relies heavily on the tongue to propel the bolus back toward the oropharynx.

The oral and pharyngeal phases of swallowing involve much of the same anatomy that is used in speaking.

Pharyngeal Phase

During the pharyngeal phase (Figure 11.2), the velum moves up to meet the rear wall of the pharynx to prevent the bolus from going into the nasal cavity. The base of the tongue and pharyngeal wall move toward one another to create the pressure needed to propel the bolus into the pharynx. The pharynx contracts and squeezes the bolus down. While this is occurring, the hyoid bone rises, bringing the larynx up and forward. The elevation of the larynx prevents the bolus from entering the trachea by closing the true and false vocal folds and lowering the epiglottis, covering the airway. The pharyngeal swallowing reflex involves contraction of superior, middle, and inferior constrictor muscles. This phase is complete when the upper esophageal sphincter opens and the food or liquid moves into the esophagus. The pharyngeal phase is under automatic neural control and occurs very quickly and is usually complete in less than 1 second (Hoit et al., 2022).

FIGURE 11.1 The oral transport phase of a normal swallow, with food depicted in green. (A) After the food is chewed and mixed with saliva during the oral preparation stage, it forms a bolus that is arranged on the back of the tongue. (B) The tongue tip moves upward and forward to contact the hard palate. (C) The back of the tongue pushes downward and backward toward the soft palate to propel the bolus into the oropharynx.

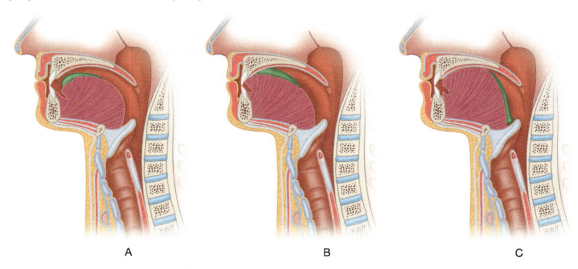

A   B   C

FIGURE 11.2 The pharyngeal phase of a normal swallow, with food depicted in green. (A) As the tongue moves upward, the velopharyngeal port closes, and the larynx begins to elevate. (B) The tongue pushes back into the pharynx, squeezing the bolus downward through the pharynx. The larynx moves upward and forward, which causes the upper esophageal segment (UES) to relax. (C) The tongue continues pushing backward, and the bolus moves through the UES into the esophagus.

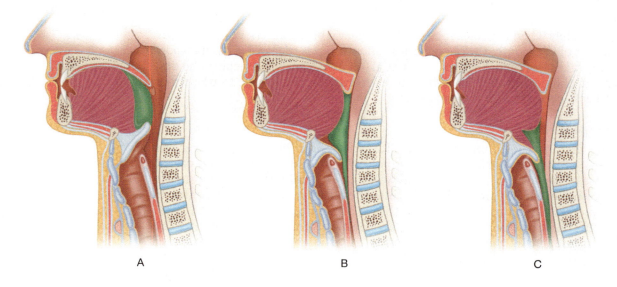

A   B   C

Esophageal Phase

The last stage of the swallowing process occurs when the muscles of the esophagus move the bolus in peristaltic, or rhythmic, wavelike contractions from the top of the esophagus into the stomach. This typically takes 3 to 20 seconds in an unimpaired individual.

Disordered Swallowing

Problems in swallowing can occur in any or all phases of the swallow. A person may have difficulty chewing food or forming a cohesive bolus. They may have difficulty moving the food or liquid from the front to the back of the mouth. Difficulties may also arise later if the person is unable to propel the bolus posteriorly in an effective manner, or if the bolus is restricted from passing from the pharynx and/or esophagus to the stomach.

Oral Preparation/Oral Transport Phase

If the lips do not seal properly, drooling can occur. Chewing may be impaired because of poor muscle tone or paralysis involving the mouth or because of missing teeth. Insufficient saliva will impede adequate bolus formation. Food may pocket or get stuck in the cheek. The muscles of the tongue might not function adequately or efficiently enough to move the food to the teeth for chewing and to transport the bolus from the front to the back of the mouth to prepare for the pharyngeal phase.

Pharyngeal Phase

Several serious problems are associated with limitations during the pharyngeal phase. If the swallow is not triggered or is delayed, material may be *aspirated*, or fall into the airway and eventually into the lungs. If the swallow is inefficient, material can remain in the pharynx after the swallow, increasing risk for aspiration of the retained material after the swallow or during a subsequent swallow. Failure to close the velopharyngeal port, the passageway to the nose, can lead to substances going into and out of the nose. Poor tongue mobility may result in insufficient pressure in the pharynx, which is needed to drive the bolus into the esophagus.

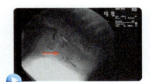

Pearson eTextbook
Video Example 11.1

In this video on videofluoroscopy, notice how the liquid bolus spills over into the airway.

> **REFLECTION QUESTION 11.2**
>
> *What similarities and differences in the physiology of swallowing and speech can you think of?*

Esophageal Phase

If peristalsis is slow or absent, the complete bolus might not be transported from the pharynx to the stomach. Residue might be left on the esophageal walls, resulting in infection and nutritional problems. Reflux from retained material in the esophagus may reach the level of the pharynx, increasing the risk of aspiration after the swallow.

The swallowing mechanism is intricately linked to respiratory coordination. The pharynx is the common pathway between the airway and the digestive tract during swallowing, requiring coordination between swallowing and breathing for successful feeding (Kamity et al., 2021).

Etiologies of Pediatric and Adult Dysphagia

Learning Objective 11.2 List and describe common etiologies of pediatric and adult dysphagia.

Feeding disorders can describe difficulties children may have accepting varied food textures or an age-appropriate diet. Swallowing disorders generally describe difficulty with eating or swallowing resulting from physiological or anatomical issues. Feeding disorders in children can develop secondary to a child's history with

FIGURE 11.3 Feeding tube being used by premature baby twin.

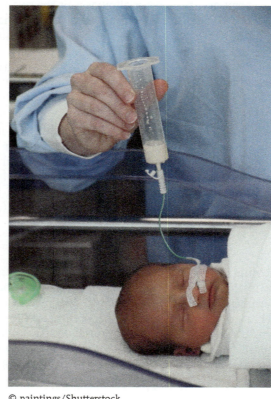

© paintings/Shutterstock

dysphagia, which may have caused uncomfortable or painful eating experiences, subsequently impacting the child's willingness to try new foods (e.g., Olson, 2012). As such, feeding and swallowing disorders are often described under the umbrella term "pediatric dysphagia." Figure 11.3 shows a premature newborn being tube fed because the infant does not yet have the coordination of sucking, swallowing, and breathing.

Infants and children with pediatric dysphagia may experience malnutrition, inadequate growth, dehydration, ill health, prolonged feeding times, fatigue, difficulty learning, and poor parent–child relationships. Children with central or peripheral nervous system deficits or immaturity, neuromuscular disease, and craniofacial anomalies are particularly vulnerable to pediatric dysphagia.

Feeding and swallowing difficulties are even more common in older individuals. One study reported a lifetime dysphagia prevalence rate of 38% in individuals between 65 and 94 years of age who were living independently (Roy et al., 2007). For adults over 50 years of age living in skilled nursing facilities, prevalence rates of dysphagia are over 60% (e.g., Suiter & Gosa, 2019).

As a result of the growing numbers of individuals experiencing dysphagia at any given time, there is an increased demand for qualified SLPs who can provide feeding and swallowing services to pediatric and adult clients in various clinical settings. Common etiologies and characteristics of feeding and swallowing disorders in pediatric and adult populations are briefly described in Table 11.1.

The high incidence and co-occurrence of dysphagia, dysarthria, and aphasia in individuals post-stroke stresses the important role of the SLP early in the stroke rehabilitation process (Stipancic et al., 2019).

TABLE 11.1

Common Etiologies of Feeding and Swallowing Disorders in Children and Adults

Etiology	Description
Disorders in Children	
Prematurity (< 37 weeks gestation)	Occurs in over 10% of live births annually. Immature, uncoordinated suck, swallow, and breathe patterns can delay successful breast- or bottle-feeding, cause difficulties with weight gain and dehydration, and increase risk of aspiration. Tube feedings may be required until sucking/swallowing development is sufficient and safe to transition to total oral feeding.
Cerebral palsy (CP)	Gastroesophageal reflux is common in infants and children with CP and ingestion of food may be painful. Reduced lip closure, drooling, poor tongue function, exaggerated bite reflex, delayed swallow initiation, and reduced pharyngeal motility are types of oral and pharyngeal problems exhibited by children with CP. In severe cases of dysphagia, children with CP require gastrostomy tube feedings.
Intellectual and developmental disability (IDD)	Delayed motor coordination skills secondary to IDD may interfere with feeding and the oral phase of swallowing. Communication disorders are common in individuals with IDD, and children may be limited in their ability to express food desires and preferences.
Autism spectrum disorder (ASD)	Feeding problems in children with ASD may result from repetitive patterns of behavior or sensory issues that restrict the types of food consumed, possibly leading to poor nutrition. Children with ASD with sensory processing deficits may be hypersensitive to sound, light, pain, smell, and touch. Avoidance is common when children with sensory disorders are introduced to new foods, with negative responses like spitting, gagging, or vomiting occurring.
Craniofacial anomalies	Infants with cleft lip and palate may have severe feeding and swallowing difficulties, including an inability to create negative intraoral pressure due to not being able to seal the nasal cavity and nasopharynx from the oral cavity and oropharynx. This can impair the ability to express milk from the nipple and cause nasopharyngeal regurgitation or milk remaining in the nose and mouth as the result of the lack of separation between the oral and nasal cavities.
Disorders in Adults	
Stroke	Oral-motor and sensory deficits are common after stroke. Tongue weakness may interfere with the ability to control the bolus or propel it posteriorly into the oropharynx. Poor awareness of food or liquid in the mouth may result in holding the bolus in the mouth for long periods. Facial weakness can lead to pocketing of food inside the cheek. Sensory deficits in the larynx and pharynx and a decreased cough reflex can cause **silent aspiration**, or aspiration with no apparent sign or response.
Head and neck cancer	Surgery, radiation, and chemotherapy are used to treat tumors of the mouth, throat, and larynx. The degree of swallowing impairment is closely related to the size and location of the original tumor(s) and the surgical procedure used to close or reconstruct the area. Radiation therapy may result in decreased salivation and dry mouth, causing decreased swallow frequency. Taste changes, swelling, and sometimes mouth sores cause pain and decrease motivation to continue an oral diet. Long-term radiation may cause tissue changes, which result in reduced mobility and can affect swallow function. Chemotherapy may cause weakness, nausea, vomiting, and loss of appetite, which also interfere with feeding and swallowing.

(Continued)

Etiology	Description
Parkinson disease (PD)	PD-related dysphagia affects all phases of swallowing. Difficulties may include reduced chewing speed and coordination, decreased bolus control and premature spilling into the pharynx, delayed initiation of the swallow, frequent swallows to clear the pharynx, slow and reduced hyolaryngeal movement, and esophageal dysmotility and reflux. Reluctance to eat in public due to embarrassment about drooling, slow eating, or fear of choking is not uncommon. Patients with more severe dysphagia have more significant drooling.
Traumatic brain injury (TBI)	Impaired attention skills and high distractibility following TBI may result in reduced intake of food or liquid and risk of malnutrition or dehydration. Motor deficits, including reduced range and control of tongue movements and/or delayed or absent swallowing, are common causes of oral-pharyngeal dysphagia. Cranial nerves may be damaged following head trauma associated with motor vehicle accidents.
Dementia	Cognitive deficits associated with dementia may impede attention and orientation to food or liquid. Forgetting to eat or eating the same meal multiple times due to memory deficits is not uncommon. Oral preparatory tongue and jaw movements may be lacking in purpose, causing drooling and poor bolus formation. Oral transport may be prolonged. Swallow initiation may be delayed and laryngeal elevation reduced.

Sources: Based on Arvedson et al. (2010, 2013); Boggs and Ferguson (2016); Broadfoot et al. (2019); Dailey (2013); Groher and Crary (2010); Kamity et al. (2021); Murray et al. (2020); Nóbrega et al. (2008); Rogus-Pulia and Robbins (2013); Rosenbek and Jones (2009); Starmer (2017); Stipancic et al. (2019).

Lifespan Issues

Lactation consultants offer supportive care for mothers and their premature infants. The SLP and lactation consultant often work together to achieve successful breastfeeding or bottle feeding between infant and caregiver (Fletcher & Ash, 2005).

Feeding and swallowing problems may occur at any point in the lifespan. Newborns may be unable to suckle and/or ingest nutriment. As they age, infants may refuse food and develop unhealthy food preferences. Neuromotor problems and structural anomalies that are congenital or acquired at any age can interfere with feeding and swallowing, as can a host of psychosocial factors. Dysphagia may be related to many diverse conditions and the causes are not mutually exclusive. For example, a medical condition such as congenital heart disease that may require prolonged hospitalization and critical care interventions can delay a child's acquisition of feeding skills, interfering with their ability to consume age-appropriate liquid or food textures (Goday et al., 2019).

Whatever the etiology, the outcomes of a swallowing disorder at any age include dehydration, malnutrition, poor health, weight loss, fatigue, frustration, respiratory infection, aspiration, and even death.

Evaluation for Swallowing

Learning Objective 11.3 List and describe the important components of the swallowing evaluation.

Not everyone with the etiologies in Table 11.1 will have a swallowing disorder. For others, swallowing problems may not be readily apparent. Patients may not report difficulties, and some may experience *silent aspiration* (lack of cough when food or liquid enters the airway). The first step in evaluation is to screen individuals at risk for dysphagia. After the screening, the SLP and dysphagia team will obtain background information and use clinical and instrumental techniques to assess swallowing. A determination is made about appropriate intervention, and treatment strategies are developed and implemented in coordination with other professionals. SLPs are advocates for their clients and help provide education and counseling to them, their families, and related others.

Screening for Dysphagia

For pediatric clients, informal screenings are conducted by pediatricians, nurses, parents, and day care providers for feeding and swallowing difficulties (Delaney, 2015). A primary indication of dysphagia in infants is **failure to thrive**. Infants in a neonatal intensive care unit are carefully monitored for weight gain and development. Full-term infants who are not accepting breast or bottle are signaling feeding problems. Such infants are observed during mealtimes to evaluate breathing and physical coordination (e.g., suck/swallow/respiratory sequence), oral-motor functioning (e.g., tongue elevation), and techniques that enable quantification of nutritive and nonnutritive sucking skill (e.g., responsive to stroking around the mouth) (Groher & Crary, 2010). Caregivers can be counseled and instrumental evaluation recommended when warranted.

For adults, the Yale Swallow Protocol (YSP) is one of many available screeners to determine aspiration risk (Suiter et al., 2014). This simple pass/fail tool consists of a brief cognitive screen, an oral mechanism examination, and a 3-ounce water challenge. The brief cognitive screen and oral mechanism examination determine if the 3-ounce water challenge should be attempted. For the cognitive screen, the patient is asked the following questions to determine their orientation to person, place, and time:

- What is your name?
- Where are you right now?
- What year is it?

They are also asked to perform the following on command: open your mouth; stick out your tongue; smile. The oral mechanism examination is then performed, which assesses lip closure, tongue range of motion, and facial symmetry during smiling and lip pucker. Only the water task determines a pass/fail outcome. The patient is provided a cup of 3 ounces of water with or without a straw and asked to drink the water slowly and steadily without stopping (Figure 11.4). A patient passes the screening if they drink the entire 3 ounces of water without stopping and without coughing, choking, or other signs of aspiration (Leder & Suiter, 2014). If they fail, it is recommended they undergo instrumental swallow examination, discussed later in this chapter.

Self-assessment checklists may be used to obtain information about feeding and swallowing difficulties from the adult patient's perspective. One such instrument is the *Eating Assessment Tool (EAT-10)*, which requires the patient to answer 10 questions on a 5-point scale, such as "swallowing solids takes extra effort" or "I cough when I eat," to provide information about dysphagia symptom severity.

Another self-report questionnaire is the *Dysphagia Handicap Index (DHI)*, which has 25 items divided into three scales: physical, functional, and emotional.

The speech-language pathologist is often the leader of the dysphagia team, which also may include a dietitian, pulmonologist, radiologist, occupational therapist, social worker, nurse, and gastroenterologist.

FIGURE 11.4 Three ounces of liquid sounds like a small amount. Do you think you could drink this amount of water nonstop without difficulty?

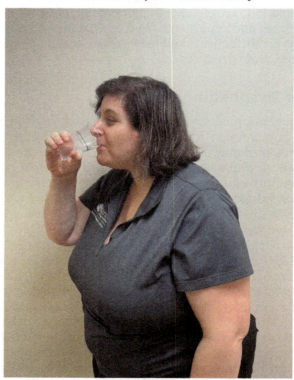

© Carolyn Abraham

Each item is rated on a 7-point scale ranging from "No difficulty" to "Presents as a severe problem." Statements such as "I feel depressed because I can't eat what I want" or "I avoid eating because of my swallowing problem" address not only dysphagia symptoms but quality of life as it pertains to eating and swallowing. Self-assessments require the individual to have adequate cognitive (intellectual) abilities. As such, these tools are not appropriate for certain clinical populations.

Dysphagia screening is an important first step in the assessment process. When feeding or swallowing difficulties are suspected based on the screening, or the patient is at risk for feeding and/or swallowing difficulties (e.g., poor weight gain in infancy; adult with dementia), additional clinical assessment is needed (Coyle, 2015). Instrumental assessment may be recommended to confirm clinical findings, determine the underlying nature of the swallowing disorder, or when pharyngeal dysphagia is suspected (Leder, 2015). Clinical evaluation of swallowing is discussed in the next section, followed by instrumental assessment.

Clinical Swallow Evaluation

Whether evaluating a child or an adult, the *clinical swallow evaluation (CSE)*, or *bedside swallow evaluation*, is an important part of the comprehensive evaluation of dysphagia. It provides the SLP with a significant amount of information about typical feeding and swallowing function, along with information about the feeding and swallowing environment (Garand et al., 2020). It also serves to establish rapport with the client and client's caregivers and provide diagnostic information about feeding and swallowing (Coyle, 2015).

The CSE has the following components:

- Case history and background information
- Cognitive-communication functioning
- Observation of environmental factors
- Oral mechanism examination
- Swallow trials

Case History and Background Information

The clinical swallow evaluation begins with a thorough case history to obtain detailed information about the chief complaint regarding the feeding and/or swallowing problem, the individual's current physical and neurological status, any medical conditions that may be present, recent surgeries, or medications the individual may be taking. A parent, caregiver, physician, nurse, or professional from an early intervention program or an adult day treatment center may make a referral to a dysphagia team, typically based on three general areas of concern:

- Difficulties have been observed related to feeding and ingestion of food or liquid.
- The client appears to be at risk for aspirating food or liquid into the lungs.
- The client appears to not be receiving adequate nourishment.

An SLP then seeks answers to questions such as those presented in Figure 11.5. The answers to these questions provide preliminary information about the location of the swallowing problem (oral, pharyngeal, or both), the kinds of food substances that are easiest and hardest to swallow, and the nature and severity of the disorder (Garand et al., 2020).

FIGURE 11.5 Important questions pertaining to swallowing.

Does the infant accept breast or bottle?	Did it worsen slowly or rapidly?
Does the problem affect solid foods or liquids?	Is there anything that relieves the symptoms?
Are there foods or liquids being avoided?	Does food seem to get stuck somewhere? If so, where?
Does food have to be modified?	What medical diagnoses or conditions may affect the swallow?
Does coughing or choking occur at mealtimes?	Has the individual had surgery that may relate to swallowing?
Do small amounts of food or liquid ever fall out of the mouth?	Is the individual using any medications?
Is the individual losing weight?	How is the individual's respiratory health?
When was the problem first observed?	How attentive is the individual?
	Is the individual able to follow directions?
	What position is the individual in when eating?

Sources: Based on Groher and Crary (2010); Murry et al. (2020).

Cognitive-Communication Functioning

Is the client alert and awake? Can they follow directions? Do they respond to questions? Do they have difficulties with attention and recall? Are they oriented to person, place, and time? Answers to these questions will determine whether it is safe to assess the client's feeding and swallowing abilities and will influence the types of interventions recommended.

Caregiver and Environmental Factors

The treating clinician will want to observe feeding as it occurs typically for the client, or caregiver and client. The clinician will pay special attention to the following:

- Is the caregiver patient and attentive?
- Does feeding take place in a reasonably quiet environment free from distractions?
- What position is the client when eating or drinking?
- How does the client express feeding preferences?

The parent or caregiver is an important part of the swallowing team. Careful observation and communication will help the SLP assess how best to improve this person's contributions. This is also an opportunity for an SLP to learn about a client's position in the family and cultural and individual factors that may influence intervention techniques. It is important to consider how treatment recommendations will influence the ability of the patient or patient's caregivers to participate in traditions. When possible, personal and cultural desires should be respected and accommodated (Riquelme, 2004).

Oral Mechanism

The integrity of the anatomy and health of a patient's mouth must be determined. Abnormalities of structure of the lips, teeth, tongue, palate, and velum are noted. Cranial nerve functioning is assessed. The SLP will look for facial symmetry and note weakness (i.e., drooping) when present. Motor difficulties such as tremor, flaccidity, excessive muscle tone (hypertonicity), and poor coordination are observed. Oral reflexes and sensation are examined. Certain reflexes such as sucking and rooting (turning to the direction of a cheek that is touched) are expected in infants but should disappear as a child matures. Checking for a strong, protective cough indirectly assesses laryngeal functioning. Poor oral hygiene, which can occur following prolonged illness, is a risk factor for aspiration and aspiration pneumonia (Murry et al., 2020).

Swallow Trials

If a client is alert and managing their saliva without any signs of aspirations or respiratory compromise, swallow trials may be conducted. The SLP will provide various foods or liquids for the patient to try and will look, listen, and feel for indications of difficulty swallowing. Overt symptoms of aspiration (e.g., coughing, throat clearing) are observed with each food or liquid trial presented. The SLP will also determine if the patient has a protective cough to keep food or liquid from entering the airway.

Patient readiness for eating or drinking is also assessed. The SLP will watch to see how well the patient eats with utensils and drinks from a cup. The SLP is interested in answering questions such as the following:

- Do the lips open and then close around the nipple, cup, or spoon?
- Is there sucking activity on the nipple?
- Is food successfully removed from the spoon?
- Is liquid or food dribbled out of the sides of the mouth?
- When the mouth opens to take in food, does the tongue cup in anticipation?
- How long does it take for the person to chew their food?
- How long is food or liquid in the mouth before it is swallowed?
- What happens after the swallow? Is there coughing?

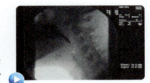

Pearson eTextbook
Video Example 11.2
Go to the link for a video of a normal swallow.

The SLP observes and feels the movement of the hyoid bone and thyroid cartilage in the neck by watching and placing a finger gently on this area. These structures should move upward during the swallow. The SLP records the number of times the client swallows while ingesting each trial of food or drink. Multiple swallows may suggest inadequate pharyngeal contraction and pharyngeal residue. Of importance are which food consistencies appear to cause difficulties and which seem to be swallowed efficiently.

Managing a Tracheostomy Tube

Some clients will have a tracheostomy tube in place to facilitate breathing. A **tracheostomy** is a surgical procedure that creates an opening through the front of the neck into the trachea where a breathing tube is inserted, providing an alternative airway. Tracheostomies can be cuffed or cuffless (Figure 11.6). The cuff is a balloon around the part of the tracheostomy tube that sits in the trachea and helps seal off the airway (Barnes & Toms, 2021). Tracheostomies may be needed because of respiratory failure requiring prolonged mechanical ventilation, a need for long-term ventilation, an inability to protect the airway, or upper airway obstruction or trauma (Saito & Morisaki, 2013).

Tracheostomized patients are at increased risk of aspiration (e.g., Bailey, 2005), so timely swallowing evaluations are critical. The swallowing evaluation for a tracheostomized patient includes all components of the clinical swallow evaluation and instrumental swallow examination when pharyngeal dysphagia is suspected. The tracheostomy cuff should be deflated and a speaking valve placed, if possible, prior to assessment.

A speaking valve is a one-way valve that allows air in through the tracheostomy during inspiration (Figure 11.7). The valve closes during expiration, forcing air up through the vocal folds and into the upper airway, enabling the possibility for speech to occur (Barnes & Toms, 2021). Speaking valves can increase swallowing efficiency and decrease aspiration risk by facilitating expiration through the upper airway after swallowing. This helps expel food or liquid that may be misdirected toward the trachea during swallowing (Prigent et al., 2012).

Instrumental Swallow Examination

Although the clinical swallow evaluation is useful in identifying the presence or absence of a swallowing problem, it cannot adequately determine the nature or severity of dysphagia of the pharyngeal phase (Leder, 2015). Complete, accurate

FIGURE 11.6 **(A) Cuffed tracheostomy tube. (B) Cuffless tracheostomy tube.**

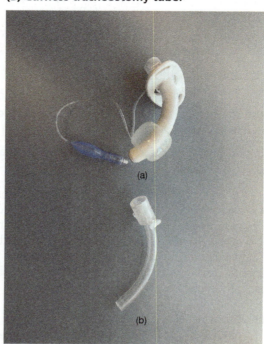

(a)

(b)

© Carolyn Abraham

FIGURE 11.7 **A speaking valve.**

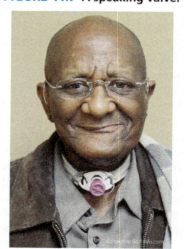

Source: Katrina M. Jensen, M.A., CCC-SLP, Advanced Head & Neck Rehabilitation Center of Texas, www.PracticalSLPinfo.com

assessment of swallowing function requires the use of instrumentation. An SLP collaborates with other team members, such as a physician, radiologist, and X-ray technician, in the use of diagnostic technology. The most common instrumental procedures to assess swallowing are described next.

Videofluoroscopic Swallowing Study

Videofluoroscopy, also referred to as a **modified barium swallow study (MBSS)**, is a video X-ray procedure performed in a radiology room. This procedure, which can be performed on children and adults, is used when clinical evaluation or screening suggests dysphagia and/or aspiration. Barium, a contrast substance that can be seen on X-rays, is prepared in different viscosities of liquids and can be added to foods such as applesauce or a cookie and ingested by the patient (Figure 11.8).

The SLP typically determines the size, texture, and consistency of the food or liquid to be presented and the head and body position of the patient during the study. A radiologist and/or X-ray technician use fluoroscopic (X-ray) equipment to record the movement of the barium throughout the swallow. These views are digitally recorded for further analysis by the physician and SLP (Figure 11.9).

Fiberoptic Endoscopic Evaluation of Swallowing

Fiberoptic (or flexible) endoscopic evaluation of swallowing (FEES) is also a type of instrumental swallow study used with pediatric or adult patients (Figure 11.10). It may be performed bedside and involves insertion of a flexible fiberoptic laryngoscope by the SLP through the patient's nose and down into the pharynx. When the scope is in place, the inside of the pharynx and larynx are clearly visible.

Accurate interpretation of videofluoroscopic swallowing studies and fiberoptic endoscopic evaluation of swallowing require a strong foundation in anatomy and physiology.

FIGURE 11.8 **A patient drinking barium during a videofluoroscopic study, also known as a modified barium swallow study.**

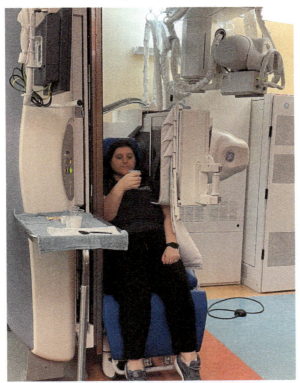

© Carolyn Abraham

Steve *(continued)*

After completing a CSE in the SLP's office, Steve was seen in radiology for an MBSS to obtain an objective measure of his swallowing function. The SLP prepared barium in various consistencies and textures for him to eat. The barium allows foods or liquids to be radiopaque, permitting visualization of the swallow on the X-ray monitor.

Steve's MBSS showed slow movements of the tongue, difficulty moving food from the front to the back of the mouth, decreased movement of the base of the tongue, and reduced hyolaryngeal elevation and excursion. Reduced pharyngeal constriction and absence of epiglottic movement were also exhibited. Pharyngeal residue was present after the swallow, especially with dry solids, requiring multiple swallows to clear. Steve exhibited laryngeal penetration of mildly thick liquids (i.e., passage of liquid into the larynx but not through the vocal folds) and silent aspiration of thin liquids. He was instructed to cough, which appeared to be helpful in expectorating material from his airway.

The patient may be asked to perform tasks such coughing and holding the breath to evaluate anatomy and physiology and swallow foods of different textures and thicknesses that have been dyed for better visualization. FEES may reveal bolus spilling into the pharynx before swallowing, and residue may be seen after the swallow. The actual swallow cannot be viewed with FEES due to a "white-out" period when the epiglottis obscures the view. Oral and esophageal phases

FIGURE 11.9 Still image from an MBSS where the patient is aspirating. The trachea can be viewed on the left and the esophagus on the right. The black material is contrast and it can be seen dripping down the trachea, indicating aspiration.

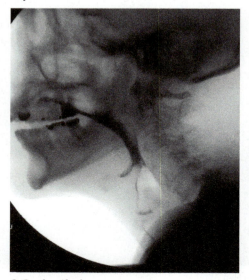

© Carolyn Abraham

FIGURE 11.10 A setup for fiberoptic endoscopic evaluation of swallowing. The sterile scope is hanging on the right side of the equipment cart.

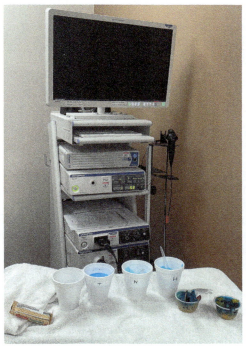

© Carolyn Abraham

of swallowing are also not visible with FEES, although reflux from the esophagus into the pharynx may be visualized. Nevertheless, observations with FEES provide valuable information about advantageous body and head posture during feeding, preferred food types, and aspiration (Figure 11.11).

FIGURE 11.11 Still image from a FEES where the patient has pharyngeal residue (blue contrast material) in the hypopharynx after the swallow.

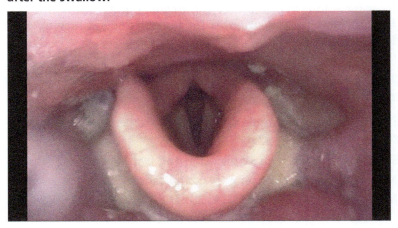

© Carolyn Abraham

The human papillomavirus, most commonly transmitted sexually, is the leading cause of cervical cancer in women. It is also a significant risk factor for head and neck cancer.

FEES may be a more effective instrumental technique than videofluoroscopy, particularly for patients with head and neck cancer who may require repeated swallow studies to minimize radiation exposure (e.g., Starmer et al., 2011). Additionally, because of its superiority in the inspection of pharyngeal anatomy and the ability to observe how a patient manages their own secretions, FEES is beneficial for those with anatomical changes following surgery or trauma or paralysis following cranial nerve damage (Groher & Crary, 2010). It is also useful for biofeedback during treatment.

Treatment of Swallowing Disorders

Learning Objective 11.4 Describe evidence-based swallowing treatments for children and adults.

Disorders of feeding and swallowing present medical, nutritional, psychological, social, and communicative problems, so many individuals are involved in working toward their resolution. As previously mentioned, the SLP is usually the dysphagia team leader, and thus the coordinator of services and the professional who is most likely to implement dysphagia treatment. Input from other team members is also essential to a satisfactory outcome.

The dysphagia team will work together to determine the most effective rehabilitation options for individuals with feeding and swallowing disorders. Generally, treatment can be divided into three categories: compensatory strategies, direct rehabilitation strategies, and indirect rehabilitation strategies. Compensatory strategies or techniques are temporary measures to maintain client safety with oral intake of food or liquids until recovery or improvement of swallowing function occurs with direct or indirect rehabilitation treatments. Direct rehabilitative techniques are those that are accomplished during swallowing, while indirect rehabilitative techniques are exercises that theoretically serve to improve swallowing (e.g., tongue strength training) without the patient having to swallow.

Compensatory strategies do not involve changes to swallowing physiology (Rogus-Pulia & Robbins, 2013). Direct and indirect rehabilitation treatments, on the other hand, are aimed at changing swallowing physiology by accelerating recovery of swallowing function after a stroke or other acquired, nonprogressive disorder. Direct and indirect treatments also help maintain swallowing function in progressive diseases for as long as possible or, in the case of pediatric disorders like prematurity, help develop the skills needed for feeding and swallowing effectiveness and efficiency.

Since patient status changes over time, ongoing assessment of feeding and swallowing function during therapy is necessary to continually update treatment goals.

Compensatory Strategies for Feeding and Swallowing Disorders

Feeding and swallowing treatments that aim to compensate for dysphagia without altering swallowing physiology address the following goals:

- Support safe and adequate nutrition and hydration
- Minimize the risk of respiratory complications
- Maximize quality of life (ASHA, 2022)

Feeding Environment

Whether the patient is an infant, young child, or adult, the environment for feeding sets the stage for a positive experience. Modifying the environment to ensure it is conducive to success during meals is important for clients with feeding and swallowing difficulties. Visual and auditory distractions should be minimized. The eating area should not contain irrelevant items. Lighting should be comfortable and noise reduced.

The caregiver should be relaxed and tuned in to the client regarding feeding speed, food preferences, and quantity. Attention and focus to the person being fed and reinforcement of healthy, effective eating behaviors are important. When possible, the goal is development of self-feeding skills.

Utensils for feeding need to be appropriate to the age and functioning of the client. For infants, a slow-flow nipple may be helpful in controlling the amount of liquid taken at a time. A Teflon or latex-covered spoon may be used for children with immature oral reflexes who may bite hard on any object placed in the mouth. Children and adults with motor coordination difficulties may benefit from using a shallow-bowled spoon. Special cutout cups may help to improve tongue positioning when drinking. Eliminating use of a straw may be helpful in managing the amount of liquid ingested. Examples of modified feeding utensils that may be helpful for children and adults with feeding difficulties are shown in Figure 11.12.

Modification of Foods and Liquids

Diet modification is a common compensatory management strategy for swallowing disorders. For certain individuals it will be a short-term solution, but for others it will represent their new "normal" to enable safe participation in oral intake of foods and liquids (Rogus-Pulia & Robbins, 2013).

FIGURE 11.12 Modified feeding utensils.

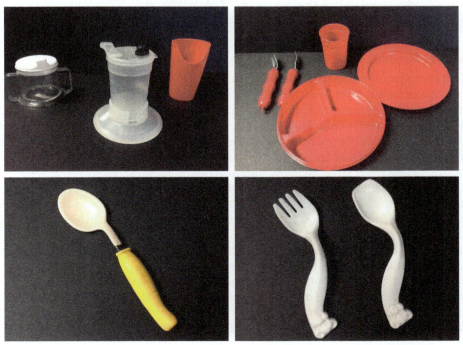

© Nikkol Anderson

Certain foods that are hard to chew, are small or slick when wet, or thick and sticky may need to be eliminated from the diet, especially for individuals with neuromotor difficulties. The elimination of certain unsafe or difficult-to-swallow diet items may be sufficient to eliminate the risk of aspiration. For others, however, a range of food consistency requirements may be recommended. Modifications to food consistency may improve chewing, thereby increasing efficiency and safety during meals (Steele et al., 2015). Increasing liquid thickness can improve control over liquids by slowing the flow of liquid through the pharynx and reduce the risk of aspiration or penetration of liquids into the airway (Newman et al., 2016).

The International Dysphagia Diet Standardization Initiative (IDDSI) is an international, standardized, culturally sensitive system to describe modifications to foods and liquids that improve the safety and efficiency of swallowing (Cichero et al., 2017). The IDDSI standardization initiative was developed to improve consistency of terminology across health care settings around the world and standardized measurement procedures to ensure correct food identification (e.g., soft and bite-sized) and liquid viscosity (e.g., slightly thick) (Rule et al., 2020). More information about the IDDSI framework can be found at ASHA's website (www.asha.org) by entering "IDDSI" into the search field.

> Providing foods of varying temperatures may increase a client's sensory awareness and improve swallowing. Cold food or drink sometimes improves tongue movement during the oral transport phase and helps to stimulate the pharyngeal swallow.

CASE STUDY   **Steve** *(continued)*

Based on the MBSS, it was recommended that Steve eat soft foods and continue with mildly thick liquids. However, he wasn't thrilled about thickening his Diet Coke. The team discussed Steve's safety while eating and drinking and concerns about his quality of life. The SLP determined that he was a good candidate for intensive swallowing treatment especially because of his motivation to return to a normal diet. At his next appointment, Steve was introduced to swallowing exercises.

Nonoral Feeding

Clients who require more than 10 seconds to swallow a liquid or food bolus or who aspirate more than 10% of either will likely require at least some nonoral feeding (Logemann, 1998). Several approaches may be used.

With **nasogastric tube (NG tube)** feeding, a tube is placed through the nose that passes through the pharynx and the esophagus, and finally into the stomach. Liquefied food and water are inserted through this tube. Unlike the more long-term procedures described later, NG tubes are usually temporary.

In **percutaneous endoscopic gastrostomy (PEG, or G-tube)**, a hole is surgically made from the abdomen to the stomach. A soft tube is placed through this hole, and blended regular food can be inserted into the tube. This procedure is used in cases of severe dysphagia and may be a permanent means for nutrition and hydration. A **jejunostomy tube (J-tube)** is like a G-tube, but it is inserted into the jejunum, or middle part of the small intestine.

Total parenteral nutrition (TPN) is a nonoral feeding method that bypasses the gastrointestinal tract and administers a specialized solution of nutrition through a vein (intravenously). All nonoral feeding methods are managed by physicians, such as a gastroenterologist, in consultation with a registered dietician.

Body and Head Positioning

Body posture and stability have a strong influence on oral-pharyngeal movements. Altering body and head positions represent compensatory treatment strategies for swallowing. An upright, symmetrical position with a 90-degree hip angle and sufficient postural support to provide stability is optimal. The individual's head and neck must be positioned and prevented from making extraneous movement, as able.

Occasionally, a child or an adult may benefit from a body posture that is not upright with a hip angle of 90 degrees. For example, some infants with severe respiratory and swallowing difficulties may feed better when placed on their sides. For some adults with pharyngeal weakness on one side, lying on their side with the stronger pharyngeal side in the down position allows gravity to assist in bolus transit toward the stronger side of the pharynx (Groher & Crary, 2010).

An SLP works closely with a physical therapist and an occupational therapist in obtaining optimum positioning for swallowing. Additional compensatory techniques include the **chin tuck** posture, which is often recommended for patients with delayed pharyngeal swallow. This position helps prevent food and liquid from entering the airway. The **head-back position** is useful for patients with poor tongue mobility if they have excellent airway closure. **Head tilt** and **head rotation** postures are used when an individual has impairment on one side. In these positions, the head may be moved in the direction of (rotation) or away from (tilt) the impairment. Compensatory positioning strategies require patient compliance, adequate intellectual abilities (cognition), and the physical capability to complete such maneuvers and manage swallowing disorders effectively in the short term (Groher & Crary, 2010).

Box 11.1 provides more specific information regarding treatment efficacy of some of these techniques with specific populations.

BOX 11.1 **Evidence-Based Practices for Individuals with Dysphagia**

General Intervention

- Involving patients and caregivers in treatment planning increases motivation and compliance with treatment recommendations and strategies.
- Ensuring that eating occurs in a familiar environment and keeping the environment free from distractions is beneficial for individuals with feeding or swallowing difficulties.

Specific Behavioral Treatment Techniques for Adults

- Postural adjustments to the body and head can facilitate safe swallowing in many patient groups. Research has shown that the chin tuck posture prevented aspiration in 55% of adult patients with mild to moderate dysphagia secondary to stroke or trauma.
- Adults with severe reflux, including those that are tube-fed, benefit from maintaining an upright posture during and after eating to prevent aspiration of stomach acids.
- The head rotation technique is effective in eliminating aspiration of liquids for some patients with dysphagia of neurological origin, as well as those with head and neck cancer post-surgery.
- Diet modification, particularly modification of thin liquids, is highly effective, at least in the short term, in patients with dysphagia associated with dementia and Parkinson disease. Thickened liquids were most effective for both patient populations, followed by thickened liquids and use of the chin tuck technique. Patient endurance must be taken into consideration when interpreting results since the benefit of thickened liquids is not maintained as patients become fatigued.
- Maintaining oral intake during radiation treatment helps prevent radiation-associated dysphagia in patients with head and neck cancer.

(continued)

- Respiratory muscle strength training targeting increased force generation of expiratory muscles, using an expiratory muscle strength training device like the one shown in Figure 11.13, improved swallowing safety and function for patients with Parkinson disease with mild dysphagia.
- Systematic lingual resistance exercise training programs increased lingual strength and swallowing ability in patients with dysphagia following stroke.
- Patients with Parkinson disease and oropharyngeal dysphagia who participated in the Lee Silverman Voice Treatment (LSVT) program demonstrated improved pharyngeal bolus transit times, reduced pharyngeal residue, and improved cough following treatment. Patients also sustained these benefits 6 months post-treatment.
- Patients with pharyngeal dysphagia who participated in a 6-week exercise program involving head-raising exercises (referred to as the *Shaker technique*) three times per day showed significant increases in swallowing functioning and reduced post-swallow aspiration.
- The supraglottic technique is difficult for many patients but is effective for some patients with dysphagia associated with neurological disease.
- The super-supraglottic swallow technique has shown positive changes in swallowing in patients with head and neck cancer.

- Studies examining the effects of neuromuscular electrical stimulation (NMES) applied to the neck via surface electrodes on functional swallowing outcomes in adults with dysphagia are promising. Well-controlled experimental trials are needed to establish the treatment efficacy of NMES procedures, however.

Specific Behavioral Treatment Techniques for Children

- Specialized feeding equipment such as bottles that reduce air intake during feeding, nipples with slower or faster flow rates, or assisted bottle-feeding delivery systems are beneficial for infants with craniofacial anomalies such as cleft lip and palate.
- Oral-motor interventions, such as non-nutritive sucking to allow sucking practice and oral stimulation to reduce hypersensitivity and improve function of the oral structures, shows positive preliminary evidence for preterm infants, including reduced hospital stays, increased alertness for feeding, and earlier transition to full oral feeding. Evidence is limited, however, and more research with larger sample sizes is needed.
- Case study research has shown that individualized swallowing programs that use principles that promote motor learning (e.g., maximized practice trials, random practice, and systematic feedback) are effective for young children with dysphagia.

Sources: Based on Arvedson (2009, 2020); Ashford et al. (2009a, 2009b); Boggs and Ferguson (2016); Clark et al. (2009); Gosa and Dodrill (2017); Logemann et al. (1989, 1997, 2008); Miles et al. (2017); Nagaya et al. (2004); Rogus-Pulia and Robbins (2013); Shaker et al. (2002); Starmer (2017); Steele et al. (2016); Troche and Mishra (2017).

Direct and Indirect Rehabilitative Swallowing Treatments

The procedures described here are used only after clinical and instrumental assessment has demonstrated their safety and appropriateness. Clients also need to be able to follow instructions. All techniques may be practiced without food; however, the swallowing techniques are specific to improving the actual swallowing process.

Exercise-Based Therapy

The goal of exercise-based therapies is to increase muscle strength and coordination to improve swallowing function. Exercises that involve swallowing are considered direct rehabilitation techniques, whereas exercise protocols that do not involve swallowing are considered indirect. For instance, tongue exercise programs that aim to increase tongue strength through progressive resistance training may indirectly result in swallowing-related changes such as improved bolus propulsion, clearance,

FIGURE 11.13 As discussed in Chapter 3, expiratory muscle strength training—using a device like the one shown here—not only helps strengthen respiratory muscles for individuals who have weaned from a ventilator, but it may also help strengthen expiratory muscles and improve cough and swallow function in some individuals with neurodegenerative disease.

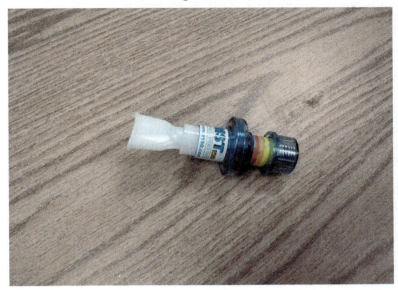

© KIMBERLY A. FARINELLA

and timing (Steele et al., 2016). Tongue exercise protocols may be paired with swallow practice to target the swallowing process more directly (Schaser, 2016). Exercise maintenance programs are needed to maintain performance gains after completion of any exercise protocol, especially in older individuals (e.g., Schaser et al., 2016). Principles of exercise science guide the development of successful direct and indirect exercise programs that may improve swallowing physiology. These principles include:

- Task specificity, or ensuring the movements involved the treatment match the motor movements to be improved with respect to speed and force
- Muscle load, or the generation of muscle force during contraction
- Resistance, or the ability of muscles to resist external pressures
- Intensity, or the strength and amount of practice of specific exercises to achieve the desired outcomes (e.g., Clark, 2012)

Swallowing-Specific Exercises

Exercises that involve a swallow have demonstrated improvement in physiological impairments of swallowing. For instance, the effortful swallow exercise, where the person is instructed to swallow while squeezing their muscles, improves retraction of the base of the tongue toward the posterior pharyngeal wall, helping propel the bolus into the oropharynx.

The supraglottic and super-supraglottic swallow exercises teach voluntary closure of the glottal area via effortful breath-holding, with the additional instruction to bear down for the super-supraglottic swallow. Both techniques may be used when the glottis doesn't fully close during swallowing or closes too late. These exercises help reduce the depth of misdirected swallows, thereby protecting the airway (Bulow et al., 2001; Rogus-Pulia & Robbins, 2013). Some evidence suggests these exercises are contraindicated in patients who have had a stroke because of potential heart abnormalities (Rogus-Pulia & Robbins, 2013).

The Mendelsohn maneuver is useful for clients who do not have adequate laryngeal elevation to protect the airway during swallowing. The patient is taught to hold the larynx manually at its highest point during the swallow (Mendelsohn & McConnel, 1987). Swallowing-specific exercises can be taught in conjunction with other potentially useful treatments such as surface electromyography and neuromuscular electrical stimulation, discussed next.

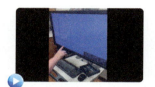

Pearson eTextbook
Video Example 11.3
This video shows sEMG during a typical swallow and an effortful swallow.

Surface Electromyography

Surface electromyography (sEMG) is a noninvasive rehabilitation tool that can provide real-time information about muscle activation during swallowing. Surface electrodes may be placed on the cheeks, the jaw, and/or the front of the neck. When muscles of the head and neck contract during movement, nerve impulses from lower motor neurons (LMNs) cause muscle fibers innervated by those LMNs to discharge, creating an electrical potential that travels in both directions toward the ends of the muscle fiber. The EMG signal represents the electrical activity generated by LMNs during muscle contraction (Stepp, 2012).

The SLP can teach patients various exercises, such as the effortful swallow exercise, and watch the patient's pattern of muscle activation on the sEMG monitor. Feedback can be provided to the patient to improve their performance with the exercise. sEMG is used as a biofeedback tool for the patient as they too can watch their muscle movements on the monitor and adjust to match the sEMG signal provided by the SLP (see Figure 11.14).

Neuromuscular Electrical Stimulation

Neuromuscular electrical stimulation (NMES) is a widely used treatment approach for swallowing despite the lack of large, randomized clinical studies to establish its efficacy (Howard & Rosario, 2019). NMES works by applying electrical stimulation to the neck area via surface electrodes, and eliciting contractions of the targeted muscles for swallowing. It is hypothesized that swallowing muscles will be strengthened, and sensory pathways for swallowing enhanced following NMES (Murry et al., 2020). Research has shown that NMES combined with swallowing-specific exercises results in better outcomes for post-stroke patients (Xia et al., 2011). Larger, randomized controlled trials are needed to confirm the benefits of NMES in swallowing rehabilitation of clinical populations with dysphagia.

A list and description of dysphagia therapy apps for clinicians and patients can be found at the National Foundation for Swallowing Disorders website.

During the assessment process, the SLP determines which of these exercises and techniques are appropriate for a particular client. Modifications in treatment approaches are often made as treatment proceeds.

Prostheses and Surgical Procedures

Patients who lack an intact swallowing mechanism because of malformation, surgery, or another cause may benefit from using a prosthetic device. For example, individuals who had oral cancer and have had a significant portion of the soft palate excised may have a palatal obturator (mentioned in Chapter 9), a permanent or removable plate that helps close this area during speaking or eating. Patients requiring a partial or

FIGURE 11.14 A surface electromyography signal that the patient is using as a biofeedback tool. The patient's signal on the left is trying to match the SLP's signal on the right. The peak in the signal represents optimal laryngeal muscle activation during swallowing.

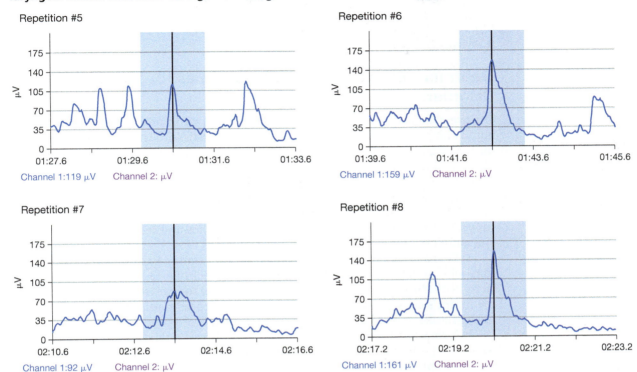

Source: Carolyn Abraham.

CASE STUDY   Steve *(continued)*

Swallowing exercises were recommended to Steve, specifically the effortful swallow and Mendelsohn maneuver. These techniques were trialed during the MBSS and determined to address his specific difficulties with tongue movements and bolus transit, hyolaryngeal elevation and excursion, and airway protection. NMES of neck muscles was combined with the swallow exercises. Surface electromyography was used for biofeedback also. Steve participated in swallow treatment with the SLP one time per week for 1-hour sessions for 12 weeks. He was also asked to complete a home exercise program daily with the goal of completing approximately 100 therapeutic swallows (i.e., about 20 effortful swallows and 10 Mendelsohn maneuvers three times per day). A repeat MBSS was scheduled in 6 weeks to ensure Steve's progress with treatment.

complete glossectomy (removal of the tongue) due to oral cancer may be fitted with a tongue prosthesis. Additional treatment strategies provided by the SLP are needed to optimize the use of a tongue prosthetic device, however (Murry et al., 2020).

If less invasive approaches have been unsuccessful, surgery to improve swallowing and prevent aspiration is sometimes needed. Some techniques attempt to correct organic defects. For example, if a patient has bony growths on the cervical vertebrae that displace the rear pharyngeal wall, these may be reduced surgically. Other surgical procedures are used to increase the dimensions of the vocal folds or elevate the larynx (Logemann, 1998).

Treatment Effectiveness and Outcomes for Swallowing Disorders

The overriding objectives of swallowing treatment are improved intake of food and liquid and prevention of aspiration of these materials into the lungs. The potential for treatment success is determined largely by the cause of the disorder, the severity of aspiration, and the onset of treatment. Early identification and successful intervention for swallowing disorders reduces the risk of aspiration and death, shortens the length of time patients need to stay in the hospital, and improves quality of life. Box 11.1, earlier in this chapter, provides a brief overview of the research evidence supporting the use of various treatment approaches and techniques for pediatric and adult clients with dysphagia.

SLPs are successful in preventing dysphagia in some cases. Caregivers of youngsters who are at risk are instructed in feeding techniques soon after the child's birth, including positioning that is most optimal for breastfeeding, attending to the infant's cues regarding readiness to eat, and paced bottle feedings to facilitate slower intake and reduce over- or underfeeding.

Information for the older population is also valuable. Among older adults, swallowing disorders are sometimes related to poor dentition, which might be corrected by appropriate dental care. SLPs can also provide education and training to caregivers who assist elderly individuals with feeding to prevent malnutrition and dehydration. Overly restrictive diets can lead to poor oral intake and reduced quality of life. As such, more liberal diets that are still safe are recommended for older adults (Dorner & Friedrich 2018).

Summary

Speech-language pathologists who want to focus their careers on treating patients with dysphagia become specially trained to assess and treat swallowing disorders in pediatric and adult populations. They work with infants who are unable to nurse adequately, children with feeding problems, and adults with oral-pharyngeal dysphagia secondary to progressive and nonprogressive medical conditions. The oral preparation, oral transport, pharyngeal, and/or esopharyngeal phases of swallowing may be impaired. Causes include congenital or acquired neurological problems, stroke, cancer, developmental disability, dementia, and trauma. Swallowing affects not only nutrition and health but also social and personal aspects of life.

A team approach is used for both assessment and intervention. Evaluation includes a careful history and direct observation of a client while they are feeding. Instrumental swallow evaluation techniques such as videofluoroscopy, also known as modified barium swallow study, and fiberoptic endoscopic evaluation of swallowing are essential for diagnostic accuracy of swallowing disorders and help determine beneficial treatment options. Compensatory and rehabilitative treatment procedures address the feeding environment, food textures and liquid consistencies, body and head positioning, oral-motor function, and specific swallowing techniques. Medical, prosthetic, and surgical approaches are used when necessary. Nonoral feeding may be required in severe cases.

Epilogue | Case Study: Steve

Steve made significant gains in his swallowing function while in therapy. His diet was advanced to thin liquids, and he started eating more regular foods, although he still required at least two swallows to clear drier foods from his throat. Occasionally, small sips of water after bites of regular food (like toast) to clear his throat were also helpful. Steve no longer had difficulties like lengthy mealtimes or coughing after meals. He felt like his swallow was "normal" again. Steve was most excited to be able to enjoy his beloved Diet Coke without the addition of a thickener.

Reflections | from a Patient Who Underwent Therapy for Swallowing

When I started with speech therapy, getting back to eating was the most important part. I didn't realize my swallow was as bad as it was back then. I would choke a lot, things would get stuck, and I was afraid to eat. But all I wanted to do was eat, and I couldn't. Had I not worked with speech therapy, I would have never gotten back to eating.

I learned how to take little bites and do exercises to make my swallow stronger. I got back to eating, but swallowing, for me, can still be difficult. I have to use my strategies and I have learned what to do. Without speech therapy, I probably would still be using my feeding tube. I now eat everything.

I am so blessed to have the people that were put before me to help me get to where I am today. I wouldn't be here without you.

Suggested Readings/Sources

Arvedson, J., Brodsky, L., & Lefton-Greif, M. (2020). *Pediatric feeding and swallowing: Assessment and management* (3rd ed.). Plural Publishing.

Homer, E. (2015). *Management of swallowing and feeding disorders in schools.* Plural Publishing.

Murry, T., Carrau, R., & Chan, K. (2020). *Clinical management of swallowing disorders* (5th ed.). Plural Publishing.

12 Audiology and Hearing Loss

David A. DeBonis, PhD

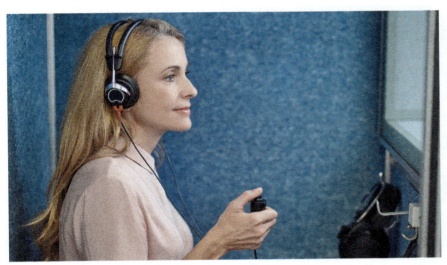

© Dmytro Zinkevych/Shutterstock

Learning Objectives

When you have finished this chapter, you should be able to:

12.1 Describe the effects of hearing loss on children and adults.

12.2 Describe the role of the audiologist.

12.3 Describe the required elements for sound to be produced and perceived.

12.4 Summarize the transmission of sound through the three main sections of the ear.

(Continued on next page)

> During my clinical fellowship year, which was more than 35 years ago, I remember seeing a 3-year-old-male whose parents brought him into the audiology clinic for comprehensive hearing testing due to his need to have things repeated. He also demonstrated delayed speech and language development. It was clear during the case history interview that Martin was not hearing well and audiological testing verified that he had a flat moderate sensorineural hearing loss in each ear. These kinds of losses are not generally addressed with medical intervention so after sharing the diagnosis with Martin's parents, my supervisor and I talked briefly with them about the fact that Martin would need hearing aids.
>
> A few days later, I received a call from Martin's parents. They reported that they had just one question: "Would Martin be able to go to college?" As I discussed this with my supervisor, it became clear that this question most likely reflected a much broader concern on the parents' part, and perhaps one shared by many parents: "Would my child be able to have a full and rewarding life?" Once fit with hearing aids and the appropriate speech, language, hearing, and academic services were put in place, Martin thrived, both in and out of the classroom, and the parents could see that their son would be able to live his life fully.
>
> It is interesting to think back to this case. As much as we were able to provide good support for Martin at the time, I am struck by how much more we can do today. The existence of newborn hearing screening programs allows for diagnosis of hearing loss so much sooner than before. Hearing aids are so much more technologically advanced and can be connected to so many other sources of information (e.g., phone, video). Also, advances in genetic testing allow for greater understanding of the nature of hearing loss and whether it might be accompanied by other medical or developmental challenges. It is truly exciting to be in a profession where so much progress has been made in helping people.
>
> *—David A. DeBonis*

12.5 Compare and contrast the three different types of hearing loss and related disorders.

12.6 Compare and contrast behavioral and non-behavioral methods of audiological assessment.

12.7 Describe three major ways people with hearing loss can be helped.

Those of you who are unfamiliar with the topic of hearing loss may have the misconception that it is a disorder that primarily affects the elderly population and is caused by age. In reality, hearing loss is common in people of all ages—from newborns to school-age children, from teenagers and young adults to seniors—and it can be caused by a number of factors. You might also think that hearing loss is a disorder that simply affects your ability to hear. In fact, hearing loss can affect the overall quality of your life. It can have a very negative impact on speech and language development, reading skills, educational achievement, job performance, social interactions, and psychological well-being. It can also have a significant negative impact on your family members and close friends. In this chapter, we provide an introductory overview of how hearing loss occurs, the many ways it impacts people's lives, how it is diagnosed, and how it is treated.

Incidence, Prevalence, Classification, and Impact of Hearing Loss: Children and Adults

Learning Objective 12.1 Describe the effects of hearing loss on children and adults.

One of the first questions that comes to mind when introducing students to the topic of hearing loss is, How many people are we talking about? Although this question is difficult to answer precisely, a general estimate is that approximately 20% of Americans, 48 million people, report some degree of hearing loss (Hearing Loss Association of America, 2018) This number has doubled since the mid-1980s and is expected to reach 40 million by 2025.

Approximately 3 in every 1,000 births results in a child with hearing loss, making it the most frequently occurring birth defect (Centers for Disease Control and Prevention [CDC], 2019). Also, approximately 1.7 in every 1,000 births results in a child with a severe to profound degree of hearing loss. Approximately 83 in every 1,000 children in the United States exhibit what is termed an "educationally significant" hearing loss that can have lifelong consequences (National Dissemination Center for Children with Disabilities, 2003).

The World Health Organization (WHO; 2017) provides important and alarming statistics regarding hearing loss worldwide in 2017. It reports that 360 million people worldwide have disabling hearing loss, including 32 million children. Approximately one-third of individuals who are older than 65 years of age have disabling hearing loss, and the majority of hearing loss that impacts children could be prevented. The WHO urges the following to prevent hearing loss: immunizing children to prevent disease and screening to identify disease early, greater access to medications to treat infections, improved hygiene practices, avoidance of medications that damage inner ear structures, early hearing testing, and providing better information to young people regarding noise-induced hearing loss. The WHO predicts that 1.1 billion individuals between the ages of 12 and 35 years are at risk of developing hearing loss from their recreational activities.

Classification of Impairment, Disability, and Handicap

When it comes to describing the effects of hearing loss, terminology can be confusing, especially for those who are new to the subject. Terms such as *impaired*, *disabled*, and *handicapped* can seem to overlap in meaning. The International Classification of Functioning (ICF; www.who.int/classifications/icf/en/) provides a system that defines and distinguishes these terms.

Impairment is defined as a loss of structure or function. As related to audiology, examples of impairments could include trauma to the eardrum, damage to the bones of the middle ear, or damage to the sensory cells in the inner ear. Do all impairments lead to a disability? The answer is no. *Activity limitation* is the term used to refer to the functional consequences associated with a particular impairment, and **disability** is a broad term that includes the impairment as well as the environmental factors that interfere with functioning. For those with hearing loss, examples of disability could include an inability to understand speech in the presence of background noise, difficulty understanding conversations on the phone, or difficulty hearing low-intensity speech sounds. When audiologists guide their clients with treatment recommendations, they are often addressing the person's hearing disability.

Finally, impairment and disability may lead to *participation restriction*, which is defined as restriction of the ability of a person to participate in life situations. Examples here could include hearing loss that makes employment impossible or that interferes with the ability to maintain positive social relationships.

It is important to remember that many individuals who have hearing loss do not have a hearing handicap because their loss does not interfere with their ability to participate in life situations. For example, despite problems hearing on the phone or understanding conversations in noisy settings, many people who have hearing loss are well-adjusted, independent, fully participating members of society.

Effects of Hearing Loss

Knowing that hearing loss can negatively impact access to speech and language and knowing how critical speech and language are to all aspects of development, we now examine the broader effects of hearing loss on individuals.

Children

It is relatively easy to understand that a profound hearing loss (i.e., thresholds of 90 dB or greater) would have a very negative impact on speech and language development. An individual demonstrating such a loss would have no access to the speech sounds in our language without amplification. What is perhaps less broadly understood is that all degrees of hearing loss, including mild losses, can interfere with speech and language. In addition, all degrees of hearing loss in children can interfere with their ability to succeed in school. This includes not only their academic abilities but also the development of their social interaction skills.

A review of the literature on this topic reveals a number of broad principles that may serve as the foundation for understanding the important relationships that exist between hearing loss, speech and language development, and school success. Some of the themes noted are:

- Children with mild hearing loss typically perform well on basic auditory tasks presented in favorable acoustic environments. However, when the task becomes more challenging and/or the environment becomes less favorable (e.g., due to noise), the negative effects of the hearing loss become more obvious. In addition, because of the added burden of hearing loss, children must rely more on their memory and attention abilities than their hearing peers. Over time, this additional effort can be difficult for the child to maintain, resulting in reduced academic performance.

- Because word endings are perceptually subtle compared to other language structures, children with hearing loss are at great risk for delays in their morphological development. Use of hearing aids to increase the child's access to these subtle grammatical markers can promote the age-appropriate development of morphemes.

- Even though children with unilateral hearing loss have normal hearing in one ear, they are still at risk for academic difficulties due to their loss. This includes difficulty in both localizing sound and hearing in noise. In addition, because of the impact of their hearing loss, these children must work harder in school to receive and understand incoming information; therefore, they become more fatigued than their peers throughout the day. The use of assistive devices, such as an FM system, may be helpful.

- Hoffman et al. (2015) compared the social interaction skills of two groups of children, all between the ages of 2.5 and 5.3 years. One group all had profound hearing loss, and the other all had normal hearing. As expected, the children without hearing loss performed better than those who were diagnosed with deafness. The researchers also found that the social competence of the children could be predicted (using statistics) by the child's hearing status and the child's degree of language development. Other factors related to social competence in the group of children who were diagnosed with deafness included the age at which the hearing loss was diagnosed and the age at which they started using amplification. In both cases, the earlier these things occurred, the better for the development of social interaction abilities.

Think for a moment about the following surprising statistic: Approximately 95% of children who have hearing loss are born to parents with typical hearing (Mitchell & Karchmer, 2004). Now think about the implications of this for the parents of these children. Most of them have little knowledge or experience related to hearing loss and the challenges it presents when raising a child. The understandable joy, hopefulness, and optimism that parents feel at the birth of a child can quickly turn to feelings of fear and helplessness when their newborn baby is identified as having significant hearing loss. Parents may feel as if their lives are suddenly spiraling out of control as they face the reality of raising a child who has a disorder. The stages of grief that are usually associated with the dying process are

CASE STUDY   Terrence

Terrence, who is 2 months old, is at the audiology clinic after having failed two hearing screenings administered at 1 and 2 days of age. These screenings were part of the hospital's newborn hearing screening program. Because there was no evidence that there was any blockage in the outer or middle ear that would be causing the failed screenings, the audiologist overseeing the program referred Terrence to the audiology clinic for further testing in order to confirm and expand the findings. Terrence was born at 39 weeks (full term) and weighed 6 pounds, 5 ounces. Parents reported that the pregnancy was uneventful and he received good prenatal care. APGAR scores, which reflect the overall condition of the child at 1 minute and 5 minutes after birth, were all normal, giving Terrence a total score of 10, which is excellent. When asked if parents had any insights into their child's responsiveness to sounds or voices, parents noted that they had not yet observed such responses. They also indicated that they were not aware of any history of hearing loss in the family.

As you read the chapter, think about the following:

- How might the parents feel after their child has failed two consecutive hearing screenings?
- Why do you think information about the pregnancy and birth are important in this case?
- Considering Terrence's very young age, what are some of the challenges that exist for the audiologist who needs to assess this child's hearing?

also applicable to those dealing with hearing loss. Parents of children with hearing loss often experience shock, denial, anger, and depression before they are finally able to accept the reality of the situation.

Adults

Although adults do not have the same kinds of challenges as children who are receiving new information on a daily basis, they still rely on their hearing to meet their own unique challenges at home and at work and to foster their physical and emotional health. The Better Hearing Institute (www.betterhearinginstitute.org) summarizes themes related to the effects of untreated hearing loss among adults, including:

- Increased irritability and fatigue due to the extra cognitive effort required to receive needed information
- Increased stress
- Greater likelihood of becoming isolated due to difficulty participating successfully in conversations
- Increased risk of injury related to being less auditorily aware of surroundings
- Reduced earning power and less confidence in ability to perform job duties
- Reduced self-esteem
- Overall reduced psychological health

In medical fields, the term *comorbidity* refers to the presence of one other condition or more that exists at the same time as the primary condition. A growing body of research supports that hearing loss has many comorbidities, making it a chronic health condition in adults. In an excellent review of the literature on this topic, Abrams (2017) identifies seven such conditions, which are summarized in Table 12.1.

TABLE 12.1

Summary of Research on Hearing Loss Comorbidities

Comorbidity	Findings
Social isolation and loneliness	Hearing loss at younger ages was significantly related to greater loneliness (Sung et al., 2016).
	Those with brain changes common in Alzheimer disease were seven times more likely to report being lonely (Donovan et al., 2016).
Depression	The likelihood of reporting being depressed increased as degree of hearing loss increased (Mener et al., 2013).
	The prevalence of moderate to severe depression is twice as high in people who report difficulty hearing compared to those who do not (Lin et al., 2011).
Falls	A significant relationship was noted between degree of hearing loss and risk of falling (Lin & Ferrucci, 2012).
Cardiovascular disease	Low frequency and flat hearing losses were strongly correlated with cardiovascular disease. Risk of stroke was associated with these hearing losses (Friedland et al., 2009).
Diabetes	People with hearing loss were much more likely to have diabetes (Bainbridge et al., 2008).
	People with diabetes were twice as likely to have hearing loss compared to those without diabetes (Horikawa et al., 2013).
Cognitive impairment and dementia	As hearing loss increased, the risk of these two conditions increased. Compared to those with normal hearing, people with a moderate hearing loss have three times greater risk of developing these conditions and those with severe losses have almost five times greater risk (Lin, 2011).

Source: Abrams (2017).

In 2016, the American Academy of Audiology (AAA) requested that the CDC officially change the classification of hearing loss in the adult population to a chronic medical condition in the hopes that it would lead to greater numbers of individuals receiving the care they need through greater referrals from health care providers and improved insurance coverage. It has been suggested that because hearing loss is not routinely included in the traditional medical model of service delivery (i.e., annual physical), individuals who have hearing loss are being underserved.

Deafness, the Deaf Community, and Deaf Culture

Our discussion of impairment and disability leads us to a brief discussion about individuals who are diagnosed with deafness. As you will learn in more detail later in this chapter, when a person's hearing loss reaches 90 dB or greater, the loss is categorized as profound; that is, we say the person is diagnosed with **deafness**. We often talk about "hearing loss," but this term does not carry a perspective shared by everyone. Consider the person who views deafness not as a disability but rather as a cultural trait. Individuals who have this perspective make up what is referred to as the **Deaf community** and often see their hearing status as a cultural difference, not a disability. They belong to a group who views deafness with a sense of pride that serves to unite its members and positively shape their sense of self-identity.

There are many cultural groups around the world and culture is created when a group of people share a common background of language, traditions, and values. Those who identify with Deaf culture in the United States share a common language, **American Sign Language (ASL)**, which is considered the natural language of the Deaf that serves to foster group cohesion. **Deaf culture** is further characterized by its rich history, traditions, folklore, and various contributions to the arts, including poetry, dance, and theater. At this point, an important distinction needs to be made between the labels *deaf* with a lowercase *d* and *Deaf* with an uppercase *D*. Individuals who are "deaf" share a common physiological condition: severe to profound hearing loss. In contrast, "Deaf" refers to individuals who are members of the Deaf community.

Think for a moment about recent technological advances that have occurred that allow individuals who are diagnosed with deafness to receive cochlear implants via a surgical procedure discussed in detail later. This surgery has allowed many individuals to receive speech and language information and to develop oral language skills. Although this can be viewed as a positive development for those individuals who choose to pursue it, the literature has described concerns about the effect this might have on Deaf culture. As fewer and fewer individuals attend schools for the deaf and greater numbers choose to get cochlear implants, learn oral English, and integrate more fully with hearing individuals, some people fear that the future of the Deaf community and culture is threatened. Possibly for this reason, leaders in the Deaf community were originally quite forceful in their opposition to the use of cochlear implants. But as Hossain (2012) notes, as the benefits of cochlear implants have become clearer, the Deaf community has become more accepting of the device and more open to the fact that this is a personal choice that should be respected.

Living and working in today's culturally diverse society, it is important for professionals in the fields of speech-language pathology and audiology to develop an awareness and understanding of Deaf culture and to think carefully about the complex and hard-to-answer questions surrounding deafness. Even though many academic training programs have traditionally seen all hearing impairments from a pathological perspective that assumes they need to be treated, those who are considering a career in speech-language pathology or audiology should be aware that this is not the only perspective. Also, in order to use evidence-based practice, we must value and respect the beliefs and preferences of our clients. Our role is not to tell our clients what to do, but rather to listen to their goals and priorities and coach them in ways that are consistent with those beliefs and with their culture. We certainly can expose clients to new information and perhaps new ways of thinking, but they must make the final decisions about their communication goals and how to achieve them.

Visual Communication Modality

As just mentioned, there are clients who choose to use a visual system of communication. These clients often have hearing loss that is in the severe to profound range. This choice could be based on cultural factors related to an allegiance to the Deaf community. For example, some caregivers who are diagnosed with deafness believe that the use of ASL with their child diagnosed with deafness will help that child gain acceptance into the Deaf community, which will be beneficial to the child's social-emotional development. In other cases, this choice may be made

FIGURE 12.1 Sign language continuum.

Manually Coded English Signing Systems	⟶	*American Sign Language*
Signed Exact English	Pidgin Signed English	
Word meaning is *not* considered (e.g., the word *right* will have the same sign regardless of context)	Signs used are more conceptual. One word may have many signs depending on meaning.	Has its own vocabulary, grammar, and sentence structure. One sign may represent an entire thought.
All grammatical markers (articles, auxiliary verbs, plurals, etc.) are signed.	Grammatical markers may or may not be signed.	Does not have specific signs for grammatical markers.
	Facial expressions and gestures are incorporated.	Facial expressions, body positions, space, and repetition are used extensively.

because the client's hearing loss is so great that they are not able to learn oral English sufficiently for it to be a functional and efficient communication system. As noted earlier, audiologists and speech-language pathologists (SLPs) must respect the choices that their clients make.

A helpful tool for understanding the options and differences among the visual approaches is the continuum found in Figure 12.1. Note that manually coded English signing systems are at one end and ASL is at the other. ASL is a language unto itself, with its own unique set of grammatical rules; it is not a visual form of English. ASL is often described as a conceptual language because a single sign can convey an entire thought. Unlike ASL, which is a natural language, forms of **manually coded English (MCE)** were developed for use in educational settings with children who are diagnosed with deafness to expose them to certain grammatical markers such as *-ed* and *-ing*. Some believe that this exposure to English language structures, which are not explicitly used in ASL, support the development of English literacy skills and overall academic achievement. In MCE much of the vocabulary comes from ASL, but the word order is the same as it is in oral English. Because of this, English can be modeled using both visual and auditory modalities at the same time.

Signed English is a dialect of sign language that is designed to promote language development by providing equivalent signs for spoken words. This often allows children to begin the process of communicating much earlier than if they relied on spoken language alone. Having a signed vocabulary can promote the onset of spoken English. (You can learn more at the Signed English website, www.sign.com.au.)

Signed English was developed by Bornstein (1974) and was originally designed for use with preschool-age children with signs that were intended to be easier to produce compared to other systems. Bornstein also noted that because most parents of children diagnosed with deafness have hearing, the signs were created to be easily learned to facilitate greater communication between child and parent. Another possible advantage of this system is in improving reading. Wilson and Hyde (1997) found that students diagnosed with deafness who were provided with Signed English reading books (i.e., sign pictures and printed text) demonstrated significantly better comprehension and story-retelling ability compared to those who had the text only.

Pidgin Signed English (PSE) is usually the type of manual communication taught in basic sign curricula for hearing people interested in learning to sign. New users of PSE tend to communicate using a structure that is more English-like, whereas experienced users tend to incorporate more features of ASL. One final popular form of manual communication to be mentioned is **fingerspelling**, which consists of hand shapes used to visually represent each of the 26 letters of the English alphabet. Although this would not be a very efficient way to communicate, fingerspelling is very helpful when used in conjunction with ASL, PSE, or MCE systems to communicate proper names, technical vocabulary, and other English words that have no known signs.

To find samples of ASL in action, visit the Signing Online website at www .signingonline.com. Go to the dictionary tab on the left and enter a word of your choice. Then, on the right side of the page, is a video of that word being signed.

REFLECTION QUESTION 12.1

Do you believe that deafness is a cultural difference, or do you view it as a disability?

What Do Audiologists Do?

Learning Objective 12.2 Describe the role of the audiologist.

The American Speech-Language-Hearing Association (ASHA) defines **audiology** as the discipline involved in "the prevention of and assessment of auditory, vestibular, and related impairments as well as the habilitation/rehabilitation and maintenance of persons with these impairments" (2004, p. 2). Note that audiology consists of work related to both assessment *and* habilitation/rehabilitation. Often, people perceive audiology as a discipline that deals strictly with the diagnosis of hearing loss. Although assessment is a critical part of audiology, treatment and management of a client diagnosed with a hearing problem are equally important (Figure 12.2).

According to the AAA Scope of Practice (2004) document, the primary responsibilities of audiologists include the following: (1) conducting hearing screenings; (2) conducting comprehensive hearing assessments; (3) providing a range of intervention services, including the fitting of hearing aids, cochlear implants, and other assistive devices and counseling, aural rehabilitation, and service on a balance team; (4) creating and implementing hearing conservation programs; and (5) conducting research on issues related to hearing and balance.

There are two kinds of doctoral degrees that audiologists typically obtain: the AuD, which is a clinical doctoral, and the PhD, which is a research doctorate. Individuals who pursue a PhD focus on developing their skills in research. These degrees often require 4 to 6 years of education beyond the bachelor's degree.

FIGURE 12.2 **Audiologist demonstrates for the parent placement of a behind-the-ear hearing aid with earmold into child's ear.**

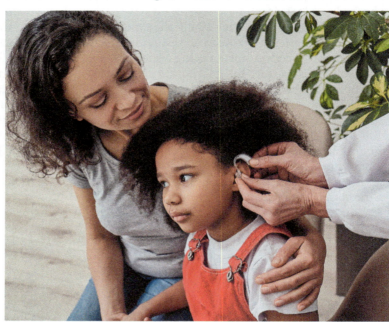

© Peakstock/Shutterstock

In many cases these degrees also involve gaining experience in teaching at the college level. ASHA notes that most of the people who complete a PhD in communication disorders choose employment at a college or university to do some combination of teaching, research, and student mentoring.

Clinical doctorates, which are much newer than research doctorates, focus on enhancing clinical skills and using research evidence to make good decisions for clients. Since 2007, the AuD has been the entry-level degree for audiologists to practice and requires 4 years of study beyond the bachelor's degree. Most audiologists with this degree do clinical work and supervision of students but some also work at colleges and universities, teaching and participating in research.

ASHA (n.d.) uses the term *speech, language, and hearing scientist* to describe professionals who study the biological, physical, and psychological processes of communication and use research to develop better ways to diagnose and treat individuals with speech, language, and hearing problems. Typically, a PhD is required for this role and the degree could be in audiology, speech pathology, or a related field, such as linguistics or psychology.

Speech-language pathologists work closely with audiologists and have very important roles in helping people with hearing loss. These include working with children who are born with hearing loss or with individuals who develop hearing loss later in life. In addition to providing language and articulation therapy, SLPs also often provide aural habilitation to young children, provide information to teachers and other school personnel for school-age children with hearing loss, and aural rehabilitation services to adults.

Listening and spoken language (LSL) specialists, also sometimes referred to as auditory-verbal therapists (AVT), are professionals who study techniques designed to promote the development of spoken language in individuals with significant hearing loss. They also study auditory skill development and hearing aids/hearing technology. These individuals believe that early identification of hearing loss and early intervention are critical to the child's development and that family members are an essential part of the intervention process.

Audiologists also regularly interact with ear, nose, and throat physicians, also referred to as otolaryngologists. These physicians are surgeons who diagnose and treat a variety of medical conditions, including chronic ear disease, hearing loss, sinus issues, allergies, swallowing disorders, breathing issues, voice challenges, balance concerns, and tumors of the head and neck. After completing their bachelor's degree, ENTs attend 4 years of medical school that is typically followed by a 5-year residency in order to gain the specific knowledge related to their practice. ENTs typically work in private practice, hospitals, or clinics.

Fundamentals of Sound

Learning Objective 12.3 Describe the required elements for sound to be produced and perceived.

Several conditions must exist in order for sound to occur and be perceived. For the purpose of this discussion, let's focus specifically on the speech signal. The following must be available: (1) an energy source, such as exhalation of air from the lungs; (2) an object capable of vibrating, such as the vocal folds of the larynx, for the energy source to act on; (3) a medium, such as air, that is capable of conducting the resulting vibrations; and (4) a receptor to receive and interpret the resulting sound.

How is it that sound is able to travel great distances through the air to reach our ears? Let's take a step back and first consider how an object, such as a simple guitar string, vibrates. Vibration can be thought of as a series of rhythmic back-and-forth movements. As the guitar string is plucked, it vibrates to and fro. As it moves in one direction, an increase in pressure occurs as air molecules that are close to each other are displaced and become compressed or packed together tightly. As the guitar string reverses and moves in the opposite direction, the air molecules that were initially compressed begin to rebound or spread apart, creating a decrease in pressure referred to as rarefaction. Sound, then, is a series of **compressions** and **rarefactions** that move outward from a vibrating source. It is important to realize that the individual air molecules themselves do not travel from their original position to the listener's ear, but their movement creates the sound wave that travels to the ear.

A vibrating object that moves back and forth from its normal resting position has special qualities. First, the vibrating object travels a measurable distance in either direction. This is referred to as the *amplitude* of the vibration. The amplitude of a sound determines its **intensity**, which is measured in decibels (dB). Second, this back-and-forth movement regularly repeats itself, resulting in a certain number of complete cycles during a specified period of time. This is referred to as the **frequency** of the vibration and is expressed in cycles per second, or hertz (Hz). Every sound, therefore, can be described in terms of its unique intensity and frequency characteristics. This information is decoded or interpreted by the auditory system, allowing the listener to differentiate the infinitesimal number of sounds they are exposed to throughout the course of a day.

Anatomy and Physiology of the Auditory System

Learning Objective 12.4 Summarize the transmission of sound through the three main sections of the ear.

Before we can begin our discussion of the various types and causes of hearing loss, a general understanding of the anatomy and physiology of the auditory system is essential. Anatomically, the auditory system can be divided into several general areas. They include the outer ear, the middle ear, the inner ear, the vestibulocochlear nerve, the auditory brainstem, and the auditory cortex of the brain. The first four areas (Figure 12.3) are commonly referred to as the **peripheral auditory system**; the latter two are part of the **central auditory system**. Typically, when we say that someone has a hearing loss, we are referring to a peripheral problem. When someone has a deficit in the central auditory system, we usually say that this person has a processing or an auditory processing problem.

The Outer Ear

Your **outer ear** is comprised of the **pinna**, or auricle, and the **external auditory meatus**, or external auditory canal. The pinna is the most visible structure of the auditory system and is made of cartilage covered with skin. If you take a look at someone's pinna, you will note various ridges and depressions; these are important because they provide a natural boost to certain sounds as they enter the ear. The pinna also collects and funnels sound into the ear canal and helps the listener to identify where sound originates in space, a process called **localization**.

Your external auditory meatus, which is also called the ear canal, is a tube lined with skin that extends from the bowl-like depression of the pinna, known as

FIGURE 12.3 **The peripheral auditory system.**

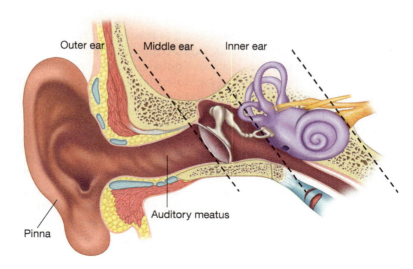

the **concha**, to the **tympanic membrane**, or **eardrum**. The ear canal is approximately 1 inch in length in adults and has a slight "S-shaped" curve as it progresses toward the eardrum. The outer region of the canal contains hair follicles and glands that produce **cerumen**, more commonly known as earwax. Similar to the pinna, the ear canal also enhances certain high-frequency sounds as they travel to the eardrum.

The Middle Ear

Your external auditory canal leads to the tympanic membrane, which marks the boundary between your outer ear and the **middle ear**. Your tympanic membrane is a thin concave-shaped structure that vibrates in response to sound waves that travel down your ear canal. Most of the surface area of your tympanic membrane is composed of three distinct layers of tissue. The middle layer is made of fibrous tissue that provides both the strength and elasticity of the eardrum. A healthy eardrum is often described as appearing "pearl gray" in color. Because your eardrum is semitransparent, it is possible to view some of the structures of the middle ear when conducting a visual examination of the eardrum.

Located behind your tympanic membrane is the **middle ear space**. This air-filled cavity is lined with a mucous membrane and includes the opening to your **Eustachian tube**. This important tube connects your middle ear with the **nasopharynx**, the space located behind the nose and above the roof of the mouth. Your Eustachian tube is normally closed but opens periodically, providing a passageway for air to ventilate the middle ear space and equalize air pressure on each side of the eardrum.

Also located in your middle ear space is a chain formed by three small bones. These bones, called the **malleus, incus,** and **stapes**, are collectively referred to as the **ossicles**, or **ossicular chain** (see Figure 12.4). The first bone in the chain, the malleus, is the largest of the three and is embedded in the fibrous layer of the

FIGURE 12.4 Structures of the middle ear.

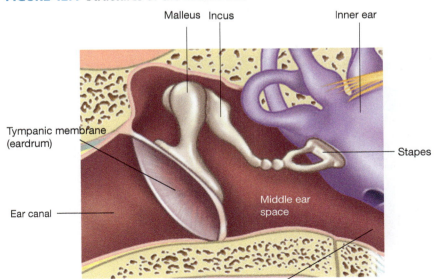

eardrum. The upper portion of the malleus makes contact with the incus, which makes contact with the stapes, the smallest bone in the human body. The footplate of the stapes rests against the **oval window**, a thin membrane that marks the entrance to the inner ear.

The Inner Ear

At this point, you should be able to begin to think about how you hear. We now know that sound waves travel through the air, down the ear canal, and cause the eardrum to vibrate. These vibrations are then carried across the ossicular chain to the footplate of the stapes, which makes contact with the oval window, which is the entry point to the inner ear. The **inner ear** is a complex structure that serves two important roles. One major component, the **cochlea**, is responsible for providing auditory input to the central auditory system. The other major component, the **vestibular system**, is responsible for supplying information regarding balance.

Let's turn our attention first to your cochlea, a structure the size of a pea that resembles a snail's shell. Your cochlea is the portion of the inner ear that contains special nerve cells designed to respond to auditory stimuli (see Figure 12.5). The **organ of Corti** sits on the basilar membrane, a structure that is narrower,

FIGURE 12.5 **The inner ear.**

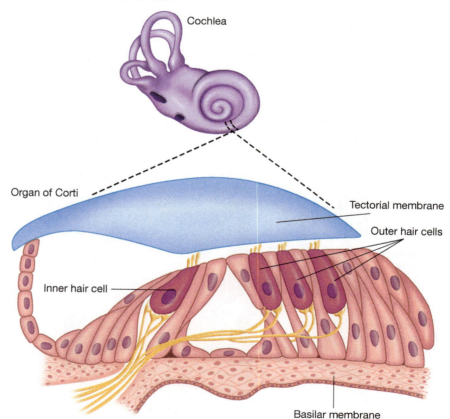

thinner, and stiffer at the base and wider, thicker, and more flaccid at the apex. Think for a moment about a guitar string; the thinner, stiffer strings produce high-frequency sounds and the thicker, looser strings produce low-frequency sounds. Although the process is not completely understood, we know that these anatomical differences of your **basilar membrane** enable it to respond differently to sounds of different frequencies. That is, the portion of the basilar membrane closest to the stapes responds best to high-frequency sounds, and the portion nearest the tip or apex of the cochlea responds best to low-frequency sounds.

Located on your basilar membrane are thousands of tiny **hair cells**, which are considered to be your sensory receptor cells of the auditory system. Located on the top of each cell are small hairlike projections called **stereocilia**. Also, forming the roof of the organ of Corti is a structure called the **tectorial membrane**. The tectorial membrane is fixed at one end, while the opposite end is free to move up and down in response to movement of the surrounding fluid.

At this point, take a look back at the pathway of sound from the sound wave in the air to movement of the stapes in the oval window, just described. Now add to that understanding the following: As your stapes rocks in and out of the oval window, fluid is displaced. As the stereocilia are bent through the movement of the tectorial and basilar membranes, chemical transmitters are released from the cochlear hair cells, and neuroelectric energy is generated and transmitted to auditory nerve fibers that form the acoustic branch of the **vestibulocochlear** or **VIIIth cranial nerve**. This information is then directed to your brainstem and eventually the brain.

CASE STUDY   Terrence *(continued)*

At this point, think back to Terrence who was introduced earlier in the chapter. You will remember that he failed his hearing screening twice and there was no indication that there was any obstruction of the outer or middle ear. You now know that the outer ear includes the ear canal. After the birth process, some babies' bodies are covered with a white substance called **vernix**, which is there to protect the babies' delicate skin. If some of this substance is in the ear canal, it can cause a failed hearing screening. Also, you now know that fluid can develop in the middle ear; this can also cause a failed screening. In the case of Terrence, both of these factors were ruled out, which means that the source of the hearing loss that Terrence has may be the inner ear.

Before we end our discussion of the inner ear, a brief mention of your vestibular system should be made. Your vestibular system also contains sensory receptor cells that sense head movement. Nerve fibers innervating the sensory cells of the vestibular system form the vestibular branch of the VIIIth nerve. The anatomical connections that exist between the balance and hearing mechanisms help explain why both balance testing and nonmedical intervention of balance disorders are included in the audiologist's scope of practice (ASHA, 2004).

The Central Auditory System

Pearson eTextbook
Video Example 12.1
In this video, a summary of how sound is created and its basic pathway from the outer ear to the brain is provided. Is this information consistent with what you read?
https://youtu.be/FADhL9xdR3E

Your central auditory system, which consists of nuclei, nerve fibers, and nerve tracts, includes pathways that carry auditory information to your brain (ascending pathway) and pathways that receive information from your brain (descending pathways). Although it may appear that the anatomical structures leading to your brain simply send neural impulses, they actually play a key role in ensuring that information about the frequency, intensity, and duration of the auditory stimuli remains intact until it reaches the highest brain regions of the auditory cortex for interpretation. Further exploration of the central auditory system is typically presented to students in anatomy and physiology and audiology courses.

Types of Hearing Loss and Auditory Disorders

Learning Objective 12.5 Compare and contrast the three different types of hearing loss and related disorders.

The previous section described the ear from an anatomical and physiological standpoint. The outer and the middle ear serve to collect, amplify, and conduct sound to the cochlea. The outer and middle ear, therefore, are referred to as the **conductive system**. The cochlea is the actual sensory organ of hearing, and the auditory branch of the VIIIth nerve is responsible for transmitting the resulting neural signal to the brainstem and eventually to the auditory cortex for processing. The cochlea and auditory nerve, therefore, make up the **sensorineural system**. When audiologists describe peripheral hearing loss, they typically use terms like *conductive* and *sensorineural*. When deficits are noted in the central auditory system, these are typically described in terms of how they impact a person's auditory processing abilities.

Conductive Hearing Loss

If you had a **conductive hearing loss**, the cause would most likely be the result of a deformation, a malfunction, or an obstruction of the outer or middle ear. Not all disorders of the outer and middle ear result in a loss of hearing. In many cases, however, problems in these areas reduce or eliminate the ear's natural conduction of sound as it travels to the cochlea. As a result, the intensity of sound arriving at the inner ear is reduced. This usually prevents low- to moderate-intensity sounds from being heard at all, and higher-intensity sounds are perceived as much softer than normal. It is important to remember that the primary consequence of conductive hearing loss is a loss of loudness or audibility. As long as the sensorineural system remains intact, sound can be heard without difficulty if it is made loud enough for the individual, such as by turning up the volume of a radio or TV or by raising the level of one's voice.

There are a few other key things you should remember about conductive hearing loss. First, it does not result in a total loss of hearing. In other words, a person who is diagnosed with deafness would not have lost hearing solely as a result of a conductive deficit. Second, most conductive losses are not permanent. Some resolve without any treatment, and most others are medically treatable. In rare cases when medical treatment cannot be given or when the client prefers not to pursue it, a hearing aid or hearing aids may be possible if medical clearance is given by the physician.

Disorders of the Outer Ear

Several conditions of the outer ear can occur due to the malformation of structures during embryonic development. If you had anotia, your pinna would be absent on one or both sides; if you had **microtia**, you would have a small malformed pinna. These conditions alone do not result in a loss of hearing, but with microtia there is an increased likelihood that you would also have some other congenital condition, such as *atresia*. **Atresia** is a disorder in which there is complete closure of the external auditory meatus; because sound cannot travel through the ear canal in the usual manner, hearing loss results. Stenosis, a severe narrowing of the external canal, may occur in some individuals. Unlike atresia, however, stenosis does not result in significant hearing loss unless debris or earwax becomes trapped in the narrow opening. These conditions most frequently occur in conjunction with other craniofacial disorders (see Chapter 11).

A much more common cause of conductive hearing loss in the outer ear and one that you may have experienced is impacted wax (cerumen) or a foreign object. Although many people view cerumen as a problem, it actually protects the ear, at least to some degree, from insects and other foreign bodies entering the canal. It also traps dirt and debris, naturally cleansing the external canal as it migrates outward. Cerumen acts as a lubricant to prevent the skin that lines the canal from drying out and serves as a chemical barrier to bacterial and fungal infection. In view of these positive attributes of wax, you should not use cotton swabs or other tools to remove cerumen. In fact, aggressive use of cotton swabs often pushes more wax further into your ear canal, which can create a wax blockage that needs to be removed by a physician. In many states cerumen management (removal) is within the audiologist's scope of practice, although it should be conducted with caution and only after proper training.

Overuse of cotton swabs can cause two additional disorders of the outer ear. The first, and one that you or someone you know may have experienced, is external otitis, more commonly known as swimmer's ear. This can occur when too much wax has been removed from the ear canal, making the canal more vulnerable to infection by bacteria or fungus. This condition is typically painful as the ear canal begins to swell. In some cases, drainage from the ear is noted. External otitis is typically treated by an **ear, nose, and throat physician (ENT)**, also referred to as an *otolaryngologist*. This physician will examine the ear canal carefully, clean it, and apply medication. Often, the physician will provide you with medicated eardrops to use at home.

Aggressive use of cotton swabs can also result in a perforation, or hole in the tympanic membrane, if the swab is pushed too deeply into the canal. Another possible cause of this condition is a blow to the head or a rupture caused by excessive fluid pressing against the eardrum. Symptoms of a perforated eardrum can be subtle or extreme, ranging from slight discomfort to significant pain and bleeding. The degree of conductive hearing loss resulting from this condition can also be subtle or significant, depending on size and location. Perforations can be identified by the ENT physician through examination of the eardrum using an otoscope and in some cases also a high-powered microscope. Perforations may heal spontaneously without any treatment but often need to be repaired by the ENT. The physician typically uses tissue from the outer ear to patch the perforated area.

Disorders of the Middle Ear

Several conditions can occur due to problems in the middle ear. For example, **oto-sclerosis** is a disorder that affects primarily young adults, particularly females, and in the majority of cases is linked to genetic factors. If you had this condition, healthy bone would be replaced with spongy bone in the area of the stapes footplate, most likely causing reduced mobility of the stapes and hearing loss. If your hearing loss was interfering with your ability to understand speech at school, at work, or in social situations, you could pursue surgery to remove all or part of the stapes footplate followed by insertion of a prosthetic device that acts as an artificial stapes.

Another middle ear condition involving the ossicles is ossicular discontinuity, which refers to a break somewhere in the ossicular chain. This condition can be caused by head trauma and typically creates a large conductive hearing loss in the affected ear. Surgical repair for this condition is done by the ENT, who examines the condition of the ossicles, identifies where the break has occurred, and either repairs the ossicle or replaces it with a prosthetic one.

One of the most common causes of conductive hearing loss, particularly in children, is **otitis media**, an inflammation of the mucous membrane lining the middle ear cavity. Otitis media generally results from **Eustachian tube dysfunction**, which prevents proper ventilation of the middle ear cavity. A normally functioning Eustachian tube opens and closes regularly as you chew, yawn, or swallow, allowing for the equalization of air pressure between your middle ear and the external environment. In children the Eustachian tube is less efficient than it is in adults and therefore is less effective in ventilating the middle ear. Another factor that can interfere with Eustachian tube function and middle ear ventilation is enlarged adenoids.

When the middle ear is not consistently ventilated, oxygen within the cavity is absorbed into the mucous membrane lining, forming a partial vacuum. This, in turn, results in a condition known as *negative middle ear pressure*, which causes your eardrum to retract into the middle ear cavity, reducing its ability to vibrate freely. If this situation goes untreated or does not respond to treatment, the secretion of fluid may occur in the middle ear; this is a condition referred to as **otitis media with effusion (OME)**. As fluid fills the cavity, sound must be conducted through fluid, instead of the usual air-filled environment. If the fluid is sterile, the condition is classified as **serous otitis media**. However, when bacteria are present, pus may form within the middle ear cavity, causing a condition referred to as **purulent (or suppurative) otitis media**. In these cases, in addition to conductive hearing loss you may also experience restlessness, irritability, ear pain, fever, and vomiting. During this process your tympanic membrane may appear reddish in color or bulging. In some cases, the eardrum may rupture due to the pressure created by the fluid behind it.

Otitis media is not rare. In fact, it is the most frequently diagnosed disorder in the United States in children younger than 15 years. More than 90% of children experience at least one episode by the age of 7 years, with peak incidence generally occurring during the period from 6 months to 2 years of age (Jung & Hanson, 1999).

Treating otitis media is a complex process because no one treatment works best for everyone. In some cases, your physician may recommend that you wait and monitor the condition because a number of these cases resolve without treatment. In other cases, use of a decongestant or an antihistamine helps resolve the underlying problem of inadequate Eustachian tube function. If you had acute otitis media with infected fluid, antibiotics such as amoxicillin would likely be used, but this must be done carefully because some people have difficulty tolerating antibiotics and there is concern among medical professionals about the overuse of antibiotics.

Some treatment options cannot be pursued by a child's pediatrician and require a referral to an ENT. When nonsurgical treatments have been ineffective, ENTs often perform a surgical treatment that research and clinical observation have shown to restore hearing and reduce the likelihood of further middle ear pathology. The procedure, called a **myringotomy**, involves making an incision into the tympanic membrane in order to drain fluid from the middle ear cavity. This is frequently followed by insertion of a **pressure equalization (PE) (or tympanostomy) tube** into the tympanic membrane. These tubes serve the same purpose as the Eustachian tube, allowing air to pass into the middle ear space. However, instead of passing from the nasopharynx in the usual manner, air enters the middle ear from the external auditory canal via the open PE tube situated in the eardrum.

The treatment of otitis media in children can be stressful for both parents and professionals because resolving the problem is often not an efficient process. From a physician's point of view, it certainly makes sense to choose treatment options that are more conservative first and to gradually move to more aggressive options. But in cases where the treatment is not working, the hearing loss that accompanies the otitis media can remain unresolved for many months in a child who is in a very critical period for speech and language development. This can be of great concern to parents, SLPs, and audiologists. In addition, the fact that some treatment options are only available through an ENT can add more waiting time to this process.

At this time, there is disagreement in the literature regarding whether early otitis media with hearing loss has negative effects on a child later in life. For example, Zumach et al. (2010) found that the early negative effects on receptive and expressive language from otitis media that were measured in children who were 27 months of age disappeared by the time the same children were 7 years old. In contrast, Shapiro et al. (2009) found that children who had a history of otitis media prior to the age of 2 years performed more poorly at 9 years of age on measures of reading and phonological awareness than did those who did not have this history and those who had otitis media after the age of 2 years. This question of the possible long-term impact of early hearing loss is an important one. If long-term effects do exist, greater efforts to quickly resolve early hearing loss in children who have otitis media will have to become part of our treatment protocols.

Pearson eTextbook
Video Example 12.2
In this video, the ENT physician is inserting a PE tube into the eardrum. What steps were necessary before this procedure could occur?

https://youtu.be/-PYCybiCfNA

Sensorineural Hearing Loss

A second general type of hearing loss is **sensorineural hearing loss**. If you had this type of loss, it would most often be due to the absence or malformation of, or damage to the structures of, the inner ear, including the hair cells within the cochlea. Sensorineural hearing loss may be present at birth or may develop over the course of one's life. It may be sudden in onset, occurring over a matter of hours, or gradual, occurring over a period of years. Some forms of sensorineural hearing loss have a genetic basis; other forms are acquired. Some cases of sensorineural hearing losses may remain stable, some become worse, and some fluctuate. Unlike conductive hearing losses, which are most commonly temporary, sensorineural losses are usually permanent.

Although sensorineural hearing loss may affect hearing sensitivity for any range of frequencies, in most cases the higher frequencies are affected. Unlike conductive hearing loss, where the problem stems from sound not being loud enough, sensorineural hearing loss can involve both a lack of loudness and a lack of clarity. Not only are certain sounds inaudible or difficult to hear but sounds that are audible are often perceived as being distorted. To illustrate this point, consider the following example. Talking on your cell phone at a low volume level simulates a conductive hearing loss. That is, sound is softer than normal, making it difficult to perceive. If, however, the volume is increased (i.e., the conductive disorder is resolved), the signal not only becomes easier to hear but the signal also becomes clear. If we now take the same phone but add distortion or static, the signal remains audible but is harder to understand. Increasing the volume sometimes makes the distorted signal louder, but it is still not clear.

As you might expect, sensorineural hearing loss can have a negative impact on speech, language, and cognitive development. Factors that influence the effects of the loss on these aspects of development include (1) the degree of the loss; (2) the age of the person when the loss occurred, referred to as *age of onset*; (3) the age of the person when the loss was identified; and (4) the age of the person when appropriate intervention was begun.

Age of onset is usually described as **congenital** (present at birth) or acquired (occurring sometime after birth). Another way of looking at this is to consider whether the hearing loss occurred **prelingually** (i.e., before speech and language skills have developed) or **postlingually** (i.e., after the person has acquired spoken language skills). There is no precise age that defines these two terms, but traditionally hearing loss that occurs prior to the age of 2 years is considered prelingual in onset, and hearing loss that occurs after the age of 5 years is considered postlingual. Think about a child who is born with a moderate hearing loss that is not detected until they are 4 or 5 years of age, compared to a child whose loss is identified when the child is a newborn. The negative effects on speech and language will be much greater for the first child. For the second child, early intervention services can be provided during a critical time of development to reduce these negative effects. Table 12.2 summarizes various terms that you will encounter when learning about sensorineural hearing loss.

> **CASE STUDY**   **Terrence** *(continued)*
>
> Thinking again about Terrence, we previously suggested that the source of the hearing loss that he has appears to be the inner ear because obstruction of the outer and middle ears was ruled out. You now know that this type of loss is referred to as a sensorineural hearing loss. You also know that the loss could be described as congenital because it is present at birth and prelingual because it has occurred prior to the development of language.

Disorders of the Inner Ear

Now that we have a general understanding of sensorineural hearing loss, let's take a look at some of the causes, starting with those that are congenital and hereditary. When a hearing loss is due to the absence or malformation of inner ear structures during embryonic development, it is referred to as **aplasia**, or **dysplasia**. There are

TABLE 12.2

Summary of Characteristics Describing Sensorineural Hearing Loss

Comparative Characteristics	Comments
Present at birth	Another term for present at birth is *congenital* and children with these losses often do not pass their newborn hearing screening. Newborn hearing screening programs increase the likelihood that these children will be diagnosed and treated early in life, both of which improve their speech, language, and developmental outcomes.
Later developing	Some hearing losses are **later developing**, which means they are not seen at birth but show up later in life. For example, a child might be born with gene mutation that causes hearing loss but the loss might not develop until some point later in life. Although children with later-developing losses are not typically diagnosed early in life, their loss has occurred after some language has been developed, which can be a positive factor. See the term *postlingual* in this table.
Acquired	In children, **acquired sensorineural hearing losses** could be due, for example, to lack of oxygen at birth or a virus. They could also occur later in life as would occur with teens who listen to very loud music.
	In adults, examples of acquired hearing losses include hearing loss caused by noise exposure or the aging process. Most adults with sensorineural hearing loss have acquired losses.
Prelingual	A child with congenital hearing loss also has a prelingual loss because the loss has occurred prior to the development of language.
Postlingual	A child with a postlingual sensorineural hearing loss already has some language in place when the hearing loss occurred.
Gradual	Gradual sensorineural hearing losses occur slowly over time, as is most often the case for people exposed to loud noise and hearing loss due to aging.
Sudden onset	In some cases, hearing loss can have a sudden onset and these losses require immediate attention. For example, a sudden sensorineural hearing loss in one ear could suggest that a virus has entered the inner ear. It could also indicate a growth on or near cranial nerve VIII. In older individuals it could be related to a change in blood supply to the brain.
Genetic	Genetic hearing loss is caused by a gene mutation and accounts for approximately half of the congenital sensorineural hearing losses.
Nongenetic	Nongenetic hearing loss (also sometimes called acquired hearing loss) refers to loss that is caused by some other factor, such as illness or injury during birth in children or the aging process in adults.
Stable	Stable sensorineural hearing losses do not change over time.
Progressive	Progressive hearing losses worsen over time. This can be very stressful for patients who fear that their loss will become so great that hearing aids will no longer help them.
Fluctuating	Fluctuating sensorineural hearing losses are rare but can occur. Meniere's disease is an example of a condition characterized by variations in hearing as well as in balance function.

several types of aplasia, depending on which part of the inner ear is affected. Very often, congenital hereditary sensorineural hearing loss is one component of a group of disorders associated with a syndrome. For example, **Usher's syndrome** is a genetic disorder characterized by significant sensorineural hearing loss as well as degenerative visual changes that result in night blindness and reduced peripheral vision. **Waardenburg's syndrome** is another genetic disorder characterized by mild to severe sensorineural hearing loss, as well as changes in the coloring of the hair, skin, and eyes. Children with **Alport's syndrome** often have sensorineural hearing loss and kidney disease.

Although sensorineural hearing loss may be present at birth, it is not always a result of genetic factors. Instead, an illness or toxic agent experienced by the mother during pregnancy may be the cause. One of the most well-known examples is hearing loss resulting from **maternal rubella** (German measles), which occurred in approximately 10,000 to 20,000 children born in the early to mid-1960s. Although a rubella vaccine is now available, other viruses, such as the human immunodeficiency virus and cytomegalovirus, continue to be major causes of congenital sensorineural hearing loss when contracted by the mother during pregnancy. Sexually transmitted bacterial infections such as syphilis can seriously damage the central nervous system of a developing fetus, leading to intellectual and developmental disabilities as well as hearing loss. Sensorineural hearing loss can occur as a result of circumstances encountered at any point during one's lifetime. Acquired hearing loss may be due to viral infections such as mumps or due to bacterial infections such as **meningitis**, an inflammation of the tissue covering the brain that can lead to a severe or profound hearing loss in young children and adults. The structures of the inner ear are vulnerable to damage either from the bacteria that caused the disease or from the high fever that often accompanies the illness. In addition, in some cases bacterial meningitis requires treatment with high doses of strong antibiotics that can be **ototoxic** (i.e., poison to the ear). Hearing loss resulting from ototoxicity may be permanent or reversible. Frequent monitoring of hearing is often recommended for individuals being treated with ototoxic medications so that drug type and dosage can be adjusted if changes in hearing are noted.

Meniere's disease is a disorder that can produce hearing loss that is rather sudden in onset. First described by Prosper Meniere in 1861, Meniere's disease is believed to be caused by pressure resulting from the buildup of **endolymph** fluid within the membranous labyrinth of the inner ear. Both the cochlear (hearing) and vestibular (balance) portions of the inner ear may be involved, or the disorder may be specific to only one region. The classic symptoms associated with Meniere's disease are fluctuating and progressive sensorineural hearing loss, tinnitus, vertigo, and a feeling of fullness in the ear. In addition, symptoms typically come and go unpredictably and may be so severe that the person must lie still until they feel better. There is no known cure for Meniere's disease, but drug therapy, surgical intervention, and changes in diet to reduce symptoms have all been used with varying amounts of success.

Another type of inner ear disorder, referred to as **auditory neuropathy spectrum disorder (ANSD)**, has received considerable attention in recent years. In general, ANSD is characterized by normal outer hair cell function (as seen in normal otoacoustic emissions) and abnormal responses from the inner hair cells or auditory nerve fibers (as seen in an abnormal auditory brainstem response). A lack of synchrony in the firing of auditory nerve fibers in response to sound appears to be the underlying problem in these cases. Individuals who have ANSD may exhibit pure tone hearing that is anywhere from within normal limits to profoundly impaired, and this pure tone hearing does not typically correlate well with their real-world difficulties or their potential to develop language. These individuals also usually have considerable difficulty understanding speech, even when their pure tone loss is not significant.

Another cause of sensorineural hearing loss is the presence of a **vestibular schwannoma**, more commonly referred to as an **acoustic neuroma**. These terms refer to a nonmalignant growth that develops on the cells near the VIII nerve. Because of the location of this tumor, symptoms that you might experience include decreased hearing, tinnitus, some type of balance difficulty, and a plugged feeling on the affected side. The particular combination of symptoms and the severity of those symptoms depend on the size of the tumor. Audiologists are trained to attempt to rule out acoustic neuroma as a diagnosis in all cases where a client demonstrates an unexplained unilateral hearing loss and to inform the client's physician when unilateral losses are seen. Diagnosis of this condition is typically made by an ENT or neurologist based on identification of the tumor using magnetic resonance imaging (MRI). For the majority of individuals who have an acoustic neuroma, surgery is recommended. In addition to removing the tumor, the surgeon's goal is to preserve the patient's hearing and avoid trauma to important surrounding structures, including the facial nerve. In a small number of cases the tumor grows very slowly; for these clients, a wait-and-watch approach may be taken rather than intervening right away.

Let's now turn our attention to a cause of sensorineural hearing loss that in most cases is avoidable: hearing loss resulting from excessive exposure to high levels of sound (noise). We live in an age where we are surrounded by ever-increasing amounts of noise. From machines at factories and construction sites to common everyday items such as power tools, motorcycles, and musical instruments, it is almost impossible to escape noise. It should come as no surprise, then, that **noise-induced hearing loss** is one of the leading causes of acquired sensorineural hearing loss in young and middle-aged adults. Now even children are at risk of noise exposure because many of today's popular toys, electronic games, and ear-level personal stereos emit sound levels that are potentially hazardous. Research now reveals some disturbing facts about personal music devices. Overwhelming majorities of both high school and college students own one, nearly 75% of the college students who own one use it every day, and young people, in general, are not well informed about listening levels that are unsafe (Danahauer et al., 2012; Punch et al., 2011; Vogel et al., 2010). Exposure to high-intensity sound exposes the delicate structures of your cochlea to considerable stress that may lead to irreversible damage.

Hearing loss that occurs from exposure to high levels of noise can be temporary or permanent. If you experience short-term exposure to a loud sound that causes a hearing loss which recovers spontaneously, you have experienced a **temporary threshold shift (TTS)**. To understand TTS better, think about the last time you went to a loud concert and later noticed a slight reduction in hearing accompanied by tinnitus (ear or head noises). After several hours of rest the ringing noise stopped and hearing returned to normal. You experienced a TTS. Although we have long believed that TTS is not a problem as long as hearing thresholds return back to normal, research by Truong and Cunningham (2011) suggest that even when hearing ability has returned to normal after TTS, permanent damage to both the cochlea and auditory nerve can be measured.

Now consider the factory worker who is exposed to loud sounds every day. Frequent exposure to high levels of noise over time may eventually lead to **permanent threshold shift (PTS)**. PTS is typically characterized by a loss of hearing sensitivity in the high-frequency range (between 3000 and 6000 Hz). As damage resulting from long-term exposure increases, more hearing is lost and the ability to understand speech decreases, particularly in the presence of background noise.

The Occupational Safety and Health Administration (OSHA) has attempted to reduce the number of individuals who are at risk for getting PTS; it has established guidelines limiting the amount of time a worker can remain in a high-noise area. In addition, OSHA has policies for the use of hearing protection for workers and the annual monitoring of hearing with hearing testing. Unfortunately, these guidelines are not practical in all cases. For example, military personnel who are exposed to sudden, unpredictable blasts of sound remain at great risk for noise-induced hearing loss.

It should be noted that clinical audiologists regularly see individuals who report considerable listening/hearing difficulties even though their pure tone hearing is normal. This is sometimes referred to as *hidden hearing loss* because the deficit is not seen on pure tone testing or speech testing done in quiet. Some theories as to why this occurs include (1) damage to the synapses that carry sound to the auditory nerve (Liberman et al., 2016); (2) undiagnosed hearing loss in the very high frequencies (Moore et al., 2017); (3) a speech-in-noise disorder (Vermiglio, 2014); or (4) a central auditory processing disorder (Musiek et al., 2018).

Finally, most of us will eventually experience some degree of sensorineural hearing loss in our lifetimes through the aging process. This hearing loss is referred to as **presbycusis** and can be due to loss of cochlear hair cells, reduced responsiveness of the hair cells, or loss of auditory nerve fibers. Because changes that occur with age can affect not just the ear but also the central auditory system, presbycusis may involve not only reduced hearing sensitivity but also deficits in auditory perception. Cruickshanks et al. (1998) estimate that approximately 45% of adults between the ages of 48 and 92 have some degree of hearing loss, with men demonstrating a higher prevalence than women. Knowing that the elderly population continues to be one of the fastest-growing segments within the United States, it is important that SLPs and audiologists have a good understanding of presbycusis and how it can impact people's lives.

REFLECTION QUESTION 12.2

What kinds of information might you provide to teenagers who are exposing themselves to very loud levels of music on a regular basis?

Mixed Hearing Loss

If you had a **mixed hearing loss**, the third general type of hearing loss, you would have the simultaneous presence of conductive and sensorineural hearing loss. For example, if the hair cells of your cochlea have been damaged by listening to loud music through a personal music device, and you have congestion in your middle ear due to a head cold, you have a mixed hearing loss. An older individual with an age-related sensorineural hearing loss who also has impacted cerumen, which temporarily decreases their hearing sensitivity even further, also has a mixed hearing loss. In most cases, the conductive component can be medically treated, leading to some improvement in overall hearing sensitivity. However, because the sensorineural component remains, the person's hearing cannot be restored to normal levels.

(Central) Auditory Processing Disorders

The three types of hearing loss described in the preceding section refer to impairment of the peripheral auditory system or the structures of the ear spanning from the pinna to the auditory nerve. The function of the peripheral auditory system is routinely assessed during a comprehensive audiological evaluation. Because what we hear needs to be processed in order to be useful, audiologists must consider the *entire* auditory system, including problems that affect the central auditory system. This can generally be thought of as the auditory structures, pathways, and neural synapses that span from the level of the brainstem to the cortex of the brain. Problems associated with the central auditory system may or may not cause hearing loss. Often, they interfere with the ability to efficiently and effectively use and interpret acoustic information. This is often reflected in problems such as difficulty hearing subtle differences between similar-sounding words and misunderstanding of speech when presented in a background of noise. These types of difficulties in an individual who has normal peripheral hearing are commonly referred to as central auditory processing deficits (CAPD) or auditory processing deficits (APD). Additional information regarding auditory processing is found on pages 420–421 and 434–436 of this chapter.

Hearing Loss Through the Lifespan

With the information covered at this point about the various types of hearing loss, it should now be clear that our hearing is something that should be attended to at all ages and stages of life, beginning immediately after birth. As discussed, newborns may be at risk for hearing loss due to a number of factors, including difficulties that occur during the birth process, genetic disorders, and syndromes. Over the past three decades, we have seen the development of **early hearing detection and intervention (EHDI) programs** in every state in the United States. All these programs are designed to identify significant hearing loss in newborn babies and follow up with prompt audiological intervention services. As of 2019, in the United States more than 98% of babies were being screened for hearing loss within the first month after birth (CDC, n.d.). The CDC also reports an increase in the number of infants identified early, from 855 in 2000 to over 6,300 in 2016. The goal is that babies who fail their newborn hearing screening and any follow-up rescreening should have a comprehensive audiological and medical evaluation before the age of 3 months to confirm or rule out the presence of hearing loss. Although the diagnosis of hearing losses that are present at birth is occurring at an earlier age in recent years due to these universal newborn hearing screening programs, this is only the first step in the audiological intervention process. It is equally important that appropriate early intervention services be planned and delivered as soon as possible after a hearing loss has been identified, preferably by 6 months. In fact, research strongly suggests that children who are diagnosed with hearing loss and receive hearing aids and early intervention by 6 months of age develop significantly better language skills than do similar children who are identified after 6 months of age (Meinzen-Derr et al., 2011; Yoshinaga-Itano et al., 1998).

Both newborns and preschoolers are particularly susceptible to hearing loss due to Eustachian tube dysfunction and otitis media, which can create a temporary, but often difficult to resolve, hearing loss that may negatively affect speech and language development. During the school-age years, students with listening difficulties often find themselves struggling to process the more complicated language structures that are part of academic learning, particularly when they are in the poor acoustic setting of the classroom. School-age, adolescent, and college-age students are all now at risk for noise-induced hearing loss due to the widespread use of ear-level music devices that can deliver very intense levels of sound directly to the ear.

By middle age, some adults with a history of early noise exposure begin to experience hearing loss as the effects of noise and aging impact their ability to understand speech. In addition, disorders such as Meniere's disease and otosclerosis are more common in middle-aged individuals. Also, some research suggests that by middle age, listeners may experience changes in their processing abilities, despite having normal hearing.

Finally, in older individuals age-related changes can affect both the cochlear hair cells and auditory nerve fibers, resulting in reduced speech understanding, sometimes even with good amplification. When these auditory changes combine with changes in memory or cognitive function, the effects on communication can be even greater.

Behavioral and Nonbehavioral Audiological Assessment Procedures

Learning Objective 12.6 Compare and contrast behavioral and nonbehavioral methods of audiological assessment.

Now that we have discussed the basic principles of sound, the anatomy and physiology of the auditory system, the various types and causes of hearing loss, and their effect on one's life, we are ready to take a look at how this knowledge is applied in the assessment of hearing. It is important to stress that no single test can accurately capture the full extent of a person's hearing loss or how that loss may be affecting the person in terms of their communication or psychological health. Instead, an audiologist must rely on a battery of tests and other measures, combined with careful questioning of and listening to the client, in order to obtain an accurate picture of an individual's hearing problem.

Before continuing, now is a good time to differentiate **assessment**, as we discuss in this section, from **screening**, referred to earlier in this chapter. Screening is the process used to determine which individuals, whether children or adults, are *likely* to have a hearing loss. If you ever had your hearing tested in school, it is likely that you participated in a screening. As previously mentioned, newborn hearing screening programs have been set up across the country in an effort to identify infants who are suspected of having a significant hearing impairment and who therefore should be referred for further testing. The screening equipment and procedures used vary with different screening programs. For example, a newborn screening performed in a hospital with automated equipment is quite different from a screening program using a traditional audiometer performed at a senior center.

In general, individuals who pass a screening are not referred for further testing, and those who fail a screening are. It is important to note that even if someone does not pass a screening, we cannot conclude that they have a hearing loss. Screenings are frequently performed in environments where background noise or distractions can interfere with the person's ability to respond accurately. It is not uncommon for students to fail their school hearing screening but have a comprehensive hearing test done in a sound-treated booth and find normal hearing. Finally, it is important to be aware that performing hearing screenings is part of the scope of practice of both an audiologist and an SLP.

The remainder of this section focuses on the types of tests that may be included in a comprehensive audiological assessment battery, as performed by an audiologist.

For students who one day hope to work as SLPs, it is important to remember that as professionals you will need to have an understanding of the hearing assessments that have been performed on your clients and how to use this information to better meet their speech and language needs.

Referral and Case History

Before conducting any tests, an audiologist spends time interviewing a client and collecting case history information. This process provides an opportunity to obtain background information from the client's perspective and helps the audiologist gain a better understanding of the client's communication challenges and goals. During this interview, the audiologist may ask questions about why the client has come in for the evaluation, whether they have been exposed to noise, whether there is a history of ear infections or ear surgery, and what communication situations are difficult for the client.

Another way to gain valuable information about a client's communication challenges and feelings about their hearing loss is by use of published self-assessment questionnaires. For example, a particular item on a questionnaire might ask the client to rate the degree of difficulty they experience when listening in a noisy restaurant. Another item might ask whether the client feels left out of social activities because of their hearing loss. Several of these questionnaires contain a companion version that can be completed by the client's significant other or a family member. Obtaining input from someone the client is close to can be very important, particularly if the client is not fully aware of how much they are missing and how much others in the family have to change their speaking pattern to accommodate the hearing loss. Finally, when these self-assessment tools are given before and after a hearing aid fitting, they can provide information about improvements that have occurred due to hearing aid use.

Otoscopic Examination

One of the first procedures performed if you were being seen for an audiological evaluation is a visual ear exam, or **otoscopic examination**. You are most likely familiar with the small handheld device that is used by an audiologist because it is the same device that physicians use to examine the ear canal and eardrum. The device is called an **otoscope**, and the otoscopic exam is an important early step in the assessment process because it alerts the audiologist to any conditions that may interfere with sound conduction during testing, such as excessive cerumen or any conditions that require immediate medical referral, such as drainage from the ear. Another version of this device, called a video otoscope, projects the image of the ear being viewed onto a television or computer monitor, allowing the client and family members to observe simultaneously. This technology allows the audiologist to print and store images that can then be shared with other medical personnel, such as the client's physician.

Electroacoustic and Electrophysiological Testing

Electroacoustic measures record acoustic signals from within the client's external auditory canal; **electrophysiological tests** record neuroelectric responses (nerve impulses) that are generated by the auditory system in response to sound. Both of these categories of tests evaluate the integrity of the peripheral and central auditory systems without requiring the client to provide any observable behavioral responses, such as repeating words or responding to tones. Because these tests do not assess a client's ability to recognize and use sound, they are not considered true hearing tests. Nevertheless, these tests do provide data that an audiologist can use to make some inferences about the functioning of the client's auditory system and their hearing.

The two types of electroacoustic measures that are commonly performed on children and adults are tests of tympanometry and otoacoustic emissions.

Tympanometry is useful in the diagnosis of conductive pathology, which would include both conductive and mixed hearing loss. Because it can be completed in a short period of time and does not require any behavioral responses, it is frequently used with children, including infants, and adults. Tympanometry is performed using a device that assesses the admittance of the middle ear as the pressure in the ear canal is changed. This process results in a graph called a **tympanogram** (see Figure 12.6). Data obtained can assist in identifying middle ear fluid, a break in the ossicular chain, or a perforation of the eardrum, for examples.

Otoacoustic emissions (OAEs) are a second type of electroacoustic measure that has received considerable attention during the past two decades. Discovered by David Kemp (1978), OAEs are low-intensity sounds, commonly referred to as "echoes," that are generated within the cochlea as a result of movement of the outer hair cells. These tiny emissions move outward from the cochlea through the middle ear to the external auditory canal, where they can be recorded by a microphone placed in the ear canal. For clinical uses, OAEs are produced by presenting a moderate-intensity acoustic stimulus to the ear canal and then determining if the emissions are present or not. Generally, when OAEs are present, hearing sensitivity is presumed to be normal or no worse than a mild loss (Glattke & Robinette, 2007). Perhaps the most important use of OAE testing is in newborn hearing screening programs. This noninvasive and quick test has provided an inexpensive and efficient way to test millions of newborns each year.

In addition to electroacoustic tests, several electrophysiological tests are available to audiologists. Recall that electrophysiological tests record neuroelectric responses (nerve impulses) generated by the auditory system in response to sound.

FIGURE 12.6 Schematic of three common tympanogram patterns: (a) normal middle ear function, (b) somewhat reduced admittance due to otosclerosis, (c) minimal admittance due to otitis media with effusion.

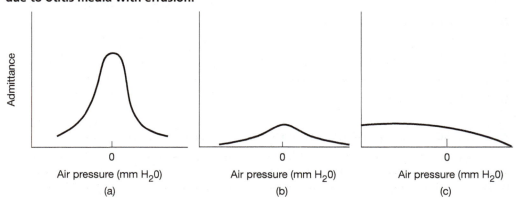

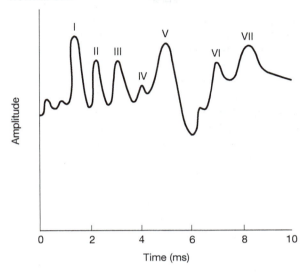

FIGURE 12.7 Schematic drawing of a typical auditory brainstem response waveform for a normal ear.

These responses are collectively referred to as **auditory evoked potentials (AEPs)**. To measure these neuroelectric responses, small electrodes would be placed on your head and sound would be delivered to your ear. These tiny responses are captured and recorded using specialized computer equipment, and the pattern that is generated would be compared to normative data. The **auditory brainstem response (ABR)** test is commonly used to assess the neuroelectric activity of the auditory nerve and structures in the lower brainstem in individuals suspected of having neurological issues, such as a tumor on the VIIIth cranial nerve or auditory neuropathy/dys-synchrony disorder. In addition, it can be used to estimate the auditory thresholds in individuals who are unable or unwilling to be evaluated using conventional behavioral techniques, such as infants, young children, and individuals who have developmental delays. Auditory brainstem testing is particularly useful for diagnosing hearing loss in infants who have failed their newborn hearing screening. Refer to Figure 12.7 for an example of an ABR wave pattern generated on a typical adult with 85 dB of stimulation.

Pearson eTextbook
Video Example 12.3

In this video, two important nonbehavioral tests are demonstrated. Under what circumstances would these tests be most helpful to the audiologist?

https://youtu.be/QvrBogzziXA

Behavioral Testing

One major limitation of electroacoustic and electrophysiological measures is that although they provide information about the integrity of the auditory system, they do not show how the individual perceives or responds to sound. For this reason, testing a person with behavioral measures is necessary to fully understand a person's ability to hear and process sound. Behavioral tests measure a person's hearing by observing some deliberate action taken by the client (e.g., raising a hand) or by noting some change in behavior (e.g., turning the head toward the sound).

Most behavioral tests are administered using a specialized piece of electronic equipment called an **audiometer**, which contains controls that allow an audiologist to select, manipulate, and present various stimuli, such as tone and speech, to assess hearing. Testing is usually carried out in a specially treated sound booth that limits the amount of external and internal noise that can interfere with hearing; this supports the reliability of the test results.

Behavioral Observation

The most basic form of behavioral assessment used with infants is a process referred to as **behavioral observation (BO)**. As the term implies, an audiologist presents a stimulus such as speech or tones through a loudspeaker and observes the child's reaction. Basic responses to sound that the audiologist looks for are gross body movements such as startling, widening of the eyes, and facial grimacing. Although fairly simple to administer, BO has been criticized for its poor reliability and validity (Hicks et al., 2000). Audiologists often have difficulty making judgments about whether a child's bodily movement was in response to a stimulus or was just a random movement. In addition, a child may quickly habituate to the task, losing interest in it after only a few presentations of the stimulus. For these reasons, electroacoustic and electrophysiological measures are preferred over BO when assessing children younger than 5 months of age.

CASE STUDY   Terrence *(continued)*

Assessment and Results: Part 1

The assessment carried out of Terrence's hearing follows the recommendations provided by the American Academy of Audiology in their Clinical Guidance Document on Assessment of Hearing in Infants and Young Children (2020). Although it had been done previously after the first failed screening, nondiagnostic otoscopy was repeated and the audiologist checked to determine that the ear canals were free of any wax or debris that might interfere with testing. She also assessed whether there was evidence of any malformations of the ear (e.g., absence or missing cartilage) and whether both ears were in the correct position on the head.

Next, to gain an idea of Terrence's overall responsiveness to sound, the audiologist performed behavioral observation testing in a sound-treated booth using speech and noise stimuli presented from speakers. To assess the pressure and admittance of the outer/middle ear system, tympanometry was performed in each ear. This test is sensitive to anything that might interfere with the transmission of sound energy through the outer and or middle ears (e.g., a perforated eardrum, middle ear fluid). Although already done in the hospital, the audiologist repeated the otoacoustic emissions testing, this time in the sound-treated booth to ensure that ambient noise was not a factor. This test assesses the function of the cochlear hair cells and is

typically normal when hearing is within normal limits or if a mild cochlear loss is present.

Nondiagnostic otoscopy confirmed that both ear canals were free of any blockage and there was no evidence of anything atypical regarding the shape or position of Terrence's ears. Behavior observation in the sound-treated booth revealed that even when speech and noise stimuli were presented at levels up to 85 dB, Terrence did not provide any observable response. Middle ear pressure and admittance values were age-appropriate, suggesting that any hearing loss that might be found would most likely not be conductive or mixed. Otoacoustic emissions continued to be absent in each ear at all frequencies.

Assessment and Results: Part 2

Because findings from the above-noted tests did not allow the audiologist to rule out significant sensorineural hearing loss, assessment of the auditory brainstem response was performed to estimate Terrence's hearing thresholds. While he was sleeping, the audiologist presented low- (500 Hz), mid- (1000 Hz), and high-frequency (3000 Hz) tone bursts to each ear and estimated Terrence's hearing thresholds to be between 90 and 95 dB at these frequencies. This finding, combined with normal tympanograms, suggests that Terrence has a profound sensorineural hearing loss in each ear.

Visual Reinforcement Audiometry

Once a child reaches the age of 5 to 6 months, the natural ability to localize, or turn toward a sound, has developed, and this means an audiologist can use a technique called **visual reinforcement audiometry (VRA)** to test behavioral responses to speech and frequency-specific tones. With VRA, the child is rewarded for turning toward the stimulus. As soon as the child responds, the audiologist activates an animated or lighted toy. This reinforcement helps maintain the child's interest in the task, giving the audiologist more time to collect hearing data. VRA is more reliable than BO and has been shown to be an effective tool for accurately assessing hearing sensitivity in young children (Diefendorf, 1988). Despite the value of VRA, most audiologists would combine VRA test results with an electrophysiological measure prior to fitting a child with hearing aids.

Pure Tone Audiometry

By 2½ years of age, a child should be able to perform many of the same procedures that are used with adults, but often with some modifications. For example, when testing a child's responses to pure tones, rather than ask a child to raise a hand or press a response button, **conditioned play audiometry (CPA)** is often used. This procedure involves the use of toys such as blocks, puzzle pieces, or stacking rings to engage the child in a listening game. The child is conditioned to put a block in a bucket or a ring on a post each time the test signal is heard. Conditioned play audiometry can be used until a child is able to be tested using conventional pure tone audiometry, which usually occurs somewhere around the age of 5 to 8 years.

> **Pearson eTextbook**
> Video Example 12.4
>
> In this video, an assistant is working with a young child during a hearing test. What specific test is being conducted and why is an assistant needed?
>
> https://youtu.be/xIeagA8IEh0

A great deal of information can be obtained about a person's hearing through **pure tone audiometry**. In fact, the pure tone test is considered to be one of, if not *the*, most fundamental behavioral tests in the standard audiometric assessment battery. **Pure tones** are sounds that contain energy only at a single frequency. Standard practice is to test a range of frequencies from 250 to 8000 Hz so that information is collected about the person's ability to perceive the speech sounds of the language. The purpose of pure tone testing is to determine a person's threshold at each test frequency for the right and left ears. **Threshold** is defined as the lowest (quietest) intensity level, measured in decibels, at which a person can just barely detect a given stimulus approximately 50% of the time.

An example of a blank audiogram is shown in Figure 12.8. Note that the standard test frequencies are listed on the *x* (horizontal) axis and are 250 and 500 Hz (low frequencies), 1000 Hz (a middle frequency), and 2000, 3000, 4000, 6000, and 8000 Hz (high frequencies). Also, intensity is listed on the *y* (vertical) axis and ranges from –10 dB (a very faint sound) to 110 dB (a very intense sound).

Degree of Hearing Loss

At this point, it will be helpful to discuss briefly the degree of hearing loss. As noted previously in this chapter, when describing a person's hearing loss, audiologists use terminology such as *conductive*, *sensorineural*, and *mixed* to specify the region of the auditory system affected. These terms describe the type of hearing loss a person has. Although this is a critical part of the diagnostic process, it is also important to quantify the degree of hearing loss; this is typically expressed in dB. A decibel is a mathematical unit based on the pressure exerted by a particular sound. The lowest

FIGURE 12.8 **Blank audiogram used to record patient thresholds in pure tone audiometry. Note frequency in hertz on the *x*-axis and intensity in decibels on the *y*-axis.**

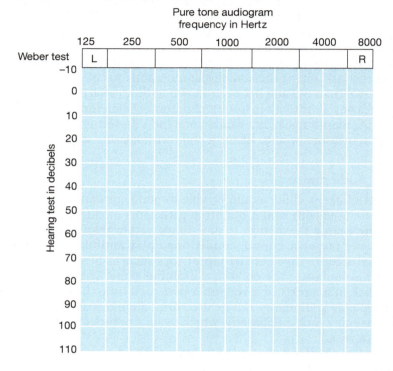

decibel level at which a given sound is barely audible represents a person's auditory threshold. The greater the decibel value required to reach a person's threshold (compared to what is considered "normal"), the greater the degree of hearing loss.

In order to assess the value of the WHO's proposed system of categorizing degrees of hearing loss in adults, Humes (2019) examined five datasets of pure tone hearing thresholds and real-world measures of speech communication from groups of older adults. The proposed system, which Humes concluded was valid, is noted in Table 12.3.

Regarding children, Lieu and colleagues (2020) proposed the following categories of hearing loss:

- Slight: hearing thresholds 16 to 25 dB
- Mild: hearing thresholds 26 to 40 dB
- Moderate: hearing thresholds 41 to 55 dB
- Moderately severe: hearing thresholds 56 to 70 dB
- Severe: hearing thresholds 71 to 90 dB
- Profound: hearing thresholds more than 90 dB

Notice that the range considered "normal" is different for children than for adults. Specifically, although adult thresholds up to 19 dB HL are considered within normal limits, the cutoff for children is set at 15 dB HL. Think for a moment about why this makes sense. What is different about the process of hearing for children

TABLE 12.3

World Health Organization's Grading System for Hearing Impairment

Degree of Hearing Loss	Hearing Thresholds in dB	Performance in Quiet	Performance in Noise
Mild	20–34	None	Some difficulty following conversation
Moderate	35–49	Difficulty with normal conversation	Difficulty with normal conversation
Moderately severe	50–64	Need loud speech to hear in quiet	Considerable difficulty, even with loud speech
Severe	65–79	Can hear speech shouted to the ear	Considerable difficulty, even with shouted speech
Profound	80–94	Cannot hear shouted speech	Cannot hear shouted speech

than for adults? Children who are in the process of developing speech and language need to have access to all of the subtle information found in the acoustic speech signal. Adults, in contrast, have more developed language and therefore have a better ability to "fill in" missing pieces of information that they did not hear. They do this by also using their prior knowledge and experience. This process is referred to as top-down processing.

In general terms, individuals whose degree of hearing loss falls within the slight/mild-to-severe range are classified as *hard of hearing* or *hearing impaired*. These individuals depend on their remaining hearing (also referred to as *residual hearing*) for receptive communication and for the learning of new concepts. For people whose auditory thresholds fall in the profound range, however, the auditory system provides limited or no access to speech without the use of amplification. As previously mentioned, these individuals are often given the diagnosis of deaf.

Finally, it should be noted that the category of "mild" hearing loss used for children can be misinterpreted as suggesting that the negative impact of the loss on the child is not great or that intervention is not necessary. This is not the case. Research has documented that children with these losses are at much greater risk for decreased abilities in reading, use of grammatical markers, and hearing in noise (Moore et al., 2020; Walker et al., 2020).

Air Conduction and Bone Conduction Testing

It is very important for students to understand that during hearing testing, pure tone thresholds are established by delivering pure tones in two different ways: through **air conduction** and **bone conduction**. Air conduction testing is administered while a client wears earphones delivering the sound to the cochlea via the outer and middle ear. This is the typical way that we hear. Hearing loss resulting from disorders in any of the three major sections of the peripheral auditory system (the outer, middle, or inner ear) will be identified with air conduction testing. Once air conduction testing is completed, the process is repeated using a bone oscillator, a small vibrating device that is positioned against the skull, behind the pinna. When a stimulus is presented through the oscillator, the bones of the skull are set into vibration, and this vibration directly stimulates the cochlea. So, with bone conduction the person is able to hear the stimulus even though it has bypassed the outer and middle ears.

By comparing the results of air conduction testing to those obtained from bone conduction testing, it is possible to identify the type of hearing loss. Take a look at the audiograms in Figures 12.9 and 12.10. In Figure 12.9, the right ear air conduction thresholds (represented by the circles) fall within the moderate to moderately severe hearing loss range. However, the bone conduction thresholds (represented by the brackets) fall within the normal range of hearing. From this, the audiologist can infer that the client has difficulty hearing sound when it is introduced in the conventional manner—that is, through the external auditory meatus. Notice, however, that the client has no difficulty hearing sound if the outer and middle ear are bypassed and the cochlea is stimulated directly. Therefore, this client has conductive hearing loss occurring in the outer or middle ear. In Figure 12.10, both the air and bone conduction thresholds fall outside the normal limits and within the moderately to severe range of hearing loss. Because the results are the same when the inner ear is stimulated by air conduction or by bone conduction, the

FIGURE 12.9 Audiogram representing a moderate to moderately severe conductive hearing loss in the right ear. (Note that the symbol used to denote bone conduction thresholds depends on the method used to assess it.)

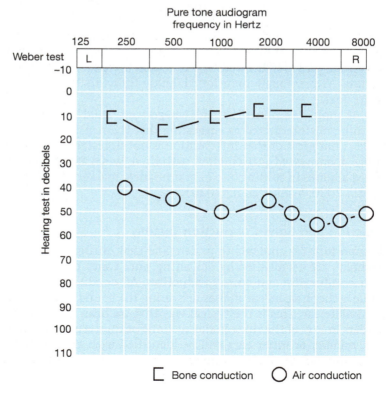

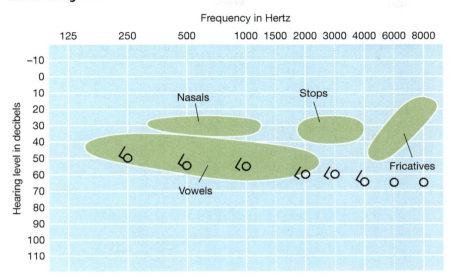

FIGURE 12.10 Audiogram representing a moderately severe to severe sensorineural hearing loss in the right ear with major speech sound categories.

audiologist can conclude that the inner ear itself must be affected. Therefore, this client has sensorineural hearing loss.

Notice also that the intensity and frequency characteristics of the four major speech sound categories are superimposed on the audiogram in Figure 12.10. This is helpful to both students who are learning about the relationships between hearing loss and speech and also to clients who want to understand their own hearing loss. Note that the person with this hearing loss has some access to vowel sounds because some of the energy of vowels is more intense than their hearing thresholds. However, this person does not have access to nasals, stops, or fricatives because these sounds are less intense than what this person can hear (i.e., their thresholds.).

In Figure 12.11, again both the air and bone conduction thresholds fall outside the normal range. However, the degree of hearing loss represented by the air conduction thresholds is greater than the degree of hearing loss represented by the bone conduction thresholds. In this case, although there is obvious damage to the inner ear, as evidenced by the bone conduction results, the person has the potential to hear better if the outer and middle ear are bypassed. Therefore, there is evidence that both sensorineural and a conductive hearing loss exist simultaneously. In other words, the client has mixed hearing loss.

Speech Audiometry

Although pure tone audiometry is often considered to be the most fundamental component of an audiological evaluation, we must keep in mind that people typically seek the services of an audiologist because they are having difficulty understanding speech, not pure tones. It is only natural, then, that we evaluate a client's ability to hear and understand speech as part of the assessment battery.

FIGURE 12.11 **Audiogram representing a moderate to profound mixed hearing loss in the right ear.**

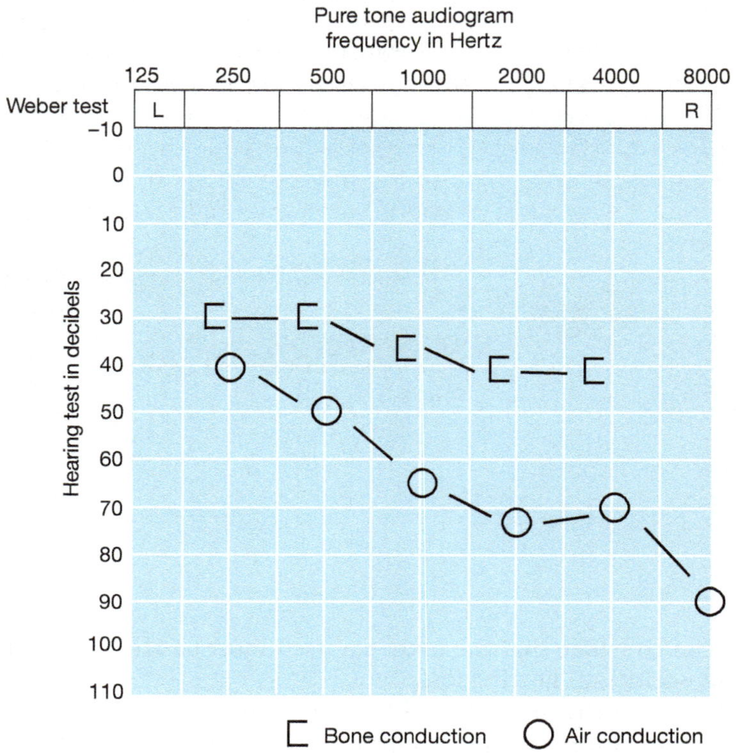

A variety of tools are available to assess a client's auditory skills for speech. Two speech audiometry measures that are typically included in routine hearing tests are the Speech Recognition Threshold and the Word Recognition Test. The **Speech Recognition Threshold (SRT)** is a measure of the lowest (softest) intensity where a person can recognize compound words, and the **Word Recognition Test (WRT)** assesses how well a client is able to identify one-syllable words presented at some level above the threshold.

Auditory Processing Assessment

According to ASHA (2005) and AAA (2010), tests of auditory processing can be used on school-age children to determine if they have a fundamental impairment of their central auditory processing system. The tests used are different from those used during the conventional hearing test and often involve testing the client's understanding of speech in challenging conditions, including in a background of noise, as well as when more than one piece of information is presented simultaneously. Sometimes nonspeech tests are also used in an effort to reduce the impact of language on the client's performance. The ASHA document states that tests of auditory processing should not be done on individuals younger than 7 years old or on those who have language or cognitive deficits that could interfere with the test results.

To understand some of the important issues related to this topic, it may be helpful to review briefly the earlier use of tests of auditory processing. Years ago, before advanced imaging techniques such as computed tomography scans and MRI were readily available, tests of auditory processing were used with patients to identify what brain regions might be impaired and to provide some information about the kinds of tasks that were challenging to them. A person, for example, with a tumor on the right side of the brain would demonstrate a different pattern of responses on these tests than would someone with a tumor on the left side. Similarly, a person with a temporal lobe problem would perform differently than someone with a frontal lobe impairment.

Today, audiologists who use tests of auditory processing typically do so not with patients with medical issues such as tumors or stroke but rather with school-age children who are experiencing difficulties functioning in the classroom. These children may be demonstrating some of the following: distractibility, difficulty comprehending rapid speech or speech in poor acoustic environments, difficulty following complex auditory directions, or difficulty paying attention.

Despite the great interest and increased awareness among professionals and the public about CAPD, the disorder remains controversial for a number of reasons. First, individuals who have deficits of the central auditory system often demonstrate a variety of different symptoms, and often those symptoms are the same as or similar to those associated with other disorders, such as learning disabilities, language impairment, and attention disorders. This raises the question as to whether the auditory processing diagnosis is truly a unique disorder.

Second, if the language and cognitive testing that are done prior to performing tests of auditory processing are not thorough, a child with language, learning, or cognitive deficits may perform poorly on the auditory processing tests and that child may be misdiagnosed as having an auditory processing disorder. Such a child would then not receive the appropriate diagnosis and resulting intervention to address their difficulties.

Third, the current literature includes greater awareness that processing of auditory stimuli involves many systems (e.g., auditory, language, cognitive) and it is difficult if not impossible to create tests that assess only auditory abilities. It is also more widely understood that although there are children who demonstrate normal peripheral hearing with reduced listening abilities, tests of auditory processing may not be the most effective tools to identify such children.

Fourth, there is a tendency for the public to believe (incorrectly) that an auditory processing deficit may be the underlying cause of other disorders, such as autism or attention deficits. The important point to note here is that even though individuals with autism and attention deficits frequently display problems in their ability to understand/process auditory information, the fundamental, underlying cause of their processing difficulty is neurological, not auditory.

Finally, this testing is controversial because there is still a lack of evidence from research regarding how to improve the way the auditory processing system works. It is understandable that this would be frustrating to parents who are seeking to help their children.

For information regarding support for children who have been diagnosed with auditory processing disorders or who are suspected of having listening difficulties, see pages 434–436 of this chapter.

Helping People Who Have Hearing Loss

Learning Objective 12.7 Describe three major ways people with hearing loss can be helped.

Aural (Audiological) Habilitation/Rehabilitation

After an audiological assessment has been completed and various tests analyzed, it is time to work with the client in creating an appropriate course of treatment in order to reduce the negative impact of the hearing loss on their communication abilities. In some cases, this requires a referral to a physician for a medical evaluation. In many cases it involves providing some form of **amplification** (e.g., hearing aids, cochlear implant, assistive listening device) combined with various therapy services; this is often referred to as *aural habilitation/rehabilitation*.

Aural habilitation refers to intervention conducted with individuals whose hearing loss occurred at an early age and therefore prevented normal development of auditory and spoken language skills. In general, this refers to services and therapies used primarily with children who are prelingually hearing impaired and also their families. One of the critical concepts related to aural habilitation with children who have hearing loss is the importance of intervening early. This is important because in order for the parts of the brain that process auditory information to develop fully, they need to receive sound. The longer a child is deprived of sound due to hearing loss, the greater the chance that these auditory areas will not efficiently respond to sound once it is provided. This relates to what is referred to as brain plasticity, the ability of the brain and central nervous system to be changed in response to sensory input (e.g., sound). Yoshinaga-Itano and colleagues (1998) compared a group of children with hearing loss, all of whom were fit with hearing aids prior to 6 months, with a similar group who were fit after 6 months. The researchers found that the group that was fit earlier had significantly better language development when tested later. In 2000, Congress authorized early hearing detection intervention (EHDI) programs, which provided funds for states to identify children with hearing loss and to receive early intervention services. Consistent with the research, the primary goal of EHDI programs is for these children to have a hearing screening by 1 month, a diagnosis by 3 months, and intervention by 6 months.

Aural rehabilitation refers to services and therapies provided to individuals who have lost their hearing later in life, after spoken language skills have at least partially developed. In this case, the focus is on preserving and restoring communication skills that have been negatively impacted by a loss of hearing. Frequently, the term *aural rehabilitation* is used to refer to both habilitative and rehabilitative aspects of intervention, as is done in the remainder of this chapter.

Whether working with adults or caregivers of children, during this process we collect detailed information about the presenting communication challenges by synthesizing information obtained from the case history interview, self-assessment questionnaires, and results of the audiometric test battery. In some cases, collaboration with medical personnel, SLPs, special education teachers, teachers of individuals with hearing loss, psychologists, and vocational rehabilitation counselors may also be needed in order for the rehabilitation plan to be strong. By identifying the specific needs of the individual and selecting treatment methods using principles of evidence-based practice, both the client and the clinician can feel confident that the rehabilitation process will be based on the best available information. Also, one of the most important things that audiologists can do in creating this intervention plan is to listen to the client and/or caregivers. When we listen to our clients, we not only learn a great deal of information about their perspective of the challenges that they face, but we also communicate respect to them and start to build a rapport with them that will enhance the effectiveness of any other recommendations we make.

Counseling

At this point, it is important to discuss briefly the critical role of counseling. Although counseling can be used from the very first minute that you meet a new client, it is introduced here because our efforts to help an individual with communication challenges related to a hearing loss (or any communication disorder) can be enhanced considerably if we use effective counseling techniques. Counseling is an essential component of all the audiological services we provide.

Counseling is usually thought of as the process of giving a client information, sometimes referred to as **informational counseling**. Some examples of this include explaining the results of individual tests, providing technical information on the anatomy of the ear, or explaining how hearing loss occurs so the client can better understand the nature of their problem. The audiologist might also present possible courses of treatment, including hearing aids and rehabilitation options, to support spoken communication. This type of counseling is critical and requires great skill on the part of the clinician so that information is communicated in a way that is easily understood and remembered. It has been reported that only 50% of the information conveyed by health care providers is actually remembered by clients and that approximately half of this information is remembered inaccurately (Kessels, 2003; Margolis, 2004). For this reason, it is a good policy to provide a written summary of information discussed so that the client can refer back to it. Some clinical providers are now providing clients access to a website where they can find information that specifically relates to their condition.

Although important, informational counseling is only one part of the counseling process. A second broad category of counseling is **personal adjustment counseling**, which involves providing assistance to the client and family in dealing with the emotional consequences of hearing loss. As noted earlier in this chapter, hearing loss can have a profound impact on a person's psychological, social, and emotional well-being. Clients may struggle as they try to come to terms with feelings of anger, anxiety, fear, frustration, and despair that are a direct result of their hearing loss. These feelings are often seen not only in the client but also in others who are in close contact with the individual, such as parents or a partner. Often, unless these individuals receive support from an empathetic clinician, they cannot move forward to address their communication problems.

Most audiologists and SLPs are comfortable providing informational counseling because they feel confident that they can provide accurate information about the factual aspects of hearing loss. Personal adjustment counseling is more intimidating to many clinicians because it involves skills that many of us believe are less well developed. It is important to note that the literature on personal adjustment counseling clearly indicates that one of the most important skills we can use as clinicians is to be good listeners. An audiologist, then, must pay close attention to what a client reports and what questions the client asks in an effort to uncover any underlying personal adjustment issues. The audiologist must try to distinguish between the client's request for factual information and the client's need for the audiologist to acknowledge some personal feelings the client is having about the hearing problem (English, 2007).

Personal adjustment counseling involves encouraging clients to "tell their stories" about what it's like to live with a hearing loss. Eventually, as a rapport develops between a client and an audiologist, the client can be helped to accept and assume ownership of the hearing loss and move forward to solving their communication challenges. Simply telling a client what they should do will not lead to progress if the client does not first acknowledge and accept the fact that a problem exists.

Some final points regarding counseling should be made. First, clinicians must attend to the client's/family's cultural background and linguistic needs so that appropriate and effective communication is used (Scott, 2000). Second, audiologists should provide counseling whenever the opportunity presents itself, not only at the conclusion of a clinical session. Finally, clinicians should always be aware of their professional boundaries. When you suspect that a client is dealing with potential psychological or mental health issues that are beyond those related to the hearing loss, a referral to a qualified professional counselor should be made.

Hearing Aids

Amplification is considered the core of most aural rehabilitation plans. For this reason, one of the first steps in the aural rehabilitation process is the selection, fitting, and evaluation of amplification. In most cases, amplification consists of **personal hearing aids**, although other amplification options, described later, are also available.

Pearson eTextbook
Video Example 12.5
Based on the information provided in this video, what are the major components of all hearing aids?
https://youtu.be/AxzVyMcmRcs

Hearing aids come in a variety of styles and sizes, ranging from tiny custom-made models that fit entirely in the ear canal to custom in-the-ear models that fit into the concha region of the pinna to slightly larger instruments that are worn behind the ear (see Figure 12.12). Regardless of the style, every hearing aid contains certain basic components: a microphone, an amplifier, a receiver, and some type of computer processor. The microphone picks up acoustic energy from the environment, converts it to an electrical signal, and sends it to the amplifier. The amplifier increases the voltage of the electrical signal and sends it to the receiver, which in turn converts it back into acoustic energy and routes it to the user's ear canal.

There have been numerous advances in hearing aid technology in recent years. Nearly all hearing aids dispensed today incorporate sophisticated digital signal processing. Sound entering the hearing aid is converted into a digital code that can be processed and manipulated in various ways to improve audibility while also reducing unwanted background noise and eliminating acoustic feedback (the annoying "whistle" that hearing aids sometimes create). Modern hearing

FIGURE 12.12 **Styles of air conduction hearing aids.**

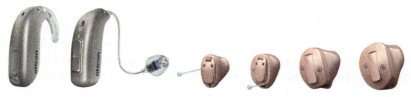

Photographs courtesy of Oticon, Inc.

aids are programmed by an audiologist using a computer and special software. The primary goal in most hearing aid fittings is to make speech audible. This is not a simple task because, unlike with eyeglasses that, in many cases, can restore a person's sight to 20/20, a hearing aid will not return hearing to normal.

Let's consider for a moment a person whose hearing loss prevents him from hearing some sounds at all and for whom other sounds are softer than usual. Obviously, this will interfere greatly with his ability to understand speech. But if audibility is the main problem, the use of hearing aids should be quite helpful because they amplify the specific sounds that he is missing. Once this person has access to those sounds, he will hopefully understand speech much more easily.

Unfortunately, however, in some cases clients report that their hearing aids have made things louder but not clearer, and they still cannot understand speech. These individuals may be experiencing distortion due to the type of damage they have to their auditory system. In this case, the audiologist may need to provide strategies and supports to be used in conjunction with the hearing aids to increase speech understanding. In some cases, an SLP can be very helpful in providing communication strategies to address these clients' needs. When a person is considering whether to purchase amplification, they must be counseled so that their expectations for improvement remain realistic. Later in this chapter we discuss the role of cochlear implants as another important option for some people who are not helped by hearing aids.

Hearing Aids in Children

Tomblin and colleagues (2015) compared language performance from 2 to 5 years of age in children with four different degrees of hearing loss (ranging from mild to severe) and children who had normal hearing. They found that the children with hearing loss demonstrated, on average, decreased language levels and the greater the degree of loss, the lower the language test score. Also, children who wore their hearing aids for greater amounts of time demonstrated better language skills. The researchers also found that the degree of hearing loss had a greater impact on the child's use of word endings (i.e., morphemes) than the development of vocabulary. This is consistent with the fact that word endings (*walk* vs. *walked*, *book* vs. *books*) tend to be high in frequency and have less intensity than other sounds. Finally, Tomblin and colleagues found that children who were fit with hearing aids earlier (i.e., before 6 months) showed overall good language skills at 2 years of age and those fit after 18 months had considerably lower levels of language and speech ability.

Hearing Aids in Adults

Picou (2020), using adult survey data, found that the public is, overall, very satisfied with their hearing aids and with the ability to pair their aids to other devices, including computers and phones. In addition, improved hearing appears to lead to improved quality of life. Think back now to the comorbidities summarized by Abrams (2017) earlier in this chapter. One of the most important and interesting questions being asked related to this research is whether hearing aids can reduce the risks of these co-occurring conditions. Although research on the impact of hearing aids is not yet sufficient to determine whether hearing aids reduce the chance of developing comorbid conditions, the findings in Table 12.4 are encouraging (Abrams, 2017).

TABLE 12.4
Preliminary Findings Regarding Hearing Aid Benefit in Adults

Comorbidity	Findings
Falls	Participants who were fit with hearing aids demonstrated increased stability compared to performance without hearing aids (Rumalla et al., 2015).
Depression	The likelihood of being diagnosed with depression or related symptoms was lower for those using hearing aids (Abrams & Kihm, 2015; Mener et al., 2013).
	Both depression in participants and stress on their caregivers were reduced during a period using hearing aids (Boi et al., 2012).
Loneliness	Significant decreases in feelings of loneliness were reported after 4–6 weeks of hearing aid use (Weinstein et al., 2016).
Cognition	Improved performance on a cognitive screener was noted after use of hearing aids for 3 months (Acar et al., 2011).

Bone Conduction Hearing Aids

We mentioned previously in the chapter that most conductive hearing losses can be treated with either medication or surgery. In cases where conductive hearing loss is not medically treatable, such as a chronically draining ear, use of a bone conduction hearing aid may be useful. Bone conduction hearing aids send sound directly to the cochlea and bypass the outer and middle ear. This is the same process that happens when audiologists test hearing with a bone oscillator.

To help understand the different bone conduction devices, we can categorize them into two broad types:

- **Extrinsic devices**: All of the components are worn outside the head and no surgery is required
- **Semi-implantable devices:** require surgery; some transmit the sound by surgically going through the skin and others do so by use of a magnet

In extrinsic devices, the components are held onto the mastoid bone by a head band or some type of adhesive. A special soft band is often used with children who are too young to have a surgically implanted device (Figure 12.13). Extrinsic devices are also used for those patients who are assessing the possible value of a bone conduction device. Because sound vibrations have to travel through the skin before stimulating the skull, these devices often do not deliver adequate amplification to high-frequency sounds and skin can sometimes break down in the mastoid area.

The bone-anchored hearing aid is one of the most popular semi-implantable devices and surgically attaches the sound processor to the skull (Figure 12.14). It delivers good high-frequency amplification, but because it involves broken skin the daily care of the surgical site can be difficult for patients to maintain.

The newest and perhaps most promising devices leave the skin intact and the external microphone and processor send signals using magnetic coils to an implanted vibrating device (i.e., transducer) under the skin that is in direct contact with the skull (Ellsperman et al., 2021).

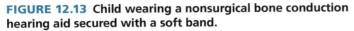

FIGURE 12.13 **Child wearing a nonsurgical bone conduction hearing aid secured with a soft band.**

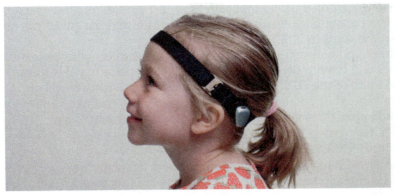

© Cochlear Limited 2022. Image courtesy of Cochlear Limited

FIGURE 12.14 **Adult with bone conduction hearing aid surgically attached to his mastoid area.**

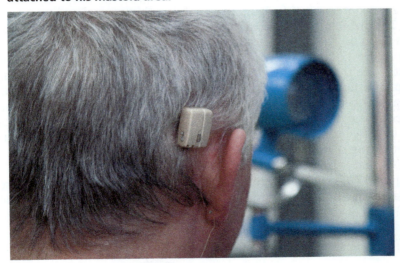

© LIFE IN VIEW/SCIENCE PHOTO LIBRARY

Over-the-Counter Hearing Aids

Because insurance coverage is rare, hearing aids are unaffordable for the large majority of individuals who could benefit from them. This, combined with the better understanding of the negative impact of hearing loss on individuals' quality of life, led Congress to authorize the Food and Drug Administration (FDA) to create a new class of hearing aids called over-the-counter (OTC) aids for adults who have mild to moderate hearing loss. These aids would be less expensive, could be obtained without having a hearing test or hearing aid fitting performed by an audiologist, and could be purchased directly in stores or online. These devices, however, would not be available for children.

In December 2012, the AAA (2020) provided its commentary on the FDA's proposed rules for OTC hearing aids. The Academy's concerns were divided into three categories: safety, efficacy, and consumer protection. For example, AAA was concerned that (1) the sound produced by the aids could damage existing hearing,

(2) the new aids might not meet appropriate performance standards, (3) the labeling information could be overwhelming for consumers, and (4) consumers may not be able to return their device and be refunded. The FDA received over 1,000 comments from the public regarding the proposed rule and the guidelines about OTC aids were finalized in 2022.

Palmer and colleagues (2022) note that consumers who are candidates for OTC aids will have to decide if they want to obtain hearing aids through the traditional route or the OTC route, which involves purchasing an aid online without the involvement of an audiologist. As an audiologist, you would have to decide if you would offer these alternative hearing aids in your practice.

Cochlear Implants

Some people with severe to profound hearing losses receive little or no benefit from traditional hearing aids because these devices fail to provide enough amplification to make sound audible. For this group of individuals, a cochlear implant may be an option. A cochlear implant is a prosthesis designed to bypass the damaged hair cells of the cochlea and directly stimulate the surviving auditory nerve fibers with electrical energy.

It may be helpful to describe the device in stages beginning with Figure 12.15. There are two items in this figure that make up the internal and external components. The first item is implanted in the skull (internal component) and the second item is worn on the ear and head.

In Figure 12.16 we see what the external components look like as worn by a patient. Note that behind the ear are the microphone and speech processor. The microphone of the cochlear implant picks up sound, converts it to electrical energy, and transmits it to the speech processor. The speech processor is a sophisticated microcomputer that is programmed for each client so that the information sent to the impaired ear includes those features of the speech signal that are critical to understanding speech. The speech processor is adhered to the side of the head by a magnet that is located inside the skull.

Figure 12.17 shows the internal components, which include the receiver-stimulator that is surgically attached to the skull and a group of electrodes that

FIGURE 12.15 Internal and external components of the cochlear implant.

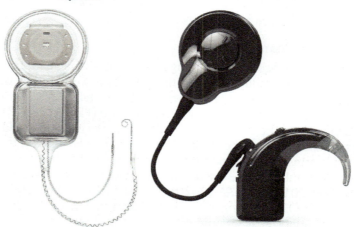

© Cochlear Limited 2022. Image courtesy of Cochlear Limited

FIGURE 12.16 External components of the cochlear implant as worn on the head.

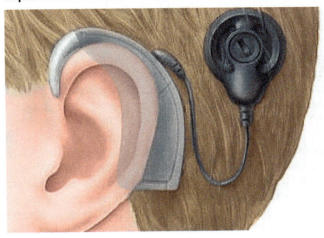

FIGURE 12.17 Internal components of the cochlear implant.

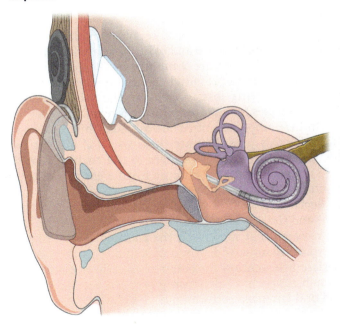

are inserted into the cochlea. These electrodes take the place of the hair cells of the cochlea and the surgeon's goal is to insert electrodes into the entire length of the cochlea so that the patient will have greater access to the various frequencies that make up speech.

To understand how all this works, read the following paragraph and then access the video in Video Example 12.6. The signal is picked up by the microphone and speech processor, which transmits the signal through a cable to the external transmitting coil that is magnetically secured to the head. Using FM radio waves, the

Pearson eTextbook

Video Example 12.6

Based on the information provided in this video, what part of the cochlear implant takes the place of the cochlear hair cells?

https://youtu.be/YdYjdYD--nk

signal is transmitted across the skin to the internal receiver–stimulator and finally to the individual electrodes implanted in the cochlea. Modern cochlear implants contain multiple electrodes that provide electrical stimulation to many sites along the basilar membrane, allowing the client to receive information of different frequencies. The resulting neural impulses are transmitted to the brain in the usual manner, by way of the ascending auditory pathways.

Bilateral implantation has become common in children and adults in an effort to improve overall hearing ability, particularly in noise, and to improve the ability to localize. Also, in some cases a client may choose to wear a cochlear implant on one ear and a hearing aid on the other ear. This might be the case when the cochlear implant is not successfully delivering certain frequency information. This is referred to as bimodal hearing because both acoustic (i.e., hearing aid) and electrical (i.e., cochlear implant) stimulation is used. Another option that now exists is a hybrid device that makes use of both hearing aid and cochlear implant technology within the same unit. Such a device can now also be used on individuals who have severe high-frequency hearing loss that cannot be addressed with hearing aids. The cochlear implant component of the device is used to address the high-frequency hearing loss, and the hearing aid component provides amplification to those frequencies where hearing is less impaired.

Cochlear Implants in Children

According to the FDA (2022) guidelines, cochlear implants are considered for children who are (1) 9 months of age and older, (2) have hearing loss that is bilaterally profound for children who are 9 months to 24 months, (3) have hearing loss that is bilaterally severe to profound for children age 24 months and older, (4) have a profound hearing loss in one ear (i.e., single-sided deafness) or asymmetrical hearing losses for children who are 5 years and older, and (5) receive minimal benefit from appropriately fitted hearing aids. Children who would typically not be candidates for this procedure are those who (1) are not healthy enough for the surgery, (2) have structural changes to the cochlea that would prevent implantation, (3) have a history of chronic middle ear pathology, and (4) have insufficient psychosocial support.

The FDA's decision to reduce both the age at which a child can obtain a cochlear implant and the degree of hearing loss that is required to be considered is consistent with research that shows that the auditory centers of the brain do not develop in the typical manner if deprived of sound. This then supports efforts to provide appropriate intervention for children as early as possible. Also, as noted previously, research supports a relationship between the age of intervention and later speech and oral language performance.

Before cochlear implants were available to children with severe to profound degrees of hearing loss, they were wearing hearing aids that, in many cases, were not providing adequate access to speech and language. Lieu and colleagues (2020) report that since implants, many of these children have been able to achieve age-appropriate expressive and receptive language skills by the time they begin school. Sharma and colleagues (2020) noted that for children whose hearing loss is profound, cochlear implantation is required if the goal is to hear and to develop speech understanding. Some of these children achieve hearing abilities and language similar to normally hearing children and many are mainstreamed in school. These outcomes were rarely possible with traditional hearing aids.

There is a lack of agreement in the literature regarding what is the optimum lowest age that a child should receive a cochlear implant. In other words, by what age would the benefit of the implants be most positive? Although no clear optimum age for implantation has been identified, there does appear to be some agreement that implantation prior to 12 months results in better outcomes in language and speech (Karltop et al., 2020).

Earlier in the chapter we discussed ANSD, which is characterized by good OAE results with absent or abnormal ABR findings, reflecting deficits somewhere at the level of the inner hair cells or fibers of the VIII. According to Berlin et al. (2010), 85% of these clients reported that hearing aids were of limited or no benefit to them. In contrast, 85% of cochlear implant recipients reported improvements in speech comprehension and language. DeSiati (2020) suggests that losses greater than moderate in those diagnosed with ANSD will often require cochlear implantation, possibly because hearing aids do not address the inconsistent transmission of the signal to the brain (i.e., dys-synchrony) that is characteristic of ANSD.

One of the primary issues related to ANSD is that the diagnosis is often not made in a timely manner because these children typically pass their newborn hearing screening. This delays initiation of the appropriate treatment plan. This is why it is important for parents to continue monitoring their child's responses to sound and their language development and have further testing done if concerns exist. Passing a newborn hearing screening does not mean that hearing is normal or that hearing loss cannot develop later in the child's life.

Demers and colleagues (2019) classify the various communication intervention approaches for children diagnosed with severe to profound hearing loss as follows:

1. Oral communication methods
   a. Auditory–verbal therapy, which focuses on access to speech sounds and processing auditory signals
   b. Auditory–oral approach, where speech sounds are a focus, along with lip and facial cues and gestures.
2. Total communication, which is a broad approach that attempts to integrate speech, lip and facial cues, gestures, and some signs.
3. Bilingual–bicultural, which attempts to promote a bilingual communicator using sign language as the first language and oral language is taught second to support reading and writing skills
4. Sign language, which involves exclusive use of some form of sign

Because the overwhelming majority of children born with severe to profound hearing loss have two hearing parents, combined with the availability of early identification and early intervention using cochlear implants, the commonly chosen approach is oral communication (Binos, 2021). Although it is not yet possible to establish cause-effect, Demers et al. (2019) found that better auditory, speech and expressive language skills appeared to be associated with oral communication methods for children with severe to profound hearing loss.

It is important to remember that, despite great progress in reducing the impact of their hearing loss, children who have significant losses often have persistent communication challenges. Nittrouer and colleagues (2018) found that although clear progress was made on grammar and vocabulary skills in a group of children with cochlear implants studied over a 4-year period, considerable deficits were still noted in the students' ability to process the sounds and syllables that make up words at sixth grade. This skill is crucial to literacy and suggests that children with significant hearing loss often need long-term educational support, even if using appropriate technology.

Mauldin (2019) interviewed 11 parents whose children had received a cochlear implant and had auditory training but were not able to achieve the goal of using spoken language as their primary communication mode. One of the themes generated from the parents was a tendency for professionals to believe that success with the cochlear implant and related therapy was possible for all children as long as parents persisted in their efforts to provide therapy and work with their child on their speech. Parents expressed concern about the considerable time, money, and effort this required. One parent reported that their child experienced loneliness and isolation due to his inability to communicate with others at school. When his parents enrolled him in a school that used sign language, he learned it quickly, connected with others, and regained his social-emotional health. It is important for us all to remember that what works for many may not work for all and a successful outcome should be defined by the impact on the client and not on the expectations of the professionals.

CASE STUDY   **Terrence** *(continued)*

Intervention

After a trial period of several months using powerful behind-the-ear hearing aids in each ear, Terrence's parents chose to have their child evaluated for bilateral cochlear implants. Terrence and his parents met all of the criteria and imaging studies did not reveal any abnormalities that would suggest that the implant would not be fully functional. He was implanted at the age of 9 months and once the device was activated and programmed to his needs, he was enrolled in an aural habilitation program with an SLP. This program began with work on sound awareness and then moved to sound discrimination and comprehension. It made use of both drill-type activities as well as more informal work. The parents chose an auditory–oral approach for their child so the program focused on speech sounds but Terrence was also provided with lip and facial cues as well as gestures.

Cochlear Implants in Adults

Boisvert and colleagues (2020) summarized the impact of cochlear implants in one ear in adults and found that 82% of the adults who had hearing loss after the development of language (postlingual) and 53% of those whose hearing loss occurred prior to the development of language (prelingual) improved their ability to understand words by at least 15 points. The researchers also found that 5–8% of the recipients received poorer speech understanding after receiving the implant. Having a prelingual hearing loss or certain types of auditory tumors decreased the chances of success with the implant.

Hearing Assistive Technology/Assistive Listening Devices

Although hearing aids and cochlear implants provide benefits in many situations, clients often experience difficulty in specific environments or specific situations where their hearing aids or cochlear implants are less helpful. For example, people who receive considerable benefit from their hearing aids regularly report that they need more help when they are communicating in high levels of background noise or when they are situated at a significant distance from the person they want to hear. Another example is a client who hears speech very well except when talking on the phone. Use of various assistive devices can be helpful in overcoming these problems, collectively referred to as *hearing assistive technology (HAT)*.

One of the principles behind assistive devices is to position the microphone of the device close to the sound source. For example, an older person sitting in a noisy dining room in a nursing home where she lives can place a microphone at the center of the table so that the intensity of the speech of her conversation partners will be increased more than the unwanted noise in the background. Similarly, a person who still can't hear the television well even with his hearing aids can attach a small microphone to the TV and place receivers in his ears. The TV signal is then sent directly to the receivers in his ears so he can hear it without the need to have the TV volume increased. Although some assistive devices are still "wired," meaning that the signal is carried to the listener by a wire, many use wireless technology in which the signal is carried by some other means, such as a radio signal. In addition, often the signal can be delivered directly to the listener's hearing aids or cochlear implant.

One type of assistive device that is very popular, particularly in educational settings, is a personal **FM system**. Such a device operates on the same principle as conventional FM radio. The talker speaks into a lapel or headset microphone attached to a small body-worn transmitter that "broadcasts" on a frequency or channel. The listener receives the FM signal through a receiver tuned to the same FM radio frequency as the transmitter. In cases in which the person uses a hearing aid or cochlear implant, this receiver can be plugged directly into the hearing instrument.

Sound field amplification is similar to a personal FM, except that instead of broadcasting the signal to individual receivers, the signal is sent to loudspeakers placed around the room. With sound field systems, all students in a room can benefit from the device, including those with fluctuating hearing loss due to otitis media, those who have attending issues, and those with language impairments.

A number of other assistive devices are available for use with telephone listening. Many clients purchase amplified telephones so that they can adjust the volume of the incoming voice to meet their hearing needs. In recent years, the availability of e-mail, text messaging, synchronous chat, and videoconferencing have been very helpful for those who have difficulty using the phone. Captioning has recently become available for phone use (Figure 12.18). The telephone of the listener includes a small screen where the talker's message is displayed in written form. Shaw (2012) reports that engineers at the University of Washington have developed a new cell phone program called MobilASL that is able to broadcast communication between ASL signers. When available, the program will be able to be used "on any 3G phone and can be integrated into any mobile device that has a camera on the screen side" (p. 22).

FIGURE 12.18 **A caption telephone.**

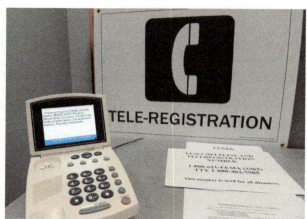

© NB/FEMA/Alamy Stock Photo

Assistive devices are also helpful for individuals who want to be alerted to sounds occurring from a distance. For example, a new parent who is concerned that even with hearing aids on they might not hear their crying infant from another room can use a system that will alert them when the baby is crying by activating a flashing light. Such devices are available to visually alert a person to a ringing phone, an alarm clock, and a smoke detector. Most of these assistive listening devices are not expensive but can make a considerable difference when people with hearing loss are communicating in noisy or dynamic environments. For a summary of commonly used communication strategies and rationales for why they are helpful, please refer to Table 12.5.

Before leaving this topic of assistive technology and devices, brief mention should be made of the term *connectivity*. On a basic level, this can refer to allowing a person who wears hearing aids to wirelessly access auditory information from a device such as a television, telephone, or computer directly into the aids. More broadly, it refers to being connected not only with other devices but also with other people in ways that were not possible in the past due to hearing loss. AAA (n.d.) notes the value of Bluetooth wireless connectivity, which allows connections between hearing aids and phones, computers, and music and video players, for examples.

Treatment and Management of (Central) Auditory Processing Disorders

Regardless of whether an audiologist accepts the view of central auditory processing described by ASHA and AAA, we do know that there are individuals who have normal peripheral hearing and difficulty understanding speech under certain difficult conditions. These conditions could involve hearing in noisy or reverberant environments as well as understanding rapid speech or speech that is presented with an accent, for example. It is the responsibility of the audiologist and SLP to attempt to help such people.

ASHA and AAA recommend that three broad areas of intervention be used in attempting to support these individuals. These areas include modifying the environment, teaching compensatory strategies, and providing direct auditory therapy.

TABLE 12.5

Rationale for Common Communication Strategies for Individuals Who Have Hearing Loss

Communication Strategy	Rationale
Reduce the distance between yourself and the person with whom you are speaking.	As sound travels it decreases in intensity, so it makes good sense to be sure that the distance between the speaker and the listener is reduced. In addition, high-frequency sounds cannot travel as far as low-frequency sounds, and many people with hearing loss have greater hearing loss in the high frequencies. Finally, most hearing aids become less effective when sound is coming from more than 4 to 6 feet away.
Use the visual modality.	Most communicators gain at least some information by watching the face and body gestures of the person with whom they are speaking. For listeners, this means that they should be attending to these nonverbal cues, and for speakers, it means that they should not be speaking with their hand in front of their face or while chewing food. Other examples of the great value of the visual modality include the use of texting and e-mail by people with hearing loss.
Reduce background noise.	One of the most common concerns expressed by individuals who have hearing loss is that they have difficulty following conversations when in a noisy or crowded environment. This most likely occurs because noise tends to cover over or "mask" important speech sounds that the listener is relying upon to understand the message. In addition, hearing in background noise requires greater attention and memory skills. Many people with hearing loss choose their social activities and the location of these activities based on the noise levels in the particular environment. For example, it would be particularly difficult for a person with a significant hearing loss to follow conversation with friends at a bowling alley, even if wearing effective hearing aids.
Use context clues.	If you are speaking with a person who has hearing loss and you begin your conversation by saying, "I'd like to talk to you about our vacation plans," you have provided that person with context. The value of this for the listener is that they now know that the vocabulary that you will be using will be related to the topic of vacation. This increases the listener's ability to predict some of what you might say and fill in some information that may be missed based on their knowledge of the topic. Another example of using context is the employee who reviews the agenda before the meeting begins. By familiarizing herself with the focus of the meeting, she can better follow the conversation even if she does not hear all of it.
Use assistive devices.	As discussed in this chapter, there are a variety of assistive listening devices that can allow individuals with hearing loss to have access to information that may be difficult to deliver using hearing aids alone. One of the problems that arises when audiologists recommend assistive devices is that some individuals with hearing loss believe that hearing aids alone (which typically are costly and not covered by insurance) should meet all of their hearing needs. Despite the additional expense involved in purchasing assistive devices, research is clear that such devices can sometimes reduce the challenges imposed by hearing loss in ways that hearing aids cannot.
Communicate your needs to your communication partners.	It is important that individuals who have hearing loss be proactive in providing to their communication partners specific suggestions that will facilitate their understanding of the spoken message. The suggestions could be related to the manner in which the partner is speaking (e.g., "Please slow down," "Please don't speak when chewing") or related to the environment ("Can we move to a quieter location?", "Please do not speak to me from another room").

Environmental accommodations refer to changes we can make to the listening environment that will improve a listener's ability to receive auditory/verbal information clearly. Some examples of environmental accommodations include adding carpeting or drapes to a classroom in an effort to reduce noise and reverberation, seating the individual closer to the sound source, fitting the individual with a personal FM or sound field system, or providing written notes to supplement verbal information. Accommodations may also include instructional techniques such as speaking clearly at a moderate rate, providing clear and concise directions, using familiar vocabulary and age-appropriate sentence structure, breaking multistep directions into smaller segments, and use of hands-on activities that include visual supports.

Work on compensatory strategies is designed to strengthen other broader cognitive areas, such as attention and language. This could include work on using memory and organizational techniques, using linguistic and contextual cues, and developing problem-solving strategies.

Finally, direct therapy consists of intensive auditory training, designed to attempt to strengthen the specific auditory deficits identified during the assessment. Although some authorities believe that this formal training of specific deficit areas has great potential, currently there is a lack of evidence that such training alone can result in changes in the functional communication abilities of students who have CAPD. For this reason, many of the recommendations made by audiologists focus on improving the listening environment and building other cognitive areas.

One final point should be made about CAPD. The role of an SLP in working with children who have or are suspected of having a listening or processing disorder is critical because students' challenges frequently show up at school where complex messages need to be understood and listening environments tend to be poor. In addition, even if the auditory processing diagnosis is valid and does apply to a student, one of the primary methods of supporting their listening and learning will be by increasing their language competence. For example, increasing their vocabulary and understanding of sentence structure will decrease the likelihood that they will experience communication breakdowns. In an article addressing students diagnosed with CAPD disorders, Kamhi (2011) states that our approach to helping these students should be the same as that used with students who have language and learning disabilities. In addition, thorough testing of these students' speech, language, and literacy skills is urged, including higher-level language abilities such as problem solving and inferencing. In addition, Kamhi states that testing should be completed by the psychologist in order to assess areas of working memory and attention and to identify undiagnosed learning issues.

REFLECTION QUESTION 12.3

How might the recommendations that we might make for a person with a hearing loss be similar to those that we might make for a person with unexplained listening deficits?

Box 12.1 summarizes some of the evidence-based research that validates the exciting progress being made in audiology for the benefit of children and adults with hearing and balance difficulties.

> ### BOX 12.1   Evidence-Based Practice in Audiology
>
> **Telepractice**
>
> Studies of the effectiveness of telepractice to deliver early intervention to families of children with hearing loss revealed positive impressions of remote service delivery in nearly 80% of the studies (McCarthy et al., 2018).
>
> Hughes and colleagues (2018) found that hearing testing results of young children with significant hearing loss using telepractice technology were not statistically different from data obtained using in-person methods.
>
> **Cochlear Implants**
>
> Research suggests that although the risk of surgical complications during or following cochlear implantation is greater for children, the risk level is still very low and within national standards established for surgeries (Karltop et al., 2020).
>
> Myers and Nicholson's (2021) review of research suggests that "children with ANSD and cochlear implants can perform equally as well as children with permanent sensorineural hearing loss and cochlear implants on speech, language and auditory behavioral outcomes" (p. 786). The researchers add that both early diagnosis and intervention can increase the chance of positive outcomes of these important skills in the future.
>
> Goudey and colleagues (2021) identified the following factors as potentially reducing the benefit from the cochlear implant: (1) longer periods of hearing loss prior to implantation, (2) hearing that was present before the development of language (prelingual loss), and (3) poorer hearing before implantation.
>
> Binos and colleagues (2021) review of the effectiveness of Auditory Verbal Therapy on language development in children who have cochlear implants led them to conclude that AVT caused statistically significant improvements in auditory comprehension and expressive language.
>
> **Hidden Hearing Loss**
>
> Research by Resnick and Polley (2021) provides some preliminary evidence suggesting that hidden hearing loss may be due to the presence of internal noise at the highest levels of the brain that is triggered by damage or degeneration to cochlear/neural structures.
>
> **Medical Solutions to Hair Cell Loss**
>
> Foster and colleagues (2022) suggest that over the next decade great progress will be made in addressing hearing losses that presently require the use of hearing aids. This is based on greater understanding of the types of drugs that can address loss of cochlear hair cells, improvements in the way these drugs can be delivered to the inner ear, and developments in gene therapy.

Summary

The profession of audiology is a diverse field that offers opportunities to work with many populations in a wide variety of settings. An audiologist has the responsibility to assess auditory and vestibular function and to provide aural (audiological) habilitation/rehabilitation services. Audiologists regularly collaborate with other professionals on behalf of their clients. A hearing loss is caused by an interruption at one or more points along the auditory pathway from the outer ear to the brain and can have a very significant negative impact on children and adults, not just on their ability to hear but on a wide range of communication, cognitive, and social skills The three types of hearing loss that affect the peripheral auditory system are conductive, sensorineural, and mixed. Audiologists are also concerned with problems affecting the central auditory system, including the auditory areas of the brainstem and brain. Problems along these pathways generally result in challenges in using and interpreting auditory information efficiently and effectively. Research suggests that the ability to process incoming information is impacted by other factors, including language, attention, and memory.

The degree of hearing loss that a person has is measured in decibels. Individuals with hearing loss in the slight/mild to moderately severe range are often referred to as hard of hearing or hearing impaired and depend as much as possible on the use of residual hearing for communication. For people with profound hearing loss, often referred to as deafness, the auditory system provides little or no access to sound without proper amplification.

When evaluating the auditory system, audiologists rely on both behavioral and nonbehavioral measures. They administer a battery of tests to identify the presence of a hearing loss, determine its type, quantify its degree, and assess its impact on communication. Aural (audiological) habilitation/rehabilitation refers to the devices, services, and procedures that are designed to minimize and resolve communication difficulties presented by a hearing loss. Both children and adults have been helped with hearing aids and for those individuals with severe to profound hearing loss, cochlear implants have been very effective. Aural habilitation refers to therapies that are used primarily with children to teach missing communication skills, and aural rehabilitation refers to services provided to those who have lost their hearing later in life, after some degree of spoken communication has been established. The focus of aural rehabilitation is to help the person recover lost skills and to use compensatory strategies effectively. Areas typically considered in creating an individual aural rehabilitation program are the evaluation and fitting of amplification and hearing assistive technology, auditory training, communication strategy training, and determination of an appropriate mode of communication. Research now indicates that due to our increased knowledge about hearing loss and intervention methods, combined with advances in technology, individuals of all ages, degrees of hearing loss, and communication preferences can successfully participate in the essential act of communication.

Epilogue   Case Study: Terrence

One year after the cochlear implant was activated, we find Terrence discriminating not only environmental sounds but also some speech sounds. He has developed a receptive vocabulary that is highly related to his everyday routines, including feeding, sleeping, playing, and bath time. In addition, expressively he can say *mama*, *dada, ball no,* and *bye.*

Reflections   from a Veterans' Hospital Audiologist: Diane Flynn, AuD

1. *Did you always want to be an audiologist or did you consider other careers?*
   After I completed my associate's degree and was thinking about what path I wanted to take for my bachelor's degree, I had to decide among several areas that were appealing to me, including psychology, English, and communication disorders. I took one class in each of them and ended up choosing to pursue a degree in communication disorders.

2. *What do you think led you to make that choice?*
   I think it was a combination of factors. I wanted to help people and growing up I knew a girl who was diagnosed with deafness who lived in my neighborhood. I took a particular interest in her situation.

3. *In your audiology program were there any particular courses that you really enjoyed or that really had an impact on how you practice?*
   The "hands-on" courses were not only my favorites but also most useful to me. I find that in my daily work as an audiologist I use many of the techniques and strategies that I learned in those courses. Also, I have always liked equipment and technology so those courses were very engaging for me.

4. *How do you spend most of your time on a typical day and what parts are most rewarding?*
   Certainly, a large part of the day is spent doing hearing testing and hearing aid fittings. Fitting people with hearing aids has always been rewarding to me. People often do not realize how good hearing aids are now and how much they have been missing. Hearing aids really do change their quality of life.

   I also have been very involved in providing service to my patients through the Progressive Tinnitus Management Program. This program was developed at the National Center for Rehabilitative Auditory Research through research grants provided by the Department of Veterans Affairs Rehabilitation Research and Development Service and has really had a positive impact on the veterans who believed that there was no hope of getting relief from their tinnitus. This is a stepped-care program that involves coordinated care between audiology and behavioral health. Delivering this program is one of most rewarding parts of my work. I have other ideas that I hope to implement in the future that address patient challenges from a whole health perspective.

5. *What would you like to say to students studying communication disorders who may want to become audiologists?*
   I would highlight how important it is to get a good foundation of knowledge and then, as you gain experience, combine it with your own insights and creativity. I think those of us who are in the helping professions have to be willing to listen to our patients, be flexible, and often "think outside the box" in order to help them.

Suggested Readings/Sources

DeBonis, D., & Donohue, C. (2020). *Survey of audiology: Fundamentals for audiologists and health professionals.* 3rd ed. NJ: Slack Incorporated.

Demers, D., & Bergeron, F. (2019). Effectiveness of rehabilitation approaches proposed to children with severe-to-profound prelinguistic deafness on the development of auditory, speech, and language skills: A systematic review. *Journal of Speech Language Hearing Research, 62*(11), 4196–4230.

Lieu, J., Kenna, M., Anne, S., & Davidson, L. (2020). Hearing loss in children: A review. *Journal of the American Medical Association, 324*(21), 2195–2205.

Meinzen-Deer, J., Wiley, S., & Choo, D. (2011). Impact of early intervention on expressive and receptive language development among young children with permanent hearing loss. *American Annals of the Deaf, 155*(5), 580–591.

Moore, D., Zabay, O., & Ferguson, M. (2020). Minimal and mild hearing loss in children: Association with auditory perception, cognition, and communication problems. *Ear and Hearing, 41*(4), 720–732.

13 Augmentative and Alternative Communication

Kelly Fagan, MS, CCC-SLP

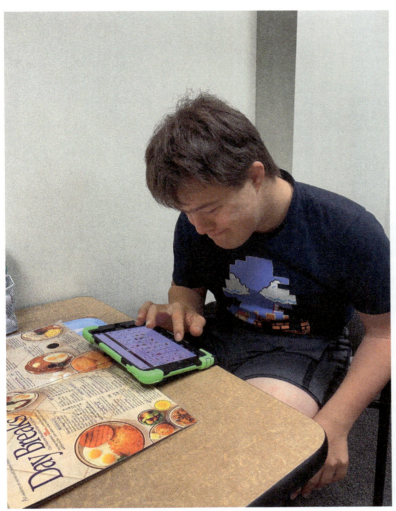

© Kelly Fagan

Learning Objectives

When you have finished this chapter, you should be able to:

13.1 Define augmentative and alternative communication (AAC).

13.2 Explain how interprofessional practice and involvement of communication partners are critical for success.

13.3 Describe various types of aided and unaided AAC systems, access methods, and AAC output and input.

13.4 Dispel myths surrounding AAC.

13.5 Explain how an AAC assessment is dynamic, collaborative, and ongoing.

13.6 Apply communicative competencies to intervention practices with individuals with complex communication needs and their communication partners.

13.7 Describe how intervention can foster language development and independence through use of supportive prompt hierarchies, adaptive play skills, focused and functional intervention, and development of literacy skills.

13.8 Understand how the Communication Bill of Rights guides advocacy and goals for AAC.

❝ What's your why?

My first question to you, as you sit taking this introductory course, is "What's your why?" Why are you here? Why are you taking this course? If you want to be a speech-language pathologist (SLP), why does it appeal to you?

It is likely you have been drawn to the helping professions. Maybe you've considered nursing, physical therapy, occupational therapy, or teaching. Maybe you've decided to change professions. You may have had a family member who needed intervention to help them communicate. You've had some experience that has brought you to be curious about the field of speech-language pathology. I am glad you are here. The world needs people who are passionate and can strive to learn how to help others. Speech-language pathology is challenging, but very rewarding. There are so many people in the world of all ages that need our help.

Ikigai is a Japanese concept that means "reason for being" (Garcia & Miralles, 2017) (Figure 13.1). As you see in the illustration, Ikigai is in the center of overlapping ideas of what the world needs, what you love, what you are good at, and what you can be paid for. As you take college classes and explore options for majors, you might reflect on this idea of what's your reason for being, what's your why? For some, the field of speech-language pathology might be the center of what might fulfill you in your professional life.

This chapter highlights my "why." It is what I love and am passionate about, it is what the world needs, I get paid to do what I love, and it is what I strive to be good at for my clients and my students. Working with individuals with complex communication needs and training clinicians to help these individuals is my passion, mission, profession, and vocation. I see their capabilities and strive to help them overcome the hurdles to connect with those around them. I have learned something from every one of the families and clients I have served. I celebrate every milestone with them and strive to open their worlds to make connections and help them develop relationships.

FIGURE 13.1 Ikigai.

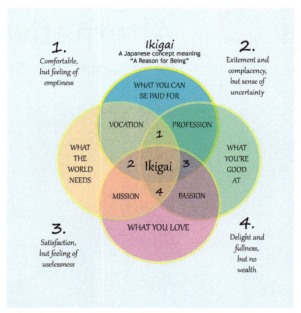

(Image created by Daniel Fagan, based on Garcia and Miralles [2017].)

As you read and study these pages, I hope it helps you find your "why?" and define your Ikigai.

I am passionate about the field of speech-language pathology primarily because of the people and families I have served. Augmentative and alternative communication has opened the doors for developing language, connections with others, and allows an individual to have their personalities shine through. I see the capabilities and am always excited by the breakthroughs that happen when someone is given the power to communicate. As you read this chapter, I introduce you to people I have met that have benefited from the use of augmentative and alternative communication.

—*Kelly Fagan*

Defining Augmentative and Alternative Communication (AAC)

Learning Objective 13.1 Define augmentative and alternative communication (AAC).

Previous chapters have highlighted a particular communication disorder and its field of research. AAC is not a disorder; rather, it is the many ways to address the disorders that might affect a person's ability to communicate. The American

Speech-Language-Hearing Association (ASHA; 2005a) defines AAC in terms of the area of practice in our profession as follows:

> *Augmentative and alternative communication* (AAC) refers to an area of research, clinical, and educational practice. AAC involves attempts to study and when necessary, compensate for temporary or permanent impairments, activity limitations, and participation restrictions of individuals with severe disorders of speech-language production and/or compensation, including spoken and written modes of communication.

ASHA also states the following on its website in response to the question "What is AAC?":

> *Augmentative and alternative communication* (AAC) includes all forms of communication (other than oral speech) that are used to express thoughts, needs, wants, and ideas. We all use AAC when we make facial expressions or gestures, use symbols or pictures, or write. (www.asha.org)

To state it simply: AAC means all of the ways someone communicates besides talking. (ASHA, 2022)

This definition recognizes that communication takes place in many different forms. A *multimodal* approach to communication incorporates all the different ways a person can communicate vocalizations, gestures, facial expressions, sign language, writing, texting, or using a symbol to convey meaning. Each of us uses *multimodal communication* every day, be it a facial expression that might mean you did not understand something, sending an email, or texting an emoji to a friend, and all can convey meaning and all are ways we use AAC. Multimodal communication can be visually based (text, writing, sign, symbols, facial expressions), auditory based (vocalizations, speech), tactile based (touch, sensory objects, Braille), or gestural (body movements, body language, head nods). Multimodal communication allows for all forms of communication including AAC.

Use of the term *augmentative* refers to situations in which a system of communication is needed to supplement existing speech. Speech might be present but ineffective so an individual might need to augment or supplement that ability with another means of communicating.

An *alternative* means of communication would be necessary in situations where natural speech may be nonfunctional or not present. Elsahar et al. (2019) described three classes of AAC users: *alternative-language* users; *augmentative-language* users, who may have difficulties in varying degrees in both receptive and expressive language; and *temporary* users, who might only need AAC for a limited period of time.

When students and others think about the field of AAC, they often just think about the devices or technology related to AAC—*speech-generating devices* (SGDs); however the focus of the field is about the people—individuals with *complex communication needs (CCN)* who require a system of communication to help them express themselves.

AAC is about helping the people who have a permanent or temporary condition that is hindering their ability to connect with others. A condition that creates a barrier that needs to be bridged by an augmentative or alternative means, through development of a multimodal system of communication.

Again, AAC is not about the things or devices, it's about the people, so let's learn first about the people involved in AAC, the individuals with complex communication needs, their families and communication partners, and the teams of professionals that serve them.

In referring to those with the need for AAC, we would refer to them as an individual with *complex communication needs*. This term is used rather than defining someone as "nonverbal" because that would assume the individual cannot produce vocalizations, which is not always an accurate representation of their capabilities.

Who Can Benefit from the Use of AAC?

Who are the people that can benefit from AAC? A wide range of people across the age span who have expressive language needs can benefit from AAC. In reviewing the chapters of this book, many of the people you already learned about with conditions that lead to difficulties with receptive or expressive language could benefit from AAC.

Individuals with language disorders (discussed in Chapter 4); poor intelligibility/speech sound disorders (Chapter 5); acquired conditions such as traumatic brain injury, stroke, or progressive neurological conditions (Chapter 7); temporary loss of voice (Chapter 9); and people with sensory/perceptual differences including those who are blind, Deaf, or hard of hearing. (Chapter 12) could benefit from a multimodal system of communication that includes AAC.

In thinking about who could benefit from AAC, consider the need for AAC might be *temporary* or permanent depending on the nature of the condition impacting the individual. Someone on vocal rest following surgery might need a temporary means of communicating and might use a text-to-speech application. A child with Down syndrome might learn language skills through a combination of unaided (sign language, head nods, gestures) and aided AAC (speech output device). Individuals across the lifespan can have conditions that cause them to have limited abilities to communicate and require AAC to help.

Those born with **congenital** conditions, such as autism spectrum disorders, Down syndrome, other genetic disorders, or developmental disabilities might require AAC approaches as part of their **habilitation** to build language skills and learn to communicate. Those with **acquired** conditions, such as a traumatic brain injury, stroke, or a degenerative disease like ALS, who may have lost the ability to communicate may have AAC intervention as part of their **rehabilitation** (Table 13.1). AAC can be of significant importance for those who due to an acquired condition like **locked-in syndrome** retain full consciousness but do not have the voluntary ability to move any muscles but their eyes.

TABLE 13.1

Conditions That Can Benefit from Use of AAC

Congenital conditions/developmental	Acquired conditions	Temporary conditions
Developmental delays or genetic syndromes	Traumatic brain injury	Intubated patient in hospital
Autism spectrum disorder	Stroke	Vocal rest/temporary loss of voice
Down syndrome	Amyotrophic lateral sclerosis	
Cerebral palsy	Alzheimer disease	
Dual sensory impairments—deaf-blind	Brainstem stroke	
Childhood apraxia of speech	Locked-in syndrome	

It is estimated that 5 million Americans and over 97 million people worldwide cannot meet their daily communication needs using natural speech (Beukleman & Light, 2020). To visualize what that means, 5 million people would be more than the entire population of the city of Los Angeles or the country of Ireland.

According to ASHA's National Joint Committee for the Communication Needs of Persons with Severe Disabilities (2021), "[B]y recent estimates, well over 2 million persons who present with significant expressive language impairment use AAC." Of concern is the gap between those who could benefit from AAC and those who are currently using AAC.

Early access to AAC can be vital for children to develop language skills and critical for adults with degenerating conditions to be able to utilize **voice banking** in time to record their own voice for their device.

One way to reach more of the people who need AAC is to ensure students in the field of communication sciences and disorders and SLPs possess the competencies to participate in collaborative teams to assess and treat those with CCN across the lifespan. This is why I do what I do, to help reach those people who need us most. As you read and study this chapter, think about the role you are preparing for and the lives that would be impacted.

CASE STUDY   Naveen

Naveen is a 6-year-old boy with Angelman syndrome, a genetic disorder that causes delays in development, possible seizures, limited or no speech, and poor balance. He has an engaging smile and lives at home with his older sister and his parents. The language of the home is Bengali.

When Naveen was between the ages of 2 and 3 years old, his parents bought a tablet and purchased a core vocabulary category-based communication app to give him a means to communicate. His mother had connected on social media with other parents of children with Angelman syndrome and had purchased the iPad and app after reading about other families using communication apps with their children.

Naveen's mother stated to the SLP that they were told by the teacher to "only speak English" to Naveen at home. She is the primary person in the home who works with him to use his communication boards; she prompts him and uses hand over hand to help him find the keys to press. Naveen was beginning to learn some modified signs including clapping his hands together for "more," waving his hand up and down as a modified sign for "yes," and tugging on his ear for "music." Due to fine motor difficulties, Naveen's ability to express

himself through sign is limited. He vocalizes vowel approximations and given models can approximate a series of "buh-buh-buh" in imitation but is unable to form true words.

Naveen has limited play skills and will throw items when he is done with them or to indicate refusal of an activity, including his device; the family has replaced his iPad twice. Naveen loves music, and during his initial evaluation he independently navigated to his preferred songs and smiled and laughed as the clinicians sang to him.

As you read this chapter, think about:

- The importance of communication partners and a team approach in the successful implementation of an AAC system
- How the assessment and treatment plan for current and future needs might change over time
- How suggestions made by the teacher to limit the home language and "only speak English" limits his ability for language development and does not demonstrate cultural competence.
- How to foster independence and the generation of spontaneous novel utterances that will lead to relationship building with a wide range of communication partners

Explain how a system of multimodal communication can benefit those with congenital and acquired communication impairments.

Interprofessional team-based assessment and intervention is critical for successful intervention and implementation of AAC with individuals with complex communication needs. A collaborative team-based model is essential.

Interprofessional Practice and the Importance of Communication Partners

Learning Objective 13.2 Explain how interprofessional practice and involvement of communication partners are critical for success.

In assessing and providing interventions for people with complex communication needs, the focus should be on individuals' needs and capabilities and how to connect them with their everyday *communication partners*. It is important to include those communication partners in the assessment and intervention process as part of the team with the individual. Again, AAC is about people developing their ability to interact and build relationships with others and creating a system of effective communication much more than it is about a particular device or piece of technology.

Given the complex nature and needs of those who can benefit from AAC, the establishment of a collaborative team of professionals, working together with the individual and their families insures positive outcomes (ASHA, 2022). ASHA has emphasized the importance of collaboration in our scope of practice and the need for interprofessional education and interprofessional practice. Building an effective team takes time, communication, and establishment of mutual respect, applying resources and principles that can lead to enhanced team functioning, and ultimately leads to improved patient outcomes (Miller et al., 2018).

The teams working with an individual with complex communication needs could have a significant number of people involved, each with their own areas of expertise, skills, and knowledge. It is important to coordinate care within these teams for the best outcomes, rather than each member doing their part without communication and collaboration with others.

One way for teams to increase their ability to provide interdisciplinary practice is to have a shared way to communicate, assess, and create goals. The World Health Organization's (2001) International Classification of Functioning, Disability and Health (WHO-ICF) was developed to support interprofessional team-based care in health systems throughout the world. The WHO-ICF model has many advantages in its use with those with complex communication needs; studies have demonstrated the importance of training in the WHO-ICF model so health care professionals, including SLPs, can implement it within the services they provide (Zerbeto et al., 2020) (Figure 13.2).

The WHO-ICF can also be utilized to help formulate client-centered goals that consider multiple needs of the client and environmental factors within an interdisciplinary model to foster success (McNeilly, 2018). Huer and Threats (2016) noted the increased need for students and professionals in the field of speech-language pathology to have an understanding of the WHO-ICF in order to assist in empowering those with complex communication needs to have increased participation in our society. The WHO-ICF can help professionals from varied fields share their information and knowledge to create team goals and priorities.

FIGURE 13.2 **WHO-ICF model.**

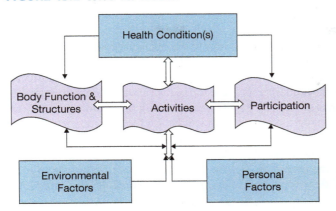

The WHO-ICF checklist can be utilized in organizing interdisciplinary assessment results to form priorities and intervention. The checklist can be found on the WHO-ICF website at www.who.int/publications/m/item/icf-checklist.

CASE STUDY **Naveen** (*continued*)

Naveen has several health conditions that affect his activity and participation. Consider Naveen's diagnosis of Angelman syndrome. Angelman syndrome is a rare genetic neurodevelopmental disorder with characteristics that include movement and balance issues—ataxia, cognitive impairments, receptive and expressive language impairments with limited ability to develop functional speech. However, individuals display positive affect, social engagement, and laughter (Calculator, 2015).

Naveen has many professionals working with him at his school, in his home, and through private outpatient clinics. Each of these professionals evaluates Naveen from their perspective and generates their own priorities and goals. Having the structure

of the WHO-ICF can help organize the team and provide a better understanding of how Naveen's health conditions influence his body functions and structures, activities, and participation. For example, given his health condition, body function, and structures he cannot talk or walk steadily. This limits his ability to participate with others.

If the team examined this information as a collaborate team, they might see that his goal to improve core strength and stability for walking would enable him to self-carry his AAC device, and then he would be able to increase his communication and participation in activities with peers and team members. Teams collaborating together with shared goals can provide better outcomes.

The Importance of Involvement of the Individual and Their Communication Partners

Involvement of the individual with complex communication needs and their families is an essential component of effective assessment and intervention. They should have active involvement in all aspects of assessment and intervention and the decision-making process (Beukleman & Light, 2020). The individual should be the center of the team and have a voice in their intervention goals and priorities.

For successful implementation of AAC systems, one cannot overlook the importance of those around the individual with complex communication needs, including their social circles of support. In fact, ensuring the communication partners are educated and have communicative competence (Light & McNaughton, 2014) in the implementation and use of AAC is critical. The day-to-day communication partners provide the opportunities for communication and will provide the foundation of support for the individual throughout their lifetime.

Pearson eTextbook
Video Example 13.1

There is a need for collaborative teams who are trained in AAC. Parents sometimes feel they are on their own to try to find solutions to their child's severe communication difficulties. Maya's mother explains in this video (Neider, 2018).

www.aac-learning-center.psu.edu/2018/07/19/the-impact-of-early-access-to-aac-dana-nieder/

CASE STUDY **Naveen** *(continued)*

Naveen's primary communication partner initially was his mother. She researched, purchased, and set up the iPad for him to begin communicating. His interaction with his sister was limited, as was his interaction with peers. The people who were paid to provide services to him were the secondary communication partners in Naveen's life and not all of them were trained on how to use AAC. Goals did not include interactions with peers or provide support for those who needed to improve their ability to operate the AAC device or know

how to teach language or literacy skills with AAC. His team was not yet working collaboratively.

When only one or two communication partners are trained within the family or school environment, Naveen is at risk of becoming dependent on them and will be less likely to interact with a wider range of communication partners (Stadsklev, 2017). Others in his home and school environment should be trained to enable them to increase their communicative competencies using AAC.

REFLECTION QUESTION 13.2

Why is collaboration important when working with someone who uses AAC to communicate?

"Alone we can do so little; together we can do so much."
—*Helen Keller*

The successful implementation of a communication system can be impacted greatly if we do not collaborate with the everyday communication partners in the individual's life. If communication partners do not know sign language or are intimidated by use of technology, if they do not realize the importance of positioning or communication strategies, or simply do not charge or take out a device, our efforts ultimately will be less effective.

Now that we have discussed the people involved in AAC, the individual with complex needs, their communication partners, and the collaborative team around them, including those closest to the individual, we can discuss the "things" that encompass the development of an AAC system. It is intentional in this chapter that the people were discussed first along with the foundations of building a team. Now let's look at the various methods we can utilize to help those with complex communication needs.

Types of Augmentative and Alternative Communication

Learning Objective 13.3 Describe various types of aided and unaided AAC systems, access methods, and AAC output and input.

The types of AAC can be categorized into *aided or unaided AAC* (Table 13.2). *Unaided AAC* involves only using your body to communicate. This could include head nods, facial expressions, body language, gestures, voluntary body movements such as finger taps or hand squeezes, vocal approximations, and sign language. Unaided AAC does not involve any external equipment other than a person's body. Unaided AAC can be used in conjunction with aided AAC for a multimodal approach. Including a combination of aided and unaided communication strategies as part of an overall AAC communication system could be beneficial especially in environments when an aided communication system might not be available. *Aided AAC* involves materials or technology that can range from low tech/no tech to high tech devices to aid in providing a means of communication. New high tech technology research on brain-computer interface technology is working toward enabling those who cannot speak to use their brain signals to control their environment and access communication systems (Brumberg et al., 2018).

An individual might also create their own signals or symbols for communication that are "read" or interpreted by communication partners that are familiar with them.

TABLE 13.2
Types of AAC

Unaided	Aided	
No-Tech	**Low-/Light-Tech**	**High-Tech**
• Gestures	• Pictures/drawings	• Single-message devices and recordable/digitized devices
• Body language	• Objects/partial objects	• AAC software or apps for communication used on a tablet, smartphone, or computer
• Manual signs (ASL, SEE)	• Photographs	• Speech-generating devices, dedicated devices with speech output, robust vocabulary
• Facial expressions	• Alphabet boards	• Direct select, eye gaze, or scanning systems that provide access to communication systems
• Vocalizations	• Writing	• Brain–computer interfaces
• Verbalizations	• Picture communication symbols	
• Body movements, eyeblinks, finger taps, hand squeezes	• Communication boards/books	

An individual without speech or any reliable AAC system might develop their own basic ways to communicate, which are interpreted by those closest to them. These signals might be anything from leading a person to what they want, use of vocalizations and facial expressions, or other behaviors to express confirmation or discontent. For those without a reliable communication system, negative behaviors or expressions of discontent could result in the most immediate attention from others. It is important to recognize as SLPs that these often negative "behaviors" are attempts at communication. We can work with individuals to give them more effective means of expression.

> **CASE STUDY**   **Naveen** (*continued*)
>
> Prior to Naveen's parents' purchasing an iPad and communication app, his attempts at communication included emotional responses, reaching toward people or objects, and facial expressions. His mother often anticipated his needs. When object choice was introduced, he initially reacted with discontent due to his perception that the delay in getting the object immediately was denying him of what he wanted, rather than realizing a choice was being given. For individuals who have had their needs anticipated for them, choice making might be a learning process.

Unaided AAC Communication Systems

Unaided AAC can range from the use of small body movements such as eyeblinks to an entire language system such as American Sign Language. We all use gestures, head nods, body language, and facial expressions to relay meaning. An individual with complex communication needs can use both unaided and aided communication strategies; it does not have to be an either–or situation, there may be certain situations where unaided communication strategies provide an effective means of communication.

Unaided AAC maximizes the capabilities an individual might have in use of their bodies to communicate meaning. Nonverbal means of communication such as head nods, thumbs-up or -down, and high-fives to represent yes and no can be understood culturally by people in the United States to affirm or refuse.

For those with acquired conditions, unaided AAC might be an initial means of communication with those who care for them in a hospital setting. The establishment of a reliable, voluntary, reproducible body movement might establish the first signals to reestablish a connection with those around them. Eyeblinks, finger movements, or hand squeezes may lead to establishment of an initial yes/no response. A person in the intensive care unit of a hospital might be **intubated**, which would limit their ability to produce speech, or could have lost the ability to speak due to a stroke or traumatic brain injury. Initial means of communication might target where that individual demonstrates voluntary movements.

Manual Sign Systems

Sign language is an unaided form of communication. In the United States, American Sign language (ASL) is the language used by the Deaf community. ASL is its own language separate from English in that it has its own distinguished grammar, syntax, semantics, and pragmatics. When working with children and adults who are Deaf, it is important to have an understanding of the Deaf community and culture. (Note that the capital *D* designates a person who identifies culturally as Deaf [ASHA, 2022; Baade, 2022].) ASL varies from spoken English in word order, in which an ASL speaker would introduce the subject or topic first. Use of signs and fingerspelling are paired with facial expressions and body language to convey meaning and can be used to vary meaning much like intonation patterns in spoken English can vary meaning to inflect humor or sarcasm. Early exposure to language is critical for children who are Deaf or hard of hearing (Goldberg, 2020; Hall, 2017; Humphries et al., 2016). ASL and fingerspelling can provide a foundation for language and literacy skills.

Fingerspelling or the manual alphabet is used within ASL and other forms of sign language (Figure 13.3). Handshapes represent letters of the alphabet and can be formed using one hand. Fingerspelling can be a part of a system of communication for those who have the fine motor abilities to form distinct handshapes.

Pearson eTextbook
Video Example 13.2
This video instructs on how to establish a yes/no response in a hospital setting.
https://nucleus.con.ohio-state.edu/media/speacs2/module8/index.html

American Sign Language is its own language with its own rules for word order, word formation, and fundamental features of language. It is separate from spoken English and is the predominant language of the Deaf population in the United States. Just like spoken language, there are varied dialects of ASL in different regional areas (National Association of the Deaf, 2022).

FIGURE 13.3 Fingerspelling.

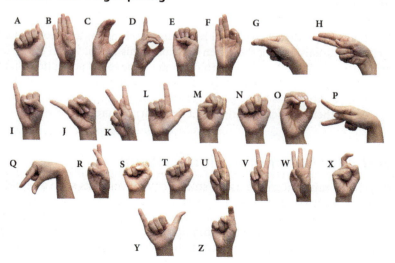

Source: Tushchakorn/Shutterstock.

FIGURE 13.4 Online resources.

> **Online Resources for Fingerspelling Practice**
> Handspell: www.handspeak.com/learn/index.php?id=413
> Fingerspell: http://fingerspell.net/#/
>
> **Online Resources for ASL**
> www.asluniversity.com
> www.signasl.org
> www.handspeak.com/word/asl-eng/

Assessment of motor abilities for unaided means of communication can include assessment of the ability to make or approximate signs.

Other forms of sign language in use in the United States are Signed Exact English (SEE) and tactile signing. Signed Exact English follows spoken English word order, translating spoken English into sign. Fingerspelling is also used in ASL and hand-shapes for beginning letters of words are used in SEE. SEE is not its own language and is not ASL, but it has been utilized in classrooms with children with developmental delays to provide a visual paired with verbal words. Sign language can be utilized by communication partners as **AAC input**, to aid in comprehension, as well as models for **AAC output** or expression. *Tactile signing* is a method of sign language used for people who are Deaf-blind or have dual sensory impairments.

Resources for ASL include online sign language dictionaries and practice for signing and reading fingerspelling (Figure 13.4). Communication partners should not only learn how to sign expressively but should also practice receptive understanding of sign language and fingerspelling.

Sign language can be used with hearing children and children with autism, Down syndrome, or other developmental disabilities to introduce language or to support understanding by supporting spoken language with a visual sign. Introduction of sign language to preverbal infants and toddlers develops responsive relationships between parent and child (Vallotton, 2012) and enables access to develop language skills.

Unaided communication systems can have drawbacks and might not be the best match for every individual. Sign language requires fine motor movements of the hands and individuals with motor limitations might not be able to use sign efficiently or effectively. Another issue with use of unaided modes of communication such as gestures, eyeblinks, and signs is that they rely heavily on the communication partners' ability to understand the meaning or intent of the communication. If those around the individual do not understand a system of eyeblinks or are not fluent in sign language, the message will not be "heard."

CASE STUDY   Naveen *(continued)*

You remember Naveen used some gestures and modified signs to communicate. He used modified signs due to his difficulties performing motor movements. Instead of using the typical sign for music, Naveen tugged on his ear. When individuals have their own modified signs, it is important for everyone around them to understand their unique ways of communicating. A personal custom "dictionary" of modified signs and other signals can be made and included in reports or training materials so staff working with the individual can understand their communication attempts.

Aided AAC Communication Systems

Aided AAC communication systems involve use of items or materials external to the individual to aid in their communication. Aided AAC can vary in the degree of technology used ranging from "no tech" to "low tech," "mid tech," and "high tech." No-tech AAC does not require a power source and could consist of printed paper communication boards with symbols or alphabet, a binder of communication symbols, object-based communication choices, or simply a whiteboard and a pen. No-tech options can also include symbol systems like the Picture Exchange Communication System (PECS; Bondy & Frost, 1994), Pragmatic Organization Dynamic Display (PODD) books (Porter & Cafiero, 2009), or core vocabulary boards. In these systems, individuals use picture symbols that can be contained in binders that can be removed to be exchanged (PECS) or pointed to (PODD and core boards) by an individual or by a communication partner using **partner-assisted scanning** to help make a selection.

Object or picture communication can be useful to provide AAC input to help an individual follow a visual schedule and are helpful in classrooms and work environments. Picture communication can be portable and wearable on a lanyard or around the wrist. No-tech AAC can also be used in environments that might not be tech friendly, like in swimming pools or on playgrounds. Picture communication boards can be laminated and attached to swim accessories like kickboards or can be enlarged to the size of a sign and placed in an accessible place on a playground or other community areas.

Low- to mid-tech AAC would involve materials that might have voice output, light indicators, or print or text output. Examples of low-tech AAC devices could include single message communicators or communication buttons that offer communication output in a series of messages. Low- to mid-tech AAC devices can be battery operated and often have recordable speech output. They usually have limited capabilities for the number of messages that can be conveyed and might offer a variety of grid sizes with multiple levels with *static* pictures that require changing picture symbols manually.

High-tech AAC devices offer *dynamic* picture or text displays with touch screen, switch, or eye gaze access. They can be dedicated devices for communication and environmental control or can be phone or tablet based with communication applications (apps) (Figure 13.5).

Symbolic Representation of Aided Symbols

The symbols used to represent the words and ideas within an aided communication system can have varying degrees of iconicity. **Iconicity** refers to the level that clearly represents the meaning of the symbol. Symbolic representation can range from *iconic* to *transparent* to *opaque*, depending on the clarity of the symbol. An example of iconic symbol representation using an unaided symbol could be demonstrated in the sign for "eat" in which a person signs by bringing their hand to their lips to symbolize eating. A photograph or object to represent an item can be iconic, such as a photo of an apple to represent an apple, which would have clear representation. Nouns are often easily represented with an iconic symbol. Other words such as adjectives, pronouns, verbs, question words, multiple-meaning words, and intangible concepts (love, hate, idea) might not be as easy to represent.

FIGURE 13.5 Continuum of aided AAC technology, with examples of each.

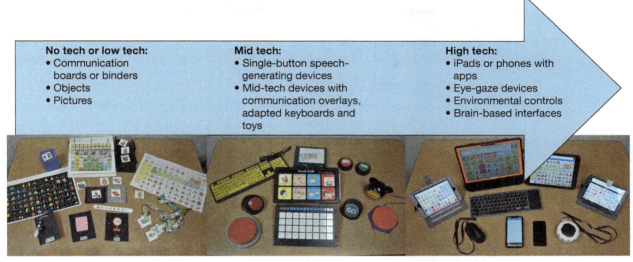

No tech or low tech:
- Communication boards or binders
- Objects
- Pictures

Mid tech:
- Single-button speech-generating devices
- Mid-tech devices with communication overlays, adapted keyboards and toys

High tech:
- iPads or phones with apps
- Eye-gaze devices
- Environmental controls
- Brain-based interfaces

© Kelly Fagan

A symbol might be *transparent* when its meaning is easily guessable, which might include line drawings representing animals or foods or an associated item such as a spoon to represent "eat." Other symbols might be *opaque* when their meaning is not easily interpreted. It is difficult to have iconic symbols for concepts that are not easy to picture. The words *help* or *more* are other examples that might have varied symbolic representation. "Help" has been represented as two hands reaching toward one another, a person helping someone get up from the floor, or a person in water being thrown a life preserver. Given an individual's background and life experience, those symbols might be difficult to interpret.

Written words and print are considered opaque symbols. Opaque symbols can be taught through modeling and practice in meaningful contexts. An individual should not be denied access to a robust vocabulary system based on assumptions of their ability to understand opaque symbols.

I challenge you, as students, to reframe thinking about the capabilities of individuals with complex communication needs. Think about the example of symbolic representation that is used in your everyday lives: You may have many apps on your phones. Their icons might not be very iconic (a circle in a square with a dot for Instagram, a triangle for Google Drive, or a ghostlike figure on a yellow background for Snapchat), but you have learned them by using them. It's likely that with the apps that you use frequently, you've even developed a motor memory for where they are on your phone and can open them based on that motor memory. Therefore, keep in mind that exposure to a robust vocabulary and meaningful practice can enable individuals with complex needs to demonstrate their capabilities even with symbols that are not very iconic. They can learn by doing.

In studies examining the selection and access to vocabulary, Sevick et al. (2018) found only "a modest difference in the ability of school aged children with developmental and language delays to learn arbitrary (opaque) versus iconic symbols when looking at known symbols and there was no differences if the vocabulary was unknown prior to the introduction of the symbols which demonstrates that the iconicity of a symbol may not be a critical factor if a target referent is not yet known." (page 274) Studies have demonstrated that a symbol does not need to be a certain level of iconicity for an individual to learn its meaningful use, which was demonstrated in a study with children as young as 18 months (Namy et al., 2004). With this in mind, let's now look at the types of symbols that can be used in an AAC communication system.

Aided Symbols: Tangible Symbols

Tangible symbols are three-dimensional (3D) objects that can be held in your hand. Sometimes they might be mounted on a surface to allow them to be on display, such as in a **visual schedule** (Figure 13.6). Tangible symbols can be miniature representations of objects (a small toy car), parts of objects or a texture representing an object (a zipper or shoelace), an associated item (key to represent car or go), 3D printed representations of items, or actual objects. Tangible symbols might be part of an overall symbol system for an individual with complex needs and they are very useful for those with vision or dual sensory (deaf-blind) impairments. Individuals with a *cortical visual impairment*, a brain-based visual impairment caused by damage either to the pathways or the vision centers in the brain (Perkins School for the Blind, 2022), might benefit from use of tangible symbols as part of a communication system.

Rowland and Schweigert's (2009) study on tangible symbol systems demonstrated the benefit of the use of tangible symbols with children who are deaf-blind; this study tracked participants for 3 years as they progressed with learning abstract symbol systems and through a multimodal approach that provided the foundation for developing speech. Rowland and Schweigert have made their Tangible Symbols Systems Primer available online (see the additional resources at the end of the chapter for more information). The Perkins School for the Blind also has a number of resources and professional education materials of use of tangible symbols. The Center for Literacy and Disabilities Project Core Program provides free templates and instructions to 3D print tangible symbols at www.project-core .com/3d-symbols/.

FIGURE 13.6 Tactile communication: objects.

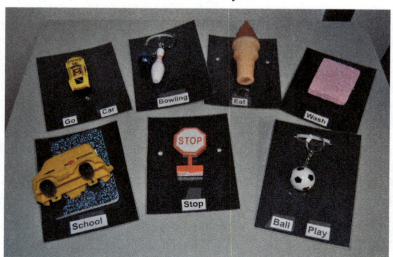

© Kelly Fagan

Aided Symbols: Pictorial Symbols

Picture-based symbols are used to represent words and ideas ranging from no-tech communication boards to high-tech voiced output systems. As discussed above, picture-based systems can have varied iconicity in the symbols they represent. Different communication apps or platforms might use differing symbol systems for concepts; for instance, the word *go* is depicted by a green arrow in one symbol set, a traffic light colored green in another, and a frog jumping in yet another symbol system. Picture-based systems can be photographs, line drawings, or representational symbols.

Picture-based communication systems can be set up in grid-based systems or *visual scene displays*. Grid systems are set up using symbols, words, or letters in a row-column-grid pattern that can be adjusted to determine total number of keys on a page. Symbols might be organized in alphabetical, category, or personalized grid configurations. Grid-based systems can be designed as low-tech communication boards or high-tech dynamic screen devices that allow access to a robust amount of vocabulary.

Visual scene displays have been shown to provide an effective mode of communication to young children given the displays have a direct connection to real-life and context-based organization. Visual scene displays can be low-tech picture scenes or high-tech apps that display photographs or video of an event, activity, or place that are then embedded with AAC hotspots to provide speech output when selected (Chapin et al., 2021). This can allow for what is called "just-in-time" programming, in which a photograph of an event in real time can be quickly programmed to create contexts for communication with immediacy (Drager et al., 2019). This type of display can be beneficial for beginning communicators of all ages as it reduces cognitive load, the symbol representation is concrete, and it can tap into motivating activities and provide immediate access to vocabulary (Holyfield et al., 2019). Visual scene displays have also been used to provide contexts for communication for individuals with aphasia (Brock et al., 2017; Hux et al., 2010).

Aided Symbols: Orthography and Orthographic Print Symbols

Orthographic symbols such as print, text, Braille, fingerspelling, and writing are all forms of AAC. Alphabetic symbols can allow an individual to generate their own unique thoughts and words. It is important to include alphabetic/orthographic symbols in any system of communication for an individual with complex needs. This is a form of literacy and literacy enables individuals with complex needs to be independent. With the ability to spell out their own words, the individual is not dependent on another person to try to predict and program the words they might need. Literacy is a critical skills for those using AAC, with literacy they can create their own messages.

As SLPs designing communication boards for others, we cannot predict what words they might need. Use of a core vocabulary approach and access to literacy-print/orthography allows individuals the independence to create their own messages.

REFLECTION QUESTION 13.3

Can you predict what words you would need for tomorrow? Divide a piece of paper into a 3 × 4 grid and use the boxes to write down the words you think you will use tomorrow. Use single- or two-word phrases only. You know yourself better than anyone else; one would think it should be easy. Can you use just those 12 words and phrases for the day?

Use of orthographic symbols or print empowers an individual to generate their own words and ideas. Having a keyboard as part of a communication system enables an individual to compose their thoughts and learn literacy. Exposure to orthographic print and a systematic approach to teaching literacy provides a foundation for providing a means for those with complex needs to have the ability to say whatever is on their minds, rather than having to rely on preprogrammed words or a limited system that cannot predict what they might need to say. Reading and writing allows for greater comprehension, expression, and overall communication. **Word prediction** paired with a text-based system can enable users to reduce the amount of effort needed to convey their message through print. Individuals with complex needs can and should be taught to read and write. As Karen Erikson and David Koppenhaver discuss in their book *Comprehensive Literacy for All: Teaching Students with Significant Disabilities to Read and Write* (2020), all children, even those with the most significant disabilities, can learn to read and write.

In reflecting back on the exercise to predict what words you would need for your day, you might have found it hard to choose words that could apply for all the situations that might occur. Having a keyboard and literacy skills would allow you to spell out words you might need, especially since one cannot predict what situations might arise in our own lives, let alone others. Our individuals with complex needs should have multiple ways to communicate available to them, including print/text that allows them greater control over their ability to compose their own unique thoughts. Teaching literacy skills opens that door. Literacy interventions, detailed in Chapter 6, can be used with individuals who use AAC.

Pearson eTextbook
Video Example 13.3
Go to this YouTube link to learn about teaching literacy skills in the classroom.
www.youtube.com/watch?v=Ti8IOEICJQc&list=PLocplddh5SSRBGRsR0tOFXIJd5wh6i89k&index=3

Multimodal Combinations of Aided and Unaided Systems

Aided and unaided communication systems do not have to be considered as an either–or decision. We all use multiple modes of communication in our daily lives: gestures, texting, writing, speaking, facial expressions, head nods, and body language. Why would we limit those with complex communication needs to only one mode of communication? Effective communication skills and communicative competence involves multiple means of communication that are used in varied situations. Again, AAC is not about a particular device of piece of technology but is about a person's ability to communicate and interact with others. Acknowledging and enabling all forms of communication can help those with complex needs have multiple strategies to communicate.

Pearson eTextbook
Video Example 13.4
This video shows Lilly's communication journey.
www.youtube.com/watch?v=9U2WZGKXHZg&t=2s

> **REFLECTION QUESTION 13.4**
>
> *Why is it important to consider various forms of aided and unaided AAC systems for people with complex communication needs?*

AAC Access Methods

At the beginning of this chapter, we reviewed the WHO-ICF and its applications to the field of AAC. A person with complex needs might have multiple health conditions that might alter body functions and structures in a way that affects their ability to participate or perform some activities. These could range from sensory-perceptual differences to motoric differences that present challenges in the ways that an individual can interact with the world around them. These challenges need to be examined by an interdisciplinary team when problem solving the most efficient and optimal *access method* for an individual to utilize when implementing an AAC approach or system. Vision specialists, audiologists, occupational therapists (OTs), physical therapists (PTs), family/caregivers, and the individual can all provide valuable information when deciding the best method of access. *Access methods* are the ways that an individual can select a message or access a symbol and are divided generally into two categories of access: direct selection and indirect selection.

Direct Selection

Direct selection involves a means of indicating via touching, taking, or pointing to an item or symbol to indicate a message. An individual might "point" in several ways, use of a finger or hand might be one way, but others include use of eye gaze, head movements, a stylus or laser pointer, or a computer mouse, trackpad, or joystick. Eye-gaze selection can be used either with low- or no-tech paper-based systems or clear plexiglass eye-gaze systems interpreted by a communication partner or high-tech voiced output devices that can track the movements of the eye. Current technology can track eye movements or head movements to allow for an individual with limited movements of their limbs to control selection of items on a screen.

Collaboration with an occupational therapist and Physical therapist can ensure proper seating and positioning to allow for *proximal stability*, which then would enable the individual to have better control of their arms, legs, and fingers for **distal mobility**. **Proximal** is a term meaning toward the center, and **distal** means away from the center. When we have a good base of support, or proximal stability, we can use our limbs and fingers and can perform movements, or distal mobility, needed to complete tasks. OTs and PTs have clinical expertise in this area and should be consulted when determining access methods. Vision specialists can also have a significant contribution in helping ensure the size, color contrast, and visual field are considered when determining access methods in an AAC system.

Direct selection methods can be difficult and slow, especially for those with severe motor-based challenges. Composing a message can take time and effort. Methods have been introduced to attempt to improve the efficiency in which an individual can compose their message, including word prediction, **semantic compaction**, and consistency of key placement to promote ease of motor planning. Semantic compaction used in some picture-based systems allows for reduced effort needed to compose messages by combining symbols to represent words and phrases. This innovative idea helps improve the efficiency of communication for those who might have previously typed out their messages letter by letter on a keyboard. In investigating access methods, the interdisciplinary team's goal is to provide the most efficient and effective means for the individual to communicate. When direct selection is not an efficient or effective method, indirect selection methods must be considered.

Indirect Selection: Scanning

Indirect selection involves use of a method of scanning through a field of items or symbols and the individual providing an indication of their selection. The methods of scanning can involve technology or utilize a communication partner to manually scan through choices, as in partner-assisted scanning. Partner-assisted scanning is a low-tech/no-tech alternative in which a communication partner might point and say selections using a communication board and the individual makes a selection by performing a voluntary, clear, repeatable signal such as an eyeblink or finger tap to indicate their selection. In either method of scanning, a visual signal highlighting choices and/or an auditory cue is provided to allow the individual to select the desired items or symbol.

Visual and/or auditory scanning allows for those with significant motor or visual perceptual challenges to have access to communication when direct selection is not a viable means for efficient communication. Selection utilizing an AAC device or system involves the use of one or more **switches** that are activated when the individual makes a selection. In auditory scanning, speech output would provide an auditory cue as options were being scanned; when the individual hears the item they want, they press their switch and the word or phrase would be spoken aloud.

Strategies can be employed to improve the efficiency of switch use and scanning. Scanning can follow patterns such as linear one by one, row-column scanning or by groups of items on a page (top-bottom, right-left groupings). An individual might use a single switch to make a selection or can have multiple switches such as one for the operation of the scanning movement and then one for the final selection.

To enable an individual's access, there are a variety of switches available to maximize efficiency and capitalize on an individual's capabilities. Interdisciplinary collaboration with the team of professionals including OTs and PTs can determine the best site for switch placement to maximize the efficiency of movement and reduce physical challenges or fatigue. Switches can be activated by touch with contact from movement of body parts (i.e., fingers, hands, head, toes, feet, elbows, knees, eyebrow, eyeblink); proximity, which involves movement toward but does not require touch or pressure; or pneumatic sip-and-puff switches operated by use of air pressure in the mouth. New technology has developed ways to use **electromyography (EMG)** to sense the electrical activity during the activation of a muscle to control a switch. Research on brain-based control of computerized devices for AAC is underway and could lead to future possibilities for those with locked-in syndrome or other severe motor impairments (Brumberg et al., 2018).

Determining the type of switch or switches to use to provide access should be determined through trials with the individual with input from the team to capitalize on evidence-based practice based on the combined clinical knowledge and the individual's preference for ease of use as well as the intrinsic evidence provided from the data collected across trials with multiple switches and access sites. It should be noted that an individual's needs and capabilities could change over time and access methods could change, especially for those with degenerative conditions. Use of switches can also enable an individual to be independent in utilizing environmental controls or access to communication via social media or the Internet, which can give them greater independence in life and development of social networks.

AAC Output

In examining an individual with complex needs to determine the features they might require in an AAC system, the output should be considered. *AAC output* is the means by which the message or content is delivered. Examples would be speech generated by a device or text. For low-tech and unaided AAC, the output method is often interpreted by the communication partner, and a sign or signal must be "read" by the listener. Mid- to high-tech AAC devices often have the capabilities for voiced or speech output, including synthesized or digitized speech.

Pearson eTextbook
Video Example 13.5
This video shows an example of switch and partner-assisted scanning.
www.youtube.com/watch?v=w-sxeiJdkyQ

Pearson eTextbook
Video Example 13.6
Tyler's two-step switch access with auditory prompts is highlighted in this video.
www.youtube.com/watch?v=3xPO1yjKGBs

Digitized speech output is recorded speech placed on the device; **synthesized speech** is computer-generated preprogrammed voice output generated by a speech synthesizer. Text-to-speech programs generate words using synthesized speech. Low- and mid-tech devices often rely on recorded digitized speech, while high-tech devices often have the capability for both digitized and synthesized speech output as well as other output such as written, text, connections to social media, or email.

When utilizing digitized speech or synthesized speech, it should be age-appropriate and matched to the individual's gender identity. The advantages of digitized speech output are that since it is recorded from a person, it sounds natural and can be easily recorded to match the individual's identity.

Digitized speech can be utilized in *voice banking* to record and preserve a person's own voice when they have been diagnosed with a degenerative disease that results in a loss of speech. A disadvantage of using digitized speech is the messages for output must be predetermined and recorded and it does not allow for spontaneous novel utterance generation, which is often the goal of AAC.

Technological advances in recent years have improved the voice output of synthesized speech to allow for choice of voices according to gender, accent or dialectical variations, and age. Synthesized voices in high-tech devices are improving in their ability to sound natural and have features to improve intelligibility of speech by adjusting volume and rate. Synthesized speech can be generated from either use of symbols or can be text to speech. This allows the individual to have greater flexibility in composing their messages. Systems that allow for both digitized and synthesized speech can be utilized to maximize message flexibility and personalization. Voiced output enhances the individual's ability to increase the number of communication partners.

AAC systems can also have output that allows for communication in the online environment. The ability to connect to social media platforms and email to communicate with friends and family or to correspond in school or work environments could be an important feature for an individual to have within their AAC system. This can have implications for the individual's ability to have independence in interacting with others for social, employment, health-related, or educational means.

AAC Input

AAC input refers to using AAC to foster comprehension, receptive abilities, or intake of a message received by the individual (Beukleman & Light, 2020). AAC input can be used with individuals who have the capabilities for speech to aid in their understanding of a message. Sign language paired with speech, visual schedules, social stories, visual supports, and **aided language stimulation** can all be forms of AAC input.

Individuals with congenital or acquired conditions could benefit from AAC input. Its use can be helpful to orient a person with acquired conditions like a traumatic brain injury, such as a whiteboard to write out key words, or providing information visually as a supplement to auditory input can support the individual's understanding. AAC input can help decrease negative behaviors by supporting increased understanding of transitions through use of visual or object schedules. Use of AAC input supports the development of language skills using AAC by providing models for language use and expansion.

Dispelling the Myths Involving AAC

Learning Objective 13.4 Dispel myths surrounding AAC.

Unfortunately, there are myths that continue to circulate regarding AAC that hinder its implementation with individuals of all ages. It is important for you as a student to know the evidence-based research that dispels these myths so you can be an informed SLP and help others realize the barriers that these myths might create. As an SLP, I have encountered parents, teachers, other SLPs, and other professionals who had attitudes and beliefs that impacted an individual's access to AAC. Some of these myths came from early thoughts or teaching on AAC believing that an individual needed certain skills to "qualify" for AAC intervention.

Myths Impacting AAC: Early Intervention

MaryAnn Romski and Rose Sevcik wrote a comprehensive article titled "Augmentative Communication and Early Intervention Myths and Realities" (2005) identifying six myths that they hoped to address through education. These myths included:

1. *AAC is a "last resort" in speech-language intervention.* This myth was based on early "decision rules" in AAC but was later debunked by researchers (Cress & Marvin, 2003; Reichle et al., 2002) who found it critical to introduce AAC before communication failure occurs. More recent research has supported intervening early with AAC to develop language in children and to help adults with acquired conditions.

2. *AAC hinders or stops further speech development.* The opposite is true. Numerous studies have shown improvement in speech skills following AAC intervention (Beukelman & Mirenda, 2013; Hall, 2017; Romski & Sevcik, 1996; Schlosser & Wendt, 2008).

3. *A person must have a certain set of skills to benefit from AAC.* This myth applies to either individuals who have cognitive disabilities or those who may have some natural speech abilities who might be precluded from access to AAC due to not fitting a specific profile. Again, access should not be denied due to a certain set of skills (Romski & Sevcik, 1988; Smith & Hustad, 2015), there are no prerequisites for AAC, and individuals do not have to prove or demonstrate symbol use prior to introduction of AAC (Cress & Marvin, 2009). Individuals do not have to "master" or use low-tech AAC before using a high-tech device.

4. *SGDs are only for those with intact cognition.* This myth was based on the erroneous idea that the technology was too sophisticated and could not be operated by someone with cognitive disabilities. Extensive research has demonstrated the more severe a communication deficit, the more likely to benefit from AAC.

5. *Children must be of a certain age to be able to benefit from AAC.* This myth was related to the misguided belief that AAC would prevent a young child from developing speech, which was disproven (Millar et al., 2000); instead, it was found AAC should be implemented as soon as possible (Branson & Demchak, 2009).

6. *There is a representational hierarchy of symbols from objects to written words.* This myth has been disproven by a number of studies (e.g., Namy et al., 2004; Sevcik et al., 2018).

Pearson eTextbook
Video Example 13.7

In the video, Genevieve, a 2-½-year-old, is interacting with her younger sibling. Think about the interaction. Would it be possible without the implementation of AAC? Genevieve is learning language and social skills and using multimodal communication so she can relate to her younger sibling without needing an adult to translate or speak for her.

www.vimeo.com/308771816?
embedded=true&source=
video_title&owner=78378989

Smith et al. in their 2016 article "AAC and Families: Dispelling Myths and Empowering Parents" continued the battle against the myths around use of AAC. The authors noted a significant change in technology happened with the onset of mobile technology and the beginnings of communication-based apps for tablets and phones (Sennott, 2011). With that increase in technology the authors noted its wider acceptance for children. Unfortunately, myths of AAC continued to persist. Smith et al. identified myths surrounding families and AAC, which included:

1. *AAC cannot be embedded in natural routines.* AAC can be embedded into everyday routines and support and training can be improved for caregivers and families.

2. *AAC systems place undo stress on families.* Support and training can provide opportunities for families to connect and use AAC.

3. *SGDs are too difficult for families to use with their child.* Support and training should be a part of every plan.

4. *AAC is only for communication partners other than the immediate family.* This is based in the erroneous idea that families do not need to use AAC because they know and can interpret or anticipate the individual's needs. Families provide opportunities for connection and growth of language skills. Instead of interpreting their nonverbal communication, families can provide natural contexts for their AAC voice to be heard.

5. *Augmentativce Communication should not be a priority for early intervention.* This myth is based on the misconceived idea that AAC can wait until the children are older.

Smith et al. also noted that despite all that is known about introducing AAC as early as possible, parents and professionals hesitate to implement AAC with very young children.

In 2022, a survey of practices of those providing early intervention services continue to show influence of these same early myths on decision making regarding use of AAC. When asked what factors influenced decision making in early intervention, SLPs surveyed rated receptive and expressive language abilities, cognitive abilities, diagnosis, and age were all factors that determined AAC use and SLPs were more likely to recommend sign language or photographs than talking switches or SGDs (Lorang et al., 2022). Further education continues to be needed to dispel myths to ensure early access to AAC as a way to provide language and the ability to interact with others. Especially for those who present with known lifelong disabilites, we should start early to support their needs.

Myths about Adult Communicators and AAC

The National Joint Committee for the Communication Needs of Persons with Severe Disabilities (2022) advocate and educate others on the needs and capabilities of those with severe disabilities. They identified several erroneous myths regarding AAC and adults with severe disabilities, including:

1. *Working on communication is not worth the effort. If expressive and receptive skills haven't developed by now, they are not going to develop.* This inaccurate statement does not factor that we all can learn throughout our lifetimes. There is no expiration date for learning.

2. *If communication, language, or literacy interventions didn't work in childhood, they won't work now.* Individuals with complex needs might not have had access to literacy approaches or technology or appropriate educational programs when they were younger.

3. *Adults with severe diabilities have simple thoughts, feelings, and understandings, so they do not need comprehensive services or supports.* This is **ableist** thinking and is harmful and discriminatory and against the Americans with Disabilities Act.

4. *Spoken communication is the only real communication.* This misconception arises from the idea that spoken speech should be the primary means of communication; however, those with complex communication needs are often unintelligibile and speech is not a reliable means of communication.

As we've stressed throughout this text, SLPs must constantly evaluate and update the methods used with clients. Myths can only be dispelled by careful research and evidence. The importance of EBP is highlighted in the discussion in Box 13.1.

BOX 13.1   **Evidence-Based Practice and Issues Concerning the Use of Facilitated Communication**

Facilitated communication (FC) was first introduced in 1992 as a technique where a "facilitator" would provide physical support to an individual with complex needs who would be presented a letter board to type while the facilitator held their finger, hand, wrist, elbow, shoulder, or other body part. Unfortunately, this technique was not evidenced based and multiple studies revealed the messages were not composed by the individual but were authored by the facilitator (Chan & Nankervis, 2014; Hemsley et al., 2018; Tostanoski et al., 2014).

ASHA (1995) responded by noting the lack of scientific validity and reliability of this technique. Three decades later, one would think this debunked technique would have gone the way of a passing fad (Wombles, 2014). Instead, the faciliated communication approach has taken on new names, including "supported typing" and "spelling to communicate (S2C)," and has shown a recent increase in users and workshops promoting its use.

With increased impact of social media and online platforms, FC, and another discredited technique, the rapid prompting method (RPM) have seen a resurgence in the past few years (Hemsley & Dann, 2014). Social media videos and misinformation have preyed upon parents and family members who are looking for a "cure" to connect with their child or loved one (Trembath, 2015). They witness via social media videos containing supposed amazing results of RPM or FC. Both of these approaches are based in pseudoscience and have been found to be unethical and damaging to the families and people involved (Tostanoski et al., 2014).

In reality, methods such as FC deny the individual AAC user their true voice and prevent or delay their ability to receive evidence-based practice in AAC (Travers et al., 2014). ASHA (2018a) strengthened the language in its recent postion statement, which stated:

> The use of FC or other "facilitator"-dependent techniques is not consistent with the communication rights of autonomy and freedom of expression and prevents access to the person's human right of communication.... It must not be assumed that messages produced via RPM or any "facilitator"-dependent technique (e.g., FC) reflect the communication of the person with a disability.

Furthermore, ASHA (American Speech-Language-Hearing Association, 2016) warned SLPs about their ethical responsiblities to provide services that provide a benefit and "do no harm." ASHA's position on facilitated communication is that it should not be used.

What are some myths about AAC and how can they be barriers to individuals getting access to the skills they need to develop language and communicate?

Assessment Considerations

Learning Objective 13.5 Explain how an AAC assessment is dynamic, collaborative, and ongoing.

One of the reasons I am so passionate about working with individuals with complex needs is the assessment process, with the focus of assessment on finding and capitalizing on an individual's *capabilities* rather than focusing on "disabilities." This involves investigating and problem solving to find solutions to bridge the gap between their receptive abilities and their ability to express themselves. The focus is on what the individuals can do and providing them with further access to reach their potential.

Due to the nature of the complex needs of individuals assessed, each AAC assessment is tailored to variables that present due to underlying etiologies and personal factors such as age, life experiences, and onset of difficulties communicating. With this variability in mind, guidance for the AAC assessment process has taken the form of assessment models or frameworks such as the Participation Model (Beukelman & Mirenda, 2013). Lund et al. (2017) noted AAC assessment models can provide a theoretical framework for the design of the assessment process but noted a need for more specific assessment protocols or research into the decision-making process used by teams experienced with AAC. They noted AAC specialists had similar procedures that included review of information and case histories in preparation of the evaluation, the areas or domains assessed, and the methods of assessment, as well as parent/caregiver education and counseling as part of the assessment process. AAC assessments can incorporate methods such as interviews, observations, adaptations to formal tests, informal testing, and dynamic assessment (Lund et al., 2017).

> Assessment in the domain of AAC needs to include all members of the team, consider current communication status, include families/significant others, understand potential barriers, recognize the individual's strengths and potential, plan for future needs, and continue as an ongoing process.

The Assessment Process

Two models of assessment discussed here are the Participation Model and communicative competencies.

The Participation Model

The Participation Model (Beukelman & Mirenda, 2013) is a widely used and foundational guide to performing a comprehensive assessment of the opportunity and access barriers and facilitators involved. The Participation Model examines the environment and participation patterns of the individual as well as peers to determine supports provided and needed. Not only does it provide a framework for assessing the individuals' capabilities and *access barriers*, but it also examines the *opportunity barriers* that hinder the individuals' abilities to participate that exist relating to policies, practice, knowledge, skills, or the attitudes of others (Beukleman & Light, 2020). Beukelman and Light (2020) emphasize the importance of examining the communication partners and environments surrounding the individual and their influence as a potential barrier to address or a positive facilitator to support.

Assessment and treatment planning for the individual can include an examination of the social networks that exist around the individual. The Social Networks Communication Inventory (Blackstone & Hunt Berg, 2012) helps to create a profile of the individual and their relationships with communication partners extending out from the families or life partners to friends and acquaintances, to those who are paid to work with the individual, to people in the community (Blackstone, 2019). Examining the social networks around an individual can yield information for treatment planning and identify areas of capabilities and potential. When an individual only has a limited social network, oftentimes comprised of one to two family members and those that are paid to work with them, we need to think about how AAC and our goals can help them widen their connections with others.

Successful communication involves more than the individual themselves, therefore our assessment of communicative competence and the individual's capabilities needs to consider the communication partners, contexts, and environments in their everyday life. Utilizing the framework of the Participation Model paired with Light's communicative competencies can provide insight into the skills and competencies of the individual with complex communication needs and those around them.

Communicative Competencies

Communicative competencies (Light & McNaughton, 2014) can be useful in assessment and planning for intervention. A profile of competencies can be created to highlight the individual's capabilities as well the competencies of support people and potential needs for education. Light's framework for AAC assessment includes five competencies that relate to an individual with complex communication needs and their communication partners: *linguistic competence, operational competence, social competence, strategic competence,* and *psychosocial competence.*

Linguistic competence describes an individual's language ability across all components of language including receptive and expressive language ability, language of the home and community, and the language involved in the use of an AAC system. Linguistic competence could apply in an unaided AAC system if the individual communicated via ASL. Their linguistic competence could be assessed by their linguistic abilities to express and understand sign language in natural contexts. Opportunity barriers might arise in the areas of knowledge and skills if the communication partners in the individual's home and community lack the linguistic competence to communicate via sign language. The language and culture of the home and community are also factors in linguistic competence. Individuals with complex communication needs should be provided with a system of AAC that includes the ability to communicate in their home language.

Culturally and linguistically diverse families are often erroneously told to forgo speaking the language of the home in favor of the dominant language of the community or language used in the school system with the idea that it would be too "confusing" for the child with complex needs to learn more than one language. Research shows that "[i]n cases where children primarily hear/speak one language at home (L1), learning another language (L2) will build on concepts established in their L1, especially during early stages of language proficiency (at the lexical

CASE STUDY   **Naveen** (*continued*)

Naveen's mother stated at the initial evaluation the family only speaks English to him. She had been told to do so by other professionals so he "would not get confused."

Unfortunately, attitudes that underestimate individuals with complex communication needs are far too common. Devaluing the language of the home in favor of the language of the academic environment or community can be a problem. As noted above, Wagner described language as learned through experiences with fluent speakers. Telling a parent to stop speaking the language of the home to the child can produce a barrier to establishing L1 language proficiency and would not be demonstrating cultural competence in service delivery.

Consider that the family most certainly speaks their home language to each other and are the people who make up the core of the individual's social network. They are the people who will be there to support the individual for their lifetimes. Narrowing the potential communication partners by limiting exposure could lead to Naveen not being able to communicate with grandparents, aunts and uncles, and other relatives.

Naveen's mother was reluctant to have their home language added to his device because of what she was told by other professionals. After several sessions of parent education and counseling, she added their home language to his device. Work will continue to ensure Naveen has the opportunities to participate in his home, school, and community environments.

level), where translated equivalents are connected to each other in the brain" (Wagner, 2018, p. 173). Wagner (2018) noted that robust AAC systems have rules for language that need to be learned, and language is learned through experiences with fluent speakers. Children with complex needs require opportunities using their AAC system to use and learn the language of the home and the language of the community to ensure they can participate in both environments. This can be applied to the language of the AAC system as it is applied to learning another language. Linguistic competency develops over time, given exposure through meaningful activities, and proficiency in two or more languages depends on frequent opportunities to use them (Soto & Yu, 2014).

Operational competence refers to the knowledge and skills needed to operate or use an AAC system. This can include how to turn the system on or set it up, learning to navigate to folders or pages to find vocabulary, developing skills for switch use and timing to make selections, or learning to search or customize the system with new vocabulary. As in all the competencies, communication partners play a role in developing their competence so adequate support is given to the individual requiring the system. If they are dependent on a communication partner to set up or charge the system, that support person's operational competence to perform those skills is imperative to the success of the individual.

Social competence relates to the social interactional aspects of communication, which can include pragmatic usage such as turn taking, topic maintenance, and use of reciprocal interactions. Social competence highlights how an individual and their communication partner relate to each other. Social competence of a communication partner might highlight some of the needed aspects of how to be a good communication partner, including ensuring the partner speaks directly to the individual rather than to an aide or caregiver pushing their wheelchair. The

> Communicative competence does not just pertain to the individual with complex needs, it also applies to the communication partners in their life. Training for communication partners is an important part of AAC intervention.

social competence of the individual with complex communication needs could include their use of phrases for socially accepted communication; for a teen, this could include slang terms that allow them to communicate using trending phrases with their peers. Social competence can include aided or unaided communication skills such as eye contact, positive affect, facial expressions, and body language for multimodal communication. Social competence allows for the individual's personally to shine through.

Strategic competence relates to problem-solving measures taken by the individual with complex communication needs or the communication partners. The learning and use of strategies to prevent or reverse communication breakdowns are included in strategic competence. Individuals who use AAC systems might use a preset communication with untrained partners that educates them to be patient listeners to the messages the individual is composing, for example, statements such as " I have something to say," " I understand everything you are saying," "Please talk directly to me," or "Please be patient, it takes me a minute to say what I want to say." Strategic competence comes into play when an AAC device might not be available and other modalities are used to maintain the interactions such as gestures or head nods.

Psychosocial competence refers to factors including attitudes, motivation, and levels of resilience that can either foster success with AAC or be a barrier to developing skills for AAC. Attitudes about AAC can be shaped by positive or negative experiences. It is important for the SLP to consider the psychosocial factors influenced by communication partners or the individual's prior experiences. Addressing negative "can't do it" attitudes will ensure the individual is supported to develop to their potential. An individual who is motivated to use their device to communicate, has people around them who have positive attitudes about AAC, and who feels supported can have a higher level of success and demonstrate psychosocial competence.

An additional area of competency—not part of Light's communicative competencies but important for independence in communication and interactions—is *literacy*. Competency in literacy is an area that can enable an individual greater independence to communicate their own novel thoughts without having to rely on words to be programmed into a device. Individuals with complex communication needs can and should be taught to read and write (Erikson & Koppenhaver, 2020). Assessment and intervention in literacy for those with complex needs can provide a foundation for their future abilities for independence and self-advocacy.

REFLECTION QUESTION 13.6

How might the success in using AAC for communication rely on both the communication partner's and the individual's development of communicative competencies?

Specific Assessment Considerations

Planning for assessment begins with collecting initial background information through a case history and parent/caregiver interview. To assess the communicative competencies of the individual and their communication partners, AAC assessments ideally include multiple contextual observations and interviews with those within their social networks. Observations, paired with criterion-based assessments, adapted standardized assessments, and dynamic assessments, can be utilized to create a comprehensive capabilities profile of the individual.

Examining a client's current communication skills provides a baseline. Understanding their motivation and desire to communicate or situations where their ability to communicate breaks down can guide treatment planning. Gaining an understanding of the intention and signals an individual might use to communicate is an initial step in the process. Their intentions might not be readily recognized by all communication partners or may be confused as inappropriate behaviors rather than attempts at communication.

An assessment of AAC starts with the individuals' current levels of ability for all modes of communication including natural speech, gestures, their own personal idiosyncratic signals, signs, and aided and unaided communication. An individual might not yet be a symbolic communicator and may use actions or emotions to express themselves. They might lead a caregiver to what they want or use other behaviors to get attention or communicate their needs.

Assessment documents the individual's status across domains including natural speech, cognitive skills, linguistic skills, literacy, gross and fine motor skills, and sensory and perceptual skills like vision and hearing (Beukleman & Light, 2020). The team of professionals working together can develop a comprehensive understanding of skills in each domain. Collaboration with family members, caregivers, the individual with complex communication needs, and other professionals is imperative to collect an accurate assessment of skills.

Dynamic assessment incorporates scaffolding, prompting, and teaching withing the assessment procedures to observe the individual with complex communication needs's learning process and capabilities (King et al., 2015). Given the limited experience with AAC and introduction of AAC techniques in the assessment process, the dynamic assessment approach can yield information on how the individual best responds or provide an understanding of the level of scaffolded support that might be used in treatment. A dynamic assessment can examine learning potential and capabilities (King Bamford et al., 2022).

Specific criterion-based assessments are available for a variety of domains. Rating scales that use interviews or direct observation of skills can provide a profile of strengths and needs prior to intervention and could be helpful in feature matching based on the individual's capabilities. Criterion-based assessments allow for collection of baseline measurements for understanding the individual's communicative intent and variety of communicative functions expressed. Specific assessments relating to the AAC assessment process include:

> Standardized assessments often need to be modified to allow for a response, so norms cannot be applied to individuals with complex needs. Dynamic assessment and criterion-based profiles might yield more descriptive information for treatment planning.

- The Augmentative and Alternative Communication Profile measures subjective, functional skills for developing communication competence using AAC systems (Kovach, 2009).

- The Dynamic AAC Goals Grid (DAGG-2) assesses communication skill level and communicative competence and assists teams in determining functional goals (Clarke & Schneider, 2015).

- An online tool, the Communication Matrix is used to assess stages of communication development and methods or behaviors used to communicate. It can be used with those with severe communication difficulties that utilize alternate methods of communication (Roland, 2012).

- The Functional Communcation Profile Revised provides a profile of an individual's communication abilities, mode of communication (e.g., verbal, sign, nonverbal, augmentative), and level of independence (Klieman, 2003).
- An assessment and intervention planning tool, the Social Networks Inventory evaluates interactions between an individual and communication partners to define strengths and areas of need (Blackstone, 2019).
- The Pragmatics Profile for People who use AAC (Martin et al., 1995) is a tool for professionals to assess communicative means and profile how an individual uses intentional communication in everyday situations.
- The Communication Supports Inventory–Children and Youth (CSI-CY), used for those who rely on AAC (Rowland et al., 2009), is a profile of strengths and needs and their effect on participation, guided by the principles of the WHO-ICF.
- The Language Sample Analysis is for those using an AAC system or language and can be utilized to gather baseline data and ongoing analysis (Van Tatenhove, 2014).

Use of standardized tests are not valid for this population, as the adaptions needed for their response invalidate standardization and norms generally do not apply (Beukleman & Light, 2020). However, standardized tests can yield information to determine a capabilities profile for the individual. Adaptations in selection, either through direct selection or partner-assisted scanning, can be utilized to determine current levels of functioning. Tests that measure receptive language, literacy, and cognitive skills can be adapted to provide a method of response for the individual to indicate their abilities. Results of adapted standardized testing, criterion-based profiles, and dynamic assessment procedures can be utilized to create profiles of strengths and needs of the individual and their communication partners. This information is then used to prepare a treatment plan that encompasses multimodal communication including aided and unaided communication interventions.

Areas of Assessment for Access to AAC

The AAC assessment team works together to determine the individual's capabilities in relation to use of AAC systems. Determining physical and perceptual capabilities involves collaboration with professionals who specialize in those areas. OTs and PTs are valued members of the team who can help assess best positioning and methods of access and determine placement or size of symbols based on motor abilities. Depending on the individual's capabilities, their ability to access an AAC system is assessed by trialing direct selection or scanning methods using varied grid layouts and key sizes, which are determined based on motor and visual abilities.

Sensory capabilities such as vision and hearing determine features the AAC team would want to have in an AAC system. Determining visual capabilities can require consultation with a vision specialist or medical professional. Given the complex health needs of the population of people who use AAC, knowledge of visual abilities such has visual field, visual acuity, or the involvement of cortical vision impairment determine features that one would include in the design of an AAC system. This could include high-contrast symbols, changing size, use of auditory cues, or use of tangible symbols depending on the degree of visual impairment. Since aided and unaided AAC systems rely on visual information, one must have an understanding of how an individual's ability to process visual information may be affected (Blackstone et al., 2021).

CASE STUDY   **Naveen** *(continued)*

Naveen had various members of the team creating activity-specific communication boards, which complicated his ability to find words without prompts from his communication partners. Placement of keys of core words were changed on newly created boards, so he had to search for the content words that were not consistently placed. Naveen did quite well navigating to words he was familiar with and could expand his utterances using AAC. He also had the need to access a growing number of words for academic, literacy, and social purposes.

After discussions with the parents and team, it was determined Naveen could benefit from a trial with a communication app that was motor based and capitalized on his skills with navigation by giving access to thousands of words within two to three key hits. This reassessment of skills examined the features needed to capitalize on Naveen's skills and find a better match. He benefited from consistent placement of symbols. Think about your keyboard when you type; the consistent placement of keys allows you to type based on motor memory.

Hearing assessment and understanding of capabilities would necessitate consultation with professionals such as an audiologist or teacher of the Deaf, as well as the individual and family. Results provide information on needed features of their AAC system to include aided or unaided input (i.e., ASL) to ensure the individual can comprehend messages from communication partners. Training and education on visual and auditory supports for communication partners can be a component of the treatment plan.

Including the individual themselves and their caregivers/family in the assessment and decision-making process provides information on preferences, motivation, likes/dislikes, and needed vocabulary. Strengths and barriers can be identified that can prevent **device abandonment**.

Factors shown to contribute to device abandonment, where a system is no longer used by the individual, include poor fit, attitude, not maintaining or adjusting the system, lack of training, lack of support, and attitudes of those around the individual (Johnson et al., 2009). These factors show that the team should be diligent in the assessment process to ensure a good fit is attained through trials and feedback from all involved. It also shows that support and training are essential for successful use of an AAC system. The AAC assessment process reassesses factors and updates the system when necessary to respond to the changing needs of the individual.

As an SLP, it can be frustrating to have gone through the process to get a device fully funded and delivered and work with the individual to get them to use it in therapy, only to have the device either not used in other settings or abandoned altogether. Knowing these factors can aid in the mindset to ensure that the individual can be set up for success.

AAC System Selection or Feature Matching

Determining the best fit for an AAC system involves a process of matching the features needed by the individual to the methods of communication that will allow them to gain communicative competence. Think about the individual's needs first and not the features of a particular device. In considering options, the solutions can be a combination of aided and unaided, low- and high-tech options depending on needs and varying contexts or environments.

The individual's needs should drive decision making on the best fit for an AAC system. For instance, if the individual is a child in a school setting, they would require access to robust vocabulary that can support their academic growth. Depending on their physical and sensory needs, they might use a switch to scan through selections or be able to directly select symbols from a visual scene or grid-based display. They would need speech output to be able to communicate their messages to peers and unfamiliar adults. They and their communication partners would need training and support to develop competencies in all areas (linguistic, operational, social, psychosocial, strategic, and literacy). They might use facial expressions, gestures, signs, and vocalizations as multimodal communication.

If the individual is an adult with an acquired degenerative condition such as amyotrophic lateral sclerosis, they might voice-bank in the early stages. They might use writing, gestures, and voice amplifiers initially, then move to a switch and speech output communication system, progressing further to an eye-gaze or switch-activated system using eye movements (Koch Fager, 2017). Features of the system would be matched to the individual's current and projected capabilities; AAC systems should be selected with a plan for the future in mind.

Features to consider include:

- Access to vocabulary: robust core vocabulary, progressive introduction of vocabulary, organization into categories, or motor-based organization. Access to vocabulary is an important factor to consider in planning for growth in language skills and ability to generate messages.
- Message characteristics including design of display/symbol system:
  1. Decisions regarding displays include visual scene displays versus grid-based displays, dynamic versus static displays.
  2. Type of symbols used could vary from photographs to symbols that have multiple meanings for categories of words. Symbols could have single-word messages or phrases and sentences that might be prestored for quick use.
  3. Color-coding and consistency of placement of symbols can be features to consider. Fitzgerald Key and Modified Fitzgerald Key use placement based on sentence word order and color-coding based on parts of speech (i.e., pronouns = yellow, verbs = green) (Tobii Dynavox, 2018).
- Portability and mobility: based on individual's capabilities, features such as weight and size, and ability to self-carry or mount on a wheelchair.
- Access method: touch, eye tracking, switch use, direct selection or scanning capabilities.
- Output method: voiced output, text to speech, print, email, social media capabilities.
- Access to literacy: keyboard, word prediction, phonemic awareness keyboard.

REFLECTION QUESTION 13.7

What are some major considerations in AAC assessment?

If the purpose of the evaluation was to determine a particular system to purchase, a report is written to justify it. Funding can be provided either through Medicaid, Medicare, or private insurance. In some cases, communication devices are purchased by the school system to provide access to the educational environment as part of the child's individualized education plan. There are also several grant programs from nonprofit charitable organizations that will assist in funding.

After the evaluation is complete, the SLP's justification report would be sent to the physician for approval as durable medical equipment and to obtain a prescription for the SGD. Companies that sell communication devices help with the funding process and can supply guidance for completing the process; they submit the paperwork to the insurance company for funding when the order is placed (Sennott et al., 2016). Acquisition of a device or setup of a system is not the end of the assessment process; it should be ongoing to ensure that the individual's needs continue to be met and adjustments are made as the needs change.

Intervention: Creating Communicative Competence

Learning Objective 13.6 Apply communicative competencies to intervention practices with individuals with complex communication needs and their communication partners.

Where to Start?: Team-Based Intervention and Communication Partners

Intervention in AAC should be team based, use natural contexts, and be centered on the individual's identified needs and priorities (Beukleman & Light, 2020). Interventions can be based on improving the linguistic, operational, social, psychosocial, and strategic competencies of the individual using AAC and their communication partners. Ensuring the team of professionals, families, caregivers, and the individual receive training and support to implement the use of AAC is needed to prevent device abandonment and maximize success. The members of the team and the individual should be supported to improve their communicative competence with AAC.

Communication partners are critical to the success of AAC intervention. It is crucial to include them in the assessment and plan for education and collaboration with the communication partners around the individual with complex needs.

Introducing AAC to an individual and their communication partners is like introducing a new language. AAC provides the means for language to develop for those with congenital conditions and gives the capacity for language back to those who lost the ability due to acquired conditions. Training and support are needed to develop communicative competence with a new system of language.

Think about AAC was a way to learn language. If you were trying to learn French, you would do so best if language learning was targeted in meaningful contexts, embedded throughout the day, and your communication partners spoke to you and coached you to learn French. If you are the only person speaking French and everyone around you is speaking English, you won't learn as quickly or have meaningful contexts to apply your learning. You would need to know the important words that affect your daily life and that would motivate you to speak to others. It is the same with learning the language of AAC. If those around the individual use AAC and model language by "speaking AAC," the individual will have more opportunities in a variety of contexts to learn. AAC intervention needs to target meaningful vocabulary/language, in functional

Research supports that intervention should *always start* with the instruction of communication partners to ensure those who use AAC are provided with meaningful opportunities to communicate and a supportive environment (Ball & Lasker, 2013).

contexts, and involve multiple communication partners throughout the individual's day. Use of AAC within daily family interactions provides a greater degree of natural opportunities and support language and literacy development (Granlund et al., 2008).

Training communication partners to interact with the individual has supported positive outcomes. The team, including families and caregivers, working with the individual should not be expected to know exactly what to do when a new device or AAC system is introduced. Training and support needs to be provided. Strategies for how to be a good communication partner, techniques for embedding use of AAC in daily routines, and support for building communicative competencies can be taught.

As an SLP who has worked in the school-based setting, I found it beneficial to work closely with paraprofessionals, one-to-one aides who spend their day with students with complex needs. Listening to them about their concerns and observations made me more informed and a better SLP, and I was able to target priorities that were important to the student by training the paraprofessional in strategies for interaction and communication. Expectant pause time was one of the communication strategies taught to aides to improve the independence of the student in interactions. Valuing input from all members of the team will capitalize on areas of expertise from each person. As was highlighted at the start of the chapter, collaboration and teamwork makes for greater success. As they say, "Teamwork can make the dream work."

What to Do?: Direct and Indirect Intervention Using AAC

Individuals learning to use AAC need direct interventions to increase their communicative competencies to become effective communicators. Indirect interventions involve the setup of the environment, training of communication partners, or actions taken by the SLP or communication partners to provide instruction such as aided language stimulation. See Table 13.3 for suggested means of direct and indirect techniques targeting each skill or competency.

Supporting Language Development and Independence

Learning Objective 13.7 Describe how intervention can foster language development and independence through use of supportive prompt hierarchies, adaptive play skills, focused and functional intervention, and development of literacy skills.

Pearson eTextbook
Video Example 13.8
This video contains an animated short about implementing aided language stimulation.
www.youtube.com/
watch?v=flFNMky22-U

Strategies that promote language development can also promote language development with AAC. Use of open-ended questions, language expansion, and applying the knowledge you have of language development and language intervention all apply to intervention with AAC. Just as verbal modeling is provided for development of speech, *aided language stimulation* can provide the modeling of AAC in the "language" of the individual. A core vocabulary approach can give the individual access to the most frequently used words in conversation. Teaching use through meaningful contexts can be done through aided language stimulation and focused lessons.

TABLE 13.3
Direct and Indirect Intervention Strategies

Competency targets	Direct intervention strategies	Indirect intervention strategies
Operational	Practice navigation to new vocabulary and use of access method (switch, eye gaze, direct selection) in functional or fun activities Teach operation (power on, search features, message delivery)	Communication partner training in aided and unaided means of communication, operation, and navigation. Teach how to add and search for vocabulary
Linguistic	Customize vocabulary and system to include interests, needs, and culture Use of hierarchy of prompts Use core vocabulary Teach language using AAC method, aided and unaided, multimodal approach Consider gestalt language processing and use of scripts; include phrases in AAC	Use of aided language stimulation provided by communication partners/team members Provide naturalistic contexts to elicit communication Teach language expansion techniques Teach least to most prompts to foster independence Train communication partners in the use of scripts and possible meaningful use of delayed echolalia
Social	Use of scripts and language-based routines to teach pragmatic skills Increase opportunities for interactions with peers and community Provide social language and practice with social vocabulary	Provide access to a variety of communicative means; make it functional Make language/interaction about more than requests (greetings, comments, jokes, complaints/refusals, informational, social closeness ["I love you"])
Psychosocial	Embed AAC into functional contexts to provide rationale and motivation Foster positive environment, positive feedback for AAC use Practice mindfulness and include sensory regulation and feelings	Collaboration with team to dispel myths and attitudes, use encouragement and positive feedback and support, provide opportunities to widen social networks, increase variety of communication partners and use of peers
Strategic	Teach strategies for interacting with others, including use of scripts to self-advocate (i.e., "Please give me a minute, I have something to say," " I understand everything you are saying," "Please speak directly to me") Use multimodal approach; teach a variety of ways to communicate	Teach and practice strategies to improve communication partner's interactions including use of expectant pause, open-ended questions, AAC modeling, and responsiveness to communication attempts (Kent-Walsh & Rosa-Lugo, 2006) Teach how to be a good communication partner
Literacy	Teach letters and letter-sound correspondence Use adapted books Provide access to keyboard and writing activities Provide structured opportunities for literacy instruction	Increase exposure to books and model AAC during reading Increase interaction with print Provide systematic instruction in reading and writing (Erikson & Koppenhaver, 2020)

Use of Prompt Hierarchy

Use of prompts can support learning and teach skills, but we must be diligent to not use prompts to control or create prompt dependency. The goal of AAC is communication, not compliance. We want an individual to use AAC as a tool to generate their own novel communication.

Hand-over-hand prompts can inadvertently teach the child or individual use of aided or unaided AAC and involves the adult or communication partner controlling their movements. Caution should be used with any use of physical, hand-over-hand, or hand-under-hand prompting This can lead to prompt dependency or control of the individual's message rather than their own intent. It also could lead a child or new communicator to believe the use of the adult's hands is needed or expected to complete the task.

Those working with beginning communicators can learn how to use a hierarchy of prompts that supports independence.

Use of least-to-most (LTM) prompts have been found to facilitate language learning and generation of multiple-symbol messages (Finke et al., 2017). When using a least-to-most prompting technique you strive to elicit the highest level of independence by setting up the natural environment for the individual to succeed. Creating a lesson with a motivating activity that is aligned with the individual's interests and providing a clear introduction of expectations/instruction, use of visual supports, and setting up a situation that elicits a targeted response can all provide a foundation to promote independence using the least restrictive prompts.

In Figure 13.7, the LTM prompting strategy would follow the arrow on the left and down the page, moving from teaching and setting up the natural enviroment to elicit communication, to use of an expectant pause, to providing a visual or gestural prompts, to then providing verbal prompts. Note there is an embedded hierarchy of LTM within tbe various types of verbal prompts that can be given as well.

When an individual is using AAC, we must allow for pause time between each prompt to allow for them to respond and compose their message. Use of models to demonstrate the expected response of the targeted behavior might be needed for new skills.

Play and Access to Adapted Toys and Books

Children learn language through play. Toys, games, and books can be adapted for children with complex needs. Giving a child the ability to activate and play with a toy via a switch can be the first step to teaching them they have the power to control their world. I have used simple cause-and-effect toys such as bubble machines, or character toys that play songs or have movement to motivate and create opportunities for switch use. This can give the child opportunities to practice initial operational and social competency skills that provide a foundation for communication.

Customizing and Updating

Whether an individual has a current system or they have just received a new system or device following an evaluation, I always take the time to customize it to their needs, interests, and culture. I also teach family members and the individual

FIGURE 13.7 Prompt hierarchy.

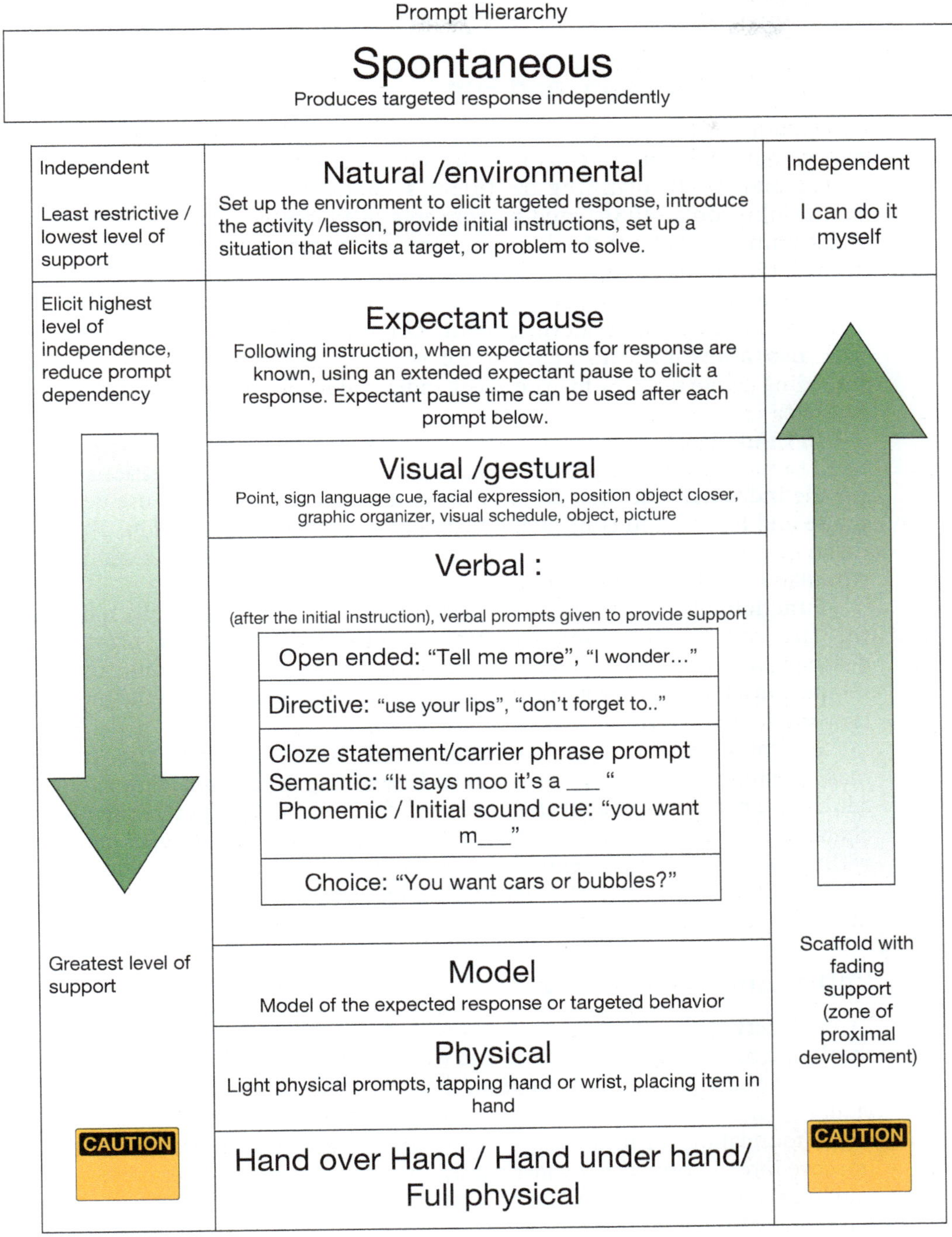

Prompt Hierarchy

Spontaneous
Produces targeted response independently

Independent Least restrictive / lowest level of support	**Natural /environmental** Set up the environment to elicit targeted response, introduce the activity /lesson, provide initial instructions, set up a situation that elicits a target, or problem to solve.	Independent I can do it myself
Elicit highest level of independence, reduce prompt dependency	**Expectant pause** Following instruction, when expectations for response are known, using an extended expectant pause to elicit a response. Expectant pause time can be used after each prompt below.	
	Visual /gestural Point, sign language cue, facial expression, position object closer, graphic organizer, visual schedule, object, picture	
	Verbal : (after the initial instruction), verbal prompts given to provide support Open ended: "Tell me more", "I wonder..." Directive: "use your lips", "don't forget to.." Cloze statement/carrier phrase prompt Semantic: "It says moo it's a ___ " Phonemic / Initial sound cue: "you want m___" Choice: "You want cars or bubbles?"	
Greatest level of support	**Model** Model of the expected response or targeted behavior	Scaffold with fading support (zone of proximal development)
	Physical Light physical prompts, tapping hand or wrist, placing item in hand	
CAUTION	**Hand over Hand / Hand under hand/ Full physical**	**CAUTION**

Source: Fagan, Kelly 2022.

themselves to add the vocabulary important to them. As discussed, we cannot predict what words someone might need for every situation that might arise but giving them the ability to type or add their own symbols is empowering.

Fit, Focus, Function, and Fun

Intervention with individuals with complex communication needs can be guided by foundational work in treatment for language disorders (like those discussed in Chapter 4). In planning treatment sessions with AAC, I always think of Judith Johnston's (1986) guiding concepts of fit, focus, and functionality, and I add "fun" to that list. Looking at planning for and treating individuals with complex communication needs, you want to make sure you have a good developmental fit in your goals and choice of activities, taking into consideration their zone of proximal development. Understanding the developmental fit can also allow for the appropriate scaffolding of prompts for support, providing opportunities for the most independent levels. Remember to teach, not test.

In thinking about focus, I always have clinicians set up the natural environment to elicit targets and provide an introduction that sets up expectations not only for the individual but their communication partners as well and use descriptive praise and feedback to continually highlight the focus of the session. This might mean targeting a certain number of core words and providing for aided language stimulation and repetition over time.

Functionality helps with the rationale and can be a factor in motivation for the individual. Using functional activities and goals provides for development of skills that benefit the individual with real-life communication and interactions. For adults, working on functional goals can provide all the motivation they need.

For children, you might have to also make sure you add in the "fun" and make the interactions with you as fun and rewarding as you can. With children or adults, listen and learn about their likes and dislikes and incorporate their favorite characters or topics. Connect with them. Be enthusiastic to see them and engage with them. Remember that children learn through play; be playful in your sessions. You can be a motivator in the way you interact with the individual and make the interactions valued. Don't forget to make it fun.

Importance of Literacy

Literacy is an essential part of AAC intervention. Literacy enables individuals to compose their own independent thoughts and communicate without the need for others to dictate their access to words.

In my interventions and interactions with the individuals I serve, I am always thinking about the future for them and what I can do today that can improve their tomorrows. Literacy is an intervention that can ensure a better tomorrow for individuals with complex communication needs; it can help them academically, provide a foundation for future employment, ensure access to improved health care, improve interactions with a wider community to build relationships (both online and in person), and improve their overall independence. In the past, attitudes that have prevented those with complex communication needs from having structured literacy as part of their education have limited some from their potential. You can make a difference by providing the foundational skills that open the door to literacy for those you serve in the future.

Advocacy: Communication Bill of Rights

Learning Objective 13.8 Understand how the Communication Bill of Rights guides advocacy and goals for AAC.

Communication is a basic human right (McLeod, 2018). For nearly 5 million Americans and 97 million people worldwide, that right is not easily attainable without the support of interventions to aid in their communication. SLPs can make a difference.

In thinking about our intervention and advocacy for individuals with complex communication needs, we should know and teach the Communication Bill of Rights. I think about these rights when I review goals for individuals; it can help us design intervention plans that promote self-determination and self-advocacy.

In 2016, the National Joint Commission for the Communication Needs of People with Severe Disabilities reviewed and updated the *Communication Bill of Rights*. It noted that all people with a disability of any extent or severity have a basic right to effect, through communication, the conditions of their existence. Beyond this general right, a number of specific communication rights should be ensured in all daily interactions and interventions involving persons who have severe disabilities.

To participate fully in communication interactions, each person has the fundamental communication rights in Figure 13.8.

Pearson eTextbook
Video Example 13.9

In this video on literacy skills, you learn about teaching phonemic awareness. See the recommended readings at the end of the chapter for more information on specific strategies for providing reading and writing instruction for individuals with complex needs.
https://youtu.be/Ti8IOEICJQc

FIGURE 13.8 The Communication Bill of Rights.

The Communication Bill of Rights

1. The right to interact socially, maintain social closeness, and build relationships
2. The right to request desired objects, actions, events, and people
3. The right to refuse or reject undesired objects, actions, events, or choices
4. The right to express personal preferences and feelings
5. The right to make choices from meaningful alternatives
6. The right to make comments and share opinions
7. The right to ask for and give information, including information about changes in routine and environment
8. The right to be informed about people and events in one's life
9. The right to access interventions and supports that improve communication
10. The right to have communication acts acknowledged and responded to even when the desired outcome cannot be realized
11. The right to always have access to functioning AAC (augmentative and alternative communication) and other AT (assistive technology) services and devices
12. The right to access environmental contexts, interactions, and opportunities that promote participation as full communication partners with other people, including peers
13. The right to be treated with dignity and addressed with respect and courtesy
14. The right to be addressed directly and not be spoken for or talked about in the third person while present
15. The right to have clear, meaningful, and culturally and linguistically appropriate communications

Source: Brady et al. (2016).

BOX 13.2   Evidence-Based Practice in Augmentative and Alternative Communication

Overall/General

- AAC has a strong positive effect on overall communication.
- AAC interventions can be used to foster early language skills; it does not hinder speech development.
- AAC is effective in managing challenging behaviors.
- Use of AAC can reduce the gap between comprehension and production of speech.
- Use of meaningful relevant interactions with family and significant others builds language; therefore, it is important to involve families in assessment and intervention.
- Instruction in literacy can improve outcomes and autonomy.
- Non-English-speaking individuals and members of nondominant communities have less access to information about AAC and face obstacles of discrimination and poverty and less resources for support.

Communication Partners

- AAC is most effective when those in the environment are an integral part of intervention.
- Interventions that involve communication partners providing aided language stimulation have been shown to promote growth in expressive and receptive vocabulary, pragmatics, and expressive syntax.
- Communication partner interventions were found to be highly effective across a range of participants using AAC, with aided AAC modeling, expectant delay, and open-ended questions the most frequently targeted communication partner interaction skills.
- Research indicates untrained communication partners frequently exhibit actions that restrict the communication of children using AAC.

Children and AAC

- Very young children respond to pictures arranged by visual scenes rather than categories or parts of speech.

- In preschoolers, use of AAC by peers to provide augmented input (aided language stimulation) was associated with stronger language growth; use of question asking and prompting by teachers was associated with weaker language growth.
- AAC is most effective when those in the environment are an integral part of intervention.

Adults and AAC

- Adults with aphasia can benefit from AAC with visual scene displays.
- Individuals with degenerative diseases benefit from beginning AAC support before they lose their ability to speak.
- Adults with developmental disabilities can learn to use AAC to communicate even if they had no prior exposure.

AAC System Characteristics

- Consistent symbol location improves motor learning for target words on displays and minimizes operational demands.
- Size of keys and grid should be determined by motoric and visual capabilities, not assumptions regarding cognitive skills.
- Use of core vocabulary and access to a keyboard allows for generation of novel utterances.
- The Picture Exchange Communication System may increase requesting and decrease problem behaviors, but there are maintenance and generalization questions.
- High-tech AAC is effective for most clients with intellectual and developmental disabilities to improve communication skills.
- Speech-generating devices are more effective for improving overall communication and interactions with others than low-tech picture communication.

Sources: Based on Allen et al. (2017); Barker et al. (2013); Beuklelman and Light (2020); Biggs et al. (2018); Douglas et al. (2013); Erikson and Koppenhaver (2020); Kent-Walsh et al. (2015); National Joint Committe for the Communication Needs of Persons with Severe Disabilities (2022); Romski and Sevcik (2005); Soto (2012); Thistle et al. (2018).

Summary

Given the variability of the population with complex communication needs, student clinicians and SLPs often lack confidence and self-efficacy in their belief in their capacity to provide AAC evaluations (Sanders et al., 2021) and intervention. Simluation experiences similar to those used within other health care fields show potential to increase skills within graduate school AAC courses (Gutmann, 2016). An increasing number of graduate schools are including an AAC class and ASHA requires hours of clinical training in treatment and assessment of augmentative and alternative communication for children and adults. Continuing education and mentoring are other potential areas to increase the number of SLPs who feel confident in assessment of individuals with complex needs.

The world needs more people who are trained in AAC, and with experience and practice you can develop skills to help make a difference for those with complex needs. I sincerely hope this introduction to communication disorders has spurred your interest in the field of speech-language pathology. I am hoping, like me, you have found your passion, mission, vocation, and profession within the field of speech-language pathology and you are ready to dedicate your life's work to helping those with complex needs. It's what the world needs, and you will meet, work with, and learn from every individual with complex communication needs. They are the most amazing people.

Epilogue   Case Study: Naveen

Given Naveen's diagnosis of Angelman syndrome, he will need AAC supports throughout his lifetime. He has made good progress in his trial with the motor-based communication app and is demonstrating emerging literacy skills.

As Naveen transitions to a new school and classroom in the fall, a team-based focus and training with his communication system including aided and unaided methods will be needed. His grandparents have come to visit, allowing him to practice using words and phrases in his home language. Naveen continues to enjoy music and has begun to increase his interactions with books, knows letters, and is beginning to spell three-letter words. He now has a keyguard and can rest his hand on the screen without activating keys; this has helped reduce the amount of physical supports his communication partners give. His mother and respite worker have faded back supports and use visual or verbal prompts with him.

Naveen will continue to need his AAC system to grow with him; he continues to learn to use new words and navigates well to find the words he uses most frequently. Phrases have been added to allow him to self-advocate and educate his communication partners to give him the time he needs to talk. Naveen continues to use multimodal communication, combining use of his AAC device with signs, vocalizations, body language, and facial expressions. His personality shines through with his smiles, laughter, and jokes. The foundation of building language and literacy through the use of AAC has just begun, but with use of evidence-based practice Naveen is developing skills that will help him throughout his lifetime.

Reflections | **from a Speech-Language Pathologist Specializing in AAC: Colby Keyser, MA, CCC-SLP**

Let me introduce you to one of my colleagues, Colby Keyser. She shares my passion for helping those with complex communication needs and volunteered to answer a few questions.

1. *Why did you become a speech-language pathologist?*
   When I was paging through college catalogs in high school, looking for possible majors, I came across speech pathology. I had never heard of it before. When I read the description, something clicked inside of me, and I knew this was my path. Once I started classes, everything was confirmed because there wasn't one course that I didn't enjoy.

2. *What clinical setting do you work in, and what types of patients do you primarily evaluate and treat?*
   I work in a school with a full caseload of students in life skills classrooms. Most students have been diagnosed with autism; some are nonspeaking, some have no language or are not yet using functional language, and some are verbal.

3. *How did you become a speech-language pathologist who specializes in augmentative and alternative communication? How did your career evolve?*
   In between undergraduate and graduate school, I took 2 years off and worked as a speech aide at a United Cerebral Palsy Residential Center for adults. The SLP who oversaw the speech aides had us carry out programming for clients. This ranged from teaching clients how to use AAC to fully conversing with others who used AAC. I got to work closely with the AAC vendor who would bring new devices to show us. I learned how to program and fix devices and converse with AAC companies when there were problems. When I started grad school, I continued to work for the state of Washington with two clients and their families to teach them to program and learn how to use their devices. I got to work with individuals with a range of AAC skills. It was where I learned to presume competence and what was possible for people using AAC. I continued this work with my first job out of graduate school.

4. *What coursework during your undergraduate and graduate programs do you feel was most important for your area of expertise?*
   In the 1990s we did not receive any coursework in AAC in either undergraduate or graduate school. Because I knew the AAC vendor, he and I actually taught a 3-hour seminar for my fellow grad students as an introduction to AAC. All of my training was on the job and then later through continuing education courses.

5. *What is the best part of your job?*
   I love watching my students discover the power of communication. I love to be a part of helping them to find their words and express their thoughts and feelings. It is a very long process but when it happens, there is nothing like it. I also really enjoy working with families and helping them to understand the importance of AAC and how to consistently use it in the home.

6. *How has the COVID-19 pandemic changed your work as an SLP, for better and for worse?*

   COVID-19 was hard, but it also allowed me to work directly with the parents using AAC at home and because our assignments included a lot of AAC homework embedded in with the academic work, parents learned a new perspective of what is possible with AAC.

7. *What advice to you have for students considering the field of speech-language pathology, particularly those considering working with people who use AAC?*

   Always presume competence with your students who are nonspeaking or even those with speech but not yet using functional language. There are so many reasons why a student is unable to access their full verbal language. AAC can open so many doors if it is taught and consistently integrated into the classroom. It is important to try to establish a good relationship with the teachers of your students and teach them all of the ways AAC can be brought into the curriculum. Teach the teachers to program and model with it; teach paraprofessionals to program and expect AAC use from their students. Teach through initial modeling in all environments and situations. Provide a rich and full vocabulary for students.

8. *What experience stands out to you as something that has shaped your passion for your career as an SLP?*

   Working with students who have become communicators and have been able to get their wants and needs met and are able to express feelings and have conversations has been so amazing. This can be a long and slow process, but our students have the right to communicate, and we must provide them with proper training to succeed. This core belief keeps me going in my career.

Suggested Readings/Sources

Beukelman, D. R., & Light, J. (2020). *Augmentative and alternative communication: Supporting children and adults with complex communication needs* (4th ed.). Brookes.

Beukelman, D. R., Yorkston K. L., & Garrett, K. M. (Eds). (2007) *Augmentative communication strategies for adults with acute or chronic medical conditions*. Brookes.

Erikson, K. A., & Koppenhaver, D. A. (2020). *Comprehensive literacy for all: Teaching students with significant disabilities to read and write*. Brookes.

AFTERWORD

We've reached the end of this text and maybe of your first course or first year. We hope that as you've proceeded through both, you've found some topics that have excited your interest and stimulated your intellect. The best part is that there is more to come—much more.

For example, the chapter on language disorders in children will blossom into an entire course, and then, hopefully at the graduate level, into a course on birth through 5 years and another on school-age children. This will be followed by at least one clinical placement with children, most likely more.

The best advice we can give you—and remember that we began where you are beginning—is to approach all your courses with the recognition that you are learning to become a professional. Unlike some majors, which are more topical, doing poorly in one course in communication disorders will most likely affect those that follow. Each course builds on the next. So, treat each one with the importance and seriousness it deserves, even when the topic seems uninteresting at first.

Will every course grab your interest? Unfortunately, no. Both of your authors have areas of the field they love and others not so much. The important thing is to give it your all. We have seen students who say they have no interest in one area who later become stars in working with that population or disorder. The only way to know is to dive in.

Never lose sight of your goal to become a professional, an SLP or audiologist. Stretch yourself, shadow an SLP or audiologist, take an extra course, engage in research with a faculty member, volunteer during the summer in a hospital or as a camp counselor. Do all that you can to become the best, most knowledgeable professional you can be.

We wish you success and hope that our paths may cross again, possibly at an ASHA convention or a professional workshop. The number of communication disorder professionals is relatively small, and you never know when you'll be in an elevator, stuck between floors—as Bob was when he was a student—with one of the big names in the field. While we don't wish to meet you in that manner, we hope to shake your hand someday as a communication disorder professional. Best of luck!

Professional Organizations

American Speech-Language-Hearing Association (ASHA)

ASHA (www.asha.org) is a nonprofit organization of speech-language pathologists, audiologists, and speech and hearing scientists that was founded in 1925. As of 2022, ASHA represents 212,534 speech-language pathologists, audiologists, and speech, language, and hearing scientists from throughout the United States and the world. It is the largest association for those concerned with communication disorders. ASHA's mission is to empower and support speech-language pathologists, audiologists, and speech, language, and hearing scientists through:

- Advancing science
- Setting standards
- Fostering excellence in professional practice
- Advocating for members and those they serve

Scientific Study of the Processes and Disorders of Human Communication

ASHA encourages study of typical and disordered communication by mandating a curriculum of study for prospective speech-language pathologists and audiologists. In addition, ASHA provides financial grants to individuals who are engaged in research that furthers our knowledge of communication and assessment, treatment, and prevention of pathologies. ASHA works closely with governmental agencies that sponsor relevant scientific investigation.

To dispense knowledge among professionals, ASHA publishes several scholarly periodicals: *Journal of Speech, Language, and Hearing Research*; *Language, Speech, and Hearing Services in Schools*; *American Journal of Speech-Language Pathology*; and *American Journal of Audiology*. ASHA also holds an annual convention at which members and others share information and learn through scientific sessions, exhibits, seminars, and short courses. Additional institutes, workshops, conferences, and teleseminars are held throughout the year. ASHA fosters continuing education for professionals through these activities.

Clinical Service in Speech-Language Pathology and Audiology

Programs that provide clinical services to people with communicative disorders may be accredited by ASHA. This means that representatives of ASHA will review the procedures that are used in diagnosis and treatment. A site visit will ensure that equipment, materials, and record keeping adhere to the highest professional standards. Clinical service will be the responsibility of individuals who meet ASHA standards for the Certificate of Clinical Competence in Speech-Language Pathology (CCC-SLP) or Certificate of Clinical Competence in Audiology (CCC-A). More information can be found at www.asha.org/certification/.

Maintenance of Ethical Standards

To ensure that the highest moral and ethical principles are followed in the professions of speech-language pathology and audiology, ASHA provides a code of ethics, which is found on the ASHA website (www.asha.org/siteassets/publications/et2016-00342.pdf). The basic principles are as follows:

1. The welfare of the persons served by communication disorders specialists is paramount.

2. Each professional must achieve and maintain the highest level of professional competence. The ASHA Certificates of Clinical Competence (CCC) are considered the minimal achievement for independent professional practice. Clinicians should provide service only within their own areas of competence. Professional development and continuing education should be ongoing. New technology requires that speech-language pathologists and audiologists continually update their skills in order to safely and accurately address patient needs.

3. Professionals must promote understanding and provide accurate information in statements to the public.

4. Professionals are responsible for ensuring that ethical standards are maintained by themselves, colleagues, students, and members of allied professions. All members of ASHA are responsible for the monitoring and maintenance of ethical standards throughout the profession (ASHA, 2010).

Advocacy for Individuals with Communicative Disabilities

ASHA is active in encouraging members of Congress and state legislatures to pass legislation that provides for appropriate services for communication-impaired individuals. Bills such as the Individuals with Disabilities Education Act and the Americans with Disabilities Act became law in part because of the extensive promotional activities of ASHA and other organizations.

The needs and characteristics of people with speech, language, and hearing disabilities are clarified and publicized by ASHA through a variety of media. In May, which is Better Speech and Hearing Month, you are especially likely to encounter public service announcements that advocate for understanding, prevention, and treatment of communication disorders. More information can be found at www.asha.org/advocacy/.

Related Professional Associations

Although ASHA is the largest organization for communication disorder professionals, other groups are also active and worthwhile. Some speech-language pathologists and audiologists belong to several associations. Table A.1 lists some of the

TABLE A.1

Selected Professional Associations Relevant to Communication Disorders

Academy of Dispensing Audiologists	American Speech-Language-Hearing Association	National Hearing Conservation Association
Academy of Rehabilitative Audiology	Audiology Foundation of America	National Student Speech-Language-Hearing Association
American Academy of Audiology	Canadian Association of Speech-Language Pathologists	Orton Dyslexia Society
American Academy of Otolaryngology—Head and Neck Surgery	Council on Education of the Deaf	Stuttering Foundation of America
American Auditory Society		

ones that are most closely affiliated. Prospective speech-language pathologists and audiologists are advised to take courses in biology, psychology, and sociology to better understand their clients and to work more effectively with professionals from other disciplines.

AAC input When communication partners use of a form of augmentative or alternative communication (gestures, sign language, pictures, visual schedule, communication app, or device) to supplement verbal words to enhance comprehension or understanding. AAC input helps foster receptive language skills. Signing or use of aided language modeling by communication partners can be a form of AAC input. This can also be called augmented input.

AAC output The use of a form of augmentative or alternative communication for expression. It is use of signs, pictures, or a device as a means to express oneself.

Abdominal aponeurosis A broad sheet of connective tissue covering the front of the abdominal wall.

Abduction When the vocal folds open or spread apart during vibration.

Ableist Fostering discrimination or bias against people who are disabled or regarding those who are disabled as damaged, incomplete, or less than others.

Acoustic neuroma Common name of a vestibular schwannoma, a benign growth that develops on cranial nerve VIII and can impact both balance and hearing.

Acquired Occurring after birth.

Acquired sensorineural hearing loss Hearing loss that is not inherited and not present at birth.

Acute laryngitis Temporary swelling of the vocal folds, resulting in a hoarse voice quality.

Addition In articulation, the insertion of a phoneme that is not part of the word.

Adduction When the vocal folds close or come together during vibration.

Affricate A combination of a stop and fricative phoneme.

Aided language stimulation A communication strategy to teach language by using augmentative or alternative communication, in which communication partners model language using the same system of communication as the individual or child. Also known as "natural aided language" or "aided language modeling."

Air conduction A method of evaluating hearing by transmitting sound to the inner ear via the outer ear and middle ear.

Allophone A phonemic variation.

Alport's syndrome A hereditary disorder characterized by kidney disease and bilateral progressive sensorineural hearing loss.

Alveolar Related to the alveolar, or gum, ridge of the mouth. In speech, alveolar consonants are those produced with the tongue on the alveolar ridge.

Alveolar pressure Pressure inside the lungs.

Alveoli Tiny air sacs in the lungs where oxygen and carbon dioxide are exchanged.

Alzheimer disease (AD) A cortical pathology that affects primarily memory, language, or visuospatial skills as a result of diffuse brain atrophy; presenile dementia.

American Sign Language (ASL) A complex nonvocal language that contains elaborate syntax and semantics. Proficiency in its use is one of the primary methods by which a deaf individual becomes part of the Deaf community.

Amplification In the context of hearing, this term refers to enhancement of the auditory signal, either through use of hearing aids, assistive devices or cochlear implants.

Amyotrophic lateral sclerosis (ALS) Most common degenerative motor neuron disease, characterized by progressive loss of both upper and lower motor neurons; often called Lou Gehrig's disease after the baseball player who was diagnosed with it. Results in fatigue, muscle weakness and atrophy (muscle wasting), involuntary contractions, and reduced muscle tone. Speech in the later stages is labored and slow with short phrasing, long pauses, hypernasality, and severely impaired articulation.

Anatomy The study of the structures of the body and the relationship of these structures to one another.

Aneurysm A type of hemorrhagic stroke that results from the rupture of a saclike bulge in a weakened artery wall.

Angular gyrus Portion of the cortex responsible for work recall.

Anomic aphasia A fluent aphasia characterized by naming difficulties and mild to moderate auditory comprehension problems.

Aphasia An impairment due to localized brain injury that affects understanding, retrieving, and formulating meaningful and sequential elements of language.

Aphonia A complete loss of voice.

Aplasia (or dysplasia) Hearing loss due to the absence of the inner ear structures during embryonic development.

Apraxia of speech A disorder in the planning or programming of movements for speech production.

Arteriovenous malformation A poorly formed tangle of arteries and veins that may result in a rare type of stroke in which arterial walls are weak and give way under pressure.

Articulation Rapid and coordinated movement of the tongue, teeth, lips, and palate to produce speech sounds.

Aspiration Inhalation, especially the inhalation of fluid or food into the lungs; in phonology, a puff of air that is released in the production of various allophones.

Aspiration pneumonia A respiratory infection that occurs when foreign material (e.g., food, saliva, liquids) enters the lungs.

Assessment As related to hearing loss, a comprehensive testing process to identify the nature of the loss, make a diagnosis, and provide recommendations for intervention.

Assessment of communication disorders The systematic process of obtaining information from many sources through various means and in different settings to verify and specify communication strengths and weaknesses, identify possible causes, and make plans to address them.

Assistive listening devices (ALDs) The general term applied to electronic devices designed to enhance the reception of sound by those whose hearing is impaired.

Ataxic dysarthria A motor speech disorder involving problems with muscle coordination; the problem involves the accuracy, timing, and direction of movement. Speech is characterized by irregular articulatory breakdowns, slowness, excessive and equal stress, and imprecise articulation.

Atresia A congenital disorder resulting in complete closure of the external auditory meatus.

Atrophy Wasting-away or loss of cells.

Attention-deficit/hyperactivity disorder (ADHD) Hyperactivity and attentional difficulties in children who do not manifest other characteristics of learning disabilities.

Audible nasal emission Perception of nasal air flow during speech. Commonly occurs in individuals with cleft palate.

Audiologist A professional whose distinguishing role is to identify, assess, manage, and prevent disorders of hearing and balance.

Audiology Professional discipline involving the assessment, remediation, and prevention of disorders of hearing and balance.

Audiometer A device used to regulate and deliver pure tone and speech stimuli during audiometric testing.

Auditory brain stem response (ABR) A type of electrophysiological test that records neural responses along the ascending auditory pathways occurring within the first 5–6 milliseconds following stimulus presentation.

Auditory evoked potentials (AEPs) Small neuroelectric responses to auditory stimulation by the ascending auditory pathways leading from the cochlea to the cortex of the brain.

Auditory neuropathy spectrum disorder (ANSD) Condition characterized by normal outer hair cell function with abnormal cranial nerve VIII function.

Auditory processing disorders (APD) Difficulty finding meaning from incoming auditory information.

Auditory training Listening activities designed to maximize a hearing-impaired person's ability to detect, discriminate, identify, and comprehend auditory information.

Augmentative and alternative communication (AAC) Gestures, signing, picture systems, print, computerized communication, and voice production used to complement or supplement speech for persons with severe communication impairments.

Aural habilitation Intervention that is conducted with individuals whose hearing loss occurred at an early age, specifically before the development of auditory and spoken language skills.

Aural rehabilitation Services and therapies that are provided to individuals whose hearing loss occurred later in life, after spoken language skills have, at least to some degree, developed.

Authentic data Information about an individual that is based on real life.

Autism spectrum disorder (ASD) Term used to characterize individuals at the severe end of the pervasive developmental disorder (PDD) continuum; an impairment in reciprocal social interaction with a severely limited behavior, interest, and activity repertoire that has its onset before 30 months of age.

Automatic The ease with which a person uses a particular skill without apparent thought.

Babbling Single-syllable nonpurposeful consonant–vowel (CV) or vowel–consonant (VC) vocalizations that begin at about 4 months of age.

Basal ganglia Large subcortical nuclei that regulate motor functioning and maintain posture and muscle tone.

Baseline data Information about client performance before intervention begins.

Basilar membrane The membrane that separates scala media from scala tympani. Contributes significantly to our perception of frequency.

Behavior modification A systematic method of changing behavior through careful target selection, stimulation, client response, and reinforcement.

Behavioral observation (BO) A method of assessing infant hearing by presentation of different stimuli and watching for any changes in activity that signal a response.

Bilabial Pertaining to two lips, such as phonemes produced with both lips.

Blend Create a word from individual sounds and syllables.

Bolus A chewed lump of food ready for swallowing; also, the substance to be ingested when eating or drinking.

Bone conduction A method of evaluating hearing by transmitting sound to the inner ear by mechanically vibrating the bones of the skull.

Booster treatment Additional therapy, based on retesting, offered after treatment has been terminated.

Bound morpheme A morpheme that must be attached to a free morpheme to communicate meaning; grammatical morpheme.

Breathiness Perception of audible air escaping through the glottis during phonation.

Broca's aphasia A nonfluent aphasia that is characterized by short sentences with agrammatism; anomia; problems with imitation of speech because of overall speech problems; slow, labored speech and writing; and articulation and phonological errors.

Broca's area Located in the left frontal area of the brain and responsible for working memory and enabling the motor cortex for speech.

Central auditory processing disorder (CAPD) Deficits in the processing of information from audible signals; hearing is often intact but meaningful processing is difficult.

Central auditory system Part of the auditory system that includes structures beyond the auditory nerve and extending to the auditory cortex.

Central nervous system (CNS) The brain and spinal cord.

Cerebellum A lower brain structure consisting of two hemispheres that smoothly regulates and coordinates the control of purposeful movement, including very complex and fine-motor activities. The cerebellum revises the transmission from the cortex's motor strip to produce accurate, precise movements. It is also important for motor skill learning.

Cerebral arteriosclerosis A type of ischemic stroke resulting from a thickening of the walls of cerebral arteries in which elasticity is lost or reduced, the walls become weakened, and blood flow is restricted.

Cerebral palsy (CP) A heterogeneous group of neurogenic disorders that result in difficulty with motor movement; were acquired before, during, or shortly after birth; and affect one or more limbs.

Cerebrovascular accident (CVA) Stroke, the most common cause of aphasia, results when the blood supply to the brain is blocked or when the brain is flooded with blood.

Cerumen (or earwax) A substance produced by glands in the ear canal that provides lubrication and protects the ear from the invasion of insects and other foreign objects.

Chin tuck A posture with the chin down that is helpful with some patients who have a swallowing disability.

Chorea Involuntary movement disorder characterized by rapid and unpredictable movements of the limbs, face, and tongue resulting from abnormalities in basal ganglia control circuitry. Huntington disease is the most common cause of chorea in adults.

Chronic laryngitis Vocal abuse during acute laryngitis that leads to vocal fold tissue damage.

Closed syllable A syllable, or basic acoustic unit of speech, that ends in one or more consonants.

Cochlea The portion of the inner ear that contains the sensory cells of the auditory system; composed of two concentric labyrinths, the outer one is composed of bone and the inner one of membrane.

Cochlear implant An electronic amplification device that is surgically placed in the cochlea and provides electrical stimulation to the surviving auditory nerve fibers.

Code switching The process in which bilingual speakers transfer between two languages, based on the listener, context, or topic.

Cognitive impairment An umbrella term for pathological conditions and syndromes that result in a decline of memory and at least one other cognitive ability that interferes with daily life activities.

Cognitive rehabilitation A treatment regimen for individuals with traumatic brain injury that is designed to increase functional abilities for everyday life by improving the capacity to process incoming information.

Communication An exchange of ideas between sender(s) and receivers(s).

Communication disorder An impairment in the ability to receive, send, process, or comprehend concepts of verbal, nonverbal, or graphic symbol systems.

Compression Part of the sound wave where the displaced molecules are in close proximity to each other.

Concha The deep bowl-like depression on the pinna.

Conditioned play audiometry (CPA) A method of assessing the hearing of children ages 2½ to 3 years and older by instructing them to put a block in a bucket, place a ring on a peg, or carry out another action whenever they hear the test signal.

Conduction aphasia A fluent aphasia in which the individual's conversation is abundant and quick. Characterized by anomia, auditory comprehension that is impaired mildly if at all, extremely poor repetitive or imitative speech, and paraphasia.

Conductive Refers to hearing loss caused by damage to the outer or middle ear.

Conductive hearing loss A loss of auditory sensitivity due to malformation or obstruction of the outer ear and/or middle ear.

Conductive system Part of the auditory system made up of the outer and middle ears.

Congenital Present at birth.

Consonant A phoneme that is produced with some vocal tract constriction or occlusion.

Contact ulcer A benign lesion that may develop on the posterior surface of the vocal folds.

Conversion (functional) aphonia A sudden loss of voice, often in the absence of laryngeal pathology, and frequently associated with stress, anxiety, depression, or emotional conflict. The individual may whisper involuntarily; excessive contraction of laryngeal muscles may also be present.

Conversion (functional) dysphonia A voice disorder that may be characterized by a wide range of vocal abnormalities, often in the absence of laryngeal pathology, and frequently associated with stress, anxiety, depression, or emotional conflict, usually involving excessive contraction of laryngeal muscles.

Conversion disorder A condition in which emotion is suppressed and transformed into a sensory or motor disability.

Cranial nerves The 12 pairs of nerves in the peripheral nervous system that innervate the muscles of speech production as well as mediate the sensations of vision, hearing, balance, smell, and touch from the face.

Craniofacial anomalies Congenital malformations involving the head (*cranio* = above the upper eyelid) and face (*facial* = below the upper eyelid).

Criterion-referenced An evaluation of an individual's strengths and weaknesses with regard to specific skills.

Critical literacy A reader's ability to actively interpret between the lines, analyze, and synthesize information and to be able to explain content.

Cultural competence Understanding, appreciating, and responding appropriately to the full range of diverse dimensions that you and clients and families bring to an interaction.

Cultural congruency The synchrony of intervention strategies and techniques with the cultural values, beliefs, and behaviors of a community that potentially yields appropriate and effective services.

Cultural humility Recognition that learning and self-reflection of cultural differences are lifelong, that power imbalances exist and must be addressed, and that institutions must be accountable.

Deaf community A group of persons who share a common means of communication (American Sign Language) that facilitates group cohesion and identity.

Deaf culture A view of life manifested by the mores, beliefs, artistic expression, understandings, and language (ASL) that is particular to members of the Deaf community.

Deafness Hearing loss that reaches 90 db or greater; can also be defined as profound hearing loss.

Decibel (dB) A mathematically derived unit based on the pressure exerted by a particular sound vibration.

Decoding Breaking or segmenting a written word into its component sounds and then blending them together to form a recognizable word.

Decontextualized Outside a conversational context. When we write, we construct the context with our writing rather than having it constructed by our conversational partner(s).

Developmental disfluency Common pattern of disfluency found in young children as they search for words and attempt to construct sentences to convey their intent.

Developmental language disorder (DLD) Language disorder with no obvious cause, although many children with this disorder have difficulty with verbal working memory.

Device abandonment When an individual ceases to use an augmentative or alternative communication (AAC) device when they continue to benefit or require support of AAC to have effective communication.

Diagnosis A statement distinguishing an individual's difficulties from the broad range of possibilities.

Diagnostic therapy Ongoing assessment and evaluation as intervention takes place.

Dialect A linguistic variation that is attributable primarily to geographic region or foreign language background; includes features of form, content, and use.

Dialectal scoring An alternative scoring procedure that accounts for language variations and potentially decreases the number of dialectal speakers who may be misdiagnosed as having a language disorder.

Dialogic reading Picture book interactive sharing between a caregiver and a young child, in which parents try to get children involved in the reading process by asking them questions about the story or allowing a child to tell the story.

Diaphragm A large muscle that divides the torso into the thorax (upper cavity) and abdomen. The diaphragm is the principal muscle of inspiration.

Digitized speech output Recorded speech that can be placed on a device to provide voiced output.

Diphthong Two vowels said in such close proximity that they are treated as a single phoneme.

Diplophonia The perception of two vocal frequencies.

Disability A restriction in ability to perform a function as a result of an impairment.

Disability The functional consequence of an impairment.

Disorder A disruption in function do to an impairment.

Distal Away from the center.

Distal mobility The ability to move the arms and limbs.

Distortion In articulation, a deviant production of a phoneme.

Dynamic Characterized by energy or effective energy, changing over time.

Dynamic assessment A nonstandardized assessment approach that can take the form of test–teach–test to determine a child's ability to learn.

Dynamic literacy A reader's ability to interrelate content to other knowledge through both deductive and inductive reasoning.

Dysarthria One of several motor speech disorders that involve impaired articulation, respiration, phonation, or prosody as a result of paralysis, muscle weakness, or poor coordination. Motor function may be excessively slow or rapid, decreased in range or strength, and have poor directionality and timing.

Dyslexia A type of learning disability characterized by difficulties with accurate or fluent word recognition, poor spelling, and deficits in coding abilities.

Dysphagia A disorder of swallowing.

Dysphonia An impairment in normal voice production.

Dysplasia See *aplasia*.

Dystonia A form of hyperkinetic dysarthria that is characterized by a slow, sustained increase and decrease of hyperkinesia involving either the entire body or localized sets of muscles. As a result, there are excessive pitch and loudness variations, irregular articulation breakdowns, and vowel distortions.

Ear, nose, and throat (ENT) physician Medical doctor specializing in diagnosis and treatment of diseases of the ear, nose, and throat.

Eardrum See *Tympanic membrane*.

Early hearing detection and intervention (EHDI) programs Public health initiative designed to facilitate early detection of hearing loss through universal hearing screening, followed by appropriate referral for diagnostic testing and early intervention as necessary.

Edema Swelling due to an accumulation of fluid.

Effectiveness The probability of benefit to individuals in a defined population from a specific intervention applied to a given communication problem under *average everyday* clinical conditions.

Efficacy The probability of benefit to individuals in a defined population from a specific intervention applied for a given communication problem under *ideal* conditions.

Efficiency Application of the quickest intervention method involving the least effort and the greatest positive benefit, including unintended effects.

Electroacoustic measures Tools that record acoustic signals from within the client's external auditory canal.

Electrolarynx A battery-powered device that sets air in the vocal tract into vibration.

Electromyography (EMG) The measurement of electrical activity in a muscle when activated.

Electropalatography (EPG) A technique used to teach correct placement of the articulators for speech production. It uses an artificial palatal plate fitted in the client's mouth that contains electrodes. The electrodes are connected to a computer. When the tongue contacts the electrodes during speech production, the articulatory patterns can be viewed on a computer screen.

Electrophysiological tests Tools that record neuroelectric responses (nerve impulses) that are generated by the auditory system in response to sound.

Embolism A blood clot, fatty materials, or an air bubble that may travel through the circulatory system until it blocks the flow of blood in a small artery. If it travels to the brain, it may cause a stroke.

Endolymph The cochlear fluid found in the scala media.

Endoscope A lens coupled with a light source that is used for viewing internal bodily structures, including the vocal folds.

Enhanced milieu teaching (EMT) A naturalistic, conversation-based strategy that uses the child's interests and initiations as opportunities to teach language and communication skills in the early stages of speech and language development.

Esophageal speech Speech that is produced by using burping as a substitute for the laryngeal voice.

Etiology The cause or origin of a problem; also, the study of cause.

Eustachian tube The tube that connects the middle ear cavity with the nasopharynx.

Eustachian tube dysfunction Condition in which the Eustachian tube does not adequately equalize middle ear pressure; commonly results in pathology of the middle ear.

Evidence-based practice (EBP) Clinical decision making based on a combination of scientific evidence, clinical experience, and client needs.

Examination of the peripheral speech mechanism Sometimes called oral peripheral exam; assessment of the structure and function of the visible speech system.

Executive function An aspect of metacognition used in self-regulation that includes the ability to attend; to set reasonable goals; to plan and organize to achieve each goal; to initiate, monitor, and evaluate your performance in relation to that goal; and to revise plans and strategies based on feedback.

Explicit instruction Intervention technique that attempts to make a child consciously aware of an underlying language pattern.

External auditory meatus (or canal) The tubular structure that extends from the concha of the pinna to the tympanic membrane.

Extrapyramidal tract Motor tract fibers involved in unconscious modulation of motor movements and the regulation of reflexes, posture, and tone; also known as the indirect activation pathway or indirect motor system.

Extrinsic devices Bone conduction devices where all of the components are worn outside the head.

Failure to thrive The absence of healthy growth and development.

Fast mapping A process in which a child infers the meaning of a word form context and uses it in a similar context at a later time; a fuller definition evolves over time; enables preschool children to expand their vocabularies quickly by being able to use a word without fully understanding the meaning.

Figurative language Nonliteral phrases consisting of idioms, metaphors, similes, and proverbs.

Filler Utterances such as "er," "um," and "you know" that are used in productions. Sometimes characteristic of disfluent speech and/or stuttering.

Fingerspelling A form of manual communication consisting of 26 distinct handshapes that visually represent the letters of the English alphabet.

Flaccid dysarthria A speech disorder caused by weak, soft, flabby muscle tone, called hypotonia. May result in hypernasality, breathiness, and imprecise articulation.

Fluency Smoothness of rhythm and rate.

Fluent aphasia Speech characterized by word substitutions, neologisms, and often verbose verbal output; also called Wernicke's aphasia.

FM system A type of hearing assistive technology that transmits sound to a hearing-impaired person via FM radio waves. The system consists of a microphone, a transmitter, and a wireless receiver.

Free morpheme The portion of a word that can stand alone and designate meaning; root morpheme.

Frequency An acoustical term that refers to the number of sound-wave cycles that are completed within a specific time period; subjectively, perceived as the pitch of a sound.

Fricative A consonant phoneme that is produced by exhaling air through a narrow passageway.

Frontal lobe Located in the anterior portion of the brain and important in decision making, motor control, executive function, and working memory.

Fundamental frequency The lowest-frequency component of a complex vibration.

Gastroesophageal reflux (GER) Movement of food or acid from the stomach back into the esophagus.

Generative Capable of being freshly created; refers to the infinite number of sentences that can be created through the application of grammatical rules.

Glide A phoneme in which the articulatory posture changes from consonant to vowel.

Global, or mixed, aphasia A profound language impairment in all modalities as a result of brain damage.

Glottal Relating to or produced in or by the glottis, the space between the vocal folds.

Glottis The space between the vocal folds.

Grammar The rules of a language.

Granuloma A nodular lesion due to injury or infection; may occur on the vocal folds and may be caused by a breathing tube being placed through the glottis.

Habilitation A process to foster the development of new skills, abilities, and knowledge. Individuals with congenital conditions at birth would likely need habilitation to help develop skills.

Habitual pitch The basic frequency level that an individual uses most of the time.

Hair cells Auditory receptor cells located in the organ of Corti that are responsible for encoding auditory information.

Handicap A social disadvantage that accrues to an individual with an impairment or disability, often in the form of barriers that can prevent an individual from reaching a goal or full potential.

Harmonics Frequencies in a complex sound that are integer multiples of the fundamental frequency.

Head rotation A posture with the head turned toward the impairment, used for some clients with a swallowing disability.

Head tilt A posture with the head away from the impairment, used for some individuals with a swallowing disability.

Head-back position A posture with the head held back that is useful for some clients with a swallowing disability.

Hearing disorder Impaired sensitivity of the auditory or hearing system.

Hematoma Blood trapped in an organ or skin tissue due to injury or surgery.

Hemiparesis Muscle weakness on one side of the body, resulting in reduced strength and control.

Hemiplegia Paralysis on one side of the body.

Hemisensory impairment Loss of the ability to perceive sensory information on one side of the body.

Hemorrhagic stroke A type of stroke resulting from the weakening of arterial walls that burst under pressure.

Hertz (Hz) The number of complete vibrations or cycles per second.

Hesitation A pause before or between parts of utterances. If used excessively, it may be considered a sign of disfluency or stuttering.

Hoarseness A voice quality that is characterized by a rough, usually low-pitched quality.

Holistic Pertaining to the whole; multidimensional.

Huntington disease Rare, inherited degenerative disease that causes progressive loss of neurons in basal ganglia and diffuse areas of cortex; begins in the fourth or fifth decade of life, with progression to death within 10–20 years. Affects movement, thinking, and personality; dysarthria and dysphagia are also common. It is also known as Huntington chorea.

Hyoid bone Horseshoe-shaped structure that serves as the point of attachment for laryngeal and tongue muscles.

Hyperfluent speech Very rapid speech found in people with fluent aphasia and characterized by few pauses, incoherence, inefficiency, and pragmatic inappropriateness.

Hyperkinetic dysarthria A speech disorder characterized by increased movement, such as tremors and tics, and by inaccurate articulation.

Hyperlexia A mild form of pervasive developmental disorder (PDD) characterized by an inordinate interest in letters and words and by early ability to read but with little comprehension.

Hypernasality Excessive nasal resonance.

Hypokinesia Abnormally decreased motor function or activity.

Hypokinetic dysarthria A speech disorder that is characterized by a decrease in or lack of appropriate movement as muscles become rigid and stiff, resulting in monopitch and monoloudness and imprecise articulation.

Hyponasality An abnormal resonance characterized by lack of nasal air flow during production of the phonemes /m/, /n/, and / ŋ / resulting from a blockage in the nasopharynx or nasal cavity.

Iconicity The level that a visual symbol represents or resembles its meaning.

Impairment A biological or physiological condition that involves the loss of physical, social, or cognitive functioning.

Incidental teaching Use of a natural activity to train targets.

Incus The middle bone of the ossicular chain in the middle ear; articulates with the malleus at the top and has a projection that is joined to the stapes at the bottom.

Infarction Death of bodily tissue due to deprivation of the blood supply.

Informational counseling The process of imparting information to clients and their families.

Inner ear The interior section of the ear, which contains the cochlea and vestibular system; supplies information to the brain regarding balance, spatial orientation, and hearing.

Intellectual developmental disorder A neurodevelopmental disorder characterized by intellectual difficulties as well as difficulties in conceptual, social, and practical areas of living.

Intellectual disability Delays in the development of the ability to gain knowledge and/or skills which often interfere with social functions and activities of daily living.

Intelligibility The ability to understand what has been detected aurally.

Intensity A measure of the magnitude of a sound, generally expressed in decibels.

Intentionality Goal directedness in interactions, which is first demonstrated at about 8 months of age, primarily through gestures.

Interdental Between the teeth; see *Linguadental*.

Intubated Having a tube placed to maintain an airway or to foster respiration by mechanical means.

Intubation Having a tube placed to maintain an airway or to foster respiration by mechanical means.

Ischemic stroke A cerebrovascular accident resulting from a complete or partial blockage or occlusion of the arteries transporting blood to the brain.

Jargon Strings of unintelligible speech sounds with the intonational pattern of adult speech.

Jejunostomy Surgical procedure that involves creating an opening in the abdomen into the jejunum, or middle part of the small intestine, and inserting a flexible feeding tube allowing food, liquids, and medications to be put directly into the stomach.

Jejunostomy tube (J-tube) A flexible feeding tube inserted into the jejunum, or middle part of the small intestine, allowing food, liquids, and medications to be put directly into the stomach.

Kinesics The study of bodily movement and gesture. Also known as body language.

Labiodental Pertaining to lips and teeth; phonemes produced with lip and tooth contact.

Language A socially shared code for representing concepts through the use of arbitrary symbols and rule-governed combinations of those symbols.

Language disorder Impairment in comprehension and/or use of spoken, written, and/or other symbol systems.

Language sampling A systematic collection and analysis of a person's speech or writing; sometimes called a corpus; used as a part of language assessment.

Laryngeal cancer Carcinoma of supraglottal, glottal, or subglottal structures.

Laryngeal papilloma A wartlike growth on the vocal folds.

Laryngeal system Structures of the larynx used for sound production.

Laryngeal webs Results from extraneous connective tissue growing between the vocal folds.

Larynx The superior termination of the trachea that protects the lower airways and is the primary sound source for speech production.

Latent aphasia Subtle impairment of linguistic abilities without clinical evidence of aphasia.

Later-developing hearing loss Hearing loss that is not evident early in life but becomes apparent at some later age.

Learning disability Disorder characterized by perceptual difficulties affecting language in all its forms.

Lexicon An individual's personal dictionary of words and meanings.

Linguadental Pertaining to tongue and teeth; phonemes produced with tongue and tooth contact.

Liquid Refers to the oral resonant consonants /r/ and /l/.

Literacy Use of visual modes of communication, specifically reading and writing.

Localization The process of determining where sound originates in space.

Locked-in syndrome A rare acquired neurological disorder that causes complete paralysis of all voluntary muscles in the body with the exception of eye movement; caused by a stroke or other acquired impairment affecting the brainstem. Individuals have consciousness but cannot move or speak; they can communicate via eye movements.

Malleus The largest of the ossicles; fastened to the eardrum and articulates with the incus, the next bone in the chain.

Manually coded English (MCE) Sign communication systems designed to manually duplicate spoken English for teaching children who are deaf.

Maternal rubella German measles contracted during pregnancy that may result in various disorders in the developing fetus.

Mean length of utterance (MLU) The average length of utterances, measured in morphemes; in English, an important measure of preschool development because language increases in complexity as it becomes longer.

Meniere's disease A condition resulting from excessive endolymph in the inner ear, involving vertigo, tinnitus, aural fullness, and sensorineural hearing loss.

Meningitis An inflammation of the meninges, or layers of tissue covering the brain and spinal cord.

Meta-analysis Determining the best evidence from multiple studies by ranking findings according to the strength of the data and then examining to see significant statistical trends and findings.

Metacognition Knowledge about knowledge and cognitive processes, including self-appraisal.

Metalinguistic skills Abilities that enable a child to consider language in the abstract, to make judgments about the correctness of language, and to create verbal contexts, such as in writing.

Microtia A congenital disorder that results in a small malformed pinna or ear canal.

Middle ear The section of the ear containing the ossicles; bounded laterally by the tympanic membrane and medially by the cochlea.

Middle ear space (or tympanic cavity) The cube-shaped area between the outer and middle ear that contains the ossicles.

Mixed dysarthrias Motor speech disorder characterized by two or more dysarthria types.

Mixed hearing loss The simultaneous presence of conductive and sensorineural hearing loss.

Modified barium swallow study (MBSS) An X-ray procedure that is used to visualize the swallowing process; also known as videofluoroscopy.

Monoloudness A voice lacking normal variations of intensity that occur during speech.

Monopitch A voice that lacks variation in fundamental frequency and inflection during speech production.

Morpheme The smallest meaningful unit of language.

Morphology An aspect of language concerned with rules governing change in meaning at the intraword level.

Motor cortex Located in the posterior portion of the frontal lobe of the brain and responsible for signaling the muscles of motor movement.

Multiple sclerosis (MS) A progressive disease characterized by demyelinization of nerve fibers of the brain and spinal cord.

Multiview videofluoroscopy Motion picture X-rays recorded from various angles.

Muscle tension dysphonia A functional voice disturbance caused by abnormal tightening of laryngeal muscles in the absence of structural or neurological abnormalities.

Myasthenia gravis An autoimmune disease characterized by rapid weakening of muscles due to inadequate transmission of nerve impulses to the muscles, causing sudden and significant hypernasality and articulatory imprecision with continued speaking.

Myringotomy A small surgical incision made in the surface of the tympanic membrane.

Nasal A phoneme that is produced with nasal resonance.

Nasalance score A numerical score that reflects the magnitude of hypernasality measured by a nasometer.

Nasogastric tube (NG tube) A tube placed into the nose and then through the pharynx and esophagus by which liquefied food may be fed.

Nasometer A commercially available device that is used to measure nasality.

Nasopharynx The space within the skull that is behind the nose and above the roof of the mouth.

Neurogenic stuttering A disorder of fluency associated with some form of brain damage.

Neuron The basic unit of the central nervous system, consisting of the cell body, axon, and dendrites.

Noise-induced hearing loss Hearing impairment that results from exposure to high levels of occupational or recreational noise.

Nonfluent aphasia Characterized by slow, labored speech and struggle to retrieve words and form sentences.

Nonvocal Without voice.

Norm-referenced A comparison that is usually based on others of the same gender and similar age.

Occipital lobe Located in the posterior region of the cortex, important for visual processing.

Omission In articulation, the absence of a phoneme that has not been produced or replaced.

Open syllable A syllable, or basic acoustic unit of speech, that ends in a vowel.

Organ of Corti The intricate structure that runs along the center of the membranous labyrinth of the cochlea and contains the auditory sensory receptor cells.

Ossicles (or ossicular chain) The small bones—the malleus, incus, and stapes—housed within the middle ear.

Otitis media Inflammation of the middle ear.

Otitis media with effusion (OME) Inflammation of the middle ear with fluid.

Otoacoustic emissions (OAEs) Measurable low-level sounds or echoes that occur either spontaneously or in response to acoustic stimulation, due to outer hair cell motility within the cochlea.

Otosclerosis A disorder characterized by the formation of spongy bone in the region of the stapes footplate, resulting in a progressive conductive hearing loss.

Otoscope A small handheld device used to visually inspect the external auditory canal and tympanic membrane.

Otoscopic examinations Visual examination of the ear canal and eardrum using an otoscope.

Ototoxic Refers to drugs and chemical agents that are potentially damaging to the inner ear.

Outer ear The section of the ear comprised of the pinna and the external auditory meatus, or ear canal.

Oval window A small oval membrane located on the lateral wall of the cochlea, behind the stapes footplate.

Palatal Refers to the front area of the roof of the mouth; in speech, palatal consonants are produced with the tongue touching or approximating the hard palate.

Palatal lift A prosthetic device for a weak or immobile soft palate.

Palatal obturator A plate that covers a portion of the soft palate; useful for individuals who have had palatal surgery.

Parietal lobe Located in the upper portion of the cortex and primarily responsible for storage; also important for memory and language processing.

Parkinson disease A slowly progressive movement disorder caused by loss of dopaminergic neurons in the substantia nigra (located in the midbrain), resulting in abnormal functioning of dopaminergic pathways in basal ganglia important for movement. It is characterized by resting tremor, slowness of movement, and difficulty initiating voluntary movements; speech may be rapid, breathy, and reduced in loudness, pitch range, and stress.

Partner-assisted scanning A technique in which a communication partner points to selections for an individual with a communication impairment to indicate their selection when the desired item is reached. The communication partner might aid in the efficiency of communication by first scanning through the rows then when the row is selected, scanning through the items one by one.

Pedunculated polyp A polyp that appears to be attached to the vocal fold by a stalk.

Percutaneous endoscopic gastrostomy (PEG, or G-tube) A surgical procedure that involves creating an opening through the abdomen to the stomach and inserting a flexible feeding tube allowing food, liquids, and medications to be put directly into the stomach.

Peripheral auditory system Part of the auditory system that includes the outer, middle, and inner ears as well as cranial nerve VIII (the auditory nerve).

Peripheral nervous system (PNS) The cranial and spinal nerves that receive and transmit information from the brain to the body.

Permanent threshold shift (PTS) A permanent change in hearing acuity associated with exposure to high-intensity noise.

Perpetuating cause See *Maintaining cause*.

Personal adjustment counseling The process of assisting clients and their families in dealing with the emotional consequences of hearing loss.

Personal hearing aid A personal amplification device ranging from tiny completely-in-the-canal models to those worn behind the ear.

Pharyngoplasty A generic term applied to various procedures used to improve velopharyngeal closure by changing the physical structure of the velopharyngeal mechanism.

Phonation Production of sound by vocal fold vibration.

Phonemic awareness Ability to manipulate sounds, such as blending sounds to create new words or segmenting words into sounds.

Phonics Sound-letter or phoneme-grapheme correspondence.

Phonological awareness (PA) Knowledge of sounds and syllables and of the sound structure of words.

Phonology The study of the sound systems of language.

Phonotactic The study of the way in which phonemes are combined and arranged into syllables and words of a particular language or dialect.

Physiology The branch of biology that is concerned with the process and function of parts of the body.

Pidgin Signed English (PSE) A sign system that incorporates ASL signs while maintaining English word order.

Pinna The funnel-shaped outermost part of the ear that collects sound waves and channels them into the ear canal.

Pitch The perceptual counterpart to fundamental frequency associated with the speed of vocal fold vibration.

Pitch breaks Sudden, uncontrolled upward or downward changes in pitch.

Pneumotachometer A vented mask that estimates oral or nasal airflow during breathing and/or production of /pi/ sounds.

Post-therapy testing Assessment following intervention.

Postlingually After the development of speech and language.

Pragmatics The use, function, or purpose of communication; the study of communicative acts and contexts.

Precipitating cause Factors that trigger a disorder (e.g., a stroke).

Predisposing cause Underlying factors that contribute to a problem (e.g., a genetic basis).

Prelingually Prior to the development of speech and language.

Presbycusis Hearing loss incurred as a result of the aging process.

Presbyphonia Voice disorder due to aging of the larynx.

Pressure equalization (PE) (or tympanostomy) tube A small-diameter tube that is surgically placed in the eardrum to provide ventilation of the middle ear space via the external auditory meatus.

Prevalence The total number of cases of a disorder at a particular point in time in a designated population.

Primary motor cortex A 2-centimeter-wide gyrus immediately in front of the central sulcus of the brain that controls voluntary motor movements.

Primary palatoplasty A term that refers to the first and perhaps only surgical closure of the palate.

Primary progressive aphasia (PPA) A neurodegenerative disorder characterized by a progressive decline of language ability and use with initial preservation of both other mental functions and activities of daily living.

Print awareness Knowledge of the meaning and function of print, including recognition of words and letters, and terminology, such as letter, word, or sentence.

Prognosis An informed prediction of the outcome of a disorder.

Prolongation In fluency analysis, the process of holding a phoneme longer than is typical (e.g., "sssssso").

Prolonged speech A group of speech rate reduction techniques (e.g., prolonged, continuous phonation; gentle voicing onsets; light articulatory contacts) used to treat stuttering and establish stutter-free speech.

Proxemics The study of physical distance between people.

Proximal Toward the center.

Psychogenic Caused by psychological factors.

Psychogenic (functional) voice disorders General term for functional voice abnormalities, or those without an organic cause, often resulting from laryngeal hyperfunction and linked to emotional stresses such as anxiety, fear, anger, frustration, and depression; may lead to structural voice abnormalities.

Pure tone audiometry A procedure that is used to assess hearing sensitivity at discrete frequencies.

Pure tones Sounds that contain energy at only a single frequency, such as 250 Hz, 500 Hz, 1000 Hz, 2000 Hz, 4000 Hz, and 8000 Hz, used in pure tone audiometry.

Purulent (or suppurative) otitis media Pus formation and discharge by the tissue of the middle ear cavity.

Pyramidal tract Descending motor fibers that arise from the motor cortex and mediate rapid, discrete, skilled volitional movement; also known as the direct activation pathway or direct motor system.

Range of motion The extent of movement of a joint from maximum extension to maximum flexion.

Rarefaction Part of the sound wave where the displaced molecules are far from each other.

Rate The speed at which something occurs. In speech this may be the number of words or syllables in a given period of time.

Recurrent laryngeal nerve A branch of the vagus nerve (cranial nerve X) that supplies the majority of laryngeal muscles used for voice production.

Reduplicated babbling Long strings of consonant–vowel syllable repetitions, such as "ma-ma-ma-ma-ma."

Reformulation An adult response to a child's utterance in which the adult adds to the child's utterance to provide a more complex example of what the child has said.

Rehabilitation The process of regaining skills, abilities, or knowledge that might have been lost due to an acquired condition resulting in loss of skills.

Reinforces Uses a procedure that follows a response with the intent of perpetuating or extinguishing it; used in conditioning.

Repetition In fluency analysis, the process of repeating a word or a part of a word, as in "the-the-the" or "b-b-ball."

Representation The process of having one thing stand for another, such as a piece of paper used as a blanket for a doll.

Respiratory system Structures, including the lungs, bronchi, trachea, larynx, mouth, and nose, that are used in breathing for life and for speech.

Resting tidal breathing Breathing to sustain life.

Right-hemisphere damage (RHD) A group of neuromuscular, perceptual, and/or linguistic deficits that results from damage to the right hemisphere of the brain and may include epilepsy, hemisensory impairment, and hemiparesis or hemiplegia.

Screening An abbreviated testing procedure to determine who is likely to have hearing loss and need comprehensive testing.

Self-monitoring The ability to recognize one's own errors and correct them.

Semantic compaction Picture-based systems that allow for reduced effort needed to compose messages, by combining symbols to represent words and phrases.

Semi-implantable devices Bone conduction devices that require surgically housing some portion of the device in the ear or skull.

Sensorineural Refers to hearing loss involving problems with the inner ear and/or auditory nerve.

Sensorineural hearing loss Hearing problems with the inner ear and/or auditory nerve.

Sensorineural system Part of the auditory system made up of the inner ear and cranial nerve VIII.

Sensory-motor approach Articulatory training that emphasizes tactile and proprioceptive sensations and sound, syllable, and word production.

Serous otitis media Inflammation of the middle ear with sterile fluid.

Sessile polyp A polyp with a broad-based attachment to the vocal fold.

Silent aspiration The entrance of food or liquid into the airway that is not accompanied by coughing.

Social cognition The ability to process, store, and apply information about other people and social situations.

Sociolinguistics The study of influences such as cultural identity, setting, and participants on communicative variables.

Sound field amplification A type of assistive listening device that transmits sound from a microphone to loudspeakers that are strategically placed within a room.

Spasmodic dysphonia (SD) A voice disorder characterized by hyperadduction of the vocal folds, resulting in strained/strangled voice production with intermittent stoppages.

Spastic dysarthria Speech that is characterized as slow, with jerky, imprecise articulation and reduction of the rapidly alternating movements of speech because of stiff and rigid muscles.

Spasticity An exaggerated response to passive stretch at a joint that occurs in one direction. In the limbs, spasticity tends to affect the arm flexor muscles and the leg extensor muscles.

Speech bulb obturator A prosthesis that fills the velopharyngeal space, closing the velopharyngeal portal.

Speech disorder Atypical production of speech sounds, interruption in the flow of speaking, or abnormal production and/or absences of voice quality, including pitch, loudness, resonance, and/or duration.

Speech Recognition Threshold (SRT) A test procedure used in speech audiometry that measures the lowest (quietest) level at which a person can recognize approximately 50% of the spondees presented for a given number of trials.

Speech-language pathologist (SLP) A professional whose distinguishing role is to identify, assess, treat, and prevent speech, language, communication, and swallowing disorders.

Speech-language pathology assistant (SLPA) Professionals who usually have a bachelor's degree in communication sciences and disorders and can administer tests and therapy under a speech-language pathologist's direction, but cannot diagnose a disorder or provide intervention independently.

Spinal nerves Any of the 31 pairs of nerves in the peripheral nervous system, containing sensory and motor fibers that arise from each side of the spinal cord to innervate the body.

Spontaneous recovery A natural recovery process that proceeds without professional intervention.

Stapes The third and smallest of the ossicles in the middle ear.

Stereocilia Small hairlike projections situated on the top of the hair cells in the organ of Corti.

Stimulability The ability to imitate a target phoneme when given focused auditory and visual cues.

Stimulus Anything that is capable of eliciting a response.

Stop consonants A consonant phoneme produced by building air pressure behind the point of constriction.

Stridor Noisy breathing or involuntary sound that accompanies inspiration and expiration.

Stroke A cerebrovascular accident, the most common cause of aphasia, which results when the blood supply to the brain is blocked or when the brain is flooded with blood.

Stuttering A disorder of speech fluency characterized by hesitations, repetitions, prolongations, tension, and avoidance behaviors.

Substitution In articulation, the production of one phoneme in place of another.

Support group Individuals with similar problems who meet together to share feelings, information, and ideas.

Suppurative otitis media See *Purulent otitis media*.

Supramarginal gyrus Portion of the cortex responsible for morphosyntactic recall.

Switches Devices that are used to activate or deactivate an electrical circuit. Adapted switches are used by those with limitations in movements to control devices that could include augmentative or alternative communication systems, environmental controls, or switch-activated toys.

Symbolization Use of an arbitrary symbol, such as a word or sign, to stand for something.

Synapse The minuscule space between the axon of one neuron and the dendrites of the next, where "communication" between neurons occurs.

Syntax How words are arranged in sentences.

Synthesized speech Computer-generated preprogrammed voice output generated by a speech synthesizer.

Tectorial membrane The gelatinous tongue-shaped structure that forms the roof of the organ of Corti.

Telepractice Provision of communication and swallowing assessment and intervention via the Internet.

Temporal lobe Located laterally in the brain, important in incoming and outgoing language processing.

Temporary threshold shift (TTS) A temporary change in hearing acuity followed by spontaneous recovery that is associated with short-term exposure to high-intensity noise.

Threshold The lowest (quietest) presentation level (measured in decibels) at which a person can barely detect a stimulus 50% of the time it is presented.

Thrombosis The formation or presence of a blood clot within a blood vessel of the body; may result in an ischemic stroke.

Thyroid cartilage Largest of the laryngeal cartilages that forms most of the front and sides of the laryngeal skeleton and protects the inner components of the larynx.

Thyroid prominence Anterior outward projection of the thyroid cartilage that is more prominent in males than females; also called the Adam's apple.

Tics Involuntary, rapid and repetitive, stereotypic movements.

Trachea A cartilaginous membranous tube by which air moves to and from the lungs.

Tracheoesophageal puncture (TEP) or tracheoesophageal shunt A device that directs air from the trachea to the esophagus for esophageal speech.

Tracheostomy Surgical procedure that involves creating a stoma (hole) in the trachea and inserting a tube to relieve a breathing obstruction.

Traditional motor approach An articulation treatment approach that emphasizes discrete skill learning, beginning first with auditory discrimination of the error sound followed by production training of the sound in isolation, in nonsense syllables, and then in words, phrases, sentences, and conversations.

Transcortical motor aphasia A nonfluent aphasia that is characterized by impaired conversational speech, good verbal imitative abilities, and mildly impaired auditory comprehension.

Transcortical sensory aphasia A rare fluent aphasia that is characterized by word substitutions, lack of nouns and severe anomia, and poor auditory comprehension but featuring the ability to repeat or imitate words, phrases, and sentences.

Transient ischemic attack (TIA) Sometimes called a mini-stroke, a condition that occurs when blood flow to some portion of the brain is blocked or reduced temporarily.

Traumatic brain injury (TBI) Damage to the brain that results from bruising and laceration caused by forceful contact with the relatively rough inner surfaces of the skull or from secondary edema or swelling, infarction or death of tissue, and hematoma or focal bleeding.

Tremor Involuntary, rhythmic movement of a body part.

Tympanic membrane (or eardrum) The thin cone-shaped structure composed of three layers of tissue located at the end of the external auditory meatus; set into vibration as acoustic energy strikes its surface.

Tympanogram A graph generated during acoustic immittance testing that depicts compliance of the eardrum relative to changes in air pressure.

Tympanometry The process of measuring the overall middle ear function as different amounts of air pressure are introduced into the ear canal.

Unilateral Used to refer to hearing disorders that occur on one side only.

Upper airway system Subdivision of the speech and swallowing mechanism comprising the pharynx (throat), velopharynx, oral, and nasal cavities and their associated structures.

Usher's syndrome A hereditary disorder characterized by sensorineural hearing impairment and progressive blindness.

Uvula A small, pendulous structure suspended from the soft palate.

Velar Refers to the posterior area of the roof of the mouth; in speech, velar consonants are produced with the tongue touching or approximating the velum or soft palate.

Velopharyngeal closure Contact of the velum with the lateral and posterior pharyngeal walls, thus separating the oral and nasal cavities.

Velopharyngeal dysfunction (VPD) Inability of the velopharyngeal mechanism to separate the oral and nasal cavities during swallowing and speech.

Vernix A waxy protective substance that covers the skin of a fetus.

Vestibular schwannoma A benign growth that develops on cranial nerve VIII and can impact both balance and hearing, commonly referred to as an acoustic neuroma.

Vestibular system Structures of the inner ear that are responsible for supplying information to the brain regarding balance and spatial orientation.

Vestibulocochlear nerve (or VIIIth cranial nerve) The cranial nerve that runs from the base of the cochlea to the cochlear nucleus of the brainstem; composed of the vestibular and cochlear branches.

Videofluoroscopy See *Modified barium swallow study.*

Videonasendoscopy An invasive instrumental procedure involving a flexible fiberoptic nasopharyngoscope that allows direct observation of velopharyngeal function during speech production.

Videostroboscopy A technique to visualize the larynx that uses a flashing strobe light to create the illusion of the vocal folds vibrating in slow motion, providing a detailed view of the vibratory characteristics of the vocal folds during phonation. Endoscopy may be used in conjunction with videostroboscopy.

Visual reinforcement audiometry (VRA) A method of hearing assessment in which a child is rewarded for localizing to a test signal through the use of moving toys and/or flashing lights.

Visual schedule Uses objects, symbols, or words to depict a sequence of steps or a series of activities. It can help an individual prepare for transitions or follow sequences of events or tasks.

Vocal abuse Any of several behaviors, including smoking and yelling, that can result in damage to the laryngeal mechanism.

Vocal fold paralysis Immobilization of the vocal fold, usually due to nerve damage.

Vocal nodules Localized growths on the vocal folds that are associated with vocal abuse.

Vocal polyp A fluid-filled lesion of the vocal fold that results from mechanical stress.

Voice Vocal tone and resonance.

Voice banking A process that enables a person to record samples of their own voice so it can be replicated by a computer synthesizer if they lose the ability to speak. This allows an individual who may lose their ability to speak to retain a voice through augmentative or alternative communication that sounds like their natural voice.

Voice tremor Variations in the pitch and loudness of the voice that are involuntary.

Voicing Refers to what the vocal folds are doing during consonant sound production. If the vocal folds are vibrating during sound production, the consonant is said to be voiced; if the folds are not vibrating, the consonant sound is voiceless.

Vowel Any of several voiced phonemes that are produced with a relatively open vocal tract.

Waardenburg's syndrome A hereditary disorder characterized by pigmentary discoloration, particularly in the irises and hair; craniofacial malformation of the nasal area; and severe to profound hearing impairment.

Wernicke's aphasia A fluent aphasia that is characterized by rapid-fire strings of sentences with little pause for acknowledgment or turn taking. Content may seem to be a jumble and may be incoherent or incomprehensible, although fluent and well articulated.

Wernicke's area Located in the left temporal lobe of the brain and responsible for processing of language.

Word prediction Used when typing text, it suggests or attempts to predict the word being typed to allow more efficient typing of a message.

Word Recognition Test (WRT) A test procedure used in speech audiometry to measure an individual's ability to recognize single-syllable words presented at a predetermined level above their auditory threshold.

Working memory (WM) An active cognitive process that allows limited information to be held in a temporarily accessible state while cognitive processing occurs.

REFERENCES

Abitbol, J., Abitbol, P., & Abitbol, B. (1999). Sex hormones and the female voice. *Journal of Voice, 13,* 424–446.

Abrams, H. (2017). Hearing loss and associated co-morbidities: What do we know? *Hearing Review, 24*(12), 32–35.

Abrams, H. B., & Kihm, J. (2015). An introduction to MarkeTrak IX: A new baseline for the hearing aid market. *Hearing Review, 22*(6), 16–22. https://hearingreview.com/2015/05/introduction-marketrak-ix-new-baseline-hearing-aid-market

Acar B., Yurekli M., Babademez M. Karabulut H. &, Karasen R. (2011). Effects of hearing aids on cognitive functions and depressive signs in elderly people. *Archives of Gerontology and Geriatrics,* 52(3), 250–252.

Adams, C. (2005). Social communication intervention for school-age children: Rationale and description. *Seminars in Speech and Language, 26*(3), 181–188.

Adesope, O., Lavin, T., Thompson, T., & Ungerleider, C. (2010). A systematic review and meta-analysis of the cognitive correlates of bilingualism. *Review of Educational Research, 80,* 207–245.

Adler, R. (2017). The SLP as counselor for the transgender client. *Perspectives of the ASHA Special Interest Groups, 2,* 92–101.

Aikens, N. L., & Barbarin, O. (2008). Socioeconomic differences in reading trajectories: The contribution of family, neighborhood, and school contexts. *Journal of Educational Psychology, 100*(2), 235–251.

Al Otaiba, S., Gillespie Rouse, A., & Baker, K. (2018). Elementary grade intervention approaches to treat specific learning disabilities, including dyslexia. *Language, Speech, and Hearing Services in Schools, 49,* 829–842.

Allen, A., S. R., Brock, K. L., & Shane, H. C. (2017). The effectiveness of aided augmented input techniques for persons with developmental disabilities: A systematic review. *Augmentative and Alternative Communication,* 149–159. https://doi.org/10.1080/07434618.2017.1338752

Alliano, A., Herriger, K., Koutsoftas, A., & Bartolotta, T. (2016). A review of 21 iPad applications for augmentative and alternative communication purposes. *Perspectives on Augmentative and Alternative Communication, 21*(2), 60–71.

Alloway, T. P., & Alloway, R. G. (2010). Investigating the predictive roles of working memory and IQ in academic attainment. *Journal of Experimental Child Psychology, 106*(1), 20–29.

Altmann, L., Lombardino, L. J., & Puranik, C. (2008). Sentence production in students with dyslexia. *International Journal of Language & Communication Disorders, 43*(1), 55–76.

Alzheimer's Association. (2017). *Alzheimer's disease facts and figure.* http://www.alz.org/facts/overview.asp

Alzheimer's Association. (2022). *Alzheimer's disease facts and figures.* https://www.alz.org/media/Documents/alzheimers-facts-and-figures.pdf

Alzrayer, N., Banda, D. R., & Koul, R. K. (2014). Use of iPad/iPods with individuals with autism and other developmental disabilities: A meta-analysis of communication interventions. *Review Journal of Autism and Developmental Disorders, 1,* 179–191.

Ambrose, N., & Yairi, E. (2002). The Tudor study: Data and ethics. *American Journal of Speech-Language Pathology, 11,* 190–203.

Ambrose, N., Cox, N., & Yairi, E. (1997). The genetic basis of persistence and recovery in stuttering. *Journal of Speech, Language, and Hearing Research, 40,* 567–580.

Amendah, D., Grosse, S. D., Peacock, G., & Mandell, D. S. (2011). The economic costs of autism: A review. In D. Amaral, D. Geschwind, & G. Dawson (Eds.), *Autism spectrum disorders* (pp. 1347–1360). Oxford University Press.

American Academy of Audiology. (2004). *Scope of practice.* https://www.audiology.org/practice-resources/practice-guidelines-and-standards/scope-of-practice/

American Academy of Audiology. (2010). *Clinical practice guidelines: Diagnosis, treatment, and management of children and adults with central auditory processing disorder.* Author.

American Academy of Audiology. (2020). *Clinical guidance document on assessment of hearing in infants and young children.* https://www.audiology.org/wp-content/uploads/2021/05/Clin-Guid-Doc_Assess_Hear_Infants_Children_1.23.20-1.pdf

American Academy of Audiology. (2021). *Commentary on FDA's proposed rule for medical devices; Ear, nose and throat devices; Establishing over-the-counter hearing aids.* https://www.audiology.org/wp-content/uploads/2021/12/AAA-OTC-HAComments12.2021.pdf

American Academy of Audiology. (n.d.). *Assistive listening and alerting devices.* https://www.audiology.org/consumers-and-patients/managing-hearing-loss/assistive-listening-and-alerting-devices/

American Academy of Pediatrics. (2022). *Fetal alcohol spectrum disorders: FAQs of parents & families.* https://www.healthychildren.org/English/health-issues/conditions/chronic/Pages/Fetal-Alcohol-Spectrum-Disorders-FAQs-of-Parents-and-Families.aspx

American Association on Intellectual and Developmental Disabilities. (2009). *Definition of intellectual disability.* www.aaidd.org/content_100.cfm?navID=21

American Cancer Society. (2021, January 21). *Risk factors for laryngeal and hypopharyngeal cancers.* https://www.cancer.org/cancer/laryngeal-and-hypopharyngeal-cancer/causes-risks-prevention/risk-factors.html

American Psychiatric Association. (1994). *Diagnostic and statistical manual of mental disorders* (4th ed.). Author.

American Psychiatric Association. (2000). *Diagnostic and statistical manual of mental disorders* (4th ed., text rev.). Author.

American Psychiatric Association. (2013). *Diagnostic and Statistical Manual of mental disorders* (5th ed.). Author.

American Psychiatric Association. (2018, November). *What is specific learning disorder.* Accessed on August 19, 2019 at https://www.psychiatry.org/patients-families/specific-learning-disorder/what-is-specific-learning-disorder

American Speech-Language-Hearing Association (ASHA). (1994). *Functional assessment of communicative skills for adults (FACS).* Author.

American Speech-Language-Hearing Association (ASHA). (1995). *Facilitated communication [Position Statement].* Author.

American Speech-Language-Hearing Association (ASHA). (2000a). *Background information for the standards and implementation for the certificate of clinical competence in speech-language pathology.* http://professional.asha.org/library/slp_standards.htm

American Speech-Language-Hearing Association (ASHA). (2000b). *Background information for the standards and implementation for the certificate of clinical competence in audiology.* http://professional.asha.org/library/audiology_standards.htm

American Speech-Language-Hearing Association (ASHA). (2000c). *Fact sheet: Speech-language pathology.* http://professional.asha.org/students/careers/slp.htm

American Speech-Language-Hearing Association (ASHA). (2001a, December 26). Code of ethics (revised). *ASHA Leader, 6*(23), 2.

American Speech-Language-Hearing Association (ASHA). (2001b). *Standards for accreditation of graduate education programs in audiology and speech-language pathology.* http://professional.asha.org/students/caa_programs/standards.htm

American Speech-Language-Hearing Association (ASHA). (2001c). *Fact sheet: Audiology.* http://professional.asha.org/students/careers/audiology.htm

American Speech-Language-Hearing Association (ASHA). (2001d). *Roles and responsibilities of speech-language pathologists with respect to reading and writing in children and adolescents* [Position paper, technical report, and guidelines]. Author.

American Speech-Language-Hearing Association (ASHA). (2004). Scope of practice in audiology. *ASHA Supplement, 24.*

American Speech-Language-Hearing Association (ASHA). (2005a). *Augmentative and alternative communication: Knowledge and skills for service delivery* [Knowledge and skills]. https://www.asha.org/policy

American Speech-Language-Hearing Association (ASHA). (2005b). *(Central) auditory processing disorders* [Knowledge and skills]. https://www.asha.org/policy/TR2005-00043/

American Speech-Language-Hearing Association (ASHA). (2005c). *(Central) auditory processing disorders* [Technical report]. http://www.asha.org/policy

American Speech-Language-Hearing Association (ASHA). (2007). *Childhood apraxia of speech* [Position statement]. www.asha.org/policy

American Speech-Language-Hearing Association (ASHA). (2008). *Treatment efficacy summary: Cognitive-communication disorders resulting from right hemisphere brain damage.* www.asha.org/uploaded-Files/public/TESCognitiveCommunicationDisordersfromRightHemisphereBrainDamage.pdf

American Speech-Language-Hearing Association (ASHA). (2009) *About the American Speech-Language-Hearing Association (ASHA).* www.asha.org/about_asha.htm

American Speech-Language-Hearing Association (ASHA). (2010). *2010 Audiology survey summary report: Number and type of responses.* Author.

American Speech-Language-Hearing Association (ASHA). (2010). *Roles and responsibilities of speech-language pathologists in schools.* http://www.asha.org/policy/PI2010-00317/

American Speech-Language-Hearing Association (ASHA). (2016). *Code of ethics.* https://www.asha.org/policy/et2016-00342/

American Speech-Language-Hearing Association (ASHA). (2018a). *Facilitated communication [Position Statement].* https://www.asha.org/policy/ps2018-00352/

American Speech-Language-Hearing Association (ASHA). (2018b). *Rapid prompting method [Position Statement].* https://www.asha.org/policy/ps2018-00351/

American Speech-Language-Hearing Association (ASHA). (2019). *Social communication disorder.* https://www.asha.org/practice-portal/clinical-topics/social-communication-disorder

American Speech-Language-Hearing Association (ASHA). (2020a, January 1). *2020 Standards and implementation procedures for the certificate of clinical competence in audiology.* https://www.asha.org/certification/2020-audiology-certification-standards/

American Speech-Language-Hearing Association (ASHA). (2020b, January 1). *2020 Standards and implementation procedures for the certificate of clinical competence in speech-language pathology.* https://www.asha.org/certification/2020-slp-certification-standards/

American Speech-Language-Hearing Association (ASHA). (2021). *ASHA SLP Health Care Survey 2021: Caseload characteristics.* Author.

American Speech-Language-Hearing Association (ASHA). (2022a). *Using the Interprofessional Practice (IPP) Case Rubric*. https://www.asha.org/siteassets/ipp/using-the-interprofessional-practice-ipp-case-rubric.pdf

American Speech-Language-Hearing Association (ASHA). (2022b). *Interprofessional education/interprofessional practice (IPE/IPP)*. https://www.asha.org/practice/ipe-ipp/

American Speech-Language-Hearing Association (ASHA). (2022c). *Adult dysphagia*. https://www.asha.org/Practice-Portal/Clinical-Topics/Adult-Dysphagia/

American Speech-Language-Hearing Association (ASHA). (n.d.). *About speech, language, and hearing scientist careers*. https://www.asha.org/students/about-speech-language-and-hearing-scientist-careers/

American Speech-Language-Hearing Association (ASHA). (n.d.). *About the American Speech-Language-Hearing Association*. https://www.asha.org/about/

American Speech-Language-Hearing Association (ASHA). (n.d.). *Central auditory processing disorders*. https://www.asha.org/practice-portal/clinical-topics/central-auditory-processing-disorder/

American Speech-Language-Hearing Association (ASHA). (n.d.). *Right hemisphere damage*. https://www.asha.org/practice-portal/clinical-topics/right-hemisphere-damage/

American Speech-Language-Hearing Association (ASHA). (n.d.). *Using the interprofessional practice (IPP) case rubric*. https://www.asha.org/siteassets/ipp/using-the-interprofessional-practice-ipp-case-rubric.pdf

American Speech-Language-Hearing Association (ASHA). (n.d.-a). *Cultural competence*. (Practice Portal). https://www.asha.org/Practice-Portal/Professional-Issues/Cultural-Competence/

American Speech-Language-Hearing Association (ASHA). (n.d.-b). *Working with culturally and linguistically diverse (CLD) students in schools*. https://www.asha.org/slp/cldinschools/

ANCDS TBI Writing Committee. (2022). Tutorial: The speech-language pathologist's role in return to work for adults with traumatic brain injury. *American Journal of Speech-Language Pathology, 31*, 188–202.

Anderson J. (2014). Pitch elevation in transgendered patients: Anterior glottic web formation assisted by temporary injection augmentation. *Journal of Voice, 28*, 816–821.

Andreu, L., Sanz-Torrent, M., & Guardia-Olmos, J. (2012). Auditory word recognition of nouns and verbs in children with specific language impairment (SLI). *Journal of Communication Disorders, 45*, 20–34.

Andrews, C., O'Brian, S., Harrison, E., Onslow, M., Packman, A., & Menzies, R. (2012). Syllable-timed speech treatment for school-age children who stutter: A phase I trial. *Language, Speech, and Hearing Services in Schools, 43*, 359–369.

Andrews, G., Craig, A., Feyer, A. M., Hoddinott, S., Howie, P., & Neilson, M. (1983). Stuttering: A review of research findings and theories circa 1982. *Journal of Speech and Hearing Disorders, 48*, 226–246.

Andrews, G., Hoddinott, S., Craig, A., Howie, P., Feyer, A-M., & Neilson, M. (1983). Stuttering: A review of research findings and theories circa 1982. *Journal of Speech and Hearing Disorders, 48*, 226–246.

Angelo, D. (2000). Impact of augmentative and alternative communication devices on families. *Augmentative and Alternative Communication, 16*(1), 37–47.

Anthony, J. L., Davis, C., Williams, J. M., & Anthony, T. I. (2014). Preschoolers' oral language abilities: A multilevel examination of dimensionality. *Learning and Individual Differences, 35*, 56–61.

Apel, K., & Masterson, J. (2001). Theory-guided spelling assessment and intervention: A case study. *Language, Speech, and Hearing Services in Schools, 32*, 182–194.

Apel, K., & Self, T. (2003). Evidence-based practice: The marriage of research and clinical practice. *The ASHA Leader, 8*(16), 6–7.

Apel, K., & Werfel, K. (2014). Using morphological awareness instruction to improve written language skills. *Language, Speech, and Hearing Services in Schools, 45*, 251–260.

Archibald, L. M., & Joanisse, M. (2009). On the sensitivity and specificity of nonword repetition and sentence recall to language and memory impairments in children. *Journal of Speech, Language, and Hearing Research, 52*, 899–914.

Aronson, A. E. (1990a). *Clinical voice disorders*. Thieme.

Aronson, A. (1990b). Importance of the psychosocial interview in the diagnosis and treatment of "functional" voice disorders. *Journal of Voice, 4*, 287–289.

Arvedson, J. (2008). Assessment of pediatric dysphagia and feeding disorders: clinical and instrumental approaches. *Developmental Disabilities Research Review, 14*, 118–127. https://doi.org/10.1002/ddrr.17

Arvedson, J. (2009, June 19). *Pediatric feeding and swallowing disorders. Treatment efficacy summary*. www.asha.org/NR/rdonlyres/EEE3706F-215C-428B-A461-3ABFA8C0787A/0/TESPediatricFeedingandSwallowing.pdf

Arvedson, J. (2013). Feeding children with cerebral palsy and swallowing difficulties. *European Journal of Clinical Nutrition, 67*, S9–S12.

Arvedson, J., Brodsky, L., & Lefton-Greif, M. (2020). *Pediatric feeding and swallowing: Assessment and management*. Plural Publishing.

Arvedson, J., Clark, H., Lazarus, C., Schooling, T., & Frymark, T. (2010). Evidence-based systematic review: Effects of oral motor interventions on feeding and swallowing in preterm infants. *American Journal of Speech-Language Pathology, 19*, 321–340.

Ashford, J. R., Logemann, J. A., & McCullough, G. (2009a, June 19). *Swallowing disorders (dysphagia) in adults. Treatment efficacy summary.* www.asha.org/NR/rdonlyres/1EC1FFDC-CDD2-4569-AB57-319987BFB858/0/TESDysphagiainAdults.pdf

Ashford, J. R., McCabe, D., Wheeler-Hegland, K., Frymark, T., Mullen, R., Musson, N., et al. (2009b). Evidence-based systematic review: Oropharyngeal dysphagia behavioral treatments: Part III. Impact of dysphagia treatments on populations with neurological disorders. *Journal of Rehabilitation Research & Development, 46,* 195–204.

Associated Press. (2013, April 4). Study: Dementia leader in cost. *Times Union* (Albany, NY), A6.

Baade, A. (2022). Ending audism begins with education. *The ASHA Leader, 27*(3). https://leader.pubs.asha.org/do/10.1044/leader.FMP.27032022.ableism-audism.4/full/

Bacon, E. C., Osuna, S., Courchesne, E., & Pierce, K. (2018). Naturalistic language sampling to characterize the language abilities of 3-year-olds with autism spectrum disorder. *Autism.* https://doi.org/10.1177/1362361318766241

Bailey, R. (2005). Tracheostomy and dysphagia: A complex association. *Perspectives on Swallowing and Swallowing Disorders (Dysphagia), 14,* 2–7.

Bainbridge, K., Hoffman, H., & Cowie, C. (2008). Diabetes and hearing impairment in the United States: Audiometric evidence from the National Health and Nutrition Examination Survey, 1999–2004. *Annals of Internal Medicine, 149*(1), 1–10.

Baken, R., & Orlikoff, R. (2000). *Clinical management of speech and voice* (2nd ed.). Singular Press.

Ball, L. J., & Lasker, J. (2013). Teaching partners to support communication for adults with acquired communication impairment. *Perspectives on Augmentative and Alternative Communication, 22*(1), 4–15. https://doi.org/10.1044/aac22.1.4

Ball, L. J., Marvin, C. A., Beukelman, D. R., Lasker, J., & Rupp, D. (2000). Generic talk use by preschool children. *Augmentative and Alternative Communication, 16,* 145–155.

Balsamo, L., Xu, B., Grandin, C., & Petrella, J., et al. (2002). A functional magnetic resonance imaging study of left hemisphere language dominance in children. *Archives of Neurology, 59,* 1168–1174.

Bangert, K. J., Halverson, D. M., & Finestack, L. H. (2019). Evaluation of an explicit instructional approach to teach grammatical forms to children with low-symptom severity autism spectrum disorder. *American Journal of Speech-Language Pathology, 28*(2), 650–663. https://doi.org/10.1044/2018_AJSLP-18-0016

Bankson, N., & Bernthal, J. (1990). *Bankson-Bernthal test of phonology.* PRO-ED.

Barker, R. M., Akaba, S., Brady, N. C., & Thiemann-Bourque, K. (2013). Support for AAC use in preschool, and growth in language skills, for young children with developmental disabilities. *Augmentative and Alternative Communication, 29*(4), 334–346.

Barkmeier-Kraemer, J. (2012). Updates on vocal tremor and its management. *Perspectives of the ASHA Special Interest Groups, 1,* 97–103.

Barkmeier-Kramer, J. (2016, November). *How do principles of speech science inform clinical practice for voice disorders?* Oral presentation presented at the annual convention of the American Speech-Language-Hearing Association, Philadelphia.

Barnes, G., & Toms, N. (2021). An overview of tracheostomy tubes and mechanical ventilation management for the speech-language pathologist. *Perspectives of the ASHA Special Interest Groups, 6,* 885–896.

Barth, A. E., & Elleman, A. (2017). Evaluating the impact of a multistrategy inference intervention for middle-grade struggling readers. *Language, Speech, and Hearing Services in Schools, 48,* 31–41.

Bartow, C., Collins, N., Kopp, E., & Guillamondegui, O. (2018). Benefits of a multidisciplinary tracheostomy team: Acute care experience. *Perspectives of the ASHA Special Interest Groups, 3,* 89–100.

Baum, S., & Dwivedi, V. (2003). Sensitivity to prosodic structure in left- and right-hemisphere-damaged individuals. *Brain and Language, 87,* 278–289.

Baylor, C., Burns, M., McDonough, K., Mach, H., & Yorkston, K. (2019). Teaching medical students skills for effective communication with patients who have communication disorders. *American Journal of Speech-Language Pathology, 28,* 155–164.

Baylor, C., Yorkston, K., Eadie, T., Kim, J., Chung, H., & Amtmann, D. (2013). The Communicative Participation Item Bank (CPIB): Item bank calibration and development of a disorder-generic short form. *Journal of Speech, Language, and Hearing Research, 56,* 1190–1208. https://doi.org/10.1044/1092-4388(2012/12-0140)

Bear, D. R., Invernizzi, M., Templeton, S., & Johnston, F. (2000). *Words their way: Word study for phonics, vocabulary, and spelling instruction* (2nd ed.). Prentice Hall.

Bear, D. R., Invernizzi, M., Templeton, S., & Johnston, F. (2004). *Words their way: Word study with phonics, vocabulary, and spelling instruction* (3rd ed.). Merrill/Prentice Hall.

Bear, D. R., Invernizzi, M., Templeton, S., & Johnston, F. (2016). *Words their way* (6th ed.). Pearson.

Beck, D., & Fabry, D. (2011, January/February). Access America: It's about connectivity. *Audiology Today,* 24–29.

Bedore, L. M. (2010). Choosing the language of intervention for Spanish–English bilingual preschoolers with language impairment. *EBP Briefs, 5*(1), 1–13.

Bedore, L. M., & Leonard, L. B. (2001). Grammatical morphological deficits in Spanish-speaking children with specific language impairment. *Journal of Speech, Language, and Hearing Research, 44,* 905–924.

Bedore, L. M., Peña, E. D., Fiestas, C., & Lugo-Neris, M. J. (2020). Language and literacy together: Supporting grammatical development in dual language learners with risk for language and learning difficulties. *Language, Speech, and Hearing Services in Schools, 51,* 282–297.

Beecher, R., & Alexander, R. (2004). Pediatric feeding and swallowing: Clinical examination and evaluation. *Perspectives on Swallowing and Swallowing Disorders (Dysphagia), 13,* 21–27.

Behrman, A. (2007). *Speech and voice science.* Plural Publishing.

Behrman, A., Rutledge, J., Hembree, A., & Sheridan, S. (2008). Voice hygiene education, voice production therapy, and the role of patient adherence: a treatment effectiveness study in women with phonotrauma. *Journal of Speech, Language, and Hearing Research, 51,* 350–366.

Belin, P., Zatorre, R. J., Lafaille, P., Ahad, P., & Pike, B. (2000) Voice-selective areas in human auditory cortex. *Nature, 403,* 309–312.

Bellinger, L., Ouellette, N., & Robertson, J. (2021). The effectiveness of physical, occupational, and speech therapy in the treatment of patients with COVID-19 in the inpatient rehabilitation setting. *Perspectives of the ASHA Special Interest Groups, 6*(5), 1291–1298.

Belmonte. M.K., & Bourgeron, T. (2006). Fragile X syndrome and autism at the intersection of genetic and neural networks. *Nature Neuroscience, 9,* 1221–1225. https://doi.org/10.1038/nn1765

Benelli, B., Belacchi, C., Gini, G., & Lucanggeli, D. (2006). "To define means to say what you know about things": The development of definitional skills as metalinguistic acquisition. *Journal of Child Language, 33,* 71–97.

Benfer, K., Weir, K., Bell, K., Ware, R., Davies, P., & Boyd, R. (2013). Oropharyngeal dysphagia and gross motor skills in children with cerebral palsy. *Pediatrics, 131,* 1553–1562.

Bent, T., & Holt, R., (2017). Representation of speech variability. *Wiley Interdisciplinary Reviews: Cognitive Science, 8*(4), e1434.

Bergman, R. L., Piacentini, J., & McCracken, J. (2002). Prevalence and description of selective mutism in a school-based sample. *Journal of the American Academy of Child and Adolescent Psychiatry, 41,* 938–946.

Berlin, C., Hood, L., Morlet, T., Wilensky, D., Li, L., Mattingly, L., Jeanfreau, J., Keats, B., St. John, P., Montgomery, E., Shallop, J., Russell, B. & Frisch, S. (2010) Multi-site diagnosis and management of 260 patients with Auditory Neuropathy/Dys-synchrony (Auditory Neuropathy Spectrum Disorder[*]), *International Journal of Audiology,* 49:1, 30–43. https://doi.org/10.3109/14992020903160892

Bernard-Bonnin, A. C. (2006). Feeding problems of infants and toddlers. *Canadian Family Physician, 52,* 1247–1251.

Bernhardt, B. H., & Holdgrafer, G. (2001). Beyond the basics I: The need for strategic sampling from in-depth phonological analysis. *Language, Speech, and Hearing Services in Schools, 32,* 18–27.

Berninger, V. W. (2000). Development of language by hand and its connections with language by ear, mouth, and eye. *Topics in Language Disorders, 20*(4), 65–84.

Berninger, V. W., Abbott, R. D., Billingsley, F., & Nagy, W. (2001). Processes underlying timing and fluency of reading: Efficiency, automaticity, coordination, and morphological awareness. In M. Worf (Ed.), *Dyslexia, fluency, and the brain* (pp. 383–413). York.

Berninger, V. W., Vaughan, K., Abbott, R. D., Brooks, A., Begayis, K., Curtin, G., et al. (2000). Language-based spelling instruction: Teaching children to make multiple connections between spoken and written words. *Learning Disability Quarterly, 23*(2), 117–135.

Bernstein Ratner, N. (2006). Evidence-based practice: An examination of its ramifications for the practice of speech-language pathology. *Language, Speech, and Hearing Services in Schools, 37,* 257–267.

Bernthal, J., Bankson, N., & Flipsen, P. (2017). *Articulation and phonological disorders: Speech sound disorders in children* (8th ed.). Pearson Education.

Bess, F. H., Dodd-Murphy, J., & Parker, R. A. (1998). Children with minimal sensorineural hearing loss: Prevalence, educational performance, and functional status. *Ear and Hearing, 19,* 339–354.

Bessell, A., Hooper, L., Shaw, W., Reilly, S., Reid, J., & Glenny, A. (2011). Feeding interventions for growth and development in infants with cleft lip, cleft palate or cleft lip and palate. *Cochrane Database of Systematic Reviews, 2,* CD003315.

Beukelman, D. R., & Ansel, B. (1995). Research priorities in augmentative and alternative communication. *Augmentative and Alternative Communication, 11,* 131–134.

Beukelman, D. R., & Mirenda, P. (2013). *Augmentative and Alternative communication: supporting children and adults with complex communication needs* (4th ed.). Brookes.

Beukleman, D. R., & Light, J. C. (2020). *Augmentative and alternative communication: Supporting children and adults with complex communicative needs* (5th ed.). Brookes.

Bhatnagar, S., (2013). *Neuroscience for the study of communicative disorders* (4th ed.). Lippincott Williams & Wilkins.

Bhattacharyya, N. (2014). The prevalence of dysphagia among adults in the United States. *Otolaryngology-Head and Neck Surgery, 151,* 765–769.

Bhattacharyya, N. (2014). The prevalence of voice problems among adults in the United States. *The Laryngoscope, 124,* 2359–2362.

Biggs, E. E., Carter, E. W., & Gilson, C. B. (2018). Systematic review of interventions involving aided AAC modeling for children with complex communication needs. *American Journal on Intellectual and Developmental Disabilities,* 443–473. https://doi.org/10.1352/1944-7558-123.5.443

Binger, C., & Light, J. (2007). The effect of aided AAC modeling on the expression of multisymbol messages by preschoolers who use AAC. *Augmentative and Alternative Communication, 23,* 30–43.

Binos, P., Nirgianaki, E., & Psillas, G. (2021). How effective is auditory-verbal therapy (AVT) for building language development of children with cochlear implants?: A systematic review. *Life, 11,* 239.

Bishop, D. V. (2014). Ten questions about terminology for children with unexplained language problems. *International Journal of Language & Communication Disorders, 49,* 381–415.

Bishop, D. V. M., & McDonald, D. (2009). Identifying language impairment in children: Combining language test scores with parental report. *International Journal of Language & Communication Disorders, 44*(5), 600–615.

Bishop, D. V., Snowling, M. J., Thompson, P. A., Greenhalgh, T., & CATALISE-2 consortium. (2017). Phase 2 of CATALISE: A multinational and multidisciplinary Delphi consensus study of problems with language development: Terminology. *The Journal of Child Psychology and Psychiatry, 58*(10), 1068–1080.

Bitetti, D., & Scheffner Hammer, C. (2016). The home literacy environment and the English narrative development of Spanish–English bilingual children. *Journal of Speech, Language, and Hearing Research, 59,* 1159–1171. https://doi.org/10.1044/2016_JSLHR-L-15-0064

Blachman, B., Ball, E., Black, R., & Tangel, D. (2000). *Road to the code: A phonological awareness program for young children.* Brookes.

Black, L. I., Vahratian, A., & Hoffman, H. J. (2015). *Communication disorders and use of intervention services among children aged 3–17 years: United States, 2012* (NCHS Data Brief, No. 205). National Center for Health Statistics.

Black, L. I., Vahratian, A., & Hoffman, H. J. (2016, May 29). Communication disorders and use of intervention services among children aged 3–17 years: United States, 2012 (NCHS Data Brief, No. 205). National Center for Health Statistics. www.nidcd.nih.gov/health/statistics/quick-statistics-voice-speech-language

Blackstone, S. W. (2019). *Social Networks: A Communication Inventory for Individuals with Complex Communication Needs and Their Communication Partners.* Attainment Company.

Blackstone, S. W., Luo, F., Canchola, J., Wilkinson, K. M., & Roman-Lantzy, C. (2021). Children with cortical visual impairment and complex communication needs: Identifying gaps between needs and current practice. *Language, Speech, and Hearing Services in Schools, 52*(2), 612–629. https://doi.org/10.1044/2020_LSHSS-20-00088

Blackstone, S., & Hunt Berg, M. (2012). *Social Networks: A Communication Inventory for Individuals with Complex Needs and Their Communication Partners.* Attainment Company.

Blackwell, Z., & Littlejohns, P. (2010). A review of the management of dysphagia: A South African perspective. *Journal of Neuroscience Nursing, 42,* 61–70.

Blake, M. L. (2006). Clinical relevance of discourse characteristics after right hemisphere brain damage. *American Journal of Speech-Language Pathology, 15,* 255–267.

Blake, M. L. (2007). Perspectives on treatment for communication deficits associated with right hemisphere brain damage. *American Journal of Speech-Language Pathology, 16,* 331–342.

Blake, M. L. (2009). Inferencing processes after right hemisphere brain damage: Maintenance of inferences. *Journal of Speech, Language, and Hearing Research, 52,* 359–372.

Blake, M. L., & Lesniewicz, K. (2005). Contextual bias and predictive inferencing in adults with and without right hemisphere brain damage. *Aphasiology, 19,* 423–434.

Blake, M. L., Duffy, J. R., Myers, P. S., & Tompkins, C. A. (2002). Prevalence and patterns of right hemisphere cognitive/communicative deficits: Retrospective data from an inpatient rehabilitation unit. *Aphasiology, 16,* 537–548.

Bleile, K. (2020). *Speech sounds disorders* (4th ed.). Plural Publishing.

Bloodstein, O. (1995). *A handbook on stuttering.* Singular.

Bloodstein, O., & Ratner, N. (2008). *A handbook on stuttering* (6th ed.). Thomson Delmar Learning.

Blumenthal, M. (2007). Tolken bij diagnostiek van spraak-taalproblemen. Ontwikkeling cursus en richtlijnen [Interpreters in assessment of speech-language problems. Development of a course and guidelines]. *Logopedie en Foniatrie, 1,* 10–19.

Blumgart, E., Tran, Y., & Craig, A. (2014). Social support and its association with negative affect in adults who stutter. *Journal of Fluency Disorders, 40,* 83–92.

Boberg, E., & Kully, D. (1989). A retrospective look at stuttering therapy. *Canadian Journal of Speech-Language Pathology and Audiology, 13,* 5–13.

Boburg, E., & Kully, D. (1995). The comprehensive stuttering program. In C. W. Starkweather & H. F. M. Peters (Eds.), *Stuttering: Proceedings of the First World Congress on Fluency Disorder* (pp. 305–308). International Fluency Association.

Boersma, P., Black, L.I., & Ward, B.W. (2020, September 17). *Prevalence of multiple chronic conditions among US adults, 2018.* Centers for Disease Control and Prevention. https://www.cdc.gov/pcd/issues/2020/20_0130.htm

Boey, R., Van de Heyning, P., Wuyts, F., Heylen, L., Stoop, R., & De Bodt, M. (2009). Awareness and reactions of young stuttering children aged 2–7 years old towards their speech disfluency. *Journal of Communication Disorders, 42,* 334–346.

Boggs, T., & Ferguson, N. (2016). A little PEP goes a long way in the treatment of pediatric feeding disorders. *Perspectives of the ASHA Special Interest Groups, 1,* 26–37.

Boi, R., Racca, L., Cavallero, A., Carpaneto, V., Racca, M., Dall'Acqua, F., et al. (2012). Hearing loss and depressive symptoms in elderly patients. *Geriatrics and Gerontology International, 12*(3), 440–445.

Boisvert, I., Reis, M., Au, A., Cowan, R., & Dowell, R. (2020). Cochlear implantation outcomes in adults: A scoping review. *PloS ONE, 15*(5), e0232421.

Boliek, C., Hixon, T., Watson, P., & Morgan, W. (1997). Vocalization and breathing during the first year of life. *Journal of Voice, 10,* 1–22.

Bondy, A. S., & Frost, L. A. (1994). The Picture Exchange Communication System. *Focus on Autistic Behavior, 9*(3), 1–19.

Boone, D. R., & McFarlane, S. C. (2000). *The voice and voice therapy* (4th ed.). Allyn & Bacon.

Boone, D. R., McFarlane, S. C., Von Berg, S. L., & Zraick, R. I. (2010). *The voice and voice therapy.* (8th ed.). Allyn & Bacon.

Bornstein, H. (1974). Signed English: A manual approach to English language development. *Journal of Speech and Hearing Disorders, 30*(3) 330–343.

Bornstein, M. H., Hahn, C., Putnick, D. L., & Suwalsky, J. T. D. (2014). Stability of core language skill from early childhood to adolescence: A latent variable approach. *Child Development, 85,* 1346–1356.

Boswell, S. (2004). International agreement brings mutual recognition of certification. *The ASHA Leader, 9*(19), 1–22.

Bothe, A., Davidow, J., Bramlett, R., & Ingham, R. (2006). Stuttering treatment research 1970–2005: I. Systematic review incorporating trial quality assessment of behavioral, cognitive, and related approaches. *American Journal of Speech-Language Pathology, 15,* 321–341.

Boudreau, D. (2005). Use of a parent questionnaire in emergent and early literacy assessment of preschool children. *Language, Speech, and Hearing Services in Schools, 36,* 33–47.

Boudreau, D. M., & Chapman, R. (2000). The relationship between event representation and linguistic skills in narratives of children and adolescents with Down syndrome. *Journal of Speech, Language, and Hearing Research, 43,* 1146–1159.

Boudreau, D. M., & Larson, J. (2004, November). *Strategies for teaching narrative abilities to school-aged children.* Paper presented at the annual convention of the American Speech-Language-Hearing Association, Philadelphia.

Bourgeois, M. S., & Hickey, E. M. (2009). *Dementia: From diagnosis to management: A functional approach.* Psychology Press.

Boutsen, F., Cannito, M., Taylor, M., & Bender, B. (2002). Botox treatment in adductor spasmodic dysphonia: A meta-analysis. *Journal of Speech, Language, and Hearing Research, 45,* 469–481.

Boutsen, F., Park, E., Dvorak, J., & Cid, C. (2018). Prosodic improvement in persons with Parkinson disease receiving SPEAK OUT!® voice therapy. *Folia Phoniatrica et Logopaedica, 70,* 51–58.

Boyle, M. (2015). Relationships between psychosocial factors and quality of life for adults who stutter. *American Journal of Speech-Language Pathology, 24,* 1–12.

Brackenbury, T., & Pye, C. (2005). Semantic deficits in children with language impairments: Issues for clinical assessment. *Language, Speech, and Hearing Services in Schools, 36,* 5–16.

Brackenbury, T., Burroughs, E., & Hewitt, L. E. (2008). A qualitative examination of current guidelines for evidence-based practice in child language intervention. *Language, Speech, and Hearing Services in Schools, 39,* 78–88.

Brackett, K., Arvedson, J. C., & Manno, C. J. (2006). Pediatric feeding and swallowing disorders: General assessment and intervention. *Perspective on Swallowing and Swallowing Disorders (Dysphagia), 15,* 10–15. https://doi.org/10.1044/sasd15.3.10

Brady, N. C., Bruce, S., Goldman, A., Erickson, K., Mineo, B., Ogletree, B. T., Wilkinson, K. (2016). Communication services and supports for individuals with severe disabilities: Guidance for assessment and intervention. *American Journal on Intellectual and Developmental Disabilities,* 121–138. https://www.asha.org/njc/communication-bill-of-rights/

Brady, N.C., Fleming, K., Bredin-Oja, S.L., Fielding-Gebhardt, H., & Warren, S.F. (2020). Language development from early childhood to adolescence in youths with fragile X syndrome. *Journal of Speech, Language, and Hearing Research, 63,* 3727–3742.

Bramble, K. (2013, March/April). Internet hearing aid sales: Our new reality. *Audiology Today,* pp. 16–18.

Branson, D., & Demchak, M. (2009). The use of augmentative and alternative communication methods with infants with disabilities: A research review. *Augmentative and Alternative Communication, 25*(4), 274–286. https://doi.org/10.3109/07434610903384529

Brault, M. W. (2005). Americans with Disabilities, 2005. In U.S. Census Bureau, *Current Population Reports* (pp. 70–117).

Brea-Spahn, M. R., & Dunn Davison, M. (2012). Writing intervention for Spanish-speaking English language learners: A review of research. *EBP Briefs, 7*(2), 1–11.

Brignell, A., Williams, K., Jachno, K., Prior, M., Reilly, S., & Morgan, A.T. (2018). Patterns and predictors of language development from 4 to 7 years in verbal children with and without autism spectrum disorder. *Journal of Autism and Developmental Disorders, 48,* 3282–3295.

Brinton, B., & Fujiki, M. (2004). Social and affective factors in children with language impairment: Implications for literacy learning. In C. A. Stone, E. R. Silliman, B. J. Ehren, & K. Apel (Eds.), *Handbook of language and literacy: Development and disorders* (pp. 130–153). Guilford Press.

Brinton, B., Spackman, M. P., Fujiki, M., & Ricks, J. (2007). What should Chris say?: The ability of children with specific language impairment to recognize the need to dissemble emotions in social situations. *Journal of Speech, Language, and Hearing Research, 50,* 798–811.

Broadfoot, C., Abur, D., Hoffmeister J., Stepp, C., & Ciucci, M. (2019). Research-based updates in swallowing and communication dysfunction in Parkinson Disease: Implications for evaluation and management. *Perspectives of the ASHA Special Interest Groups, 4,* 825–841.

Brock, K., Koul, R., Corwin, M., & Schlosser, R. (2017). A comparison of visual scene and grid displays for people with chronic aphasia: A pilot study to improve communication using AAC. *Aphasiology, 31*(11), 1282–1306. https://doi.org/10.1080/02687038.2016.1274874

Brooks, G., Torgerson, C. J., & Hall, J. (2008). The use of phonics in the teaching of reading and spelling. *EBP Briefs, 3*(2), 1–12.

Brosnahan, S., Jonkman, A., Kugler, J., Munger, J., & Kaufman, D. (2020). COVID-19 and respiratory systems disorders: Current knowledge, future clinical, and translational research outcomes. *Arteriosclerosis, Thrombosis, and Vascular Biology, 40,* 2586–2597.

Brown, J. A., Wallace, S. E., Knollman-Porter, K., & Hux, K. (2019). Comprehension of single versus combined modality information by people with aphasia. *American Journal of Speech-Language Pathology, 28,* 278–292.

Brown, J., Ackley, K., & Knollman-Porter, K. (2021). Collaborative goal setting: A clinical approach for adults with mild traumatic brain injury. *American Journal of Speech-Language Pathology, 30,* 2394–2413.

Brown, S., Ingham, R., Ingham, J., Laird, A., & Fox, P. (2005). Stuttered and fluent speech production: An ALE meta-analysis of normal neuroimaging studies. *Human Brain Mapping, 25,* 105–117.

Brumberg, J. S., Pitt, K. M., Mantie-Kozlowski, A., & Burnison, D. J. (2018). Brain–computer interfaces for augmentative and alternative communication: A tutorial. *American Journal of Speech Language Pathology, 27*(1), 1–12. https://doi.org/10.1044/2017_AJSLP-16-0244

Brundage, S., Bernstein Ratner, N., Boyle, M., Eggers, K., Everard, R., Franken, M.-C., et al. (2021). Consensus guidelines for the assessments of individuals who stutter across the lifespan. *American Journal of Speech-Language Pathology, 30,* 2379–2393.

Brunner, M., Hemsley, B., Togher, L., Dann, S., & Palmer, S. (2021). Social media and people with traumatic brain injury: A metasynthesis of research informing a framework for rehabilitation clinical practice, policy, and training. *American Journal of Speech-Language Pathology, 30,* 19–33.

Bulow, M., Olsson, R., & Ekberg, O. (2001). Videomanometric analysis of supraglottic swallow, effortful swallow, and chin tuck in patients with pharyngeal dysfunction. *Dysphagia, 16,* 190–195.

Bunton, K., & Leddy, M. (2011). An evaluation of articulatory working space area in vowel production of adults with Down syndrome. *Clinical Linguistics & Phonetics, 25,* 321–334.

Burgess, S., & Turkstra, L. S. (2006). Social skills intervention for adolescents with autism spectrum disorders: A review of the experimental evidence. *EBP Briefs, 1*(4), 41–58.

Butler, L., Kiran, S., & Tager-Flusberg, H. (2020). Functional near-infrared spectroscopy in the study of speech and language impairment across the life span: A systematic review. *American Journal of Speech-Language Pathology, 29,* 1674–1701.

Byeon, H. (2019). The risk factors related to voice disorders in teachers: A systematic review and meta-analysis. *International Journal of Environmental Research and Public Health, 16,* 3675.

Byers, B., Bellon-Harn, M., Allen, M., Saar, K., Manchaiah, V., & Rodrigo, H. (2021). A comparison of intervention intensity and service delivery models with school-age children with speech sound disorders in a school setting. *Language, Speech, and Hearing Services in Schools, 52,* 529–541.

Byrd, C., Gkalitsiou, Z., McGill, M., Reed, O., & Kelly, E. (2016). The influence of self-disclosure on school-age children's perceptions of children who stutter. *Journal of Child and Adolescent Behavior, 4,* 1–9.

Byrd, C., McGill, M., Gkalitsiou, Z., & Cappellini, C. (2017). The effects of self-disclosure on male and female perceptions of individuals who stutter. *American Journal of Speech-Language Pathology, 26,* 69–80.

Cabré, M., Serra-Prat, M., Force, L., Almirall, J., Palomera, E., & Clavé, P. (2014). Oropharyngeal dysphagia is a risk factor for readmission for pneumonia in the very elderly persons: Observational prospective study. *Journals of Gerontology, Series A: Biological Sciences and Medical Sciences, 69*(3), 330–337.

Caccamise, D., & Snyder, L. (2005). Theory and pedagogical practices of text comprehension. *Topics in Language Disorders, 25*(1), 1–20.

Cain, K. Patson, N., & Andrews, L. (2005). Age- and ability-related differences in young readers' use of conjunctions. *Journal of Child Language, 32,* 877–892.

Cain, K., Oakhill, J. V., & Bryant, P. E. (2001). Children's reading comprehension ability: Concurrent prediction by working memory, verbal ability, and component skills. *Journal of Educational Psychology, 96,* 31–42.

Calculator, S. N. (2015). AAC Considerations for Individuals with Angelman Syndrome. *Perspectives on Augmentative and Alternative Communication, 24*(3), 106–113. https://doi.org/10.1044/aac24.3.106

Calder, S. D., Claessen, M., & Leitão, S. (2018). Combining implicit and explicit intervention approaches to target grammar in young children with developmental language disorder. *Child Language Teaching and Therapy, 34*(2), 171–189.

Calvert, D. (1982). Articulation and hearing impairments. In L. Lass, J. Northern, D. Yoder, & L. McReynolds (Eds.), *Speech, language, and hearing* (Vol. 2) 638–651. Saunders.

Campbell, T., Dollaghan, H., Rockette, H., Paradise, J., Feldman, H., & Shriberg, L., et al. (2003). Risk factors for speech delay of unknown origin in 3-year-old children. *Child Development, 74,* 346–357.

Carding, P., Roulstone, S., Northstone, K., & the ALSPAC Study Team. (2006). The prevalence of childhood dysphonia: A cross-sectional study. *Journal of Voice, 20,* 623–629.

Carew, L., Dacakis, G., & Oates, J. (2007). The effectiveness of oral resonance therapy on the perception of femininity of voice in male-to-female transsexuals. *Journal of Voice, 21,* 591–603.

Carneol, S., Marks, S., & Weik, L. (1999). The speech-language pathologist: Key role in the diagnosis of velocardio-facial syndrome. *American Journal of Speech-Language Pathology, 8,* 23–32.

Carroll, J. M., & Breadmore, H. L. (2018). Not all phonological awareness deficits are created equal: Evidence from a comparison between children with otitis media and poor readers. *Developmental Science, 21*(3), e12588.

Catten, M., Gray, S., Hammond, T., Zhou, R., & Hammond, E. (1998). Analysis of cellular location and concentration in vocal fold lamina propria. *Archives of Otolaryngology—Head & Neck Surgery, 118,* 663–666.

Catts, H. W. (1997). The early identification of language-based reading disabilities. *Language, Speech, and Hearing Services in Schools, 28,* 86–89.

Catts, H. W. (2017). Early identification of reading disabilities. In Cain, K., Compton, D. L., & Parrila, R. (Eds.), *Theories of reading development* (15th ed., pp. 311–332). Benjamins.

Catts, H. W., & Kamhi, A. (2005). Causes of reading disabilities. In H. W. Catts & A. G. Kamhi (Eds.), *Language and reading disabilities* (2nd ed., pp. 94–126). Allyn & Bacon.

Catts, H. W., Adlof, S. M., & Ellis Weismer, S. (2006). Language deficits in poor comprehenders: A case for the simple view of reading. *Journal of Speech, Language, and Hearing Research, 49,* 278–293.

Catts, H. W., Fey, M. E., Zhang, X., & Tomblin, J. B. (2001). Estimating the risk of future reading difficulties in kindergarten children: A research-based model and its clinical implementation. *Language, Speech, and Hearing Services in Schools, 32,* 38–50.

Catts, H. W., Nielsen, D. C., Bridges, M. S., Liu, Y. S., & Bontempo, D. E. (2015). Early identification of reading disabilities within an RTI framework. *Journal of Learning Disabilities, 48,* 281–297.

Catts, H. W., & Kamhi, A. G. (2017). Prologue: Reading comprehension is not a single ability. *Language, Speech and Hearing Services in Schools, 48,* 73–76.

Caute, A., Woolf, C., Wilson, S., Stokes, C., Monnelly, K., Cruice, M., et al. (2019). Technology-enhanced reading therapy for people with aphasia: Findings from a quasirandomized waitlist controlled study. *Journal of Speech, Language, and Hearing Research, 62,* 4382–4416.

Cavanaugh, R., & Haley, K. L. (2020). Subjective communication difficulties in very mild aphasia. *American Journal of Speech-Language Pathology, 29,* 437–448.

Cavanaugh, R., Kravetz, C., Jarold, L., Quique, Y., Turner, R., & Evans, W. S. (2021). Is there a research-practice dosage gap in aphasia rehabilitation? *American Journal of Speech-Language Pathology, 30,* 2115–2139.

Centers for Disease Control and Prevention (CDC). (2009). *Summary of 2009 CDC EHDI data.* www.cdc.gov/ncbddd/hearingloss/ehdi-data.html

Centers for Disease Control and Prevention (CDC). (2014, March 27). *CDC estimates 1 in 68 children has been identified with autism spectrum disorder.* https://www.cdc.gov/media/releases/2014/p0327-autism-spectrum-disorder.html

Centers for Disease Control and Prevention (CDC). (2018, April 26). *Signs and symptoms of autism spectrum disorder.* https://www.cdc.gov/ncbddd/autism/signs.html

Centers for Disease Control and Prevention (CDC). (2019). *2019 Summary of diagnostics among infants not passing hearing screening.* https://www.cdc.gov/ncbddd/hearingloss/2019-data/06-diagnostics.html

Centers for Disease Control and Prevention (CDC). (2021, December 9). *Traumatic brain injury & concussion.* https://www.cdc.gov/TraumaticBrainInjury/index.html

Centers for Disease Control and Prevention (CDC). (2022, March 2). *Data & statistics on autism spectrum disorder.* https://www.cdc.gov/ncbddd/autism/data.html

Centers for Disease Control and Prevention (CDC). (2022, March 21). *Traumatic brain injury & concussion.* https://www.cdc.gov/traumaticbraininjury/data/index.html

Centers for Disease Control and Prevention (CDC). (n.d.). *2020 Annual data Early Hearing Detection and Intervention (EHDI) program.* https://www.cdc.gov/ncbddd/hearingloss/ehdi-data2019.html

Cermak, C. A., Scratch, S. E., Reed, N. P., Bradley, K., Quinn de Launay, K. L., & Beal, D. S. (2019). Cognitive communication impairments in children with traumatic brain injury. *Journal of Head Trauma Rehabilitation, 34*(2), E13–E20.

Cha, Y. J., & Kim, H. (2013). Effect of computer-based cognitive rehabilitation (CBCR) for people with stroke: A systematic review and meta-analysis. *NeuroRehabilitation, 32,* 359–368.

Chagnon, F., & Stone, R. (1996). Nodules and polyps. In W. Brown, B. Vinsor, & M. Crary (Eds.), *Organic voice disorders: Assessment and treatment* (pp. 219–244). Singular.

Chakrabarti, S., & Fombonne, E. (2001) Pervasive developmental disorders in preschool children. *Journal of the American Medical Association, 27,* 3093–3099.

Chan, J. B., & Iacano, T. (2001). Gesture and word production in children with Down Syndrome. *Augmentative and Alternative Communication, 17*(2), 73–87.

Chan, J., & Nankervis, K. (2014). Stolen voices: Facilitated communication is an abuse of human rights. *Evidence-Based Communication Assessment and Intervention, 8*(3), 151–156. https://doi.org/10.1080/17489539.2014.1001549

Chang, S., Angstadt, M., Chow, H., Etchell, A., Garnett, E., Choo, A., et al. (2017). Anomalous network architecture of the resting brain in children who stutter. *Journal of Fluency Disorders, 55,* 46–67.

Chapin, S., McNaughton, D., Light, J., McCoy, A., Caron, J., & Lee, D. L. (2021). The effects of AAC video visual scene display technology on the communicative turns of preschoolers with autism spectrum disorder. *Assistive Technology, 34*(5), 577–587.

Chapin, S., McNaughton, D., Light, J., McCoy, A., Caron, J., & Lee, D. L. (2021). The effects of AAC video visual scene display technology on the communicative turns of preschoolers with autism spectrum disorder. *Assistive Technology.* https://doi.org/10.1080/10400435.2021.1893235

Charest, M., Skoczylas, M. J., & Schneider, P. (2020). Properties of lexical diversity in the narratives of children with typical language development and developmental language disorder. *American Journal of Speech-Language Pathology, 29,* 1866–1882.

Charity, A., Scarborough, H., & Griffin, D. (2004). Familiarity with school English in African American children and its relation to early reading achievement. *Child Development, 75,* 1340–1356.

Charman, T., Drew, A., Baird, C., & Baird, G. (2003). Measuring early language development in preschool children with autism spectrum disorder using the MacArthur Communicative Development Inventory (Infant Form). *Journal of Child Language, 30,* 213–236.

Cheng, B. B. Y., Ryan, B. J., Copland, D. A., & Wallace, S. J. (2022). Prognostication in poststroke aphasia: Perspectives of significant others of people with aphasia on receiving information about recovery. *American Journal of Speech-Language Pathology, 31,* 896–911.

Cheng, L. (1991). *Assessing Asian language performance: Guidelines for evaluating limited-English proficient students* (2nd ed.). Academic Communication Associates.

Cherney, L., & Halper, A. (1996). Swallowing problems in adults with traumatic brain injury. *Seminars in Neurology, 16,* 349–353.

Cherney, L. R., Halper, A. S., Holland, A. L., & Cole, R. (2008). Computerized script training for aphasia: Preliminary results. *American Journal of Speech-Language Pathology, 17,* 19–34.

Childes, J., Acker, A., & Collins, D. (2017). Multiple perspectives on the barriers to identification and management of pediatric voice disorders. *Perspectives of the ASHA Special Interest Groups (SIG 3), 2,* 49–56.

Chopra, M., Gable, D., Love-Nichols, J., Tsao, A., Rockowitz, S., Sliz, P., et al. (2022) Mendelian etiologies identified with whole exome sequencing in cerebral palsy. *Annals of Clinical and Translational Neurology, 9,* 193–205.

Choudhury, N., & Benasich, A. A. (2003). A family aggregation study: The influence of family history and other risk factors on language development. *Journal of Speech, Language, and Hearing Research, 46,* 261–272.

Chouinard, M. M., & Clark, E. V. (2003). Adult reformulations of child errors as negative evidence. *Journal of Child Language, 30,* 637–669.

Church, C., Alisanski, S., & Amanullah, S. (2000). The social, behavioral, and academic experiences of children with Asperger syndrome. *Focus on Autism and Other Developmental Disabilities, 15*(1), 12–20.

Cichero, J., Lam, P., Steele, C., Hanson, B., Chen, J., Dantas, R., et al. (2017). Development of international terminology and definitions for texture-modified foods and thickened fluids used in dysphagia management: The IDDSI Framework. *Dysphagia, 32*, 293–314. https://doi.org/10.1007/s00455-016-9758-y

Cirrin, F. M., & Gillam, R. B. (2008). Language intervention practices for school-age children with spoken language disorders: A systematic review. *Language, Speech, and Hearing Services in Schools, 39*, 110–137.

Civier, O., Tasko, S., & Guenther, F. (2010). Over-reliance on auditory feedback may lead to sound/syllable repetitions: Simulations of stuttering and fluency-inducing conditions with a neural model of speech production. *Journal of Fluency Disorders, 35*, 246–279.

Clare, L., & Jones, R. (2008). Errorless learning in the rehabilitation of memory: A critical review. *Neuropsychological Review, 18*, 1–23.

Clark, H. (2012). Specificity of training in the lingual musculature. *Journal of Speech, Language, and Hearing Research, 55*, 657–667.

Clark, H., Lazarus, C., Arvedson, J., Schooling, T., & Frymark, T. (2009). Evidence-based systematic review: Effects of neuromuscular electrical stimulation on swallowing and neural activation. *American Journal of Speech-Language Pathology, 18*, 361–375.

Clarke, M., Newton, C., Petrides, K., Griffiths, T., Lysley, A., & Price, K. (2012). An examination of relations between participation, communication and age in children with complex communication needs. *Augmentative and Alternative Communication, 28*(1), 44–51.

Clarke, V., & Schneider, H. (2015). *The Dynamic AAC Goals Grid (DAGG-2)*. Tobii Dynavox. http://tdvox.webdownloads.s3.amazonaws.com/MyTobiiDynavox/dagg%202%20-%20writable.pdf

Cleave, P. L., Becker, S. D., Curran, M. K., Owen Van Horne, A. J., & Fey, M. E. (2015). The efficacy of recasts in language intervention: A systematic review and meta-analysis. *American Journal of Speech-Language Pathology, 24*, 237–255.

Clendon, S., & Erickson, K. A. (2008). The vocabulary of beginning writers: Implications for children with complex communication needs. *Augmentative and Alternative Communication, 24*(4), 281–293.

Cochran D'Angelo, E., Ober, B. A., & Shenaut, G. K. (2021). Combined memory training: An approach for episodic memory deficits in traumatic brain injury. *American Journal of Speech-Language Pathology, 30*, 920–932.

Coelho, C. A., DeRuyter, F., Kennedy, M. R. T., & Stein, M. (2008). *Cognitive-communication disorders resulting from traumatic brain injury*. Treatment Efficacy Summary. www.asha.org/NR/rdonlyres/4BAF3969-9ADC-4C01-B5ED-1334CC20DD3D/0/TreatmentEfficacySummaries2008.pdf

Cohen Sherman, J., Henderson, C. R., Flynn, S., Gair, J. W., & Lust, B (2021). Language decline characterizes amnestic mild cognitive impairment independent of cognitive decline. *Journal of Speech, Language, and Hearing Research, 64*, 4287–4307.

Cohen, S., & Garrett, G. (2007). Utility in voice therapy management of vocal fold polyps and cysts. *Otolaryngology Head and Neck Surgery, 136*, 742–746.

Coleman, C., Miller, L., & Weidner, M. (2015). A clinical tutorial in stuttering: Case vignette. *Perspectives on Fluency and Fluency Disorders, 25*, 5–9.

Colenbrander, D., Ricketts, J., & Breadmore, H.L. (2018). Early identification of dyslexia: Understanding the issues. *Language, Speech, and Hearing Services in Schools, 49*, 817–828.

Colton, R. H., & Casper, J. K. (1990). *Understanding voice problems: A physiological perspective for diagnosis and treatment*. Williams & Wilkins.

Colton, R., Casper, J., & Leonard, R. (2011). *Understanding voice problems: A physiological perspective for diagnosis and treatment* (4th ed.). Lippincott, Williams & Wilkins.

Condouris, K., Meyer, E., & Tager-Flusberg, H. (2003). The relationship between standardized measures of language and measures of spontaneous speech in children with autism. *American Journal of Speech-Language Pathology, 12*, 349–358.

Conti-Ramsden, G., & Botting, N. (2004). Social difficulties and victimization in children with SLI at 11 years of age. *Journal of Speech, Language, and Hearing Research, 47*, 145–161.

Conti-Ramsden, G., & Durkin, K. (2008). Language and independence in adolescents with and without a history of specific language impairment (SLI). *Journal of Speech, Language, and Hearing Research, 51*, 70–83.

Conti-Ramsden, G., Durkin, K., & Simkin, Z. (2010). Language and social factors in the use of cell phone technology by adolescents with and without specific language impairment (SLI). *Journal of Speech, Language, and Hearing Research, 53*, 196–208.

Conti-Ramsden, G., Simkin, Z., & Pickles, A. (2006). Estimating familial loading in SLI: A comparison of direct assessment versus parental interview. *Journal of Speech, Language, and Hearing Research, 49*(1), 88–101.

Conture, E. G. (1996). Treatment efficacy: Stuttering. *Journal of Speech and Hearing Research, 39*, S18–S26.

Conture, E. G., & Guitar, B. (1993). Evaluating efficacy of treatment of stuttering: School-age children. *Journal of Fluency Disorders, 18*, 253–287.

Conture, E. G., & Yaruss, J. S. (2009, June 19). *Stuttering*. Treatment Efficacy Summary. www.asha.org/NR/rdonlyres/85BCEC0C-FBF5-43C7-880D-EF2D3219F807/0/TESStuttering.pdf

Cooper, E. B. (1984). Personalized fluency control therapy: A status report. In M. Peins (Ed.), *Contemporary approaches to stuttering therapy* (pp. 1–38). Little, Brown.

Corriveau, K., Posquine, E., & Goswami, U. (2007). Basic auditory processing skills and specific language impairment: A new look at an old hypothesis. *Journal of Speech, Language, and Hearing Research, 50*, 647–666.

Corwin, M., & Koul, R. (2003) Augmentative and alternative communication intervention for individuals with chronic severe aphasia: An evidence-based practice process illustration. *Perspectives on Augmentative and Alternative Communication, 12*(4), 11–15.

Côté, H., Payer, M., Giroux, F., & Joanette, Y. (2007). Towards a description of clinical communication impairment profiles following right-hemisphere damage. *Aphasiology, 21*, 739–749.

Cowan, N., Nugent, L., Elliott, E., Ponomarev, I., & Saults, S. (2005). The role of attention in the development of short-term memory: Age differences in the verbal span of apprehension. *Child Development, 70*, 1082–1097.

Coyle, J. (2015). The clinical evaluation: A necessary tool for the dysphagia sleuth. *Perspectives on Swallowing and Swallowing Disorders (Dysphagia), 24*, 18–25.

Craig, A., & Calvert, P. (1991). Following up on treated stutterers: Studies of perception of fluency and job status. *Journal of Speech and Hearing Research, 34*, 279–284.

Craig, A., Hancock, H., Chang, E., McCready, C., Shepley, A., McCaul, A., et al. (1996). A controlled clinical trial for stuttering in persons aged 9 to 14 years. *Journal of Speech and Hearing Research, 39*, 808–826.

Craig, H. K., & Washington, J. A. (2004). Grade related changes in the production of African American English. *Journal of Speech, Language, and Hearing Research, 47*, 450–463.

Cress, C. J. (2001). Language and AAC intervention in young children: Never too early or too late to start. *American Speech-Language Hearing Association Special Interest Division 1, Language Learning and Education Newsletter, 8*(1), 3–4.

Cress, C. J., & Marvin, C. A. (2009). Common questions about AAC services in early intervention. *Augmentative and Alternative Communication, 19*(4), 254–272. https://doi.org/10.1080/07434610310001598242

Croot, K., Nickels, L., Laurence, F., & Manning, M. (2009) Impairment- and activity/participation-directed interventions in progressive language impairment: Clinical and theoretical issues, *Aphasiology, 23*(2), 125–160.

Croot, K., Raiser, T., Taylor-Rubin, C., Ruggero, L., Ackl, N., Wlasich, E., et al. (2019). Lexical retrieval treatment in primary progressive aphasia: An investigation of treatment duration in a heterogeneous case series. *Cortex, 115*, 133–158.

Crowe, K., & McLeod, S. (2020). Children's English consonant acquisition in the United States: A review. *American Journal of Speech-Language Pathology, 29*, 2155–2169.

Crowe, L. K. (2003). Comparison of two reading feedback strategies in improving the oral and written language performance of children with language-learning disabilities. *American Journal of Speech-Language Pathology, 12*, 16–27.

Cruickshanks, K. J., Wiley, T. L., Tweed, T. S., Klein, B. E. K., Klein, R., Mares-Perlman, J. A., & Nondahl, D. M. (1998). Prevalence of hearing loss in older adults in Beaver Dam, Wisconsin: The epidemiology of hearing loss study. *American Journal of Epidemiology, 148*(9), 879–885.

Cummings, L. (2008). *Clinical linguistics*. Edinburgh University Press.

Cunningham, A., Perry, K., Stanovich, K., & Stanovich, P. (2004). Disciplinary knowledge of K–3 teachers and their knowledge calibration in the domain of early literacy. *Annals of Dyslexia, 54*, 139–167.

Cunningham, J. W., Spadorcia, A., & Erickson, K. A. (2005). Investigating the instructional supportiveness of leveled texts. *Reading Research Quarterly, 40*(4), 410–427.

Cupples, L., & Iacono, T. (2000). Phonological awareness and oral reading skill in children with Down syndrome. *Journal of Speech, Language, and Hearing Research, 43*, 595–608.

Curenton, S. M., & Justice, L. M. (2004). African American and Caucasian preschoolers' use of decontextualized language: Literate language features in oral narratives. *Language, Speech, and Hearing Services in Schools, 35*, 240–253.

Cycyk, L. M., & Huerta, L. (2020). Exploring the cultural validity of parent-implemented naturalistic language intervention procedures for families from Spanish-speaking Latinx homes. American Journal of Speech-Language Pathology, 29, 1241–1259.

Dagli, M., Sati, I., Acar, A., Stone, R. E., Dursun, G., & Eryilmaz, A. (2008). Mutational falsetto: intervention outcomes in 45 patients. *Journal of Laryngology & Otology, 122*, 277–281.

Dailey, S. (2013). Feeding and swallowing management in infants with cleft and craniofacial anomalies.

Perspectives on Speech Science and Orofacial Disorders, *23*, 62–72.

Dale, P. S., McMillan, A. J., Hayiou-Thomas, M. E., & Plomin, R. (2014). Illusory recovery: Are recovered children with early language delay at continuing elevated risk? *American Journal of Speech-Language Pathology, 23*, 437–447.

Dale, P. S., Price, T. S., Bishop, D. V. M., & Plomin, R. (2003). Outcomes of early language delay: I. Predicting persistent and transient language difficulties at 3 and 4 years. *Journal of Speech, Language, and Hearing Research, 46*, 544–560.

Dalston, R., Warren, D., & Dalston, E. (1991). A preliminary investigation concerning the use of nasometry in identifying patients with hyponasality and/or nasal airway impairment. *Journal of Speech and Hearing Research, 34*, 11–18.

Danahauer, J., Johnson, D., Young, M., Rotan, S., Snelson, T., Stockwell, J., & McLain, M. (2012). Survey of high school students' perceptions about their iPod use, knowledge of hearing health, and need for education. *Language, Speech, and Hearing Services in Schools, 43*, 14–35.

Danahy Ebert, K., & Kohnert, K. (2011). Sustained attention in children with primary language impairment: A meta-analysis. *Journal of Speech, Language, and Hearing Research, 54*, 1372–1384.

Daniels, D., Gabel, R., & Hughes, S. (2012). Recounting the K–12 school experiences of adults who stutter: A qualitative analysis. *Journal of Fluency Disorders, 37*, 71–82.

Dark, L., & Balandin, S. (2007). Prediction and selection of vocabulary for two leisure activities. *Augmentative and Alternative Communication, 23*(4), 288–299.

Davidson, M. M. (2021). Reading comprehension in school-age children with autism spectrum disorder: Examining the many components that may contribute. *Language, Speech and Hearing Services in Schools, 52*, 181–196.

Davidson, M. M., & Ellis Weismer, S. (2014). Characterization and prediction of early reading abilities in children on the autism spectrum. *Journal of Autism and Developmental Disorders, 24*, 828–845.

Davies, S., Papp, V., & Antoni, C., (2015). Voice and communication change for gender nonconfirming individuals: Giving voice to the person include. *International Journal of Transgenderism, 16*, 117–159.

Davis, S., Howell, P., & Cooke, F. (2002). Sociodynamic relationships between children who stutter and their non-stuttering classmates. *Journal of Child Psychology and Psychiatry, 43*, 939–947.

Dawson, G., Carver, L., Meltzoff, A. N., Panagiotides, H., McPartland, J., & Webb, S. J. (2002). Neural correlates of face and object recognition in young children with autism spectrum disorder, developmental delay, and typical development. *Child Development, 73*, 700–712.

Dawson, J., & Tattersall, P. (2001). *Structured Photographic Articulation Test II—Featuring Dudsberry.* Janelle.

de Beer, C., de Ruiter, J. P., Hielscher-Fastabend, M., & Hogrefe, K. (2019). The production of gesture and speech by people with aphasia: Influence of communicative constraints. *Journal of Speech, Language, and Hearing Research, 62*, 4417–4432.

De Groot, B. J., Van den Bos, K. P., Van der Meulen, B. V., & Minnaert, A. E. (2015). Rapid naming and phonemic awareness in children with reading disabilities and/or specific language impairment: differentiating processes? *Journal of Speech, Language, and Hearing Research, 58*, 1538–1548.

De Houwer, A., (2015). Harmonious bilingual development: Young families' well-being in language contact situations. *International Journal of Bilingualism, 19*, 169–184.

de Valenzuela, J. S., Copeland, S. R., Qi, C. H., & Park, M. (2006). Examining educational equity: Revisiting the disproportionate representation of minority students in special education. *Exceptional Children, 72*, 425–441.

Deacon, S. H., Benere, J., & Pasquarella, A. (2013). Reciprocal relationship: Children's morphological awareness and their reading accuracy across grades 2 to 3. *Developmental Psychology, 49*, 1113–1126. https://doi.org/10.1037/a0029474

Deacon, S. H., Tong, X., & Francis, K. (2017). The relationship of morphological analysis and morphological decoding to reading comprehension. *Journal of Research in Reading, 40*, 1–16. https://doi.org/10.1111/1467-9817.12056

Dean Qualls, C., O'Brien, R. M., Blood, G. W., & Scheffner Hammer, C. (2003). Contextual variation, familiarity, academic literacy, and rural adolescents' idiom knowledge. *Language, Speech, and Hearing Services in Schools, 34*, 69–79.

DeBonis, D., & Moncrieff, D. (2008). Auditory processing disorders: An update for speech-language pathologists. *American Journal of Speech-Language Pathology, 17*, 4–18.

DeDe, G. (2012). Effects of word frequency and modality on sentence comprehension impairments in people with aphasia. *American Journal of Speech-Language Pathology, 21*, 103–114.

DeDe, G. (2013). Reading and listening in people with aphasia: Effects of syntactic complexity. *American Journal of Speech-Language Pathology, 22*, 579–590.

DeDe, G., & Salis, C. (2020). Temporal and episodic analyses of the story of cinderella in latent aphasia. *American Journal of Speech-Language Pathology, 29*, 449–462.

Deem, J., & Miller, L. (2000). *Manual of voice therapy* (2nd ed.). PRO-ED.

DeKosky, S. T. (2008, May 13). *Alzheimer's disease: Current and future research*. Public Policy Forum, Alzheimer's Association, Washington, DC.

Delaney, A. (2015). Special considerations for the pediatric population relating to a swallow screen versus clinical swallow or instrumental evaluation. *Perspectives on Swallowing and Swallowing Disorders (Dysphagia)*, 24, 26–33.

Demers, D., & Bergeron, F. (2019). Effectiveness of rehabilitation approaches proposed to children with severe-to-profound prelinguistic deafness on the development of auditory, speech, and language skills: A systematic review. *Journal of Speech Language Hearing Research*, 62(11), 4196–4230.

Demmert, W.G., McCardle, P., & Leos, K. (2006). Conclusions and commentary. *Journal of American Indian Education*, 45(2), 77–88.

DePippo, K. L., Holas, M. A., & Reding, M. J. (1992). Validation of the 3-oz water swallow test for aspiration following stroke. *Archives of Neurology*, 49(12), 1259–1261.

DeRuyter, F., Fromm, D., Holland, A., & Stein, M. (2008). *Aphasia resulting from left hemisphere stroke*. Treatment Efficacy Summary. www.asha.org/NR/rdonlyres/4BAF3969-9ADC-4C01-B5ED-1334CC20DD3D/0/TreatmentEfficacySummaries2008.pdf

DeSiati, R., Rosenzweig, F., Gersdorff, G., Gregoire, A., Rom-Baux, P., & Deggouj, N. (2020). Auditory neuropathy spectrum disorders: From diagnosis to treatment: Literature review and case reports. *Journal of Clinical Medicine*, 9(4), 1074.

Desjardins, M., Apfelbach, C., Rubino, M., & Abbotta, V. (2022). Integrative review and framework of suggested mechanisms in primary muscle tension dysphonia. *Journal of Speech, Language, and Hearing Research*, 5, 1867–1893. https://doi.org/10.1044/2022_JSLHR-21-00575

DeThorne, L. S., Petrill, S. A., Hart, S. A., Channell, R. W., Campbell, R. J., Deater-Deckard, K., et al. (2008). Genetic effects on children's conversational language use. *Journal of Speech, Language, and Hearing Research*, 51, 423–435.

Deutsch, G. K., Dougherty, R. F., Bammer, R., Siok, W. T., Gabrieli, J. D., & Wandell, B. (2005). Children's reading performance is correlated with white matter structure measured by diffusion tensor imaging. *Cortex*, 41, 354–363.

Diefendorf, A. (1988). Pediatric audiology. In J. Lass, L. McReynolds, J. Northern, & D. Yoder (Eds.), *Handbook of speech language pathology and audiology* (pp. 1315–1338). Decker.

Diehl, S. F., Ford, C., & Federico, J. (2005). The communication journey of a fully included child with an autism spectrum disorder. *Topics in Language Disorders*, 25(4), 375–387.

Dingman, M. (2022). *2-minute neuroscience videos*. https://neuroscientificallychallenged.com/videos

Dinnes, C. R., & Hux, K (2022a). Informal written language analysis methods: Case examples of adults with traumatic brain injury. *American Journal of Speech-Language Pathology*, 31, 203–220.

Dinnes, C. R., & Hux, K. (2022b). Perceptions about writing by adults with moderate or severe traumatic brain injury. *American Journal of Speech-Language Pathology*, 31, 838–853.

Dodd, B., Hua, Z., Crosbie, S., Holm, A., & Ozanne, A. (2006). *Diagnostic Evaluation of Articulation and Phonology (DEAP)*. Pearson Education.

Dollaghan, C. A. (2004). Evidence-based practice in communication disorders: What do we know, and when do we know it? *Journal of Communication Disorders*, 37, 391–400.

Dollaghan, C. A., & Horner, E. A. (2011). Bilingual language assessment: A meta-analysis of diagnostic accuracy. *Journal of Speech, Language, and Hearing Research*, 54, 1077–1088.

Donahue, M. L., & Foster, S. K. (2004). Social cognition, conversation, and reading comprehension: How to read a comedy of manners. In C. A. Stone, E. R. Silliman, B. J. Ehren, & K. Apel (Eds.), *Handbook of language and literacy: Development and disorders* (pp. 363–379). Guilford Press.

Donoso Brown, E. V., Wallace, S. E., & Liu, Q. (2021). Speech-language pathologists' practice patterns when designing home practice programs for persons with aphasia: A survey. *American Journal of Speech-Language Pathology*, 30, 2605–2615.

Donovan, N. J., Okereke, O. I., Vannini, P., Amariglio, R. E., Rentz, D. M., Marshall, G. A., et al. (2016). Association of higher cortical amyloid burden with loneliness in cognitively normal older adults. *JAMA Psychiatry*, 73(12), 1230–1237.

Dore, J., Franklin, M., Miller, R., & Ramer, A. (1976). Transitional phenomena in early language acquisition. *Journal of Child Language*, 3, 13–28.

Dorner, B., & Friedrich, E. (2018). Position of the Academy of Nutrition and Dietetics: Individualized nutrition approaches for older adults: Long-term care, post-acute care, and other settings. *Journal of Academy of Nutrition and Dietetics*, 118, 724–735.

Douglas, J. M. (2010). Relation of executive function to pragmatic outcome following severe traumatic brain injury. *Journal of Speech, Language, and Hearing Research*, 53, 365–382.

Douglas, N. F., & Affoo, R. H. (2019). Certified nursing assistants want to use external memory aids for residents with dementia: Survey results within an implementation science framework. *American Journal of Speech-Language Pathology, 28,* 591–598.

Douglas, N. F., & MacPherson, M. K. (2021). Positive changes in certified nursing assistants' communication behaviors with people with dementia: Feasibility of a coaching strategy. *American Journal of Speech-Language Pathology, 30,* 239–252.

Douglas, S. N., Light, J. C., & McNaughton, D. B. (2013). Teaching paraeducators to support the communication of young children with complex communication needs. *Topics in Early Childhood Special Education, 33*(2), 91–101. https://doi.org/10.1177/0271121412467074

Downey, D. M., & Snyder, L. E. (2000). College students with LLD: The phonological core as risk for failure in foreign language classes. *Topics in Language Disorder, 21*(1), 82–92.

Downey, D., Daugherty, P., Helt, S., & Daugherty, D. (2004). Integrating AAC into the classroom. *The ASHA Leader, 9*(17), 6–7, 36.

Drager, K. D. R., & Reichle, J. E. (2001). Effects of age and divided attention on listeners' comprehension of synthesized speech. *Augmentative and Alternative Communication, 17,* 109–119.

Drager, K. D. R., Postal, V. J., Carrolus, L., Castellano, M., Gagliano, C., & Glynn, J. (2006). The effect of aided language modeling on symbol comprehension and production in 2 preschoolers with autism. *American Journal of Speech-Language Pathology, 15,* 112–125.

Drager, K., Clark-Serpentine, E. A., Johnson, K. E., & Roeser, J. L. (2006). Accuracy of repetition of digitized and synthesized speech for young children in background noise. *American Journal of Speech-Language Pathology, 15*(2), 155–164.

Drager, K., Light, J., Currall, J., Muttiah, N., Smith, V., Kreis, D., et al. (2019). AAC technologies with visual scene displays and "just in time" programming and symbolic communication turns expressed by students with severe disability. *Journal of Intellectual and Developmental Disability, 44*(3), 321–336. https://doi.org/10.3109/13668250.2017.1326585

Duchan, J. F. (2002). What do you know about the history of speech-language pathology? And why is it important? *The ASHA Leader, 7*(23), 4–5, 29.

Duff, D., Tomblin, J. B., & Catts, H. (2015). The influence of reading on vocabulary growth: A case for a Matthew effect. *Journal of Speech, Language, and Hearing Research, 58,* 853–864.

Duffy, J. (2020). *Motor speech disorders: Substrates, differential diagnosis, and management* (4th ed.). Elsevier.

Dyson, H., Best, W., Solity, J., & Hulme, C. (2017). Training mispronunciation correction and word meanings improves children's ability to learn to read words. *Scientific Studies of Reading, 21,* 392–407.

Easterling, C., & Robbins, E. (2008). Dementia and dysphagia. *Geriatric Nursing, 29,* 275–285.

Ebert, K., & Pham, G. (2017). Synthesizing information from language samples and standardized tests in school-age bilingual assessment. *Language, Speech, and Hearing Services in Schools, 48,* 42–55.

Eckert, M. A., Leonard, C. M., Wilke, M., Eckert, M., Richards, T., Richards, A., & Berninger, V. (2005). Anatomical signatures of dyslexia in children: Unique information from manual and voxel based morphometry brain measures. *Cortex, 41*(3), 304–315.

Edmonds, L. A., & Babb, M. (2011). Effect of verb network strengthening treatment in moderate-to-severe aphasia. *American Journal of Speech-Language Pathology, 20,* 131–145.

Edwards, J., Beckman, M.E., & Munson, B. (2015). Frequency effects in phological acquisition. *Journal of Child Language, 42,* 306–311. https://doi.org/10.1017/S0305000914000634

Ehren, B. J. (2005). Looking for evidence-based practice in reading comprehension instruction. *Topics in Language Disorders, 25,* 310–321.

Ehren, B. J. (2006). Partnerships to support reading comprehension for students with language impairment. *Topics in Language Disorders, 26,* 42–54.

Ehri, L. C. (2000). Learning to read and learning to spell: Two sides of a coin. *TLD, Topics in Language Disorders, 20*(3), 19–36.

Eigsti, L., & Cicchetti, D. (2004). The impact of child maltreatment on the expressive syntax at 60 months. *Developmental Science, 7,* 88–102.

Eisenberg, S. L., Bredin-Oja, S. L., & Crumrine, K. (2020). Use of imitation training for targeting grammar: A narrative review. *Language, Speech, and Hearing Services in Schools, 51,* 205–225. https://doi.org/10.1044/2019_LSHSS-19-00024

Eisenberg, S. L., McGovern Fersko, T., & Lundgren, C. (2001). The use of MLU for identifying language impairment in preschool children: A review. *American Journal of Speech-Language Pathology, 10,* 323–342.

Eisenberg, S. L., Ukrainetz, T. A., Hsu, J. R., Kaderavek, J. N., Justice, L. M., & Gillam, R. B. (2008). Noun phrase elaboration in children's spoken stories. *Language, Speech, and Hearing Services in Schools, 39,* 145–157.

Elbourn, E., Kenny, B., Power, E., & Togher, L. (2019). Psychosocial outcomes of severe traumatic brain injury in relation to discourse recovery: A longitudinal study up to 1 year post-injury. *American Journal of Speech-Language Pathology, 28,* 1463–1478.

Ellis Weismer, S., Plante, E., Jones, M., & Tomblin, J. B. (2005): A functional magnetic resonance imaging investigation of verbal working memory in adolescents with specific language impairment. *Journal of Speech, Language, and Hearing Research, 48,* 405–425.

Ellis, L., & Beltyukova, S. (2012). Evidence-based diagnostic treatment and treatment planning for adult stuttering: A case study. *Perspectives on Fluency & Fluency Disorders, 22,* 70–87.

Ellsperman, S., Narin, E., & Stucken, E. (2021). Review of bone conduction devices. *Audiology Research, 11*(2), 207–219.

Elsahar Y., H. S.-M. (2019). Augmentative and alternative communication (AAC) advances: A review of configurations for indivudals with a speech disability. *Sensors, EISSN 1424-8220, Published by MDPI.*

Elsahar Y., Hu, S., Bouazza-Marouf, K., Kerr, D., & Mansor, A. (2019). Augmentative and alternative communication (AAC) advannces: A review of configurations for indivudals with a speech disability. *Sensors (Basel, Switzerland), 19*(8), 1911.

Elwer, S., Keenan, J. M., Olson, R. K., Byrne, B., & Samuelsson, S. (2013). Longitudinal stability and predictors of poor oral comprehenders and poor decoders. *Journal of Experimental Child Psychology, 115,* 497–516.

Englert, C. S., Raphael, T. E., Anderson, L. M., Anthony, H. M., Fear, K. L., & Gregg, S. L. (1988). A case for writing intervention: Strategies for writing informational text. *Learning Disabilities Focus, 3*(2), 98–113.

English, K. (2007). Psychosocial aspects of hearing impairment and counseling basics. In R. L. Schow & M. A. Nerbonne (Eds.), *Introduction to audiologic rehabilitation* (5th ed., pp. 245–268). Pearson.

Erikson, K. A., & Koppenhaver, D. A. (2020). *Comprehensive literacy for all: Teaching students with significant disabilities to read and write.* Baltimore: Paul H. Brookes.

Ertmer, D. J., Strong, L. M., & Sadagopan, N. (2003). Beginning to communicate after cochlear implantation: Oral language development in a young child. *Journal of Speech, Language, and Hearing Research, 46,* 328–340.

Everhart, R. (1960). Literature survey growth and developmental factors in articulation maturation. *Journal of Speech and Hearing Disorders, 25,* 59–69.

Fabiano-Smith, L. (2019). Standardized tests and the diagnosis of speech sound disorders. *Perspectives of the ASHA Special Interests Groups, 4,* 58–66.

Fabiano-Smith, L., & Goldstein, B. (2010). Phonological acquisition in bilingual Spanish-English speaking children. *Journal of Speech, Language, and Hearing Research, 53,* 160–178.

Fabiano-Smith, L., & Hoffman, K. (2018). Diagnostic accuracy of traditional measures of phonological ability for bilingual preschoolers and kindergarteners. *Language, Speech, and Hearing Services in Schools, 49,* 121–134.

Fairbanks, G. (1960). *Voice and articulation drillbook.* Harper & Row.

Fallon, K. A., Light, J. C., & Paige, T. K. (2001). Enhancing vocabulary selection for preschoolers who require augmentative and alternative communication (AAC). *American Journal of Speech-Language Pathology, 10*(1), 81–94.

Fama, M. E., Lemonds, E., & Levinson, G. (2022). The subjective experience of word-finding difficulties in people with aphasia: A thematic analysis of interview data. *American Journal of Speech-Language Pathology, 31,* 3–11.

Faroqi-Shah, Y., & Gehman, M. (2021). The role of processing speed and cognitive control on word retrieval in aging and aphasia. *Journal of Speech, Language, and Hearing Research, 64,* 949–964.

Feeney, J., & Capo, M. (2002, November). *Using self-advocacy videos to educate staff in TBI rehabilitation.* Paper presented at the American Speech-Language-Hearing Association national convention, Atlanta.

Feinberg, M. (1997). The effects of medications on swallowing. In B. C. Sonies (Ed.), *Dysphagia: A continuum of care.* Aspen. 107–122

Feldman, H. M., Dollaghan, C. A., Campbell, T. F., Colborn, D. K., Janosky, J., Kurs-Lasky, M., et al. (2003). Parent-reported language skills in relation to otitis media during the first 3 years of life. *Journal of Speech, Language, and Hearing Research, 46,* 273–287.

Felsenfeld, S., Kirk, K., Zhu, G., Statham, D., Neale, M., & Martin, N. (2000). A study on the genetic and environmental etiology of stuttering in a selected twin sample. *Behavior Genetics, 305,* 359–366.

Ferguson, N. F., Evans, K., & Raymer, A. M. (2012). A comparison of intention and pantomime gesture treatment for noun retrieval in people with aphasia. *American Journal of Speech-Language Pathology, 21,* 126–139.

Ferré, P., Clermont, M., Lajoie, C., Côté, H., Ferreres, A., Abusamra, V., et al. (2009). Identification of communication patterns of adults with right brain profiles. *Journal of Latin-American Neuropsychology, 1,* 32–40.

Ferré, P., Ska, B., Lajoie, C., Bleau, A., & Joanette, Y. (2011). Clinical focus on prosodic, discursive and pragmatic treatment for right hemisphere damaged adults: What's right? *Rehabilitation Research and Practice,* 1–10.

Ferreri, G. (1959). Senescence of the larynx. *Italian General Review of Otorhinolaryngology, 1,* 640–709.

Fey, M. E., Long, S. H., & Finestack, L. H. (2003). Ten principles of grammar facilitation for children with specific language impairment. *American Journal of Speech-Language Pathology, 12,* 3–15.

Fey, M.E., Catts, H., Proctor-Williams, K., Tomblin, B., & Zhang, X. (2004). Oral and written story composition skills of children with language impairment. *Journal of Speech, Language, and Hearing Research, 47,* 1301–1318.

FHI 360. (2003). National Dissemination Center for Children with Disabilities. https://www.fhi360.org/projects/national-dissemination-center-children-disabilities-nichcy

Filiatrault-Veilleux, P., Bouchard, C., Trudeau, N., & Desmarais, C. (2016). Comprehension of inferences in a narrative in 3- to 6-year-old children. *Journal of Speech, Language, and Hearing Research, 59*, 1099–1110.

Finestack, L. H. (2018). Evaluation of an explicit intervention to teach novel grammatical forms to children with developmental language disorder. *Journal of Speech, Language and Hearing Disorders, 61*, 2065–2075.

Finestack, L. H., & Fey, M. E. (2009). Evaluation of a deductive procedure to teach grammatical inflections to children with language impairment. *American Journal of Speech-Language Pathology, 18*, 289–302.

Finke, E. H., Davis, J. M., Benedict, M., Goga, L., Kelly, J., Palumbo, L., & Waters, S. (2017). Effects of a least-to-most prompting procedure on multisymbol message production in children with Autism Spectrum Disorder who use augmentative and alternative communication. *American Journal of Speech-Language Pathology, 26*(1), 81–98. https://doi.org/10.1044/2016_AJSLP-14-0187

Fitzhugh, M. C., LaCroix, A. N., & Rogalsky, C. (2021). Distinct contributions of working memory and attentional control to sentence comprehension in noise in persons with stroke. *Journal of Speech, Language, and Hearing Research, 64*, 3230–3241.

Flax, J. F., Realpe-Bonilla, T., Hirsch, L. S., Brzustowicz, L. M., Bartlett, C. W., & Tallal, P. (2003). Specific language impairment in families: Evidence for co-occurrence with reading impairments. *Journal of Speech, Language, and Hearing Research, 46*, 530–543.

Fletcher, K., & Ash, B. (2005). The speech-language pathologist and the lactation consultant: The baby's feeding dream team. *The ASHA Leader, 10*(2). https://leader.pubs.asha.org/doi/10.1044/leader.FTR2.10022005.8

Florit, E., Roch, M., & Levorato, M. C. (2014). Listening text comprehension in preschoolers: A longitudinal study on the role of semantic components. *Reading and Writing: An Interdisciplinary Journal, 27*(5), 793–817.

Flurie, M., Ungrady, M., & Reilly, J. (2020). Evaluating a maintenance-based treatment approach to preventing lexical dropout in progressive anomia. *Journal of Speech, Language, and Hearing Research, 63*, 4085–4095.

Fombonne, E. (2003). The prevalence of autism. *Journal of the American Medical Association, 289*, 87–89.

Foster, A., Jacques, B., & Fabrice, P. (2022). Hearing loss: The final frontier of pharmacology. *Pharmacology Research and Perspectives, 10*(3), e00970.

Foster, W. A., & Miller, M. (2007). Development of the literacy achievement gap: A longitudinal study of kindergarten through third grade. *Language, Speech, and Hearing Services in Schools, 38*, 173–181.

Fox, C., & Boliek, C. (2012). Intensive voice treatment (LSVT LOUD) for children with spastic cerebral palsy and dysarthria. *Journal of Speech, Language, and Hearing Research, 55*, 930–945.

Fox, C., & Boliek, C. (2017). Implementation of LSVT LOUD in pediatric motor speech disorders online course. (Available from LSVT Global, 4720 N. Oracle Rd., Ste. 100, Tucson, AZ 85705)

Fox, C., Boliek, C., & Ramig, L., (2006, March). *The impact of intensive voice treatment (LSVT®) on speech intelligibility in children with spastic cerebral palsy.* Poster presented at the Conference on Motor Speech, Austin, TX.

Fox, C., Morrison, C., Ramig, L., & Sapir, S. (2002). Current perspectives on the Lee Silverman Voice Treatment (LSVT) for individuals with idiopathic Parkinson disease. *American Journal of Speech-Language Pathology, 11*, 111–123.

Fox, L. E., & Rau, M. T. (2001). Augmentative and alternative communication for adults following glossectomy and laryngectomy surgery. *Augmentative and Alternative Communication, 17*, 161–166.

Foy, J. G., & Mann, V. (2003). Home literacy environment and phonological awareness in preschool children: Differential effects for rhyme and phoneme awareness. *Applied Psycholinguistics, 24*, 59–88.

Francis, A. L., Nusbaum, H. C., & Fenn, K. (2007). Effects of training on the acoustic-phonetic representation of synthetic speech. *Journal of Speech, Language, and Hearing Research, 50*, 1445–1465.

Francis, D., Daniero, J., Hovis, K., Sathe, N., Jacobson, B., Penson, D., et al. (2017). Voice-relate patient-reported outcome measures: A systematic review of instrument development and validation. *Journal of Speech, Language, and Hearing Research, 60*, 62–88.

Franco, R., & Andrus, J. (2009). Aerodynamic and acoustic characteristics of voice before and after adduction arytenopexy and medialization laryngoplasty with GORE-TEX in patients with unilateral voice fold immobility. *Journal of Voice, 23*, 261–267. https://doi.org/10.1016/j.jvoice.2007.09.009

Franken, M.-C., Kielstra-Van der Schalk, C. J., & Boelens, H. (2005). Experimental treatment of early stuttering: A preliminary study. *Journal of Fluency Disorders, 30*, 189–199.

Frazier Norbury, C., Gooch, D., Wray, C., Baird, G., Charman, T., Simonoff, E., Vamvakas, G., & Pickles, A. (2016). The impact of nonverbal ability on prevalence and clinical presentation of language disorder: Evidence from a population study. *Journal of Child Psychology and Psychiatry, 57*, 1247–1257. https://doi.org/10.1111/jcpp.12573

Fremont A., & Hoyland, J. (2007). Morphology, mechanisms, and pathology of musculoskeletal ageing. *Journal of Pathology, 211*, 252–259.

Fridriksson, J., Moser, D., Ryalls, J., Bonilha, L., Rorden, C., & Baylis, G. (2009). Modulation of frontal lobe speech areas associated with the production and perception of speech movements. *Journal of Speech and Hearing Research, 52*, 812–819.

Fried-Oken, M., Fox, L., Rau, M. T., Tullman, J., Baker, G., Hindal, M., et al. (2006). Purposes of AAC device use for persons with ALS as reported by caregivers. *Augmentative and Alternative Communication, 22*, 209–221.

Friedland, D., Cederberg, C., & Tarima, S. (2009). Audiometric pattern as a predictor of cardiovascular status: Development of a model for assessment of risk. *Laryngoscope, 119*(3), 473–486.

Fry, R. (2007). *The changing racial and ethnic composition of U.S. public schools.* Pew Hispanic Center.

Fuchs, D., Fuchs, L. S., Thompson, A., Otaiba, S. A., Yen, L., Yang, N. J., et al. (2001). Is reading important in reading-readiness programs?: A randomized field trial with teachers as program implementers. *Journal of Educational Psychology, 93*, 251–267.

Fudala, J., & Stegall, S. (2017). *Arizona Articulation and Phonology Scale, Fourth Revision (Arizona-4).* WPS.

Galaburda, A. L. (2005). Neurology of learning disabilities: What will the future bring? The answer comes from the successes of the recent past. *Journal of Learning Disabilities, 28*, 107–109.

Gallinat, E., & Spaulding, T. J. (2014). Differences in the performance of children with specific language impairment and their typically developing peers on nonverbal cognitive tests: A meta-analysis. *Journal of Speech, Language, and Hearing Research, 57*, 1363–1382.

Garand, K., McCullough, G., Crary, M., Arvedson, J., & Dodrill, P. (2020). Assessment across the life span: The clinical swallow evaluation. *American Journal of Speech-Language Pathology, 29*, 919–933.

Garcia, H., & Miralles, F. (2017). *Ikigai: The Japanese secret to a long and happy life.* Penguin.

Gary, K. W., Sima, A., Wehman, P., & Johnson, K. R. (2019). Transitioning racial/ethnic minorities with intellectual developmental disabilities: Influence of socioeconomic status on related services. *Career Development and Transition for Exceptional Individuals, 42*(3), 158–167.

Gathercole, S. E., Alloway, T. P., Willis, C., & Adams, A. M. (2006). Working memory in children with reading disabilities. *Journal of Experimental Child Psychology, 93*, 256–281.

Gatlin, B., & Wanzek, J. (2015). Relations among children's use of dialect and literacy skills: A meta-analysis. *Journal of Speech, Language, and Hearing Research, 58*, 1306–1318.

Gelfer, M., & Schofield, K. (2000). Comparison of acoustic and perceptual measures of voice in male-to-female transsexuals perceived as female versus those perceived as male. *Journal of Voice, 14*(1), 22–23.

Georges, A., & Das, J. M. (2022). *Traumatic brain injury.* StatPearls. https://www.ncbi.nlm.nih.gov/books/NBK459300/

Gerber, A., & Klein, E. R. (2004, November). *Teacher/tutor assisted literacy learning in the primary grades, a speech-language approach to early reading: T. A. L. L. while small.* Paper presented at the annual convention of the American Speech-Language-Hearing Association, Philadelphia.

Gersten, R., & Baker, S. (2001). Teaching expressive writing to students with learning disabilities: A meta-analysis. *Elementary School Journal, 101*(3), 251–272.

Gersten, R., Compton, D., Connor, C. M., Dimino, J., Santoro, L., Linan-Thompson, S., & Tilly, W. D. (2009). *Assisting students struggling with reading: Response to Intervention and multitier intervention for reading in the primary grades. A practice guide* (NCEE 2009-4045). Institute of Education Sciences. http://ies.ed.gov/ncee/wwc/publications/practiceguides/

Gierut, J. (2007). Phonological complexity and language learnability. *American Journal of Speech-Language Pathology, 16*, 6–17.

Gierut, J. A. (1998). Treatment efficacy: Functional phonological disorders in children. *Journal of Speech, Language, and Hearing Research, 41*(1), S85–S100.

Gierut, J. A. (2001). Complexity in phonological treatment: Clinical factors. *Language, Speech, and Hearing Services in Schools, 32*, 229–241.

Gierut, J. A. (2005). Phonological intervention: The how or the what? In A. Kamhi & K. Pollock (Eds.), *Phonological disorders in children: Clinical decision making in assessment and intervention* (pp. 201–210). Brookes.

Gierut, J. A. (2009, June 19). *Phonological disorders in children.* Treatment Efficacy Summary. www.asha.org/NR/rdonlyres/F251004F-005C-47D9-8A2C-B85C818F3D33/0/TESPhonologicalDisordersinChildren.pdf

Gierut, J. A., Morrisette, M. L., Hughes, M. T., & Rowland, S. (1996). Phonological treatment efficacy and developmental norms. *Language, Speech, and Hearing Services in Schools, 27*, 215–230.

Gildersleeve-Neumann, C., Kester, E., Davis, B., & Peña, E. (2008). English speech sound development in preschool-aged children from bilingual English-Spanish environments. *Language, Speech, and Hearing Services in Schools, 39*, 314–328. https://doi.org/10.1044/0161-1461(2008/030)

Gillam, R. B., & Gorman, B. K. (2004). Language and discourse contributions to word recognition and text interpretation. In E. R. Silliman & L. C. Wilkinson (Eds.), *Language and literacy learning in schools* (pp. 63–97). Guilford Press.

Gillon, G. T. (2000). The efficacy of phonological awareness intervention for children with spoken language impairment. *Language, Speech, and Hearing Services in Schools, 31,* 126–141.

Gilmore, N., Mirman, D., & Kiran, S. (2022). Young adults with acquired brain injury show longitudinal improvements in cognition after intensive cognitive rehabilitation. *Journal of Speech, Language, and Hearing Research, 64,* 1494–1520.

Girolametto, L., Hoaken, L., Weitzman, E., & van Lieshout, R. (2000). Patterns of adult-child linguistic interaction in integrated day care groups. *Language, Speech, and Hearing Services in Schools, 31,* 155–168.

Girolametto, L., Weitzman, E., & Greenberg, J. (2003). Training day care staff to facilitate children's language. *American Journal of Speech-Language Pathology, 12,* 299–311.

Girolametto, L., Weitzman, E., & Greenberg, J. (2012). Facilitating emergent literacy: Efficacy of a model that partners speech-language pathologists and educators. *American Journal of Speech-Language Pathology, 21,* 47–63.

Glaspey, A., & Stoel-Gammon, C. (2007). A dynamic approach to phonological assessment. *Advances in Speech Language Pathology, 9,* 286–296.

Glattke, T. J., & Robinette, M. S. (2007). Otoacoustic emissions. In R. J. Roeser, M. Valente, & H. H. Dunn (Eds.), *Audiology: Diagnosis* (2nd ed., pp. 478–496). Thieme.

Glaze, L., Bless, D., Milenkovic, R., & Susser, R. (1988). Acoustic characteristics of children's voice. *Journal of Voice, 2,* 312–319.

Glennen, S. L., & DeCost, D. C. (1997). *The handbook of augmentative and alternative communication.* Cengage.

Glennen, S. L., & DeCoste, C. (1997). *Handbook of augmentative communication.* Singular.

Gliklich, R., Glovsky, R., & Montgomery, W. (1999). Validation of a voice outcome survey for unilateral vocal cord paralysis. *Journal of Otolaryngology-Head and Neck Surgery, 120,* 153–158.

Goday, P., Huh, S., Silverman, A., Lukens, C., Dodrill, P., Cohan, S., et al. (2019). Pediatric feeding disorder: Consensus definition and conceptual Framework. *Journal of Pediatric Gastroenterology and Nutrition, 68,* 124–129.

Goffman, L., & Leonard, J. (2000). Growth of language skills in preschool children with specific language impairment: Implications for assessment and intervention. *American Journal of Speech-Language Pathology, 9,* 151–161. https://doi.org/10.1044/1058-0360.0902.151

Goldberg, E. B., Meier, E. L., Sheppard, S. M., Breining, B. L., & Hillis, A. E. (2021). Stroke recurrence and its relationship with language abilities. *Journal of Speech, Language, and Hearing Research, 64,* 2022–2037.

Goldberg, K. A. (2020). Language deprivation and the impact on mental health of deaf/hard of hearing and blind/low vision children. *Journal of the American Academy of Child and Adolescent Psychiatry, 59*(10, Suppl.), S74.

Goldman, R., & Fristoe, M. (2015). *Goldman-Fristoe test of articulation-Third edition (GFTA-3).* Pearson Education.

Goldstein, B. (2007). Phonological skills in Puerto Rican and Mexican Spanish-speaking children with phonological disorders. *Clinical Linguistics & Phonetics, 21,* 93–109.

Goldstein, B., & Cintron, P. (2001). An investigation of phonological skills in Puerto Rican Spanish-speaking 2-year-olds. *Clinical Linguistics & Phonetics, 15,* 343–361.

Goldstein, B., & Iglesias, A. (2006). *Contextual Probes of Articulation Competence: Spanish (CPAC-S).* PRO-ED.

Goldstein, B., & Iglesias, A. (2013). Language and dialectal variations. In J. Bernthal, N. Bankson, & P. Flipsen (Eds.), *Articulation and phonological disorders: Speech sound disorders in children* (7th ed., pp. 326–354). Pearson Education.

Goldstein, B., & Iglesias, A. (2017). Language and dialectical variations. In J. Bernthal, N. Bankson, & P. Flipsen (Ed.), *Articulation and phonological disorders: Speech sound disorders in children* (8th ed., pp. 277–301). Pearson Education

Goldstein, B., & Pollock, K. (2000). Vowel errors in Spanish-speaking children with phonological disorders: A retrospective comparative study. *Clinical Linguistics & Phonetics, 14,* 217–234.

Goldstein, B., Fabiano, L, & Washington, S. (2005). Phonological skills in predominately English-speaking, predominantly Spanish-speaking, and Spanish-English bilingual children. *Language, Speech, and Hearing Services in Schools, 36,* 201–218.

Goldstein, H., & Prelock, P. (2008). *Child language disorders.* Treatment Efficacy Summary. www.asha.org/NR/rdonlyres/4BAF3969-9ADC-4C01-B5ED-1334CC20DD3D/0/TreatmentEfficacySummaries2008.pdf

Goodrich, J. M., Lonigan, C. J., & Farver, J. M. (2013). Do early literacy skills in children's first language promoted development of skills in their second language? An experimental evaluation of transfer. *Journal of Educational Psychology, 105,* 414–426.

Gorham-Rowan, M., & Morris, R. (2006). Aerodynamic analysis of male-to-female transgender voice. *Journal of Voice, 20*(2), 251–262.

Gorman, B. K. (2012). Relationships between vocabulary size, working memory, and phonological awareness in Spanish-speaking English language learners. *American Journal of Speech-Language Pathology, 21,* 109–123.

Gormley, J., & Light, J. (2019). Providing services to individuals with complex communication needs in the inpatient rehabilitation setting: The experiences and perspectives of speech-language pathologists. *American Journal of Speech-Language Pathology, 28,* 456–468.

Gosa, M., & Dodrill, P. (2017). Pediatric dysphagia rehabilitation: Considering the evidence to support common strategies. *Perspectives of the ASHA Special Interest Groups, 2,* 27–35.

Gottwald, S. (2010). Stuttering prevention and early intervention: A multidimensional approach. In B. Guitar & R. J. McCauley (Eds.), *Treatment of stuttering: Established and emerging interventions* (pp. 91–117). Lippincott Williams & Wilkins.

Goudey, B., Plant, K., Kiral, I., Jimeno-Yepes, A., Swan, A., Gambhir, M., et al. (2021). A multicenter analysis of factors associated with hearing outcome for 2,735 adults with cochlear implants. *Trends in Hearing, 25,* 1–7.

Gough Kenyon, S. M., Palikara, O., & Lucas, R. M. (2018). Explaining reading comprehension in children with developmental language disorder: The importance of elaborative inferencing. *Journal of Speech, Language and Hearing Disorders, 61,* 2517–2531.

Gozzard, H., Baker, E., & McCabe, P. (2004). *Single Word Test of Polysyllables.* Unpublished manuscript.

Graham, C. (2015). *The high cost of being poor in America: Stress, pain, and worry.* Brookings Institute. https://www.brookings.edu/blog/social-mobility-memos/2015/02/19/the-high-costs-of-being-poor-in-america-stress-pain-and-worry/

Graham, S. (2006). Writing. In E. Anderman, P. H. Winne, P. A. Alexander, & L. Corno (Eds.), *Handbook of educational psychology* (pp. 457–478). Routledge.

Granlund, M., Björck-ÄKesson, E., Wilder, J., & Ylvén, R. (2008). AAC interventions for children in a family environment: Implementing evidence in practice. *Augmentative and Alternative Communication, 24,* 207–219.

Gray, S. (2004). Word learning by preschoolers with specific language impairment: Predictors and poor learners. *Journal of Speech, Language, and Hearing Research, 47,* 1117–1132.

Gray, S. (2005). Word learning by preschoolers with specific language impairment: Effect of phonological or semantic cues. *Journal of Speech, Language, and Hearing Research, 48,* 1452–1467.

Gray, S., Fox, A. B., Green, S., Alt, M., Hogan, T. P., Petscher, Y., & Cowan, N. (2019). Working memory profiles of children with dyslexia, developmental language disorder, or both. *Journal of Speech, Language, and Hearing Research, 62,* 1839–1858. https://doi.org/10.1044/2019_JSLHR-L-18-0148

Greenhalgh, K. S., & Strong, C. J. (2001). Literate language features in spoken narratives of children with typical language and children with language impairments. *Language, Speech, and Hearing Services in Schools, 32,* 114–126.

Greenough, W. T. (1975). Experimental modification of the developing brain. *American Science, 63,* 37–46.

Grice, S. J., Halit, H., Farroni, T., Baron-Cohen, S., Bolton, P., & Johnson, M. H. (2005). Neural correlates of eye-gaze detection in young children with autism. *Cortex, 41,* 327–341.

Grigorenko, E. L. (2005). A conservative meta-analysis of linkage and linkage-association studies of developmental dyslexia. *Scientific Studies of Reading, 9,* 285–316.

Groher, M., & Crary, M. (2010). *Dysphagia: Clinical management in adults and children.* Mosby Elsevier.

Gross, R., Mahlmann, J., & Grayhack, J., (2003). Physiologic effects of open and closed tracheostomy tubes on the pharyngeal swallow. *Annals of Otology, Rhinology, & Laryngology, 112,* 142–152.

Grove, N., & Dockrell, J. (2000) Multisign combinations by children with intellectual impairments: An analysis of language skills. *Journal of Speech, Language and Hearing Research, 43,* 309–323.

Grunwell, P. (1987). *Clinical phonology* (2nd ed.). Chapman & Hall.

Guitar, B. (2019). *Stuttering: An integrated approach to its nature and treatment* (5th ed.). Wolters Kluwer.

Guo, L.-Y., Tomblin, J. B., & Samelson, V. (2008). Speech disruptions in the narratives of English-speaking children with specific language impairment. *Journal of Speech, Language, and Hearing Research, 51,* 722–738.

Gutierrez-Clellen, V. F., Restrepo, M. A., Bedore, L., Pena, E., & Anderson, R. (2000). Language sample analysis in Spanish-speaking children: Methodological considerations. *Language, Speech, and Hearing Services in Schools, 31,* 88–98.

Gutmann, M. (2016). Use of simulation with standardized patients in AAC pre-service training: Potentiating practical learning. *Perspectives of the ASHA Special Interest Groups SIG 12 AAC,* 38–44. https://doi.org/10.1044/persp1.SIG12.38

Guyatt, G., & Rennie, D. (Eds.). (2002). *User's guides to the medical literature: A manual for evidence-based clinical practice.* American Medical Association Press.

Haak, P., Lenski, M., Hidecker, M., Li, M., & Paneth, N. (2009). Cerebral palsy and aging. *Developmental Medicine & Child Neurology, 51*(Suppl. 4), 16–23.

Haarbauer-Krupa, J., Heggs Lee, A., Bitsko, R. H., Zhang, X., & Kresnow-Sedacca, M. (2018). Prevalence of parent-reported traumatic brain injury in children and associated health conditions. *JAMA Pediatrics, 172*, 1078–1086.

Hadley, P. A., Simmerman, A., Long, M., & Luna, M. (2000). Facilitating language development in inner-city children: Experimental evaluation of a collaborative classroom-based intervention. *Language, Speech, and Hearing Services in Schools, 31*, 280–295.

Hadley, P. A., McKenna, M. M., & Rispoli, M. (2018). Sentence diversity in early language development: Recommendations for target selection and progress monitoring. *American Journal of Speech-Language Pathology, 27*, 553–565. https://doi.org/10.1044/2017_AJSLP-17-0098

Haley, K. L., Cunningham, K. T., Barry, J., & de Riesthal, M. (2019). Collaborative goals for communicative life participation in aphasia: The FOURC model. *American Journal of Speech-Language Pathology, 28*, 1–13.

Hall, J., McGregor, K. K., & Oleson, J. (2017). Weaknesses in lexical-semantic knowledge among college students with specific learning disabilities: Evidence from a semantic fluency task. *Journal of Speech, Language, and Hearing Research, 60*, 640–653.

Hall, W. (2017). What you don't know can hurt you: The risk of language deprivation by impairing sign language development in deaf children. *Maternal Child Health, 21*(5), 961–965. https://doi.org/10.1007/s10995-017-2287-y

Hambly, C., & Riddle, L. (2002, April). *Phonological awareness training for school-age children.* Paper presented at the annual convention of the New York State Speech-Language-Hearing Association, Rochester.

Hambly, H., Wren, Y., McLeod, S., & Roulstone, S. (2013). The influence of bilingualism on speech production: a systematic review. *International Journal of Communication Disorders, 48*, 1–24.

Hamdan, A-L., Tabet, G., Fakhri, G., Sarieddine, D., Btaiche, R., & Seoud, M. (2018). Effect of hormonal replacement therapy on voice. *Journal of Voice, 32*, 116–121.

Hancock, A., & Garabedian, L. (2013). Transgender voice and communication treatment: A retrospective chart review of 25 cases. *International Journal of Communication Disorders, 48*, 54–65.

Hancock, A., & Haskin, G. (2015). Speech-language pathologists' knowledge and attitudes regarding lesbian, gay, bisexual, trans-gender, and queer (LGBTQ) populations. *American Journal of Speech-Language Pathology, 24*, 206–221.

Hancock, A., & Helenius, L. (2012). Adolescent male-to-female transgender voice and communication. *Journal of Communication Disorders, 45*, 313–324.

Hane, A. A., Feldstein, S., & Dernetz, V. H. (2003). The relation between coordinated interpersonal timing and maternal sensitivity in four-month-olds. *Journal of Psycholinguistic Research, 32*, 525–539.

Hansen, P. (2017). What makes a word easy to acquire? The effects of word class, frequency, imageability and phonological neighbourhood density on lexical development. *First Language, 37*, 205–225. https://doi.org/10.1177/0142723716679956

Hansen, P. (2017). What makes a word easy to acquire?: The effects of word class, frequency, imageability and phonological neighbourhood density on lexical development. *First Language, 37*, 205–225.

Hardin-Jones, M., Chapman, K., & Scherer, N. J. (2006, June 13). Early intervention in children with cleft palate. *The ASHA Leader, 11*(8), 8–9, 32.

Hardy, E., & Robinson, N. (1999). *Swallowing disorders treatment manual* (2nd ed.). PRO-ED.

Hardy, E., & Robinson, N. M. (1993). *Swallowing disorders treatment manual.* Imaginart.

Harlaar, N., Hayiou-Thomas, M. E., Dale, P. S., & Plomin, R. (2008). Why do preschool language abilities correlate with later reading?: A twin study. *Journal of Speech, Language, and Hearing Research, 51*, 688–705.

Harmon, T. G., Jacks, A., Haley, K. L., & Bailliard, A. (2020). How responsiveness from a communication partner affects story retell in aphasia: Quantitative and qualitative findings. *American Journal of Speech-Language Pathology, 29*, 142–156.

Harris, K. R., & Graham, S. (1996). *Making the writing process work: Strategies for composition and self-regulation.* Brookline.

Harrison, L. J., & McLeod, S. (2010). Risk and protective factors associated with speech and language impairment in a nationally representative sample of 4- to 5-year-old children. *Journal of Speech, Language, and Hearing Research, 53*, 508–529.

Hart, K. I., Fujiki, M., Brinton, B., & Hart, C. H. (2004). The relationship between social behavior and severity of language impairment. *Journal of Speech, Language, and Hearing Research, 47*, 647–662.

Hashimoto, N. (2016). The use of one or three semantic associative primes in treating anomia in aphasia. *American Journal of Speech-Language Pathology, 25*, S665–S686.

Hayden, D., & Square, P. (1999). *Verbal motor production assessment for children.* Psychological Corporation.

Hayiou-Thomas, M. E., Harlaar, N., Dale, S., & Plomin, R. (2010). Preschool speech, language skills, and reading at 7, 9, and 10 years: Etiology of the relationship. *Journal of Speech, Language, and Hearing Research, 53*, 311–332.

Hearing Loss Association of America. (2018). *Hearing loss facts and statistics*. http://hearingloss.org/content/basic-facts-about-hearing-loss

Hemsley, B., & Dann, S. (2014). Social media and social marketing in relation to facilitated communication: Harnessing the affordances of social media for knowledge translation. *Evidence-Based Communication Assessment and Intervantion, 8*(4), 187–206.

Hemsley, B., Bryant, L., Schlosser, R. W., Shane, H., Lang, R. P., Banajee, M., & Ireland, M. (2018). Systematic review of facilitated communication 2014–2018 finds no new evidence that messages delivered using facilitated communication are authored by the person with the disability. *Autism & Developmental Language Impairments, 3*. https://doi.org/10.1177/2396941518821570

Henderson, E. H. (1990). *Teaching spelling* (2nd ed.). Houghton Mifflin.

Henry, M. L., Hubbard, H. I., Grasso, S. M., Dial, H. R., Beeson, P. M., Miller, B. L., & Gorno-Tempini, M. L. (2019). Treatment for word retrieval in semantic and logopenic variants of primary progressive aphasia: Immediate and long-term outcomes. *Journal of Speech, Language, and Hearing Research, 62,* 2723–2749.

Herring, M., Putney, L., Wyatt, G., Finkbeiner, W., & Hyde, D. (2014). Growth of alveoli during postnatal development in humans based on stereological estimation. *American Journal of Physiology—Lung Cellular and Molecular Physiology, 307*(4), L338–L344.

Hewat, S., Onslow, M., Packman, A., & O'Brain, S. (2006). A phase II clinical trial of self-imposed time-out treatment for stuttering in adults and adolescents. *Disability and Rehabilitation, 28,* 33–42.

Hewetson, R., Cornwell, P., & Shum, D. H. K. (2021). Relationship and social network change in people with impaired social cognition post right hemisphere stroke. *American Journal of Speech-Language Pathology, 30,* 962–973.

Hewlett, N. (1990). The processes of speech production and speech development. In P. Grunwell (Ed.), *Developmental speech disorders: Clinical issues and practical implications* (pp. 15–38). Churchill Livingstone.

Hickok, G., Okada, K., Barr, W., Pa, J., Rogalsky, C., Donnelly, K., et al. (2008). Bilateral capacity for speech sound processing in auditory comprehension: Evidence from Wada procedures. *Brain and Language, 107,* 179–184.

Hicks, C. B., Tharpe, A. M., & Ashmead, D. H. (2000). Behavioral auditory assessment of young infants: Methodologic limitations or natural lack of auditory responsiveness? *American Journal of Audiology, 9,* 124–130.

Higginbotham, D. J., Bisantz, A. M., Sunm, M., Adams, K., & Yik, F. (2009). The effect of context priming and task type on augmentative communication performance. *Augmentative and Alternative Communication, 25*(1), 19–31.

Highnam, C.L., & Bleile, K.M. (2011). Language and the cerebellum. *American Journal of Speech-Language Pathology, 20,* 337–347.

Hill, E. L. (2001). Non-specific nature of specific language impairment: A review of the literature with regard to concomitant motor impairments. *International Journal of Language & Communication Disorders, 36,* 149–171.

Hirano, M., & Sato, K. (1993). *Histological color atlas of the human larynx.* Singular.

Hirano, M., Kurita, S., & Sakaguchi, S. (1989). Aging of the vibratory tissue of the human vocal folds. *Acta Otolaryngologia, 107,* 428–433.

Hirano, M., Vennard, W., & Ohala, J. (1970). Regulation of register, pitch, and intensity of voice. *Folia Phoniatrica, 22,* 1–20.

Hirsh, S. (2017). Combining voice, speech science, and art approaches to resonant challenges in transgender voice and communication training. *Perspectives of the ASHA Special Interest Groups, 2*(10), 74–82.

Hixon, T., & Hoit, J. (2005). *Evaluation and management of speech breathing disorders: Principles and methods.* Redington Brown.

Hixon, T., Weismer, G., & Hoit, J. (2008). *Preclinical speech science: Anatomy, physiology, acoustics, and perception.* Plural Publishing.

Hixon, T., Weismer, G., & Hoit, J. (2014). *Preclinical speech science: Anatomy, physiology, acoustics, and perception* (2nd ed.). Plural Publishing.

Hixon, T., Weismer, G., & Hoit, J. (2020). *Preclinical speech science: Anatomy, physiology, acoustics, and perception* (3rd ed.). Plural Publishing.

Hodge, S. (2007, July). Why is the potential of augmentative and alternative communication not being realized?: Exploring experiences of people who use communication aids. *Disability & Society, 22*(5). https://doi.org/10.1080/09687590701427552

Hodson, B. (2004). *Hodson assessment of phonological patterns* (3rd ed.). PRO-ED.

Hodson, B. (2007). *Evaluation and enhancing children's phonological systems: Research and theory of practice.* Thinking Publications.

Hodson, B. (2011). Enhancing phonological patterns of young children with highly unintelligible speech. *The ASHA Leader, 16*(4), 16–19.

Hodson, B. (2012). *Hodson Computerized Analysis of Phonological Patterns—4th edition (HCAPP).* PhonoComp.

Hodson, B., & Paden, E. (1991). *Targeting intelligible speech: A phonological approach to remediation* (2nd ed.). PRO-ED.

Hoepner, J. K., Sievert, A., & Guenther, K. (2021). Joint video self-modeling for persons with traumatic brain injury and their partners: A case series. *American Journal of Speech-Language Pathology, 30,* 863–882.

Hoffman, M., Quittner, A., & Cejas, I. (2015). Comparisons of social competence in young children with and without hearing loss: A dynamic systems framework. *Journal of Deaf Studies and Deaf Education, 20*(2), 115–125.

Hoffman, R., Norris, J., & Monjure, J. (1990). Comparison of process targeting and whole language treatment for phonologically delayed preschool children. *Language, Speech, and Hearing Services in Schools, 21,* 102–109.

Hogan, T., & Catts, H. W. (2004, November). *Phonological awareness test items: Lexical and phonological characteristics affect performance.* Paper presented at the annual convention of the American Speech-Language-Hearing Association, Philadelphia.

Hogikyan N., & Sethuraman G. (1999). Validation of an instrument to measure voice-related quality of life (V-RQOL). *Journal of Voice, 13,* 557–569.

Hoit, J., & Weismer, G. (2018). *Foundations of speech and hearing: Anatomy and Physiology.* Plural Publishing.

Hoit, J., Hixon, T., Watson, P., & Morgan, W. (1990). Speech breathing in children and adolescents. *Journal of Speech and Hearing Research, 33,* 51–69.

Hoit, J., Watson, P., Hixon, K., McMahon, P., & Johnson, C. (1994). Age and velopharyngeal function during speech production. *Journal of Speech and Hearing Research, 37,* 295–302.

Hoit, J., Weismer, G., & Story, B. (2022). *Foundations of speech and hearing: Anatomy and physiology* (2nd ed.). Plural Publishing.

Holland, A., & Fridriksson, J. (2001). Aphasia management during the early phases of recovery following stroke. *American Journal of Speech-Language Pathology, 10,* 19–28.

Hollien, H., Green, R., & Massey, K. (1994). Longitudinal research of adolescent voice change in males. *Journal of the Acoustical Society of America, 34,* 80–84.

Holyfield, C., Caron, J. G., Drager, K., & Light, J. (2019). Effect of mobile technology featuring visual scene displays and just-in-time programming on communication turns by preadolescent and adolescent beginning communicators. *International Journal of Speech-language Pathology,* 201–211. https://doi.org/10.1080/17549507.2018.1441440

Holyfield, C., Caron, J. G., Drager, K., & Light, J. (2019). Effect of mobile technology featuring visual scene displays and just-in-time programming on communication turns by preadolescent and adolescent beginning communicators. *International Journal of Speech-language Pathology, 21*(2), 201–211.

Homer, E. (2015). *Management of swallowing and feeding disorders in schools.* Plural Publishing.

Honjo, I., & Isshiki, N. (1980). Laryngoscopic and voice characteristics of aged persons. *Archives of Otolaryngology, 106,* 149–150.

Hoover, E., DeDe, G., & Maas, E. (2021). A randomized controlled trial of the effects of group conversation treatment on monologic discourse in aphasia. *Journal of Speech, Language, and Hearing Research, 64,* 4861–4875.

Hopper, T. (2005, November 8). Assessment and treatment of cognitive-communication disorders in individuals with dementia. *The ASHA Leader, 10*(15), 10–11.

Hopper, T., Bourgeois, M., Pimentel, J., Dean Qualls, C., Hickey, E., Frymark, T., & Schooling, T. (2013). An evidence-based systematic review on cognitive interventions for individuals with dementia. *American Journal of Speech-Language Pathology, 22,* 126–145.

Horikawa C., Kodama S., Tanaka S., Fujihara, K., Hirasawa, R., Yachi, Y., et al. (2013). Diabetes and risk of hearing impairment in adults: A meta-analysis. *Journal of Clinical Endocrinology and Metabolism, 98*(1), 51–58.

Horton J., Atwood C., Gnagi S., Teufel R., & Clemmens, C. (2018). Temporal trends of pediatric dysphagia in hospitalized patients. *Dysphagia, 33,* 655–661.

Hossain, S. (2012, June 11). *Cochlear implants and the Deaf culture: A transhumanist perspective.* http://hplusmagazine.com/2012/06/11/cochlear-implants-and-the-deaf-culture-a-transhumanist-perspective/

Houston-Price, C., Plunkett, K., & Haris, P. (2005). Word-learning wizardry at 1;6. *Journal of Child Language, 32,* 175–189.

Howard, M., & Rosario, E. (2019). A clinical approach to neuromuscular electrical stimulation for speech and swallow in an acute rehabilitation facility. *Perspectives of the ASHA Special Interest Groups, 4,* 1044–1048.

Howell, J., & Dean, E. (1994). *Treating phonological disorders in children: Metaphon—theory to practice* (2nd ed.). Whurr.

Howle, A., Baguley, I., & Brown, L. (2014). Management of dysphagia following traumatic brain injury. *Current Physical Medicine and Rehabilitation Reports, 2,* 219–230.

Hsu, H. J., & Bishop, D. V. M. (2014). Sequence-specific procedural learning deficits in children with specific language impairment. *Developmental Science, 17,* 352–365. https://doi.org/10.1111/desc.12125

Huaqing Qi, C., & Kaiser, A. P. (2004). Problem behaviors of low-income children with language delays: An observation study. *Journal of Speech, Language, and Hearing Research, 47,* 595–609.

Huckabee, M. (2009). The development of swallowing respiratory coordination. *Perspectives on Swallowing and Swallowing Disorders (Dysphagia)*, *18*(1), 19–24.

Huckvale, M. (2020). *WASP2*. https://www.speechand-hearing.net

Huer, M., & Threats, T. (2016). Shared responsibilities for full participation in society: Planning further integration of the ICF into AAC. *Perspectives in Augmentative and Alternative Communication*, *1*(3), 83–93.

Hugdahl, K., Gundersen, H., Brekke C., Thomsen, T., Rimol, L. M., Ersland, L., et al. (2004). fMRI brain activation in a Finnish family with specific language impairment compared with a normal control group. *Journal of Speech, Language, and Hearing Research*, *47*, 162–172.

Hughes, M., Sevier, J., & Choi, S. (2018). Techniques for remotely programming children with cochlear implants using pediatric audiological methods via telepractice. *American Journal of Audiology*, *27*(3, Suppl.), 385–390.

Hui, J., & Logan, J. (2019). Improving reading comprehension in the primary grades: Mediated effects of a language-focused classroom intervention. *Journal of Speech, Language, and Hearing Research*, *62*, 2812–2828.

Hulme, C., & Snowling, M. J. (2014). The interface between spoken and written language: Developmental disorders. *Philosophical Transactions of the Royal Society of London B: Biological Sciences*, *369*, 20120395.

Humes, L. (2019). The World Health Organization's hearing-impairment grading system: An evaluation for unaided communication in age-related hearing loss. *International Journal of Audiology*, *58*(1), 12–20.

Humphries, T., Cardy, J. O., Worling, D. E., & Peets, K. (2004). Narrative comprehension and retelling abilities of children with nonverbal learning disabilities. *Brain and Cognition*, *56*, 77–88.

Humphries, T., Kushalnagar, P., Mathur, G., Napoli, D., Padden, C., Rathmann, C., & Smith, S. (2016). Avoiding linguistic neglect of deaf children. *Social Service Review*, *90*, 589–619.

Hurst, M., & Cooper, G. (1983). Employer attitudes towards stuttering. *Journal of Fluency Disorders*, *8*, 1–12.

Hustad, K., Jones, T., & Dailey, S. (2003). Implementing speech supplementation strategies: Effects on intelligibility and speech rate of individuals with chronic severe dysarthria. *Journal of Speech, Language, Hearing Research*, *46*, 462–474.

Hustad, K., Mahr, T., Natzke, P., & Rathouz, P. (2021). Speech development between 30 and 119 months in typical children I: Intelligibility growth curves for single-word and multiword productions. *Journal of Speech, Language, and Hearing Research*, *64*, 3707–3719. https://doi.org./10.1044/2021_JSLHR-21-00142

Hutcheson, K. (2016). Rehabilitation of heavily treated head and neck cancer patients. In J. Bernier (Ed.), *Head and neck cancer* (pp. 783–798). Springer. https://doi.org/10.1007/978-3-319-27601-4_47

Hux, K., Buechter, M., Wallace, S., & Weissling, K. (2010). Using visual scene displays to create a shared communication space for a person with aphasia. *Aphasiology*, *24*(5), 643–660. https://doi.org/10.1080/02687030902869299

Imgrund, C. M., Loeb, D. F., & Barlow, S. M. (2019). Expressive language in preschoolers born preterm: Results of language sample analysis and standardized assessment. *Journal of Speech, Language, and Hearing Research*, *62*, 884–895.

Individuals with Disabilities Education Act, 20 U.S.C. § 1400. (2004).

Ingham, R. J., & Cordes, A. K. (1997). Self-measurement and evaluating stuttering treatment efficacy. In R. F. Curlee & G. M. Siegel (Eds.), *Nature and treatment of stuttering: New directions* (2nd ed., pp. 413–437). Allyn & Bacon.

Ingham, R. J., Ingham, J. C., Finn, P., & Fox, P. T. (2003). Towards a functional neural systems model of developmental stuttering. *Journal of Fluency Disorders*, *28*, 297–318.

Inglebret, E., Jones, C., & Pavel, D. M. (2008). Integrating American Indian/Alaska Native culture into shared storybook intervention. *Language, Speech, and Hearing Services in Schools*, *39*, 521–527.

Ingram, K., Bunta, F., & Ingram, D. (2004). Digital data collection and analysis: Application for clinical practice. *Language, Speech, and Hearing Services in Schools*, *35*, 112–121.

Insalaco, D. (2022). Primary progressive aphasia: A short review of diagnostic criteria and anomia treatments. *The Communicator*, *52*, 8–9.

Insalaco, D., Ozkurt, E., & Santiago, D. (2007). The perceptions of students in the allied health professions towards stroke rehabilitation teams and the SLP's role. *Journal of Communicatin Disorders*, *40*(3), 196–214.

Inspiration Software. (2017). What is visual learning and visual thinking? http://www.inspiration.com/visual-learning

Institute on Disability. (2021). *2021 Annual report on people with disabilities in America*. https://disability-compendium.org/sites/default/files/user-uploads/Events/2022ReleaseYear/Annual%20Report%20---%202021%20---%20WEB.pdf

Israel, H. (1968). Continuing growth in the human cranial skeleton. *Archives of Oral Biology*, *13*, 133–137.

Israel, H. (1973). Age factor and the pattern of change in craniofacial structures. *American Journal of Physical Anthropology*, *39*, 111–128.

Isshiki, N. (1964). Regulatory mechanisms of voice intensity variation. *Journal of Speech and Hearing Research, 7,* 17–29.

Isshiki, N., & von Leden, H. (1964). Hoarseness: Aerodynamic studies. *Archives of Otolaryngology, 80,* 206–213.

Iverach, L., & Rapee, R. (2014). Social anxiety disorder and stuttering: Current status and future directions. *Journal of Fluency Disorders, 40,* 69–82.

Iverach, L., Rapee, R., Wong, Q., & Lowe, R. (2017). Maintenance of social anxiety in stuttering: A cognitive-behavioral model. *American Journal of Speech-Language Pathology, 26,* 540–556.

Jacobs, B. J., & Thompson, C. K. (2000). Cross-modality generalization effects of training noncanonical sentence comprehension and production in agrammatic aphasia. *Journal of Speech, Language, and Hearing Research, 43,* 5–20.

Jacobson, B., Johnson, A., Grywalski, C., Silbergleit, A., Jacobson, G., Benninger, M., & Newman, C. (1997). The Voice Handicap Index (VHI): Development and validation. *American Journal of Speech-Language Pathology, 6,* 66–70.

Jacobson, L., & Reid, R. (2007). Self-regulated strategy development for written expression: Is it effective for adolescents? *EBP Briefs, 2*(3), 1–13.

Jarvis, J. (1989). Taking a Metaphon approach to phonological development: A case study. *Child Language Teaching and Therapy, 5,* 16–32.

Jerome, A. C., Fujiki, M., Brinton, B., & James, S. L. (2002). Self-esteem in children with specific language impairment. *Journal of Speech, Language, and Hearing Research, 45,* 700–714.

Jetté, M. (2016). Toward an understanding of the pathophysiology of chronic laryngitis. *Perspectives of the ASHA Special Interest Groups, 1,* 14–25.

Jimenez, B. (1987). Acquisition of Spanish consonants in children aged 3–5 years, 7 months. *Language, Speech, and Hearing Services in Schools, 18,* 357–363.

Jin, F., Schjølberg, S., Vaage Wang, M., Eadie, P., Bang Nes, R., Røysamb, E., & Tambs, K. (2020). Predicting literacy skills at 8 years from preschool language trajectories: A population-based cohort study. *Journal of Speech, Language, and Hearing Research, 63,* 2752–2762.

Johnson, C. J. (2006). Getting started in evidence-based practice for childhood speech-language disorders. *American Journal of Speech-Language Pathology, 15,* 20–35.

Johnson, C. J., & Yeates, E. (2006). Evidence-based vocabulary instruction for elementary students via storybook reading. *EBP Briefs, 1*(3).

Johnson, C. J., Beitchman, J. H., Young, A., Escobar, M., Atkinson, L., Wilson, B., et al. (1999). Fourteen-year follow-up of children with and without speech/language impairments: Speech/language stability and outcomes. *Journal of Speech, Language, and Hearing Research, 42,* 744–760.

Johnson, C., Danhauer, J., Ellis, B., & Jilla, A. (2016). Hearing aid benefit in patients with mild sensorineural hearing loss: A systematic review. *Journal of the American Academy of Audiology, 27*(4), 293–310.

Johnson, J. M., Inglebret, E., Jone, C., & Ray, J. (2009). Perspectives of speech language pathologists regarding success versus abandonment of AAC. *Augmentative and Alternative Communication, 22*(2), 85–99. https://doi.org/10.1080/07434610500483588

Johnson, L. W., & Hall, K. (2022). A scoping review of cognitive assessment in adults with acute traumatic brain injury. *American Journal of Speech-Language Pathology, 31,* 739–756.

Johnson, L., Basilakos, A., Yourganov, G., Cai, B., Bonilha, L., Rorden, C., & Fridriksson, J. (2019). Progression of aphasia severity in the chronic stages of stroke. *American Journal of Speech-Language Pathology, 28,* 639–649.

Johnson, W. (1948). *Speech handicapped school children.* Harper.

Johnston, J. R. (1986). Fit, focus and functionality: An essay on early language intervention. *Child Language Teaching & Therapy, 1*(2), 125–134. https://doi.org/10.1177/026565908500100201

Johnston, J. R. (2001). An alternative MLU calculation: Magnitude and variability of effects. *Journal of Speech, Language, and Hearing Research, 44,* 156–164.

Johnston, S., Reichle, J., & Evans, J. (2004). Supporting augmentative and alternative communication use by beginning communications with severe disabilities. *American Journal of Speech-Language Pathology, 13,* 20–30.

Jones, M., Onslow, M., Packman, A., O'Brian, S., Hearne, A., Williams, S., . . . Schwarz, I. (2008). Extended follow-up of a randomized controlled trial of the Lidcombe Program of early stuttering intervention. *International Journal of Language & Communication Disorders, 43,* 649–661.

Jung, T. T. K., & Hanson, J. B. (1999). Otitis media: Surgical principles based on pathogenesis. *Otolaryngologic Clinics of North America, 32,* 369–383.

Justice, L. M., & Ezell, H. K. (2002). Use of storybook reading to increase print awareness in at-risk children. *American Journal of Speech-Language Pathology, 11,* 17–29.

Justice, L. M., & Kaderavek, J. N. (2004). Embedded-explicit emergent literacy intervention I: Background and description of approach. *Language, Speech, and Hearing Services in Schools, 35,* 201–211.

Justice, L. M., & Pence, K. (2007). Parent-implemented interactive language intervention: Can it be used effectively? *EBP Briefs, 2*(1).

Justice, L. M., Logan, J., & Kaderavek, J. N. (2017). Longitudinal impacts of print-focused read-alouds for children with language impairment. *American Journal of Speech-Language Pathology, 26*(2), 383–396.

Justice, L. M., Mashburn, A., Hamre, B., & Pianta, R. (2008). Quality of language and literacy instruction in preschool classrooms serving at-risk pupils. *Early Childhood Research Quarterly, 23,* 51–68.

Kaderavek, J. N., & Justice, L. M. (2004). Embedded-explicit emergent literacy intervention II: Goal selection and implementation in the early childhood classroom. *Language, Speech, and Hearing Services in Schools, 35,* 212–228.

Kagan, A., Black, S. E., Duchan, J. F., Simmons-Mackie, N., & Square, P. (2001). Training volunteers as conversation partners using "supported conversation for adults with aphasia" (SCA): A controlled trial. *Journal of Speech, Language, and Hearing Research, 44,* 624–638.

Kagohara, D. M., van der Meera, L., Ramdoss, S., O'Reilly, M. F., Lancioni, G. E., Davis, T. N., et al. (2013). Using iPods and iPads in teaching programs for individuals with developmental disabilities: A systematic review. *Research in Developmental Disabilities, 34*(1), 147–156.

Kahane, J. (1978). A morphological study of the human prepubertal and pubertal larynx. *American Journal of Anatomy, 151,* 11–20.

Kahane, J. (1987). Connective tissue changes in the larynx and their effects on voice. *Journal of Voice, 1,* 27–30.

Kahane, J. (1988). Age-related changes in the human cricoarytenoid joint. In O. Fujimura (Ed.), *Vocal physiology: Voice production, mechanisms, and functions* (pp. 145–157). Raven Press.

Kahane, J., (1982). Growth of the human prepubertal and pubertal larynx. *Journal of Speech and Hearing Research, 25,* 446–455.

Kamhi, A. (2011). What speech-language pathologists need to know about auditory processing disorder. *Language, Speech, and Hearing Services in Schools, 42,* 265–272.

Kamhi, A. G. (2003). The role of the SLP in improving reading fluency. *The ASHA Leader, 8*(7), 6–8.

Kamhi, A. G. (2006a). Prologue: Combining research and reason to make treatment decisions. *Language, Speech, and Hearing Services in Schools, 37,* 225–256.

Kamhi, A. G. (2006b). Treatment decisions for children with speech-sound disorders. *Language, Speech, and Hearing Services in Schools, 37,* 271–279.

Kamhi, A. G., & Catts, H. W. (2005). Language and reading: Convergences and divergences. In H. W. Catts & A. G. Kamhi (Eds.), *Language and reading disabilities* (2nd ed., pp. 1–25). Allyn & Bacon.

Kamhi, A. G., & Hinton, L. N. (2000). Explaining individual differences in spelling ability. *Topics in Language Disorders, 20*(3), 37.

Kamity, R., Kapavarapu, P., & Chandel, A. (2021). Feeding problems and long-term outcomes in preterm infants—A systematic approach to evaluation and management. *Children, 8,* 1158–1174.

Kapa, L. L., & Erikson, J. A. (2020). The relationship between word learning and executive function in preschoolers with and without developmental language disorder. *Journal of Speech, Language, and Hearing Research, 63,* 2293–2307.

Karagiannis, A., Stainback, W., & Stainback, S. (1996). Historical overview of inclusion. In S. Stainback & W. Stainback (Eds.), *Inclusion: A guide for educators.* Brookes. 35–48

Karltop, E., Eklof, M., Ostlund, E., Asp, F., Tideholm, B., & Lofkvist, U. (2020). Cochlear implants before 9 months of age led to more natural spoken language development without increase surgical risks. *Acta Paediatricia, 109*(2), 332–341.

Katz, W. F. (2003). From basic research in speech science to answers in speech-language pathology. *The ASHA Leader, 8*(1), 6–7, 20.

Kaufman, N. (1995). *Kaufman Speech Praxis Test for Children.* Wayne State University Press.

Kavé, G., & Levy, Y. (2003). Morphology in picture descriptions provided by persons with Alzheimer's disease. *Journal of Speech, Language, and Hearing Research, 46,* 341–352.

Kavrie, S., & Neils-Strunjas, J. (2002). Dysgraphia in Alzheimer's disease with mild cognitive impairment. *Journal of Medical Speech-Language Pathology, 10*(1), 73–85.

Kawashima, K., Motohashi, Y., & Fujishima, I. (2004). Prevalence of dysphagia among community-dwelling elderly individuals as estimated using a questionnaire for dysphagia screening. *Dysphagia, 19*(4), 266–271.

Kay-Raining Bird, E., Cleave, P. L., White, D., Pike, H., & Helmkay, A. (2008). Written and oral narratives of children and adolescents with Down syndrome. *Journal of speech, Language, and Hearing Research, 51,* 436–450.

Keator, L. M., Basilakos, A., Rorden, C., Elm, J., Bonilha, L., & Fridriksson, J. (2020). Clinical implementation of transcranial direct current stimulation in aphasia: A survey of speech-language pathologists. *American Journal of Speech-Language Pathology, 29,* 1376–1388.

Keenan, J. M., & Meenan, C. E. (2014). Test differences in diagnosing reading comprehension deficits. *Journal of Learning Disabilities, 47*(2), 125–135.

Kelly-Hayes, M. (2010). Influence of age and health behaviors on stroke risk: Lessons from longitudinal studies. *Journal of the American Geriatric Society, 58*(2), S325–S328. doi:10.1111/j.1532-5415.2010.02915.x

Kemp, D. T. (1978). Stimulated acoustic emissions from within the human auditory system. *Journal of the Acoustical Society of American, 64*, 1386–1391.

Kemper, S., Thompson, M., & Marquis, J. (2001). Longitudinal change in language production: Effects of aging and dementia on grammatical complexity and prepositional content. *Psychology and Aging, 16*, 600–614.

Kempster, G., Gerratt, B., Abbott, K., Barkmeier-Kraemer, J., & Hillman, R. (2009). Consensus auditory-perceptual evaluation of voice: Development of a standardized clinical protocol. *American Journal of Speech-Language Pathology, 18*, 124–132.

Kendall, D. L., Oelke Moldestad, M., Allen, W., Torrence, J., & Nadeau, S. E. (2019). Phonomotor versus semantic feature analysis treatment for anomia in 58 persons with aphasia: A randomized controlled trial. *Journal of Speech, Language, and Hearing Research, 62*, 4464–4482.

Kendall, D. L., Oelke, M., Brookshire, C. E., & Nadeau, S. E. (2015). The influence of phonomotor treatment on word retrieval abilities in 26 individuals with chronic aphasia: An open trial. *Journal of Speech, Language, and Hearing Research, 58*, 798–812.

Kendeou, P., Bohn-Gettler, C. M., White, M. J., & Van den Broek, P. (2008). Children's inference generation across media. *Journal of Research in Reading, 31*, 259–272.

Kent, R. (1981). Articulatory-acoustic perspectives on speech development. In R. Stark (Ed.), *Language behavior in infancy and childhood* (pp. 105–126). Elsevier-North Holland.

Kent, R. D. (1997). *The speech sciences*. Singular.

Kent, R., & Murray, A. (1982). Acoustic features of infant vocalic utterances at 3, 6, and 9 months. *Journal of the Acoustical Society of America, 72*, 353–365.

Kent, R., & Vorperian, H. (2013). Speech impairment in Down syndrome: A review. *Journal of Speech, Language, and Hearing Research, 56*, 178–210.

Kent-Walsh, J., & Mcnaughton, D. (2009). Communication partner instruction in AAC: Present practices and future directions. *Augmentative and Alternative Communication, 21*(3), 195–204.

Kent-Walsh, J., & Rosa-Lugo, L. (2006). Communication partner interventions for children who use AAC: Storybook reading across culture and language. *ASHA Leader, 11*(3), 6–7. https://doi.org/10.1044/leader.FTR2.11032006.6

Kent-Walsh, J., Murza, K. A., Malani, M. D., & Binger, C. (2015). Effects of communication partner instruction on the communication of individuals using AAC: A meta-analysis. *Augmentative and Alternative Communication, 31*(4), 271–284.

Kerr, W., Kelly, J., & Geddes, D. (1991). The areas of various surfaces in the human mouth from nine years to adulthood. *Journal of Dental Research, 70*, 1528–1530.

Kessels, R. P. C. (2003). Patients' memory for medical information. *Journal of Royal Society of Medicine, 96*, 219–222.

Ketelaars, M. P., Alphonsus Hermans, T. S., Cuperus, J., Jansonius, K., & Verhoeven, L. (2011). Semantic abilities in children with pragmatic language impairment: The case of picture naming skills. *Journal of Speech, Language, and Hearing Research, 54*, 87–98.

Ketelaars, M., Cuperus, J., & van Daal, J. (2009). Screening for pragmatic language impairment: The potential of the Children's Communication Checklist. *Research in Developmental Disabilities 30*(5), 952–960. https://doi.org/10.1016/j.ridd.2009.01.006

Keuning, K., Wieneke, G., van Wijngaarden, H., & Dejonckere, P. (2002). The correlation between nasalance and a differentiated perceptual rating of speech in Dutch patients with velopharyngeal insufficiency. *Cleft Palate-Craniofacial Journal, 39*, 277–284.

Khan, L., & Lewis, N. (2002). *Khan-Lewis Phonological Analysis—Second Edition (KLPA-2)*. American Guidance Service.

Khan, L., & Lewis, N. (2015). *Khan-Lewis Phonological Analysis—Third Edition (KLPA-3)*. Pearson Education.

Kim, E. S., Suleman, S., & Hopper, T. (2020). Decision making by people with aphasia: A comparison of linguistic and nonlinguistic measures. *Journal of Speech, Language, and Hearing Research, 63*, 1845–1860.

Kim, H. (2020). Vocal feminization for transgender women: Current strategies and patient perspectives. *International Journal of General Medicine, 13*, 43–52.

King Bamford, C., Masso, S., Baker, E., & Ballard, K. J. (2022). Dynamic assessment for children with communication disorders: A systematic scoping review and framework. *American Journal of Speech-Language Pathology, 31*(4), 1878–1893. https://doi.org/10.1044/2022_AJSLP-21-00349

King, M. R., Binger, C., & Kent-Walsh, J. (2015). Using dynamic assessment to evaluate the expressive syntax of children who use augmentative and alternative communication. *Augmentative and Alternative Communication, 31*(1), 1–14.

Kirgezen, T., Sunter, A., Yigit, O., & Huq, G. (2017). Sex hormone receptor expression in the human vocal fold subunits. *Journal of Voice, 31*, 476–482.

Kirk, C., & Gillon, G. T. (2009). Integrated morphological awareness intervention as a tool for improving literacy. *Language, Speech, and Hearing Services in Schools, 40*, 341–351.

Kleim, J. A., & Jones, T. A. (2008). Principles of experience-dependent neural plasticity: Implications for rehabilitation after brain damage. *Journal of Speech, Language, and Hearing Research, 51,* S225–S239.

Klein, H. (1998, December 8). Book review of *Handbook of phonological disorders from the perspective of constraint-based nonlinear phonology* by B. Bernhardt and J. Stemberger. *The ASHA Leader,* pp. 23–24.

Klieman, L. (2003). *The Functional Communication Profile—Revised.* Pro-Ed.

Knollman-Porter, K., Brown, J. A., Wallace, T., & Spitz, S. (2021). First-line health care providers' reported knowledge of and referrals to speech-language pathologists for clients with mild traumatic brain injury. *American Journal of Speech-Language Pathology, 30,* 2214–2227.

Knollman-Porter, K., Wallace, S. E., Brown, J. A., Hux, K., Hoagland, B. L., & Ruff, D. R. (2019). Effects of written, auditory, and combined modalities on comprehension by people with aphasia. *American Journal of Speech-Language Pathology, 28,* 1206–1221.

Knutsen, J., Crossman, M., Perrin, J., Shui, A., & Kuhlthau, K. (2019). Sex differences in restricted repetitive behaviors and interests in children with autism spectrum disorder: An Autism Treatment Network study. *Autism, 23,* 858–868.

Koch Fager, S. (2017). Alternative access for adults who rely on augmentative and alternative communication. *Perspectives of the ASHA Special Interest Groups,* 6–12. https://doi.org/10.1044/persp3.SIG12.6

Kollara, L., Schenck, G., Jaskolka, M., & Perry, J. (2017). Examining a new method to studying velopharyngeal structures in a child with 22q11.2 deletion syndrome. *Journal of Speech, Language, and Hearing Research, 60,* 892–896.

Koppenhaver, D. A. (2000). Literacy in AAC—What should be written on the envelope we push? *Augmentative and Alternative Communication, 16,* 270–279.

Koppenhaver, D., & Erickson, K. (2003). Natural emergent literacy supports for preschoolers with autism and severe communication impairments. *Topics in Language Disorders, 23*(4), 283–292.

Koul, R. K., & Corwin, M. (2010). Augmentative and alternative communication intervention for persons with chronic severe aphasia: Bringing research to practice. *EBP Briefs, 6*(2), 1–8.

Koul, R., & Hester, K. (2006). Effects of repeated listening experiences on the recognition of synthetic speech by individuals with severe intellectual disabilities. *Journal of Speech, Language, and Hearing Research, 49,* 47–57.

Kouri, T. A., Selle, C. A., & Riley, S. A. (2006). Comparison of meaning and graphophonemic feedback strategies for guided reading instruction of children with language delays. *American Journal of Speech-Language Pathology, 15,* 236–246.

Koutsoftas, A. D., Harmon, M., & Gray, S. (2008, October 24). *The effect of Tier 2 intervention for phonemic awareness in a response-to-intervention model in low-income preschool classrooms.* American Speech-Language-Hearing Association. http://lshss.asha.org/cgi/rapidpdf/0161-1461_2008_07-0101v1?maxtoshow=&HITS=10&hits=10&RESULTFORMAT=&authorl=Koutsoftas&andorexactfulltext=and&searchid=1&FIRSTINDEX=0&sortspec=relevance&resourcetype

Kovach, T. M. (2009). *Augmentative & Alternative Communication Profile: A Continuum of Learning.* Pro-Ed.

Kridgen, S. (2019). *Patient-reported events associated with the onset of phonotraumatic and nonphonotraumatic vocal hyperfunction.* MGH Institute of Health Professions.

Kristensen, H. (2000). Selective mutism and comorbidity with developmental disorder/delay, anxiety disorder, and elimination disorder. *Journal of the American Academy of Child and Adolescent Psychiatry, 39,* 249–256.

Kuehn, D. (1991). New therapy for treating hypernasal speech using continuous positive airway pressure (CPAP) for treatment of hypernasality. *Cleft Palate-Craniofacial Journal, 39,* 267–276.

Kuehn, D., & Henne, L. (2003). Speech evaluation and treatment for patients with cleft palate. *American Journal of Speech-Language Pathology, 12,* 103–109.

Kuehn, D., Imrey, P., Tomes, L., et al. (2002). Efficacy of continuous positive airway pressure (CPAP) treatment of hypernasality. *Cleft Palate-Craniofacial Journal, 39,* 267–276.

Kully, D., Langevin, M., & Lomheim, H. (2003). Intensive treatment of stuttering in adolescents and adults. In E. Conture & R. Curlee (3rd Ed., pp. 213–232), *Stuttering and related disorders of fluency.* New York: NY: Thieme Medical Publisher.

Kumin, L. (2006). Speech intelligibility and childhood verbal apraxia in children with Down syndrome. *Down's Syndrome, Research, and Practice, 10,* 10–22.

Kumin, L., Council, C., & Goodman, M. (1994). A longitudinal study of emergence of phonemes in children with Down syndrome. *Journal of Communication Disorders, 27,* 293–303.

Kummer, A. (2011a). Perceptual assessment of resonance and velopharyngeal function. *Seminars in Speech and Language, 32,* 159–167.

Kummer, A. (2011b). Types and causes of velopharyngeal dysfunction. *Seminars in Speech and Language, 32,* 150–158.

Kummer, A. (2014a). Orofacial examination. In A. Kummer (Ed.), *Cleft palate and craniofacial anomalies: The effects on speech and resonance* (3rd ed., pp. 352–386). Cengage Learning.

Kummer, A. (2014b). Speech and resonance assessment. In A. Kummer (Ed.), *Cleft palate and craniofacial anomalies: The effects on speech and resonance* (3rd ed., pp. 324–351). Cengage Learning.

Kummer, A. (2014c). Speech and resonance disorders related to cleft palate and velopharyngeal dysfunction: A guide to evaluation and treatment. *Perspectives on School-Based Issues, 15*, 57–74.

Kummer, A., & Lee, L. (1996). Evaluation and treatment of resonance disorders. *Language, Speech, and Hearing Services in Schools, 27*, 271–281.

La Paro, K. M., Justice, L., Skibbe, L. E., & Pianta, R. C. (2004). Relations among maternal, child, and demographic factors and the persistence of preschool language impairment. *American Journal of Speech-Language Pathology, 13*, 291–303.

Lainhart, J. E. (2015). Brain imaging research in autism spectrum disorders: in search of neuropathology and health across the lifespan. *Current Opinion in Psychiatry, 28*, 76–82. https://doi.org/10.1097/YCO.0000000000000130

Langevin, M., & Narasimha Prasad, N. (2012). A stuttering education and bullying awareness and prevention resource: A feasibility study. *Language, Speech, and Hearing Services in Schools, 43*, 344–358.

Langevin, M., Packman, A., & Onslow, M. (2009). Peer responses to stuttering in the preschool setting. *American Journal of Speech-Language Pathology, 18*, 264–276.

Langford, S., & Cooper, E. (1974). Recovery from stuttering as viewed by parents of self-diagnosed recovered stutterers. *Journal of Communication Disorders, 7*, 171–181.

Language and Reading Research Consortium (LARRC), Jiang, Hui., & Logan, J. (2019). Improving reading comprehension in the primary grades: mediated effects of a language-focused classroom intervention. *Journal of Speech, Language, and Hearing Research, 62*, 2812–2828. https://doi.org/10.1044/2019_JSLHR-L-19-0015

Language and Reading Research Consortium, Jiang, H., & Davis, D. (2017). Let's know!: Proximal impacts on prekindergarten through grade 3 students' comprehension-related skills. *Elementary School Journal, 118*(2), 177–206.

Lanter, E., & Watson, L. R. (2008). Promoting literacy in students with ASD: The basics for the SLP. *Language, Speech, and Hearing Services in Schools, 39*, 33–43.

Lanzi, A. M., Saylor, A. K., & Cohen, M. L. (2022). Survey results of speech-language pathologists working with cognitive-communication disorders: Improving practices for mild cognitive impairment and early-stage dementia from Alzheimer's disease. *American Journal of Speech-Language Pathology, 31*(4), 1653–1671.

Lanzi, A., & Bourgeois, M. S. (2020). Structured external memory aid treatment for mild cognitive impairment. *American Journal of Speech-Language Pathology, 29*, 474–484.

Lapko, L., & Bankson, N. (1975). Relationship between auditory discrimination, articulation stimulability and consistency of misarticulation. *Perceptual and Motor Skills, 40*, 171–177.

Larrivee, L., & Catts, H. (1999). Early reading achievement in children with expressive phonological disorders. *American Journal of Speech-Language Pathology, 8*, 118, 128.

Larson, D., & Derkay, C. (2010). Epidemiology of recurrent respiratory papillomatosis. *APMIS, 118*, 450–454.

Larson, A. L., Cycyk, L. M., Carta, J., Hammer, C. S., Baralth, M., Uchikoshi, Y., et al. (2020). A systematic review of language-focused interventions for children from culturally and linguistically diverse backgrounds. *Early Childhood Research Quarterly, 50*(Pt. 1), 157–178.

Laska, A. C., Hellblom, A., Murray, V., Kahan, T., & Von Arbin, M. (2001). Aphasia in acute stroke and relation to outcome. *Journal of Internal Medicine, 249*(5), 413–22. https://doi.org/10.1046/j.1365-2796.2001.00812.x

Lasker, J. P., & Bedrosian, J. L. (2000). Acceptance of AAC by adults with acquired disorders. In D. Beukelman, K. Yorkston, & J. Reichle (Eds.), *Augmentative communication for adults with neurogenic and neuromuscular disabilities* (pp. 107–136). Brookes.

Lasker, J. P., & Bedrosian, J. L. (2001). Promoting acceptance of augmentative and alternative communication by adults with acquired communication disorders. *Augmentative and Alternative Communication, 17*, 141–153.

Lau, C. (2006). Oral feeding in the preterm infant. *Neonatal Reviews, 7*, e19–e27.

Laures-Gore, J. S., Dotson, V. M., & Belagaje, S. (2020). Depression in poststroke aphasia. *American Journal of Speech-Language Pathology, 29*, 1798–1810.

Law, J., Boyle, J., Harris, F., Harkness, A., & Nye, C. (2000). Prevalence and natural history of primary speech and language delay: Findings from a systematic review of the literature. *International Journal of Language & Communication Disorders, 35*, 165–188.

Law, J., Garrett, Z., & Nye, C. (2004). The efficacy of treatment for children with developmental speech and language delay/disorder: A meta-analysis. *Journal of Speech, Language, and Hearing Research, 47*, 924–943.

Law, J., Rush, R., Schoon, I., & Parsons, S. (2009). Modeling developmental language difficulties from school entry into adulthood: Literacy, mental health, and employment outcomes. *Journal of Speech, Language, and Hearing Research, 52*, 1401–1416.

Lê, K., Coelho, C., Mozeiko, J., Krueger, F., & Grafman, J. (2014). Does brain volume loss predict cognitive and narrative discourse performance following traumatic brain injury? *American Journal of Speech-Language Pathology, 23*, S271–S284.

Leaman, M. C., & Archer, B. (2022). "If you just stay with me and wait . . . you'll get an idea of what I'm saying": the communicative benefits of time for conversational self-repair for people with aphasia. *American Journal of Speech-Language Pathology, 31,* 1264–1283.

Leaman, M. C., & Edmonds, L. A. (2021a). Assessing language in unstructured conversation in people with aphasia: Methods, psychometric integrity, normative data, and comparison to a structured narrative task. *Journal of Speech, Language, and Hearing Research, 64,* 4344–4365.

Leaman, M. C., & Edmonds, L. A. (2021b). Measuring global coherence in people with aphasia during unstructured conversation. *American Journal of Speech-Language Pathology, 30,* 359–375.

Leder, S. (2015). Comparing simultaneous clinical swallow evaluations and fiberoptic endoscopic evaluations for swallowing: Findings and consequences. *Perspectives on Swallowing and Swallowing Disorders (Dysphagia), 24,* 12–17.

Leder, S., & Suiter, D. (2014). *The Yale Swallow Protocol: An evidence-based approach to decision making.* Springer International.

Lee, J., Croen, L. A., Lindan, C., Nash, K. B., Yoshida, C. K., Ferriero, D. M., et al. (2005). Predictors of outcome in perinatal arterial stroke: A population-based study. *Annals of Neurology, 58*(2), 303–308.

Lee, L. (1974). *Developmental sentence analysis.* Northwestern University Press.

Lee, S. A. S., Sancibrian, S., & Ahlfinger, N. (2013). The effects of technology-assisted instruction to improve phonological awareness skills in children with reading difficulties: A systematic review. *EBP Briefs, 8*(1), 1–10.

Lefton-Greif, M. A. (2008). Pediatric dysphagia. *Physical Medicine and Rehabilitation Clinics of North America, 19,* 837–851. https://doi.org/10.1016/j.pmr.2008.05.007

Lehman Blake, M. (2006). Clinical relevance of discourse characteristics after right hemisphere brain damage. *American Journal of Speech-Language Pathology, 15,* 255–267.

Lehman Blake, M. (2007). Perspectives on treatment for communication deficits associated with right hemisphere brain damage. *American Journal of Speech-Language Pathology, 16,* 331–342.

Lehman Blake, M., & Tompkins, C. A. (2008). *Cognitive-communication disorders resulting from right hemisphere damage.* Treatment Efficacy Summary. www.asha.org/NR/rdonlyres/4BAF3969-9ADC-4C01-B5ED-1334CC20DD3D/0/TreatmentEfficacySummaries2008.pdf

Lehman Blake, M., Frymark, T., & Venedictov, R. (2013). An evidence-based systematic review on communication treatments for individuals with right hemisphere brain damage. *American Journal of Speech-Language Pathology, 22,* 146–160.

Lehman, M. T., & Tompkins, C. (2000). Inferencing in adults with right hemisphere brain damage: An analysis of conflicting results. *Aphasiology, 14,* 485–499.

Lenell, C., Sandage, M., & Johnson, A. (2019). A tutorial of the effects of sex hormones on laryngeal senescence and neuromuscular response to exercise. *Journal of Speech, Language, and Hearing Research, 62,* 602–610.

Leonard, L. B. (2011). The primacy of priming in grammatical learning and intervention: A tutorial. *Journal of Speech, Language, and Hearing Research, 54,* 608–621.

Leonard, L. B. (2014). *Children with specific language impairment* (2nd ed.). MIT Press.

Leonard, M. A., Milich, R., & Lorch, E. P. (2011). Pragmatic language use in mediating the relation between hyperactivity and inattention and social skills problems. *Journal of Speech, Language, and Hearing Research, 54,* 567–579.

Lewis, B. A., Minnes, S., Short, E. J., Min, M. O., Wu, M., Lang, A., et al. (2013). Language outcomes at 12 years for children exposed prenatally to cocaine. *Journal of Speech, Language, and Hearing Research, 56,* 1662–1676.

Lewis, B., Freebairn, L., & Taylor, H. (2000). Follow-up of children with early expressive phonology disorders. *Journal of Learning Disabilities, 33*(5), 433–444.

Liberman, C., Epstein, M, Cleveland, S., Wang H., & Maison, S. (2016). Toward a differential diagnosis of hidden hearing loss in humans. *PloS ONE, 11*(9), e0162726.

Liberman, Z., Woodward, A. L., Keysar, B., & Kinzler, K. D. (2017). Exposure to multiple languages enhances communication skills in infancy. *Developmental Science, 20,* e12420. https://doi.org/10.1111/desc.12420

Lidz, C. S. (1991). *Practitioner's guide to dynamic assessment.* Guilford Press.

Lieu, J., Kenna, M., Anne, S., & Davidson, L. (2020). Hearing loss in children: A review. *Journal of the American Medical Association, 324*(21), 2195–2205.

Lieven, E., Behrens, H., Speares, J., & Tomasello, M. (2003). Early syntactic creativity: A usage-based approach. *Journal of Child Language, 30,* 333–370.

Light, J. (1999). Do augmentative and alternative communication interventions really make a difference?: The challenges of efficacy research. *Augmentative and Alternative Communication, 15*(1), 13–24.

Light, J. C., & Binger, C. (1998). *Building communicative competence with individuals who use augmentative and alternative communication.* Brookes.

Light, J. C., Binger, C., Agate, T. L., & Ramsay, K. N. (1999). Teaching partner-focused questions to individuals who use augmentative and alternative communication to enhance their communicative competence. *Journal of Speech, Language, and Hearing Research, 42*(1), 241–255.

Light, J. C., Roberts, B., Dimarco, R., & Greiner, N. (1998). Augmentative and alternative communication to support receptive and expressive communication for people with autism [*Special Issue: Autism: New Perspectives on Assessment and Intervention*]. *Journal of Communication Disorders, 31*(2), 153–180.

Light, J., & Drager, K. (2007). AAC technologies for young children with complex communication needs: State of the science and future research directions. *Augmentative and Alternative Communication, 23*(3), 204–216.

Light, J., & McNaughton, D. (2012). The changing face of augmentative and alternative communication: Past, present, and future challenges. *Augmentative and Alternative Communication, 28*(4), 197–204.

Light, J., & McNaughton, D. (2014). Communicative competence for individuals who require augmentative and alternative communication: A new definition for a new era of communication? *Augmentative and Alternative Communication, 30*(1), 1–18. https://doi .org/10.3109/07434618.2014.885080

Liiva, C. A., & Cleave, P. L. (2005). Roles of initiation and responsiveness in access and participation for children with specific language impairment. *Journal of Speech, Language, and Hearing Research, 48*, 868–883.

Lim, N., O'Reilly, M. F., Sigafoos, J., Ledbetter-Cho, K., & Lancioni, G. E. (2019). Should heritage languages be incorporated into interventions for bilingual individuals with neurodevelopmental disorders?: A systematic review. *Journal of Autism and Developmental Disorders, 49*, 1–26

Lin, F., & Ferrucci, L. (2012). Hearing loss and falls among older adults in the United States. *Archives of Internal Medicine, 172*(4), 369–371.

Lin, F. R., Niparko, J. K., & Ferrucci, L. (2011). Hearing loss prevalence in the United States. *Archives of Internal Medicine, 171*, 1851–1852.

Lincoln, M., & Onslow, M. (1997). Long-term outcome of early intervention for stuttering. *American Journal of Speech-Language Pathology, 6*, 51–58.

Linscheid, T. (2006). Behavioral treatments for pediatric feeding disorders. *Behavior Modification, 30*, 1–19.

Lloyd, L. L., Fuller, D., & Arvidson, H. (1997). *Augmentative and alternative communication: A handbook of principles and practices.* Allyn & Bacon.

Lloyd, L. L., & Kangas, K. A. (1994). Augmentative and alternative communication. In G. H. Shames, E. H. Wiig, & W. A. Secord (Eds.), *Human communication disorders* (4th ed.). Allyn & Bacon.

Logemann, J. A. (1997). Structural and functional aspects of normal and disordered swallowing. In C. T. Ferrand & R. L. Bloom (Eds.), *Introduction to organic and neurogenic disorders of communication: Current scope of practice.* Allyn & Bacon.

Logemann, J. A. (1998). *Evaluation and treatment of swallowing disorders* (2nd ed.). PRO-ED.

Logemann, J., Gensler, G., Robbins, J., Lindblad, J., Brandt, D., Hind, J. A., et al. (2008). A randomized study of three interventions for aspiration of thin liquids in patients with dementia or Parkinson's disease. *Journal of Speech, Language, and Hearing Research, 51*, 173–183.

Logemann, J., Kahrilas, P., Kobara, M., & Vakil, N. (1989). The benefit of head rotation on pharyngoesophageal dysphagia. *Archives of Physical Medicine Rehabilitation, 70*, 767–771.

Logemann, J., Pauloski, B., Rademaker, A., & Colangelo, L. (1997). Super-supraglottic swallow in irradiated head and neck cancer patients. *Journal of the Sciences and Specialties of the Head and Neck, 19*, 535–540. https://doi.org/10.1002/(SICI)1097-0347(199709)19:6<535::AID-HED11>3.0.CO;2-4

Lorang, E., Maltman, N., Venker, C., Eith, A., & Sterling, A. (2022). Speech-language pathologists' practices in augmentative and alternative communication during early intervention. *Augmentative and Alternative Communication, 38*(1), 41–52. https://doi.org/10.1080/07434618.2022.2046853

Losh, M., & Capps, L. (2003). Narrative ability in high-functioning children with autism or Asperger's syndrome. *Journal of Autism and Developmental Disorders, 33*, 239–251.

Louise-Bender, P. T., Kim, J., & Weiner, B. (2002). The shaping of individual meanings assigned to assistive technology: a review of personal factors. *Disability and Rehabilitation 24*(1–3), 5–20.

Love, R., & Webb, W. (2001). *Neurology for the speech-language pathologist* (4th ed.). Butterworth–Heinemann.

Lubinski, R., & Masters, M. G. (2001). Special populations, special settings: New and expanding frontiers. In R. Lubinski & C. Frattali (Eds.), *Professional issues in speech-language pathology and audiology* (2nd ed.). Singular.

Lucas, R., & Frazier Norbury, C. (2015). Making inferences from text: It's vocabulary that matters. *Journal of Speech, Language, and Hearing Research, 58*, 1224–1232.

Ludwig, L., Pasman, J. A., Nicholson, T., Aybek, S., David, A. S., Tuck, S., et al. (2018). Stressful life events and maltreatment in conversion (functional neurological) disorder: Systematic review and meta-analysis of case-control studies. *The Lancet Psychiatry, 5*, 307–320.

Lum, J. A., Powell, M., Timms, L., & Snow, P. (2015). A meta-analysis of cross sectional studies investigating language in maltreated children. *Journal of Speech, Language, and Hearing Research, 58*, 961–976.

Lund, N., & Duchan, J. (1993). *Assessing children's language in naturalistic contexts* (3rd ed.). Prentice Hall.

Lund, S. K., Quach, W., Weissling, K., McKelvey, M., & Dietz, A. (2017). Assessment with children who need augmentative and alternative communication (AAC): Clinical decisions of AAC specialists. *Language Speech and Hearing Services in the Schools, 48*(1), 56–68. https://doi.org/10.1044/2016_LSHSS-15-0086

Lund, S., & Light, J. (2006). Long-term outcomes for individuals who use augmentative and alternative communication: Part I—What is a good outcome? *Augmentative and Alternative Communication, 22*, 284–299.

Lund, S., & Light, J. (2007). Long-term outcomes for individuals who use augmentative and alternative communication: Part II—What is a good outcome? *Augmentative and Alternative Communication, 23*, 1–15.

Lundgren, K., Brownell, H., Cayer-Meade, C., Milione, J., & Kearns, K. (2011). Treating metaphor interpretation deficits subsequent to right hemisphere brain damage: Preliminary results. *Aphasiology, 25*, 456–474.

Lyon, G. R., Shaywitz, S. E., & Shaywitz, B. A. (2003). Defining dyslexia, comorbidity, teachers' knowledge of language and reading: A definition of dyslexia. *Annals of Dyslexia, 53*, 1.

Maas, E., & Farinella, K. (2012). Random versus blocked practice in treatment for childhood apraxia of speech. *Journal of Speech, Language, and Hearing Research, 55*, 561–578.

Maas, E., Butalla, C., & Farinella, K. (2012). Feedback frequency in treatment for childhood apraxia of speech. *American Journal of Speech-Language Pathology, 21*, 239–257.

Maas, E., Robin, D. A., Austermann Hula, S. N., Freedman, S. E., Wulf, G., & Ballard, K. J. (2008). Principles of motor learning in treatment of motor speech disorders. *American Journal of Speech-Language Pathology, 17*, 277–298.

MacArthur, C. A. (2000). New tools for writing: Assistive technology for students with writing difficulties. *Topics in Language Disorders, 20*, 85–100.

Mach, H., Baylor, C., Hunting Pompon, R., & Yorkston, K. (2021). Beyond the patient: A mixed-methods inquiry into family members' involvement in the treatment of Parkinson's disease to target third-party disability. *American Journal of Speech-Language Pathology, 30*, 169–185.

Machalicek, W., Sanford, A., Lang, R., Rispoli, M., Molfenter, N., & Mbeseha, M. K. (2010). Literacy interventions for students with physical and developmental disabilities who use aided AAC devices: A systematic review. *Journal of Developmental and Physical Disabilities, 22*(3), 219–240.

Mackie, C., & Dockrell, J. (2004). The nature of written language deficits in children with SLI. *Journal of Speech, Language, and Hearing Research, 47*, 1469–1483.

MacSwan, J., & Rolstad, K. (2006). How language proficiency tests mislead us about ability: Implications for English language learner placement in special education. *Teachers College Record, 108*, 2304–2328. https://doi.org/10.1111/j.1467-9620.2006.00783.x

MacWhinney, B. (2022). *Tools for analyzing talk part 2: The CLAN Program.* https://talkbank.org/manuals/CLAN.pdf

Magaziner, J., German, P., Itkin Zimmerman, S., Hebel, J. R., Burton, L., Bruber-Baldini, A. L., et al. (2000). The prevalence of dementia in a statewide sample of new nursing home admissions aged 65 and older: Diagnosis by expert panel. *The Gerontologist, 40*(6), 663–672.

Mainela-Arnold, E., Evans, J. L., & Coady, J. A. (2008). Lexical representations in children with SLI: Evidence from a frequency-manipulated gating task. *Journal of Speech, Language, and Hearing Research, 51*, 381–393.

Mainela-Arnold, E., Evans, J. L., & Coady, J. A. (2010). Explaining lexical-semantic deficits in specific language impairment: The role of phonological similarity, phonological working memory, and lexical competition. *Journal of Speech, Language, and Hearing Research, 53*, 1742–1756.

Makdissi, H., & Boisclair, A. (2006). Interactive reading: A context for expanding the expression of causal relations in preschoolers. *Written Language & Literacy, 9*, 177–211.

Manikam, R., & Perman, J. A. (2000). Pediatric feeding disorders. *Journal of Clinical Gastroenterology, 30*, 34–46. https://doi.org/10.1097/00004836-200001000-00007

Mann, V., & Singson, M. (2003). Linking morphological knowledge to English decoding ability: Large effects of little suffixes. In E. Assink & D Sandra (Eds.), *Reading complex words: Cross-language studies* (pp. 1–25). Kluwer.

Mann, W., & Lane, J. (1991). *Assistive technology for persons with disabilities: The role of occupational therapy.* American Occupational Therapy Association.

Mansson, H. (2000). Childhood stuttering: Incidence and development. *Journal of Fluency Disorders, 25*, 47–57.

Margolis, R., Killion, M., Bratt, G., & Saly, G. (2016). Validation of the Home Hearing Test. *Journal of the American Academy of Audiology, 27*(5), 416–420.

Marini, A., Boewe, A., Caltagirone, C., & Carlomagno, S. (2005). Age-related differences in the production of textual descriptions. *Journal of Psycholinguistic Research, 34*, 439–464.

Markel, N., Meisels, M., & Houck, J. (1964). Judging personality from voice quality. *Journal of Abnormal Social Psychology, 69*, 458–463.

Marshall, C. R., Hardy, C. J. D., Volkmar, A., Russell, L. L., Bond, R. L., Fletcher, P. D., et al. (2018). Primary progressive aphasia: A clinical approach. *Journal of Neurology, 265*, 1474–1490.

Martin, G. E., Bush, L., Klusek, J., Patel, S., & Losh, M. (2018). A multimethod analysis of pragmatic skills in children and adolescents with fragile X syndrome, autism spectrum disorder, and Down syndrome. *Journal of Speech, Language and Hearing Disorders, 61*, 3023–3037.

Martin, R. E., Neary, M. A., & Diamant, N. E. (1997). Dysphagia following anterior cervical spine surgery. *Dysphagia, 12*(1), 2–10.

Martin, R., & Lindamood, L. (1986). Stuttering and spontaneous recovery: Implications for the speech-language pathologist. *Language, Speech, and Hearing Services in Schools, 17*, 207–218.

Martin, S., Small, K., & Stevens, R. (1995). *The Pragmatics Profile for people who use AAC*. Ace Centre. https://aaclanguagelab.com/resources/pragmatics-profile

Martins, R., do Amaral, H., Tavares, E., Martins, M., Gonçalves, T., & Dias, N. (2016). Voice disorders: Etiology and diagnosis. *Journal of Voice, 16*, 761.e1–761.e9.

Martins, R., Pereiera, E., Hidalgo, C., & Tavares, E. (2014). Voice disorders in teachers. A review. *Journal of Voice, 28*, 716–724.

Marvin, C. A., & Wright, D. (1997). Literacy socialization in the homes of preschool children. *Language, Speech, and Hearing Services in Schools, 28*, 154–163.

Masterson, J. J., & Apel, K. (2000). Spelling assessment: Charting a path to optimal intervention. *Topics in Language Disorders, 20*(3), 50–65.

Masterson, J. J., & Bernhardt, B. (2001). *Computerized Articulation & Phonology Evaluation System (CAPES)*. Pearson.

Matsuo, K., & Palmer, J. (2009). Coordination of mastication, swallowing, and breathing. *Japanese Dental Science Review, 45*, 31–40.

Mauldin, L. (2019). Don't look at it as a miracle cure: Contested notions of success and failure in family narratives of pediatric cochlear implantation. *Social Science & Medicine, 228*, 117–125. https://doi.org/10.1016/j.socscimed.2019.03.021

Max, L., & Caruso, A. J. (1997). Contemporary techniques for establishing fluency in the treatment of adults who stutter. *Contemporary Issues in Communication Science and Disorders, 24*, 45–52.

Mayo Clinic. (2022). *Persistent post-concussive symptoms*. https://www.mayoclinic.org/diseases-conditions/post-concussion-syndrome/symptoms-causes/syc-20353352

McAleer, P., Todorov, A., & Belin, P. (2014). How do you say "hello"?: Personality impressions from brief novel voices. *PLoS One, 9*, e90779. https://doi.org/10.1371/journal.pone.0090779

McCabe, A., & Bliss, L. S. (2004–2005). Narratives from Spanish-speaking children with impaired and typical language development. *Imagination, Cognition, and Personality, 24*, 331–346.

McCarthy, J., & Light, J. (2001). Instructional effectiveness of an integrated theatre arts program for children using augmentative and alternative communication and their nondisabled peers: Preliminary study. *Augmentative and Alternative Communication, 17*, 88–98.

McCarthy, M., Leigh, G., & Kelly, M. (2018). Telepractice delivery of family-centered early intervention for children who are deaf or hard of hearing: A scoping review. *Journal of Telemedicine and Telecare, 24*(4), 249–260.

McCauley, R., & Strand, E. (2008). A review of standardized tests of nonverbal oral and speech motor performance in children. *American Journal of Speech-Language Pathology, 17*, 81–91.

McCoy, K. F., Bedrosian, J. L., Hoag, L. A., & Johnson, D. E. (2007). Brevity and speed of message delivery trade-offs in augmentative and alternative communication. *Augmentative and Alternative Communication, 23*, 76–88.

McCullough, K. C., Bayles, K. A., & Bouldin, E. D. (2019). Language performance of individuals at risk for mild cognitive impairment. *Journal of Speech, Language, and Hearing Research, 62*, 706–722.

McDonald, E. T. (1964). *Articulation testing and treatment: A sensory-motor approach*. Stanwix House.

McFadden, T. U. (1998). Sounds and stories: Teaching phonemic awareness in interactions around text. *American Journal of Speech-Language Pathology, 7*(2), 5–13.

McFarland, C., & Cacase, T. (2006). Current controversies in CAPD: From Procrustes bed to Pandora's box. In T. K. Parthasarathy (Ed.), *An introduction to auditory processing disorders in children* (pp. 247–263). Erlbaum.

McGillion, M., Herbert, J. S., Pine, J., Vihman, M., dePaolis, R., Keren-Portnoy, T. & Matthews, D. (2017). What paves the way to conventional language? The predictive value of babble, pointing, and socioeconomic status. *Child Development, 88*, 156–166. https://doi.org/10.1111/cdev.12671

McGinty, A. S., & Justice, L. M. (2006). Classroom-based versus pull-out interventions: A review of the experimental evidence. *EBP Briefs, 1*(1).

McGinty, A., & Justice, L. M. (2009). Predictors of print knowledge in children with specific language impairment: Experiential and developmental factors. *Journal of Speech, Language, and Hearing Research, 52*, 81–97.

McGregor, K. K. (2000). The development and enhancement of narrative skills in a preschool classroom: Toward a solution to clinician-client mismatch. *American Journal of Speech-Language Pathology, 9*, 55–71.

McGregor, K. K., Goffman, L., Owen Van Horne, A., Hogan, T. P., & Finestack, L. (2020). Developmental Language Disorder: Applications for Advocacy, Research, and Clinical Service. *Perspectives of the ASHA Special Interest Groups, 5*(1), 38–46.

McGregor, K. K., Newman, R. M., Reilly, R. M., & Capone, N. C. (2002). Semantic representation and naming in children with specific language impairment. *Journal of Speech, Language, and Hearing Research, 45,* 998–1014.

McGregor, K. K., Sheng, L., & Smith, B. (2005). The precocious two-year-old: Status of the lexicon and links to the grammar. *Journal of Child Language, 32,* 563–585.

McLaughlin, T. F., Weber, K. P., & Derby, M. (2013). Classroom spelling interventions for students with learning disabilities. In H. L. Swanson, K. R. Harris, & S. Graham (Eds.), *Handbook of learning disabilities* (2nd ed., pp. 439–447). Guilford Press.

McLeod, S. (2018). Communication rights: Fundamental human rights for all. *International Journal of Speech Language Pathology, 20*(1), 3–11. https://doi.org/10.1080/17549507.2018.1428687

McLeod, S., & Baker, E. (2017). *Children's speech: An evidence-based approach to assessment and intervention.* Pearson Education.

McLeod, S., & Crowe, K. (2018). Children's consonant acquisition in 27 languages: A cross-linguistic review. *American Journal of Speech-Language Pathology, 27*(4), 1546–1571.

McLeod, S., & Searl, J. (2006). Adaptation to an electropalatograph palate: Acoustic, impressionistic, and perceptual data. *American Journal of Speech-Language Pathology, 15,* 192–206.

McLeod, S., & Verdon, S. (2014). A review of 30 speech assessments in 19 languages other than English. *American Journal of Speech-Language Pathology, 23,* 708–723.

McLeod, S., Harrison, L. J., & McCormack, J. (2012a). *Escala de la Inteligibilidad en Contexto: Español* [Intelligibility in Context Scale: Spanish] (R. Prezas, R. Rojas, & B. A. Goldstein, Trans.). Charles Sturt University. http://www.csu.edu.au/research/multilingual-speech/ics

McLeod, S., Harrison, L. J., & McCormack, J. (2012b). *Intelligibility in Context Scale.* Charles Sturt University. http://www.csu.edu.au/research/multilingual-speech/ics

McMaster, K. L., Kunkel, A., Shin, J., Jung, P. G., & Lembke, E. (2017). Early writing intervention: A best evidence synthesis. *Journal of Learning Disabilities, 51*(4), 363–380.

McNaughton, D., Light, J., & Groszyk, L. (2001). "Don't give up": Employment experiences of individuals with amyotrophic lateral sclerosis who use augmentative and alternative communication. *Augmentative and Alternative Communication, 17,* 179–195.

McNeilly, L. (2005). HIV and communication. *Journal of Communication Disorders, 38,* 303–310.

McNeilly, L. (2016 March). Rise in speech-language disorders in SSI-supported children reflects national trends: A new national report reviews the prevalence and implications of speech-language disorders for children living in poverty. *The ASHA Leader, 21.* https://doi.org/10.1044/leader.PA2.21032016.np

McNeilly, L. G. (2018). Using the International Classification of Functioning, Disability and Health framework to achieve interprofessional functional outcomes for young children: A speech-language pathology perspective. *Pediatric Clinics of North America, 65*(1), 125–134.

McSwan, J., & Rolstad, K. (2006). How language proficiency tests mislead us about ability: Implications for English language learner placement in special education. *Teachers College Record, 108,* 2304–2328.

Medwetsky, L. (2011). Spoken language processing model: Bridging auditory and language processing to guide assessment and intervention. *Language, Speech, and Hearing Services in Schools, 42,* 286–296.

Mei, C., Reilly, S., Reddihough, D., Mensah, F., & Morgan, A. (2014). Motor speech impairment, activity, and participation in children with cerebral palsy. *International Journal of Speech-Language Pathology, 16,* 427–435.

Meilijson, S. R., Kasher, A., & Elizur, A. (2004). Language performance in chronic schizophrenia: A pragmatic approach. *Journal of Speech, Language, and Hearing Research, 47,* 695–713.

Meinzen-Deer, J., Wiley, S., & Choo, D. (2011). Impact of early intervention on expressive and receptive language development among young children with permanent hearing loss. *American Annals of the Deaf, 155*(5), 580–591.

Mendelsohn, M., & McConnel, F. (1987). Function in the pharyngoesophageal segment. *The Laryngoscope, 97,* 483–489.

Mener, D., Betz, J., Genther, D., Chen, D., & Lin, F. (2013). Hearing loss and depression in older adults. *Journal of the American Geriatric Society, 61*(9), 1627–1629.

Mental Health Research Association. (2007). *Childhood schizophrenia.* www.narsad.org/dc/childhood_disorders/schizophrenia.html

Menzies, G., Onslow, M., Packman, A., & O'Brian, S. (2009). Cognitive behavior therapy for adults who stutter: a tutorial for speech-language pathologists. *Journal of Fluency Disorders, 34,* 187–200.

Menzies, R., Packman, A., Onslow, M., O'Brian, S., Jones, M., & Helgadóttir, F. (2019). In-clinic and stand-alone internet cognitive behavior therapy treatment for social anxiety in stuttering: A randomized trial of iGlebe. *Journal of Speech, Language, and Hearing Research, 62,* 1614–1624.

Meulenbroek, P., & Cherney, L. R. (2019). The voicemail elicitation task: Functional workplace language assessment for persons with traumatic brain injury. *Journal of Speech, Language, and Hearing Research, 62,* 3367–3380.

Miccio, A. W., & Ingrisano, D. (2000). The acquisition of fricatives and affricates: Evidence from a disordered phonological system. *American Journal of Speech-Language Pathology, 9,* 214–229.

Miccio, A. W., Elbert, M., & Forrest, K. (1999). The relationship between stimulability and phonological acquisition in children with normally developing and disordered phonologies. *American Journal of Speech-Language Pathology, 8,* 347–363.

Mihai, A., Butera, G., & Friesen, A. (2017) Examining the use of curriculum to support early literacy instruction: A multiple case study of head start teachers. *Early Education and Development, 28,* 323–342.

Miles, A., Jardine, M., Johnston, F., de Lisle, M., Friary, P., & Allen, J. (2017). Effect of Lee Silverman Voice Treatment (LSVT LOUD®) on swallowing and cough in Parkinson's disease: A pilot study. *Journal of the Neurological Sciences, 15,* 180–187.

Millar, D. C., Light, J. C., & Schlosser, R. W. (2006). The impact of augmentative and alternative communication intervention on the speech production of individuals with developmental disabilities: A research review. *Journal of Speech, Language, and Hearing Research, 49,* 248–264.

Millar, D., Light, J. A., & Schlosser, R. (2000, July). The impact of AAC on natural speech development: A metaanalysis. *Proceedings of the 9th Biennial Conference of the International Society for Augmentative and Alternative Communication,* pp. 740–741.

Millard, S., & Davis, S. (2016). The Palin parent rating scales: Parents' perspectives on childhood stuttering and its impact. *Journal of Speech, Language, and Hearing Research, 59,* 950–963.

Miller, C. A., Kail, R., Leonard, L. B., & Tomblin, J. B. (2001). Speed of processing in children with specific language impairment. *Journal of Speech, Language, and Hearing Research, 44,* 416–433.

Miller, C. A., Leonard, L. B., Kail, R. V., Zhang, X., Tomblin, J. B., & Francis, D. J. (2006). Response time in 14-year-olds with language impairment. *Journal of Speech, Language, and Hearing Research, 49,* 712–728.

Miller, C. J., Kim, B., Silverman, A., & Bauer, M. S. (2018). A systematic review of team-building interventions in non-acute healthcare settings. *BMC Health Services Research, 18*(1), 146. https://doi.org/10.1186/s12913-018-2961-9

Miller, C., & Madhoun, L. (2016). Feeding and swallowing issues in infants with craniofacial anomalies. *Perspectives of the ASHA Special Interest Groups, 1,* 13–26.

Miller, J., & Iglesias, A. (2015). *Systematic Analysis of Language Transcripts* (SALT; Research Version 2012) [Computer software]. SALT Software.

Minga, J., Fromm, D., Williams-DeVane, C., & MacWhinney, B. (2020). Question use in adults with right-hemisphere brain damage. *Journal of Speech, Language, and Hearing Research, 63,* 738–748.

Miniutti, A. (1991). Language deficiencies in inner-city children with learning and behavioral problems. *Language, Speech, and Hearing Services in Schools, 22,* 31–38.

Mitchell, R. E., & Karchmer, M. A. (2004). Chasing the mythical ten percent: Parental hearing status of deaf and hard of hearing students in the United States. *Sign Language Studies, 4,* 138–163.

Moats, L., & Foorman, B. (2003). Measuring teachers' conversational knowledge of language and reading. *Annals of Dyslexia, 53,* 23–45.

Mok, P. L. H., Pickles, A., Durkin, K., & Conti-Ramsden, G. (2014). Longitudinal trajectories of peer relations in children with specific language impairment. *Journal of Child Psychology & Psychiatry, 55,* 516–527.

Mol, L., Krahmer, E., & van de Sandt-Koenderman, M. (2013). Gesturing by speakers with aphasia: How does it compare? *Journal of Speech, Language, and Hearing Research, 56,* 1224–1236.

Mol, S. E., & Bus, A. G. (2011). To read or not to read: A meta-analysis of print exposure from infancy to early adulthood. *Psychological Bulletin, 137,* 267–296.

Montgomery, J. W. (2006). Real-time language processing in school-age children with specific language impairment. *International Journal of Language & Communication Disorders, 41,* 275–291.

Montgomery, J. W., & Evans, J. L. (2009). Complex sentence comprehension and working memory in children with specific language impairment. *Journal of Speech, Language, and Hearing Research, 52,* 269–288.

Montgomery, J. W., & Leonard, L. B. (2006). Effects of acoustic manipulation on the real-time inflectional processing of children with specific language impairment. *Journal of Speech, Language, and Hearing Research, 49,* 1238–1256.

Montgomery, J. W., Gillam, R. B., & Evans, J. L. (2016). Syntactic versus memory accounts of the sentence comprehension deficits of specific language impairment: Looking back, looking ahead. *Journal of Speech, Language, Hearing research, 59,* 1491–1504. https://doi.org/10.1044/2016_JSLHR-L-15-0325

Montgomery, J., Evans, J., Fargo, J., Schwartz, S., & Gillam, R. (2018). Structural relationship between cognitive processing and syntactic sentence comprehension in children with and without developmental language disorder. *Journal of Speech, Language, and Hearing Research, 61*(12), 2950–2976.

Moore, D., Hunter, L., & Munro, K. (2017). Benefits of extended high-frequency audiometry for everyone. *The Hearing Journal, 70*(3), 50.

Moore, D., Zabay, O., & Ferguson, M. (2020). Minimal and mild hearing loss in children: Association with auditory perception, cognition, and communication problems. *Ear and Hearing, 41*(4), 720–732.

Moran, C., & Gillon, G. (2005). Inference comprehension of adolescents with traumatic brain injury: A working memory hypothesis. *Brain Injury, 19,* 743–751.

Morford, J. P., Grieve-Smith, A. B., & MacFarlane, J. (2008). Effects of language experience on the perception of American sign language. *Cognition, 109*(1), 41–53.

Morgan, P. L., Scheffner Hammer, C., Farkas, G., Hillemeier, M. M., Maczuga, S., Cook, M., & Morano, S. (2016). Who receives speech/language services by 5 years of age in the United States? *American Journal of Speech-Language Pathology, 25,* 183–199.

Mortimer, J., & Rvachew, S. (2010). A longitudinal investigation of morpho-syntax in children with speech sounds disorders. *Journal of Communication Disorders, 43,* 61–76.

Mullins, T. (2004). Depression in older adults with hearing loss. *The ASHA Leader, 21,* 12–13, 27.

Murphy, K. A., & Diehm, E. (2020). collecting words: a clinical example of a morphology-focused orthographic intervention. *Language, Speech, and Hearing Services in Schools, 51,* 544–560.

Murphy, K. A., Justice, L. M., O'Connell, A. A., Pentimonti, J. M., & Kaderavek, J. N. (2016). Understanding risk for reading difficulties in children with language impairment. *Journal of Speech, Language, and Hearing Research, 59,* 1436–1447.

Murphy, S. M., Faulkner, D. M., & Farley, L. R. (2014). The behaviour of young children with social communication disorders during dyadic interaction with peers. *Journal of Abnormal Child Psychology, 42*(2), 277–289.

Murray, D. S., Ruble, L. A., Willis, H., & Molloy, C. A. (2009). Parent and teacher report of social skills in children with autism spectrum disorder. *Language, Speech, and Hearing Services in Schools, 40,* 109–115.

Murray, E., McCabe, P., & Ballard, K. (2014). A systematic review of treatment outcomes for children with childhood apraxia of speech. *American Journal of Speech-Language Pathology, 17,* 1–19.

Murray, E., McCabe, P., Heard, R., & Ballard, K. (2015). Differential diagnosis of children with suspected childhood apraxia of speech. *Journal of Speech, Language, and Hearing Research, 58,* 43–60.

Murray, J., & Schutte, B. (2004). Cleft palate: players, pathways, and pursuits. *Journal of Clinical Investigation, 113,* 1676–1678.

Murray, L. L. (2012). Attention and other cognitive deficits in aphasia: presence and relation to language and communication measures. *American Journal of Speech-Language Pathology, 21,* 51–64.

Murry, T., Carrau, R., & Chan, K. (2020). *Clinical management of swallowing disorders* (5th ed.). Plural Publishing.

Musiek, F. E., Chermak, G. D., Bamiou, D. E., & Shinn, J. (2018). CAPD: The most common "hidden hearing loss." *The ASHA Leader, 23*(3), 6–9.

Mustofa, K. (2010). The effect of cognitive behavioral therapy on stuttering. *Social Behavior and Personality, 38,* 301–310.

Muter, V., Hulme, C., Snowling, M. J., & Stevenson, J. (2004). Phonemes, rimes, vocabulary, and grammatical skills as foundations of early reading development: Evidence from a longitudinal study. *Developmental Psychology, 40,* 665–681.

Myers, K., & Nicholson, N. (2021). Cochlear implant behavioral outcomes for children with auditory neuropathy spectrum disorder: A mini-systematic review. *American Journal of Audiology, 30,* 777–789.

Myers, P. S. (2001). Toward a definition of RHD syndrome. *Aphasiology, 15,* 913–918.

Nagaya, M., Kachi, T., Yamada, T., & Sumi, Y. (2004). Videofluorographic observations on swallowing in patients with dysphagia due to neurodegenerative diseases. *Nagoya Journal of Medical Sciences, 67,* 17–23.

Naglieri, J., & Rojahn, J. (2001). Gender differences in planning, attention, simultaneous, and successive (PASS) cognitive processes and achievement. *Journal of Educational Psychology, 93,* 430–437.

Nam, S. (2018). Surgical treatment of velopharyngeal insufficiency. *Archives of Craniofacial Surgery, 19,* 163–167.

Namy, L. L., Campbell, A. L., & Tomasello, M. (2004). The changing role of iconicity in non-verbal symbol learning: A U-shaped trajectory in the acquisition of arbitrary gestures. *Journal of Cognition and Development, 5*(1), 37–57.

Narayanan, S., & Kalappa, N. (2017) Speech, language and swallowing difficulties in a child with AIDS. *Acta Oto-Laryngologica Case Reports, 2,* 34–42.

Narayanan, U. (2012). Management of children with ambulatory cerebral palsy: An evidence-based review. *Journal of Pediatric Orthopedics, 32,* S172–S181.

Naremore, R. C. (2001). *Narrative frameworks and early literacy.* Seminar presented for Rochester Hearing and Speech Center and Nazareth College, Rochester, NY.

Narne, J., Prabhu, P., Chandan, H., & Deepthi, M. (2016). Gender differences in audiological findings and hearing aid benefit in 255 individuals with auditory neuropathy spectrum disorder: A retrospective study. *Journal of the American Academy of Audiology*, *27*(10), 839–845.

Nathan, L., Stackhouse, J., Goulandris, N., & Snowling, M. J. (2004). The development of early literacy skills among children with speech difficulties: A test of the "critical age hypothesis." *Journal of Speech, Language, and Hearing Research, 47*, 377–391.

Nation, K., & Norbury, C. F. (2005). Why reading comprehension fails: Insights into developmental disorders. *Topics in Language Disorders, 25*(1), 21–32.

Nation, K., & Snowling, M. J. (2004). Beyond phonological skills: Broader language skills contribute to the development of reading. *Journal of Research in Reading, 27*, 342–356.

Nation, K., Clarke, P., Marshall, C. M., & Durand, M. (2004). Hidden language impairment in children: Parellels between poor reading comprehension and Specific Language Impairment. *Journal of Speech, Language, and Hearing Research, 47*, 199–211.

Nation, K., Snowling, M. J., & Clarke, P. J. (2007). Dissecting the relationship between language skills and learning to read: Semantic and phonological contributions to new vocabulary learning in children with poor reading comprehension. *Advances in Speech-Language Pathology, 9*, 131–139.

National Aphasia Association. (n.d.). *Aphasia FAQs.* aphasia.org/aphasia-faqs/

National Assessment of Educational Progress. (2022). National Center for Educational Statistics. https://www.nationsreportcard.gov/reading/states/achievement/?grade=4

National Assessment of Educational Progress. (2022). *Nation's Report Card.* https://www.nationsreportcard.gov/reading/states/achievement/?grade=4

National Association of the Deaf. (2022). *Position Statement on American Sign Language.* Author.

National Center for Education Statistics (NCES). (2022, June 6). *National Assessment of Educational Progress.* https://nces.ed.gov/nationsreportcard/

National Center for Education Statistics (NCES). (2022a, May). English learners in public schools. *Condition of Education.* U.S. Department of Education, Institute of Education Sciences. https://nces.ed.gov/programs/coe/indicator/cgf

National Center for Education Statistics (NCES). (2022b, May). Racial/ethnic enrollment in public schools. *Condition of Education.* U.S. Department of Education, Institute of Education Sciences. https://nces.ed.gov/programs/coe/indicator/cge

National Center for Injury Prevention and Control. (2009). *What is traumatic brain injury?* www.cdc.gov/ncipc/tbi/TBI.htm.

National Clearinghouse for English Language Acquisition. (2018, April). *Fast facts: English learner (EL) populations by local educational agency.* https://ncela.ed.gov/files/fast_facts/LEAs_Fact_Sheet_2018_Final.pdf

National Dysphagia Diet Task Force. (2002). *National Dysphagia Diet: Standardization for optimal care.* American Dietetic Association.

National Institute of Deafness and Other Communication Disorders. (2017, September 13). *Specific language impairment.* https://www.nidcd.nih.gov/health/specific-language-impairment

National Institute on Deafness and Other Communication Disorders. (2021, March 25). *Quick statistics about deafness.* https://www.nidcd.nih.gov/health/statistics/quick-statistics-hearing

National Joint Committee for the Communication Needs of Persons with Severe Disabilities. (2022, June 16). *Myths About Adult Communicators With Severe Disabilities.* https://www.asha.org/njc/myths-about-adult-communicators-with-severe-disabilities/

National Reading Panel. (2000). *National Reading Panel progress report.* Author.

Neel, A. (2021). Promoting cultural and linguistic competence in speech science courses. *Perspectives of the ASHA Special Interest Groups, 6*(1), 207–213.

Neider, D. (2018, 07 19). The impact of early access to AAC. https://aac-learning-center.psu.edu/2018/07/19/the-impact-of-early-access-to-aac-dana-nieder/

Neils-Strunjas, J., Groves-Wright, K., Mashima, P., & Harnish, S. (2006). Dysgraphia in Alzheimer's disease: A review for clinical and research purposes. *Journal of Speech, Language, and Hearing Research, 49*, 1313–1330.

Nel, E., & Ellis, A. (2012). Swallowing abnormalities in HIV infected children: an important cause of morbidity. *BMC Pediatrics, 12*, 1–4.

Nelson Bryen, D. (2006). Job-related social networks and communication technology. *Augmentative and Alternative Communication, 22*, 1–9.

Nelson Bryen, D. (2008). Vocabulary to support socially-valued adult roles. *Augmentative and Alternative Communication, 24*, 294–301.

Nelson, N. W., & Van Meter, A. (2003, June). *Measuring written language abilities and change through the elementary years.* Poster session presented at the annual meeting of the Symposium for Research in Child Language Disorders, Madison, WI.

Nelson, N. W., & Van Meter, A. M. (2002). Assessing curriculum-based reading and writing samples. *Topics in Language Disorders, 22*(2), 35–59.

New York State Department of Health. (2002). *Clinical Practice Guideline* (Publication No. 4218). www.asha.org/members/ebp/compendium/

Newman, R., Vilardell, N., Clavé, P., & Speyer, R. (2016). Effect of bolus viscosity on the safety and efficacy of swallowing and the kinematics of the swallow response in patients with oropharyngeal dysphagia: White paper by the European Society for Swallowing Disorders (ESSD). *Dysphagia, 31,* 232–249.

Nguy, B., Quique, Y. M., Cavanaugh, R., & Evans, W. S. (2022). Representation in aphasia research: An examination of U.S. treatment studies published between 2009 and 2019. *American Journal of Speech-Language Pathology, 31,* 1424–1430.

Nicolson, R., Lenane, M., Singaracharlu, S., Malaspina, D., Giedd, J. N., Hamburger, S. D., et al. (2000). Premorbid speech and language impairments in childhood-onset schizophrenia: Association with risk factors. *American Journal of Psychiatry, 157,* 794–800.

Nigam, R., Schlosser, R. W., & Lloyd, L. L. (2006). Concomitant use of the matrix strategy and the mand-model procedure in teaching graphic symbol combinations. *Augmentative and Alternative Communication, 22,* 160–177.

Nilsen, E. S., Mangal, L., & MacDonald, K. (2013) Who receives speech/language services by 5 years of age in the United States? *Journal of Speech, Language, and Hearing Research, 56,* 590–603.

Nippold, M. (2014). Language intervention at the middle school: Complex talk reflects complex thought. *Language, Speech, and Hearing Services in Schools, 45,* 153–156.

Nippold, M. (2017). Reading comprehension deficits in adolescents: Addressing underlying language abilities. *Language, Speech, and Hearing Services in Schools, 48*(2), 125–131.

Nippold, M., & Packman, A. (2012). Managing stuttering beyond the preschool years. *Language, Speech, and Hearing Services in the Schools, 43,* 338–343.

Nippold, M., & Sun, L. (2008). Knowledge of morphologically complex words: A developmental study of older children and young adolescents. *Language, Speech, and Hearing Services in Schools, 39,* 365–373.

Nippold, M., Hesketh, L., Duthie, J., & Mansfield, T. (2005). Conversational vs. expository discourse: A study of syntactic development in children, adolescents, and adults. *Journal of Speech, Language, and Hearing Research, 48,* 1048–1064.

Nippold, M., Mansfield, T., & Billow, J. (2007). Peer conflict explanations in children, adolescents, and adults: Examining the development of complex syntax. *American Journal of Speech-Language Pathology, 16,* 179–186.

Nippold, M., Ward-Lonergan, J., & Fanning, J. (2005). Persuasive writing in children, adolescents, and adults: A study of syntactic, semantic, and pragmatic development. *Language, Speech, and Hearing Service in Schools, 36,* 125–138.

Nittrouer, S., Muir, M., Tietgens, K., Moberly, A., & Lowenstein, J. (2018). Development of phonological, lexical, and syntactic abilities in children with cochlear implants across elementary grades. *Journal of Speech, Language, and Hearing Research, 16*(10), 2561–2577.

Nóbrega, A., Rodrigues, B., Torres, A., Scarpel, R., Neves, C., & Melo, A. (2008). Is drooling secondary to a swallowing disorder in patients with Parkinson's disease? *Parkinsonism & Related Disorders, 14,* 243–245. https://doi.org/10.1016/j.parkreldis.2007.08.003

Nordberg, A., Miniscalco, C., Lohmander, A., & Himmelmann, K. (2013). Speech problems affect more than one in two children with cerebral palsy: Swedish population-based study. *Acta Paediatrica, 102,* 161–166.

Nuttall, E. V., Romero, I., & Kalesnik, J. (1992). *Assessing and Screening Preschoolers.* Allyn & Bacon.

Nye, C., Vanryckeghem, M., Schwartz, J., Herder C., Turner, H., & Howard, C. (2013). Behavioral stuttering interventions for children and adolescents: A systematic review and meta-analysis. *Journal of Speech, Language, and Hearing Research, 56,* 921–932.

O'Neal-Pirozzi, T. M. (2009). Feasibility and benefit of parent participation in a program emphasizing preschool child language development while homeless. *American Journal of Speech-Language Pathology, 12,* 229–242.

O'Neil-Pirozzi, T. M. (2003). Language functioning of residents in family homeless shelters. *American Journal of Speech-Language Pathology, 12,* 229–242.

Obermeyer, J., Reinert, L., Kamen, R., Pritchard, D., Park, H., & Martin, N. (2022). Effect of working memory load and typicality on semantic processing in aphasia. *American Journal of Speech-Language Pathology, 31,* 12–29.

Oetting, J. B. (2019). Variability within varieties of English profiles of typicality and impairment. In T. Ionin & M. Rispoli (Eds.), *Three streams of generative language acquisition research. Selected papers from the 7th meeting of Generative Approaches to Language Acquisition – North America, University of Illinois at Urbana–Champaign.* Benjamins. 59–82

Oetting, J. B., Berry, J. R., Gregory, K. D., Rivière, A. M., & McDonald, J. (2019). Specific language impairment in African American English and Southern White English: Measures of tense and agreement with dialect-informed probes and strategic scoring. *Journal of Speech, Language, and Hearing Research, 62,* 3443–3461.

Office of Technology Assessment. (1978). *Assessing the efficacy and safety of medical technologies* (OTA-H-75). U.S. Government Printing Office.

Olazarán, J., Reisberg, B., Clare, L., Cruz, I., Peña-Casanova, J., Del Ser, T., et al. (2010). Nonpharmacological therapies in Alzheimer's disease: A systematic review of efficacy. *Dementia and Geriatric Cognitive Disorders, 30,* 161–178.

Olivier, C., Hecker, L., Klucken, J., & Westby, C. (2000). Language: The embedded curriculum in postsecondary education. *Topics in Language Disorders, 21*(1) 15–29.

Oller, J., Kim, K., & Choe, Y. (2001). Can instructions to nonverbal tests be given in pantomime? Additional applications of a general theory of signs. *Semiotica, 133,* 15–44.

Olson, G. (2012). *Swallowing disorders vs. feeding disorders in children.* http://nspt4kids.com/parenting/swallowing-disorders-vs-feeding-disorders-in-children/

Olswang, L. B., Svensson, L., & Astley, S. (2010). Observation of classroom communication: Do children with Fetal Alcohol Syndrome Disorders spend their time differently than their typically developing peers? *Journal of Speech, Language, and Hearing Research, 53,* 1687–1703.

Ors, M., Ryding, E., Lindgren, M., Gustafsson, P., Blennow, G., & Rosén, I. (2005). SPECT findings in children with specific language impairment. *Cortex, 41,* 316–326.

Orton, S., & Travis, L. (1929). Studies in stuttering: IV. Studies of action currents in stutterers. *Archives of Neurology and Psychiatry, 21,* 61–68.

Owens, R. E. (2012). *Language development: An introduction* (8th ed.). Pearson Education.

Owens, R. E. (2014). *Language disorders: A functional approach to assessment and intervention* (5th ed.). Allyn & Bacon.

Owens, R. E. (2016). *Language development: An Introduction* (9th ed.). Pearson Education.

Owens, R. E. (2018). *Early communication intervention.* Pearson Education.

Owens, R. E. (2020). *Language development: An introduction* (10th ed.). Pearson Education.

Owens, R. E., & Kim, K. (2007, November). *Holistic reading and semantic investigation intervention with struggling readers.* Paper presented at the annual convention of the American Speech-Language-Hearing Association, Boston.

Owens, R. E., & Pavelko, S. L. (2021). *Sugar (Sampling Utterances and Grammatical Analysis Revised).* https://www.sugarlanguage.org

Özçalskan, S., & Goldin-Meadow, S. (2010). Sex differences in language first appear in gesture. *Developmental Science, 13*(5), 752–760.

Packman, A. (2012). Therapy and therapy in stuttering: A complex relationship. *Journal of Fluency Disorders, 37,* 225–233.

Packman, A., Onslow, M., Webber, M., Harrison, E., Arnott, S., Bridgman, K., et al. (2015). *The Lidcombe Program treatment guide.* http://sydney.edu.au/health-sciences/asrc/docs/lp_treatment_guide_2015.pdf

Paek, E. J., & Murray, L. L. (2021). Quantitative and qualitative analysis of verb fluency performance in individuals with probable Alzheimer's disease and healthy older adults. *American Journal of Speech-Language Pathology, 30,* 481–490.

Paek, E. J., & Yoon, S. I. (2021). Partner-specific communication deficits in individuals with Alzheimer's disease. *American Journal of Speech-Language Pathology, 30,* 376–390.

Palardy, G. J. (2008). Differential school effects among low, middle, and high social class composition schools: A multiple group, multilevel latent growth curve analysis. *School Effectiveness and School Improvement, 19*(1), 21–49

Palasik, S., & Hannan, J. (2013). The clinical applications of acceptance and commitment therapy with clients who stutter. *Perspectives on Fluency and Fluency Disorders, 23,* 54–69.

Palasik, S., Gabel, R., Hughes, C., & Rusnak, E. (2012). Perceptions of people who stutter about occupational experiences. *Perspectives on Fluency and Fluency Disorders, 22,* 22–33.

Palmer, C., Findlen, U., & Rauterkus, E. (2022, July/August). Advent of over-the-counter hearing aids: How to be prepared. *Audiology Today.* https://www.audiology.org/news-and-publications/audiology-today/articles/advent-of-over-the-counter-hearing-aids-how-to-be-prepared/

Papaliou, C. F., & Trevarthen, C. (2006). Prelinguistic pitch patterns expressing "communication" and "apprehension." *Journal of Child Language, 33,* 163–178.

Papsin, B. K., Gysin, C., Picton, N., Nedzelski, J., & Harrison, R. V. (2000). Speech perception outcome measures in prelingually deaf children up to four years after cochlear implantation. *Annals of Otology, Rhinology & Laryngology Supplement, 185,* 38–42.

Paradis, J. (2005). Grammatical morphology in children learning English as a second language: Implications of similarities with specific language impairment. *Language, Speech, and Hearing Services in Schools, 36,* 172–187.

Paradis, J., Schneider, P., & Sorenson Duncan, T. (2013). Discriminating children with language impairment among English-language learners from diverse first-language backgrounds. *Journal of Speech, Language, and Hearing Research, 56,* 971–981.

Paratore, J. R. (1995). Assessing literacy: Establishing common standards in portfolio assessment. *Topics in Language Disorders, 16*(1), 67–82.

Parham, D., Buder, E., Oller, D., & Boliek, C. (2011). Syllable -related breathing in infants in the second year of life. *Journal of Speech, Language, and Hearing Research, 54,* 1039–1050.

Park, S., & Sarkar, M. (2007). Parents attitudes toward heritage language maintenance for their children and their efforts to help their children maintain the heritage language: A case study of Korean Canadian immigrants. *Language, Culture and Curriculum, 20,* 223–235.

Pasricha, N., Dacakis, G., & Oates, J. M. (2008). Communicative satisfaction of male-to-female transsexuals. *Logopedics, Phoniatrics, Vocology, 33,* 25–34.

Pataraia, E., Simos, P. G., Castillo, E. M., Billingsley-Marshall, R. L., McGregor, A. L., Breier, J. I., et al. (2004). Reorganization of language-specific cortex in patients with lesions or mesial temporal epilepsy. *Neurology, 63,* 1825–1832.

Patel, R., Awan, S., Barkmeier-Kraemer, J., Courey, M., Deliyski, D., Eadie, T., et al. (2018). Recommended protocols for instrumental assessment of voice: American Speech-Language-Hearing Association expert panel to develop a protocol for instrumental assessment of vocal function. *American Journal of Speech-Language Pathology, 27,* 887–905.

Patterson, J. L. (2000). Observed and reported expressive vocabulary and word combinations in bilingual toddlers. *Journal of Speech, Language, and Hearing Research, 43,* 121–128.

Pauls, L. J., & Archibald, L. M. (2016). Executive functions in children with specific language impairment: A meta-analysis. *Journal of Speech, Language, and Hearing Research, 59,* 1074–1086.

Pavelko, S. (2010). Pre-literacy interventions for preschool students. *EBP Briefs, 5*(3), 1–9.

Pavelko, S. L., & Owens, R. E. (2017). Sampling Utterances and Grammatical Analysis Revised (SUGAR): New normative values for language sample analysis measures. *Language, Speech and Hearing Services in Schools, 48,* 197–215.

Pavelko, S. L., & Owens, R. E. (2019). Diagnostic accuracy of the SUGAR measures for identifying children with language impairment. *Language, Speech, and Hearing Services in Schools, 50*(2), 211–223.

Pavelko, S. L., Lieberman, R. J., Schwartz, J., & Hahs-Vaughn, D. (2018). The contributions of phonological awareness, alphabet knowledge, and letter writing to name writing in children with specific language impairment and typically developing children. *American Journal of Speech-Language Pathology, 27,* 166–180.

Pavelko, S. L., Owens, R. E., Ireland, M., & Hahs-Vaughn, D. L. (2016). Use of language sample analysis by school-based SLPS: Results of a nationwide survey. *Language, Speech and Hearing Services in Schools, 47,* 246–258.

Peña, E. D., Gillam, R. B., & Bedore, L. M. (2014). Dynamic assessment of narrative ability in English accurately identifies language impairment in English language learners. *Journal of Speech, Language, and Hearing Research, 57,* 2208–2220.

Peña, E. D., Gillam, R. B., Malek, M., Ruiz-Felter, R., Resendiz, M., Fiestas, C., & Sabel, T. (2006). Dynamic assessment of school-age children's narrative ability: An experimental investigation of classification accuracy. *Journal of Speech, Language, and Hearing Research, 49,* 1037–1057.

Peña, E., Gutierrez-Clellen, V., Iglesias, A., Goldstein, B., & Bedore, L (2018). *Bilingual English-Spanish Assessment (BESA).* Brookes.

Peña, E., Gutierrez-Clellen, V., Iglesias, A., Goldstein, B., & Bedore, L., (2018). *Bilingual Input-Output Survey (BIOS) (English and Spanish Edition).* Brookes.

Peña, E., Iglesias, A., & Lidz, C. S. (2001). Reducing test bias through dynamic assessment of children's word learning ability. *American Journal of Speech-Language Pathology, 10,* 138–154.

Peach, R. K. (2001). Further thoughts regarding management of acute aphasia following stroke. *American Journal of Speech-Language Pathology, 10,* 29–36.

Pedersen, P.M., Vinter, K., & Olsen, T.S. (2004). Aphasia after stroke: type, severity and prognosis. *Cerebrovascular Disorders, 17*(1), 35–43. https://doi.org/10.1159/000073896

Pei, Y., & O'Brien, K. H. (2021). Reading abilities post traumatic brain injury in adolescents and adults: A systematic review and meta-analysis. *American Journal of Speech-Language Pathology, 30,* 789–816.

Peijnenborgh, J. C., Hurks, P. M., Aldenkamp, A. P., Vles, J. S., & Hendriksen, J. G. (2016). Efficacy of working memory training in children and adolescents with learning disabilities: A review study and meta-analysis. *Neuropsychological Rehabilitation, 26*(5–6), 645–672.

Pell, M. (2006). Cerebral mechanisms for understanding emotional prosody in speech. *Brain and Language, 96,* 221–234.

Pena-Brooks, A., & Hedge, M. (2007). *Assessment and treatment of articulation and phonological disorders in children* (2nd ed.). PRO-ED.

Pence, K. L., Justice, L. M., & Wiggins, A. K. (2008). Preschool teachers' fidelity in implementing a comprehensive language-rich curriculum. *Language, Speech, and Hearing Services in Schools, 39,* 329–341.

Pennington, B. F., & Lefly, D. L. (2001). Early reading development in children at family risk for dyslexia. *Child Development, 72,* 816–833.

Perkins School for the Blind. (2022). *What is CVI?* https://www.perkins.org/what-is-cvi/

Perrault, A., Chaby, L. Bigouret, F., Oppetit, A., Cohen, D., Plaza, M., & Xavier, J. (2018). Comprehension of conventional gestures in typical children, children with autism spectrum disorders and children with language disorders. *Neuropsychiatrie de l'Enfance et de l'Adolescence, 67,* 1–9.

Perry, J., & Schenck, G. (2013). Instrumental assessment in cleft palate care. *Perspectives on Speech Science and Orofacial Disorders, 23,* 49–61.

Persky, H. R., Daane, M. C., & Jin, Y. (2003, July). *The Nation's Report Card: Writing 2002.* National Center for Education Statistics. https://nces.ed.gov/nationsreportcard/pdf/main2002/2003529.pdf

Pestana, P., Vaz-Freitas, S., & Manso, M. (2017). Prevalence of voice disorders in singers: Systematic review and meta-analysis. *Journal of Voice, 31,* 722–727.

Peterson, E., & Galgano, J. (2019). *Spread of effects of LSVT LOUD: More than increased loudness* [Webinar]. http://4ujv31qo92b4af8hc17c9xtr-wpengine.netdna-ssl.com/wp-content/uploads/2019/02/Webinar-Handout_LSVT-LOUD-Spread-of-Effects_2-20-19.pdf

Peterson, R., Pennington, B., Shriberg, L., & Boada, R. (2009). What influences literacy outcome in children with speech sound disorder? *Journal of Speech. Language. and Hearing Research, 52,* 1175–1188.

Peterson-Falzone, S. J., Trost-Cardamone, J., Karnell, M., & Hardin-Jones, M. (2006). *The clinician's guide to treating cleft palate speech.* Mosby.

Peterson-Falzone, S., Hardin-Jones, M., & Karnell, M. (2010). *Cleft palate speech* (4th ed.). Mosby.

Peterson-Falzone, S., Trost-Cardamone, J., Karnell, M., & Hardin-Jones, M. (2017). *The clinician's guide to treating cleft palate speech* (2nd ed.). Mosby.

Pettemeridou, E., & Constantinidou, F. (2021). The association between brain reserve, cognitive reserve, and neuropsychological and functional outcomes in males with chronic moderate-to-severe traumatic brain injury. *American Journal of Speech-Language Pathology, 30,* 883–893.

Pham, G., & Tipton, T. (2018). Internal and external factors that support children's minority first language and English. *Language, Speech, and Hearing Services in Schools, 49,* 595–606.

Pickering, J. (2015). Transgender voice and communication: Introduction and international context. *Perspectives on Voice and Voice Disorders, 25,* 25–31. https://doi.org/10.1044/vvd25.1.25

Picou, E. (2020). MarkeTrak 10 (MT10) survey results demonstrate high satisfaction with and benefits from hearing aids. *Seminars in Hearing, 41*(1), 21–36.

Pijnacker, J., Davids, N., van Weerdenburg, M., Verhoeven, L., Knoors, H., & van Alphen, P. (2017). Semantic processing of sentences in preschoolers with specific language impairment: Evidence from the N400 effect. *Journal of Speech, Language, and Hearing Research, 60,* 627–639.

Pindzola, R. (1993). Materials for use in vocal hygiene programs for children. *Language, Speech, and Hearing Services in the Schools, 24,* 174–176.

Plante, E., Ogilvie, T., Vance, R., Aguilar, J. M., Dailey, N. S., Meyers, C., et al. (2014). Variability in the language input to children enhances learning in a treatment context. *American Journal of Speech-Language Pathology, 23,* 530–545.

Plexico, L. W., Manning, W. H., & DiLollo, A. (2010). Client perceptions of effective and ineffective therapeutic alliances during treatment for stuttering. *Journal of Fluency Disorders, 35,* 333–354.

Pollock, K., & Berni, M. (2003). Incidence of non-rhotic vowel errors in children: Data from the Memphis Vowel Project. *Clinical Linguistics & Phonetics, 17,* 393–401.

Pontes, P., Brasolotto, A., & Behlau, M. (2005). Glottic characteristics and voice complaint in the elderly. *Journal of Voice, 19,* 84–94.

Porter, G., & Cafiero, J. (2009). Pragmatic Organization Dynamic Display (PODD) communication books: A promising practice for individuals with autism spectrum disorders. *Perspectives on Augmentative & Alternative Communication,* 121–129.

Postma, A., & Kolk, H. H. J. (1993). The covert repair hypothesis: Prearticulatory repair processes in normal and stuttered disfluencies. *Journal of Speech and Hearing Research, 36,* 472–487.

Potocki, A., & Laval, V. (2019). Comprehension and inference: Relationships between oral and written modalities in good and poor comprehenders during adolescence. *Journal of Speech, Language, and Hearing Research, 62,* 3431–3442.

Prelock, P. A. (2008). *Autism spectrum disorders.* Treatment Efficacy Summary. www.asha.org/NR/rdonlyres/4BAF3969-9ADC-4C01-B5ED-1334CC20DD3D/0/TreatmentEfficacySummaries2008.pdf

Prelock, P. A., Beatson, J., Bitner, B., Broder, C., & Ducker, A. (2003). Interdisciplinary assessment of young children with autism spectrum disorder. *Language, Speech, and Hearing Services in Schools, 34,* 194–202.

Pressley, M., & Hilden, K. R. (2004). Cognitive strategies: Production deficiencies and successful strategy instruction everywhere. In D. Kuhn & R. Siegler (Eds.), *Handbook of child psychology: Vol. 2. Cognition, perception, and language* (6th ed.). Wiley.

Price, J. R., & Jackson, S. C. (2015). Procedures for obtaining and analyzing writing samples of school-age children and adolescents. *Language, Speech, and Hearing Services in Schools, 46,* 277–293.

Price, J. R., Roberts, J. E., Hennon, E. A., Berni, M. C., Anderson, K. L., & Sideris, J. (2008). Syntactic complexity during conversation of boys with fragile X syndrome and Down syndrome. *Journal of Speech, Language, and Hearing Research, 51,* 3–15.

Pringent, H., Lejaille, M., Terzi, N., Annane, D., Figere, M., Orlikowski, D., & Lofas, F. (2012). Effect of a tracheostomy speaking valve on breathing-swallowing interaction, *Intensive Care Medicine, 38,* 85–90.

Prins, D., & Ingham, R. (2009). Evidence-based treatment and stuttering—Historical perspective. *Journal of Speech, Language, and Hearing Research, 52,* 254–263.

Prizant, B. M., Schuler, A. L., Wetherby, A. M., & Rydell, P. (1997). Enhancing language and communication: Language approaches. In D. Cohen & F. Volkmar (Eds.), *Handbook of autism and pervasive developmental disorders* (2nd ed., pp. 572–605). Wiley.

Pry, R., Petersen, A., & Baghdadli, A. (2005). The relationship between expressive language level and psychological development in children with autism 5 years of age. *International Journal of Research and Practice, 9,* 179–189.

Pugh, S., & Klecan-Aker, J. S. (2004, November). *Effects of phonological awareness training on students with learning disabilities.* Paper presented at the annual convention of the American Speech-Language-Hearing Association, Philadelphia.

Puig, V. (2010). Are early intervention services placing home languages and cultures "at risk?" *Early Childhood Research and Practice, 12.* https://ecrp.illinois.edu/v12n1/puig.html

Pulvermuller, F. B., Neininger, B., Elbert, T., Mohr, B., Rockstroh, B., Koebbel, P., et al. (2001). Constraint-induced therapy of chronic aphasia after stroke. *Stroke, 32,* 1621–1626.

Punch, J., Elfenbein, J., & James, R. (2011). Targeting hearing health messages for users of personal listening devices. *American Journal of Audiology, 20,* 69–82.

Puranik, C. S., Lombardino, L. J., & Altmann, L. J. (2007). Writing through retellings: An exploratory study of language impaired and dyslexic populations. *Reading and Writing: An Interdisciplinary Journal, 20,* 251–272.

Qi, C. H., Kaiser, A. P., Milan, S. E., Yzquierdo, Z., & Hancock, T. B. (2003). The performance of low-income African American children on the Preschool Language Scale-3. *Journal of Speech, Language, and Hearing Research, 46,* 576–590.

Quinn, A. (2012). A person-centered approach to multicultural counseling competence. *Journal of Humanistic Psychology, 53,* 202–251.

Quique, Y. M., Evans, W. S., & Walsh Dickey, M. (2019). Acquisition and generalization responses in aphasia naming treatment: A meta-analysis of semantic feature analysis outcomes. *American Journal of Speech-Language Pathology, 28,* 230–246.

Rackensperger, T. (2012). Family influences and academic success: The perceptions of individuals using AAC. *Augmentative and Alternative Communication, 28*(2), 106–116.

Rainforth, B., York, J., & MacDonald, C. (1992). *Collaborative teams for students with severe disabilities: Integrating therapy and educational services.* Brookes.

Raju, T., Higgins, R., Stark, A., & Leveno, K. (2006). Optimizing care and outcome for late-preterm (near-term) infants: A summary of the workshop sponsored by the National Institute of Child Health and Human Development. *Pediatrics, 118,* 1207–1214.

Ramig, L. (2002). The joy of research. *The ASHA Leader, 7*(8), 6–7, 19.

Ramig, L. O., & Verdolini, K. (2009, June 19). *Laryngeal-based voice disorders.* Treatment Efficacy Summary. www.asha.org/NR/rdonlyres/5B211B91-9D44-42D2-82C7-55A1315D8CD6/0/TESLaryngealBasedVoiceDisorders.pdf

Ramig, L., & Verdolini, K. (1998). Treatment efficacy: Voice disorders. *Journal of Speech-Language-Hearing Research, 41,* S101–S116.

Ramsey, A., & Lehman Blake, M. (2020). Speech-language pathology practices for adults with right hemisphere stroke: What are we missing? *American Journal of Speech-Language Pathology, 29,* 741–759.

Rassameehiran, S., Klomjit, S., Mankongpaisarnrung, C., & Rakvit, A. (2015). Postextubation dysphagia. *Baylor University Medical Center Proceedings, 28*(1), 18–20.

Rauterkus, E., & Palmer, C. (2014). The hearing aid effect. *Journal of the American Academy of Audiology, 25*(9), 893–903.

Raymer, A. M., Beeson, P., Holland, A., Kendall, D., Mahe, L. M., Martin, N., et al. (2008). Translational research in aphasia: From neuroscience to neurorehabilitation. *Journal of Speech, Language, and Hearing Research (Neuroplasticity Supplement), 51,* S259–S275.

Reardon-Reeves, N., & Yaruss, J. (2013). *School-age stuttering therapy: A practical guide.* Stuttering Therapy Resources.

Redmond, S. M. (2003). Children's production of the affix -ed in past tense and past participle contexts. *Journal of Speech, Language, and Hearing Research, 46,* 1095–1109.

Redmond, S. M., & Rice, M. L. (2001). Detection of irregular verb violations by children with and without SLI. *Journal of Speech, Language, and Hearing Research, 44,* 655–669.

Redmond, S. M. (2011). Peer victimization among students with specific language impairment, attention-deficit/hyperactivity disorder, and typical development. *Language, Speech, and Hearing Services in Schools, 42,* 520–535.

Reed, H. C., Hurks, P. P. M., Kirschner, P. A., & Jolles, J. (2015). Preschoolers' causal reasoning during shared picture book storytelling: A cross-case comparison descriptive study. *Journal of Research in Childhood Education, 29*(3), 367–389.

Reed, V. A. (2018). *An introduction to children with language disorders* (5th ed.). Pearson.

Regan, K., & Joshi, A. (2019). A tutorial of the current treatment modalities and voice management in laryngeal cancer, *Perspectives of the ASHA Special Interest Groups, 4,* 805–813.

Reichle, J., Beukelman, D., & Light, J. (2002). *Implementing an augmentative communication system: Exemplary strategies for beginning communicators*. Brookes.

Rescher, B., & Rappelsberger, P. (1996). EEG changes in amplitude and coherence during a tactile task in females and males. *Journal of Psychophysiology, 10*, 161–172.

Rescorla, L. (2005). Age 13 language and reading outcomes in late talking toddlers. *Journal of Speech, Language, and Hearing Research, 48*, 459–473.

Rescorla, L. A. (2009). Age 17 language and reading outcomes in late-talking toddlers: Support for dimensional perspective on language delay. *Journal of Speech, Language, and Hearing Research, 52*, 16–30.

Rescorla, L., & Alley, A. (2001). Validation of the Language Development Survey (LDS): A parent report tool for identifying language delay in toddlers. *Journal of Speech, Language, and Hearing Research, 44*(2), 434–445. https://doi.org/10.1044/1092-4388(2001/035)

Rescorla, L., & Turner, H. L. (2015). Morphology and syntax in late talkers at age 5. *Journal of Speech, Language, and Hearing Research, 58*, 434–444.

Resnik, J., & Polley, D. (2021). Cochlear neural degeneration disrupts hearing in background noise by increasing auditory cortex internal noise. *Neuron, 109*(6), 984–996.

Restrepo, M. A., Morgan, G. P., & Thompson, M. S. (2013). The efficacy of a vocabulary intervention for dual-language learners with language impairment. *Journal of Speech, Language, and Hearing Research, 56*, 748–765.

Reynolds, M., E., & Jefferson, L. (1999). Natural and synthetic speech comprehension: Comparison of children from two age groups. *Augmentative and Alternative Communication, 15*(3), 174–182.

Ribot, K. M., & Burridge, A. (2018). Language use contributes to expressive language growth: Evidence from bilingual children. *Child Development, 89*, 929–940.

Ribot, K. M., Hoff, E. & Burridge, A. (2017). Language use contributes to expressive language growth: Evidence from bilingual children. *Child Development, 89*(3), 929-940. https://doi.org/10.1111/cdev.12770

Rice, M. L. (2012). Toward epigenetic and gene regulation models of specific language impairment: Looking for links among growth, genes, and impairments. *Journal of Neurodevelopmental Disorders, 4*, 27.

Rice, M. L., & Hoffman, L. (2015). Predicting vocabulary growth in children with and without specific language impairment: A longitudinal study from 26 to 21 years of age. *Journal of Speech, Language, and Hearing Research, 58*, 345–359.

Rice, M. L., Cleave, P. L., & Oetting, J. B. (2000). The use of syntactic cues in lexical acquisition by children with SLI. *Journal of Speech, Language, and Hearing Research, 34*, 582–594.

Rice, M. L., Hoffman, L., & Wexler, K. (2009). Judgments of omitted BE and DO in questions as extended finiteness clinical markers of Specific Language Impairment (SLI) to 15 years: A study of growth and asymptote. *Journal of Speech, Language, and Hearing Research, 52*, 1417–1433.

Rice, M. L., Redmont, S. M., & Hoffman, L. (2006). Mean length of utterance in children with specific language impairment and in younger control children shows concurrent validity and stable and parallel growth trajectories. *Journal of Speech, Language, and Hearing Research, 49*, 793–808.

Rice, M. L., Tomblin, J. B., Hoffman, L., Richman, W. A., & Marquis, J. (2004). Grammatical tense deficits in children with SLI and nonspecific language impairment: Relationships with nonverbal IQ over time. *Journal of Speech, Language, and Hearing Research, 47*, 816–834.

Rice, M. L. (2012). Toward epigenetic and gene regulation models of specific language impairment: Looking for links among growth, genes, and impairments. *Journal of Neurodevelopmental Disorders, 4*, 27. https://doi.org/10.1186/1866-1955-4-27

Richels, C., & Conture, E. (2010). Indirect treatment of childhood stuttering: Diagnostic predictors of treatment outcome. In B. Guitar, & R. McCauley (Eds.), *Treatment of stuttering: Established and emerging interventions* (pp. 18–55). Lippincott Williams & Wilkins.

Ricketts, J., Davies, R., Masterson, J., Stuart, M., & Duff, F. J. (2016). Evidence for semantic involvement in regular and exception word reading in emergent readers of English. *Journal of Experimental Child Psychology, 150*, 330–345.

Ricketts, J., Nation, K., & Bishop, D. V. M. (2007). Vocabulary is important for some, but not all reading skills. *Scientific Studies of Reading, 11*, 235–257.

Rieber, R. W., & Wollock, J. (1977). The historical roots of the theory and therapy of stuttering. *Journal of Communication Disorders, 10*, 3–24.

Riley, E. A., & Owora, A. (2020). Relationship between physiologically measured attention and behavioral task engagement in persons with chronic aphasia. *Journal of Speech, Language, and Hearing Research, 63*, 1430–1445.

Riley, G. (2009). *Stuttering Severity Instrument for Children and Adults—Fourth Edition (SSI-4)*. PRO-ED.

Riley, J. (2002). *Client-centered therapy: Its current practice, implications, and theory*. Constable.

Riquelme, L. (2004). Cultural competence in dysphagia. *The ASHA Leader, 9*. 8–22

Rispoli, M. (2005). When children reach beyond their grasp: Why some children make pronoun case errors and others don't. *Journal of Child Language, 32*, 93–116.

Ritchie, K., & Lovenstone, S. (2002). The dementias. *The Lancet, 360*, 1759–1766.

Rivera G., & Morell F. (2021). *Laryngeal papillomas.* StatPearls. https://www.ncbi.nlm.nih.gov/books/NBK562327/

Roark, B., Fried-Oken, M., & Gibbons, C. (2015). Huffman and linear scanning methods with statistical language models. *Augmentative and Alternative Communication, 31*(1), 37–50.

Roberts J., Price J., & Malkin, C. (2007). Language and communication development in Down Syndrome. *Mental Retardation and Developmental Disabilities Research Reviews 13*, 26–35.

Roberts, J. E., Long, S. H., Malkin, C., Barnes, E., Skinner, M., Hennon, E. A., et al. (2005). A comparison of phonological skills with fragile X syndrome and Down syndrome. *Journal of Speech, Language, and Hearing Research, 48*, 980–995.

Roberts, J., Mirrett, P., & Burchinal, M. (2001). Receptive and expressive communication development in young males with fragile X syndrome. *American Journal of Mental Retardation, 106*, 216–231.

Roberts, J., Rosenfield, R., & Zeisel, S. (2004). Otitis media and speech and language: A meta-analysis of prospective studies. *Pediatrics, 113*, e238–e248.

Roberts, M. Y., & Kaiser, A. P. (2011). The effectiveness of parent-implemented language interventions: A meta-analysis. *American Journal of Speech-Language Pathology, 20*, 180–199.

Roberts, M. Y., Kaiser, A. P., Wolfe, C. E., Bryant, J. D., & Spidalieri, A. M. (2014). Effects of the teach-model-coach-review instructional approach on caregiver use of language support strategies and children's expressive language skills. *Journal of Speech, Language, and Hearing Research, 57*, 1851–1869.

Robey, R. R., & Schultz, M. C. (1998). A model for conducting clinical-outcome research: An adaptation of the standard protocol for use in aphasiology. *Aphasiology, 12*(9), 787–810.

Robin, N., & Shprintzen, R. (2005). Defining the clinical spectrum of deletion 22q11.2. *Journal of Pediatrics, 147*, 90–96.

Roche Chapman, L., & Hallowell, B. (2021). The unfolding of cognitive effort during sentence processing: Pupillometric evidence from people with and without aphasia. *Journal of Speech, Language, and Hearing Research, 64*, 4900–4917.

Roden, D. F., & Altman, K. W. (2013). Causes of dysphagia among different age groups: A systematic review of the literature. *Otolaryngologic Clinics of North America, 46*(6), 965–987.

Rodermerk, K., & Galster, J. (2015). The benefits of remote microphones using four wireless protocols. *Journal of the American Academy of Audiology, 26*(8), 724–731.

Rogus-Pulia, N., & Robbins, J. (2013). Approaches to rehabilitation of dysphagia in acute poststroke patients. *Seminars in Speech and Language, 34*, 154–169.

Roitsch, J., Prebor, J., & Raymer, A. M. (2021). Cognitive assessments for patients with neurological conditions: A preliminary survey of speech-language pathology practice patterns. *American Journal of Speech-Language Pathology, 30*, 2263–2274.

Roland, C. (2012). *Communication Matrix: Description, Research Basis and Data.* https://www.communicationmatrix.org/

Romeo, R. R., Leonard, J. A., Robinson, S. T., West, M. R., Mackey, A. P., Rowe, M. L., & Gabrielli, J. D. (2018). Beyond the 30-million-word gap: Children's conversational exposure is associated with language-related brain function. *Psychological Science, 29*, 700–710.

Rommel, N., Davidson, G., Cain, T., Hebbard, G., & Omari, T. (2008). Videomanometric evaluation of pharyngooesophageal dysmotility in children with velocardiofacial syndrome. *Journal of Pediatric Gastroenterology and Nutrition, 46*, 87–91.

Romski, M. A., & Sevcik, R. A. (1996). *Breaking through the speech barrier: Language development through augmented means.* Baltimore: Paul H. Brookes.

Romski, M., & Sevcik, R. A. (1988). Augmentative and alternative communication systems: Considerations for individuals with severe intellectual disabilities. *Augmentative and Alternative Communication, 4*(2), 83–93.

Romski, M., & Sevcik, R. A. (2005). Augmentative communication and early intervention myths and realities. *Infants and Young Children, 18*(3), 174–185.

Romski, M., Sevcik, R., Barton-Hulsey, A., & Whitmore, A. S. (2015). Early intervention and AAC: What a difference 30 years makes. *Augmentative and Alternative Communication, 31*(3), 181–202.

Rosa-Lugo, L. I., Mihai, F. M., & Nutta, J. W. (2012). *Language and literacy development: An interdisciplinary focus on English learners with communication disorders.* Plural Publishing.

Rosenbaum, P., Paneth, N., Leviton, A., Goldstein, M., Bax, M., Damiano, D., et al. (2007). A report: The definition and classification of cerebral palsy April 2006. *Developmental Medicine & Child Neurology, 49*, 8–14.

Rosenbek, J. C., Lemme, M., Ahern, M., Harris, E., & Wertz, R. (1973). A treatment for apraxia of speech in adults. *Journal of Speech and Hearing Disorders, 43*, 462–472.

Rosenbek, J., & Jones, H. (2009). *Dysphagia in movement disorders.* Plural Publishing, Inc.

Ross, K. B., & Wertz, R. T. (2003). Discriminative validity of selected measures of differentiating normal from aphasic performance. *American Journal of Speech-Language Pathology, 12*, 312–319.

Roth, F. P. (2000). Narrative writing: Development and teaching with children with writing difficulties. *Topics in Language Disorders, 20*(4), 15–28.

Roth, F. P. (2004). Word recognition assessment framework. In C. A. Stone, E. R. Silliman, B. J. Ehren, & K. Apel (Eds.), *Handbook of language and literacy: Development and disorders* (pp. 461–480). Guilford Press.

Roth, F. P. (2011). *Treatment resource manual for speech-language pathology* (4th ed.). Delmar Learning.

Rowe, M. L., Leech, K. A., & Cabrera, N. (2017). Going beyond input quantity: *Wh*-questions matter for toddlers' language and cognitive development. *Cognitive Science, 41*, 162–179. https://doi.org/10.1111/cogs.12349

Rowland, C., & Schweigert, P. (2009). Tangible symbols, tangible outcomes. *Augmentative and Alternative Communication, 16*(2), 61–78. https://doi.org/10.1080/07434610012331278914

Rowland, C., Fried-Oken, M., & Steiner, S. A. (2009). *Communication Supports Inventory-Children and Youth (CSI-CY)*. Design to Learn Projects, Oregon Health & Science University.

Roy, N. (2004). Functional voice disorders. In R. D. Kent (Ed.), *MIT encyclopedia of communication disorders* (pp. 27–30). MIT Press.

Roy, N. (2008). Assessment and treatment of musculoskeletal tension in hyperfunctional voice disorders. *International Journal of Speech-Language Pathology, 10*, 195–209.

Roy, N., Gray, S., Simon, M., Dove, M., Dove, H., Corbin-Lewis, K., et al. (2001). An evaluation of the effects of two treatment approaches for teachers with voice disorders: A prospective randomized clinical trial. *Journal of Speech, Language, and Hearing Research, 44*, 286–296.

Roy, N., Merrill, R. M., Thibeault, S., Parsa, R. A., Gray, S. D., & Smith, E. M. (2004). Prevalence of voice disorders in teachers and the general population. *Journal of Speech, Language, and Hearing Research, 47*, 281–293.

Roy, N., Merrill, R., Gray, S., & Smith, E. (2005). Voice disorders in the general population: Prevalence, risk factors, and occupational impact. *The Laryngoscope, 115*, 1988–1995.

Roy, N., Stemple, J., Merrill, R., & Thomas, L. (2007). Dysphagia in the elderly: Preliminary evidence of prevalence, risk factors, and socioemotional effects. *Annals of Otology, Rhinology, & Laryngology, 116*, 858–865.

Rubin, K. H., Burgess, K. B., & Coplan, R. J. (2002). Social withdrawal and shyness. In P. K. Smith & C. H. Hart (Eds.), *Blackwell handbook of childhood social development* (pp. 329–352). Blackwell.

Rudolph, C. D., & Link, D. T. (2002). Feeding disorders in infants and children. *Pediatric Clinics of North America: Pediatric Gastroenterology and Nutrition, 49*(1), 97–112.

Rudolph, J. M. (2017). Case history risk factors for specific language impairment: A systematic review and meta-analysis. *American Journal of Speech-Language Pathology, 26*, 991–1010.

Rule, D., Kelchner, L., Mulkern, A., Couch, S., Silbert, N., & Weldena, K. (2020). Implementation strategies for the International Dysphagia Diet Standardisation Initiative (IDDSI), Part I: Quantitative analysis of IDDSI performance among varied participants. *American Journal of Speech-Langauge Pathology, 29*, 1514–1528.

Rumalla K., Karim A. & Hullar T. (2015). The effect of hearing aids on postural stability. *Laryngoscope. 125*(3):720–723. http://onlinelibrary.wiley.com/doi/10.1002/lary.24974/abstract

Russell, M., & Abrams, M. (2019). Transgender and nonbinary adolescents: The role of voice and communication therapy. *Perspectives of the ASHA Special Interest Groups, 4*, 1298–1305.

Russo, M. J., Prodan, V., Meda, N. N. Carcavallo, L., Muracioli, A., Sabe, L., et al. (2017) High-technology augmentative communication for adults with post-stroke aphasia: A systematic review. *Expert Review of Medical Devices, 14*(5), 335–370.

Rvachew, S. (2006). Longitudinal predictors of implicit phonological awareness skills. *American Journal of Speech-Language Pathology, 15*, 165–176.

Rvachew, S. R., & Grawburg, M. (2006). Correlates of phonological awareness in preschoolers with speech sound disorders. *Journal of Speech, Language, and Hearing Research, 49*, 74–87.

Rvachew, S., Gaines, B. R., Cloutier, G., & Blanchet, N. (2005). Productive morphology skills of children with speech delay. *Canadian Journal of Speech-Language Pathology and Audiology, 29*, 83–89.

Ryan, B. P. (1974). *Programmed therapy for stuttering children and adults*. Charles C. Thomas.

Ryan, B. P., & Van Kirk Ryan, B. (1995). Programmed stuttering treatment for children: Comparisons of two established programs through transfer, maintenance, and follow-up. *Journal of Speech and Hearing Research, 38*, 61–75.

Saint-Exupéry, A. de (1968). *The little prince*. Harcourt Brace.

Saito, K., & Morisaki, H. (2013). Percutaneous dilatational tracheostomy: Collaborative team approach for safe airway management. *Journal of Anesthesia, 27,* 161–165.

Salis, C., & DeDe, G. (2022). Sentence production in a discourse context in latent aphasia: A real-time study. *American Journal of Speech-Language Pathology, 31,* 1284–1296.

Sandberg, C. W., Nadermann, K., Parker, L., Kubat, A. M., & Conyers, L. M. (2021). Counseling in aphasia: Information and strategies for speech-language pathologists. *American Journal of Speech-Language Pathology, 30,* 2337–2349.

Sandberg, C., Gray, T., & Kiran, S. (2020). Development of a free online interactive naming therapy for bilingual aphasia. *American Journal of Speech-Language Pathology, 29,* 20–29.

Sander, E. (1972). When are speech sounds learned? *Journal of Speech and Hearing Disorders, 37,* 55–63.

Sanders, E. J., Page, T. A., & Lesher, D. (2021). School-based speech-language pathologists: Confidence in augmentative and alternative communication assessment. *Language, Speech, and Hearing Services in Schools, 52*(2), 512–528. https://doi.org/10.1044/2020_LSHSS-20-00067

Sanders, I., Rai, S., Han, Y., & Biller, H. (1998). Human vocalis contains distinct superior and inferior subcompartments: Possible candidates for the two masses of vocal fold vibration. *Annals of Otology, Rhinology, and Laryngology, 197,* 826–833.

Sanders, L. D., & Neville, H. J. (2000). Lexical, syntactic, and stress-pattern cues for speech segmentation. *Journal of Speech, Language, and Hearing Research, 43,* 1301–1321.

Santo Pietro, M. J., Marks, D. R., & Mullen, A. (2019). When words fail: Providing effective psychological treatment for depression in persons with aphasia. *Journal of Clinical Psychology in Medical Settings, 26*(4), 483–494.

Sasaki, C., Levine, P., Laitman, J., & Crelin, E. (1977). Postnatal descent of the epiglottis in man. *Archives of Otolaryngology, 103,* 169–171.

Sauder, C., Roy, N., Tanner, K., Houtz, D., & Smith, M. (2010). Vocal function exercises for presbylaryngitis: A multidimensional assessment of treatment outcomes. *Annals of Otology, Rhinology & Laryngology, 119,* 460–467.

Sawyer, D. J. (2006). Dyslexia: A generation of inquiry. *Topics in Language Disorders, 26,* 95–109.

Sawyer, J., Matteson, C., Ou, H., & Nagase, T. (2017). The effects of parent-focused slow relaxed speech intervention on articulation rate, response time latency, and fluency in preschool children who stutter. *Journal of Speech, Language, and Hearing Research, 60,* 794–809.

Saxena, R., Lehmann, A., Hight, A., Darrow, K., Remenschneider, A., Kozin, E., & Lee, D. (2015). Social media utilization in the cochlear implant community. *Journal of the American Academy of Audiology, 26*(2), 197–204.

Saxton, J., Morrow, L., Eschman, A., Archer, G., Luther, J., & Zuccolotto, A. (2009). Computer assessment of mild cognitive impairment. *Postgrad Medicine, 121*(2), 177–185.

Scarborough, H. S. (1990). Index of productive syntax. *Applied Psycholinguistics, 11,* 1–22.

Scarpino, S., & Goldstein, B. (2012). Analysis of the speech of multilingual children with speech sound disorders. In S. McLeod & B. A. Goldstein (Eds.), *Multilingual aspects of speech sound disorders in children* (pp. 196–206). Multilingual Matters.

Schölderle, T., Staiger, A., Lampe, R., Strecker, K., & Ziegler, W. (2016). Dysarthria in adults with cerebral palsy: Clinical presentation and impacts on communication. *Journal of Speech, Language, and Hearing Research, 59,* 216–229.

Schaser, A. (2016). Emerging scientist: Examining exercise-based therapies for voice and swallow disorders with a neuroplastic eye. *Perspectives of the Special Interest Groups (SIG 13), 1,* 33–38.

Schaser, A., Ciucci, M., & Conner, N. (2016). Cross-activation and detraining effects of tongue exercise in aged rats. *Behavioral Brain Research, 297,* 285–296.

Scheffner Hammer, C., Morgan, P., Farkas, G., Hillemeier, M., Bitetti, D., & Maczuga, S. (2017). Late talkers: A population-based study of risk factors and school readiness consequences. *Journal of Speech, Language, and Hearing Research, 60,* 607–626.

Schlosser, R. W. (2003). Outcomes measurement in AAC. In J. C. Light, D. R. Beukelman, & J. Reichle (Eds.), *Communicative competence for individuals who use AAC: From research to effective practice* (pp. 479–508). Brookes.

Schlosser, R. W., & Koul, R. K. (2015). Speech output technologies in interventions for individuals with autism spectrum disorders: A scoping review. *Augmentative and Alternative Communication, 31*(4), 285–309.

Schlosser, R. W., & Raghavendra, P. (2004). Evidence-based practice in augmentative and alternative communication. *Augmentative and Alternative Communication, 20*(1), 1–21.

Schlosser, R. W., & Wendt, O. (2008). Effects of augmentative and alternative communication intervention on speech production in children with autism: A systematic review. *American Journal of Speech-Language Pathology, 17*(3), 212–230. https://doi.org/10.1044/1058-0360(2008/021)

Schlosser, R. W., Laubscher, E., Sorce, J., Koul, R., Flynn, S., Hotz, L., et al. (2013). Implementing directives that involve prepositions with children with autism: A comparison of spoken cues with two types of augmented input. *Augmentative and Alternative Communication*, 29(2), 132–145.

Schlosser, R. W., Walker, E., & Sigafoos, J. (2006). Increasing opportunities for requesting in children with developmental disabilities residing in group homes through pyramidal training. *Education and Training in Developmental Disabilities*, 41(3), 244–252.

Schmitt, M. B. (2020). Children's active engagement in public school language therapy relates to greater gains. *American Journal of Speech-Language Pathology*, 29, 1505–1513.

Schneider, F., Marcotte, K., Brisebois, A., Martins Townsend, S. A., Dick Smidarle, A., Loureiro, F., et al. (2021). Neuroanatomical correlates of macrolinguistic aspects in narrative discourse in unilateral left and right hemisphere stroke: A voxel-based morphometry study. *Journal of Speech, Language, and Hearing Research*, 64, 1650–1665.

Schneider, S. (2019). Update: Behavioral management of unilateral vocal fold paralysis and paresis. *Perspectives of the ASHA Special Interest Groups (SIG 3)*, 4, 474–482.

Schow, R. L., & Nerbonne, M. A. (2007). *Introduction to audiologic rehabilitation*. Pearson.

Schuele, C. M. (2001). Socioeconomic influences on children's language acquisition. *Journal of Speech-Pathology and Audiology*, 25(2), 77–88.

Schuele, C. M., & Boudreau, D. (2008). Phonological awareness intervention: Beyond the basics. *Language, Speech, and Hearing Services in Schools*, 39, 3–20.

Schwartz, J. B., & Nye, C. (2006). Improving communication for children with autism: Does sign language work? *EBP Briefs*, 1(2).

Schwichtenberg, A. J., Kellerman, A. M., Young, G. S., Miller, M., & Ozonoff, S. (2019). Mothers of children with autism spectrum disorders: Play behaviors with infant siblings and social responsiveness. *Autism*, 23, 821–833.

Scott, C. M. (2000). Principles and methods of spelling instruction: Applications for poor spellers. *Topics in Language Disorder*, 20(3), 66–82.

Scott, C. M. (2014). One size does not fit all: Improving clinical practice in older children and adolescents with language and learning disorders. *Language, Speech, and Hearing Services in Schools*, 45, 145–152.

Scott, C. M., & Windsor, J. (2000). General language performance measures in spoken and written narrative and expository discourse of school-age children with language learning disabilities. *Journal of Speech, Language, and Hearing Research*, 43, 324–339.

Sebat, J., Lakshmi, B., Malhotra, D., Troge, J., Lese-Martin, C., Walsh, T., et al. (2007, April 20). Strong association of de novo copy number mutations with autism. *Science*, 20, 445–449.

Secord, W., & Donohue, J. (2014). *Clinical Assessment of Articulation and Phonology—Second Edition (CAAP-2)*. Pro-Ed.

Segebart DeThorne, L., & Watkins, R. V. (2001). Listeners' perceptions of language use in children. *Language, Speech, and Hearing Services in Schools*, 32, 142–148.

Segebart DeThorne, L., Hart, S. A., Petrill, S. A., Deater-Deckard, K., Thompson, L. A., Schatschneider, C., et al. (2006). Children's history of speech-language difficulties: Genetic influences and association with reading-related measures. *Journal of Speech, Language, and Hearing Research*, 49, 1280–1293.

Segebart DeThorne, L., Petrill, S. A., Schatschneider, C., & Cutting, L. (2010). Conversational language use as a predictor of early reading development: Language history as a moderating variable. *Journal of Speech, Language, and Hearing Research*, 53, 209–223.

Seikel, J., King, D., & Drumright, D. (2010). *Anatomy and physiology for speech, language, and hearing* (4th ed.). Delmar, Cengage Learning.

Sellars, C., Bowie, L., Bagg, J., Sweeney, M. P., Miller, H., Tilston, J., et al. (2007). Risk factors for chest infection in acute stroke: A prospective cohort study. *Stroke*, 38, 2284–2291.

Sencibaugh, J. M. (2007). Meta-analysis of reading comprehension interventions for students with learning disabilities: Strategies and implications. *Reading Improvement*, 44(1), 6–22.

Sennott, S. (2011). An introduction to the Special Issue on New Mobile Technologies. *Perspectives on Augmentative and Alternative Communication*, 20(1), 3–6. https://doi.org/10.1044/aac20.1.3

Sennott, S. C., Ferrari, R., McLernon, G., Lesher, D. (2016). The three definitions of application for AAC intervention. *Perspectives on Augmentative and Alternative Communication*, 1(12), 99–107. https://doi.org/10.1044/persp1.SIG12.99

Serra-Prat, M., Hinojosa, G., López, D., Juan, M., Fabré, E., Voss, D. S., et al. (2011). Prevalence of oropharyngeal dysphagia and impaired safety and efficacy of swallow in independently living older persons. *Journal of American Geriatrics Society*, 59(1), 186–187.

Seung, H., & Chapman, R. (2000). Digit span in individuals with Down syndrome and in typically developing children: Temporal aspects. *Journal of Speech, Language, and Hearing Research*, 43, 609–620.

Sevcik, R. A., Barton-Hulsey, A., Romski, M., & Hyatt Fonseca, A. (2018). Visual-graphic symbol aquistiion in school age children with developmental and language delays. *Augmentative and Alternative Communication, 34*(4), 265–275. https://doi.org/10.1080/07434618.2018.1522547

Seymour, H. N., Roeper, T. W., & de Villiers, J. (2018). *Diagnostic Evaluation of Language Variance – Norm Referenced* (DELV-NR). Ventris Learning.

Shadden, B. B., & Toner, M. A. (Eds.). (1997). *Aging and communication: For clinicians by clinicians.* PRO-ED.

Shaker, R., Easterling, C., Kern, M., Nitschke, T., Massey, B., Daniels, S., et al. (2002). Rehabilitation of swallowing by exercise in tube-fed patients with pharyngeal dysphagia secondary to abnormal UES opening. *Gastroenterology, 122*, 1314–1321.

Shapiro, L., Hurry, J., Masterson, J., Wydell, T., & Doctor, E. (2009). Classroom implications of recent research into literacy development: From predictors to assessment. *Dyslexia, 15*, 1–2.

Sharma, G., & Goodwin, J. (2006). Effect of aging on respiratory system physiology and immunology. *Clinical Interventions in Aging, 1*(3), 253–260.

Sharma, S., Cusing, S., Papsin, B., & Gordon, K. (2020). Hearing and speech benefit of cochlear implantation in children: A review of the literature. *International Journal of Pediatric Otorhinolaryngology, 133*,

Shaw, G. (2012). Sign of the times: ASL comes to mobile phones. *The Hearing Journal, 65*(10), 22–26.

Sheffield, S., Jahn, K., & Gifford, R. (2015). Preserved acoustic hearing cochlear implantation improves speech perception. *Journal of the American Academy of Audiology, 26*(2), 145–154.

Shekim, L. (1990). Dementia. In L. L. LaPointe (Ed.), *Aphasia and related neurogenic language disorders* (pp. 210–220). Thieme.

Sheng, L., & McGregor, K. A. (2010). Object and action naming in children with specific Language Impairment. *Journal of Speech, Language, and Hearing Research, 53*, 1704–1719.

Shipley, K., & McAfee, J. (2016). *Assessment in speech-language pathology: A resource manual* (5th ed). Cengage Learning.

Shire, S. Y., & Jones, N. (2015). Communication partners supporting children with complex communication needs: A systematic review. *Communication Disorders Quarterly, 37*(1), 3–15.

Shprintzen, R. J. (1995). A new perspective on clefting. In R. J. Shprintzen & J. Bardach (Eds.), *Cleft palate speech management: A multidisciplinary approach.* Mosby.

Shriberg, L. (1993). Four new speech and prosody-voice measures for genetics research and other studies in developmental phonological disorders. *Journal of Speech and Hearing Research, 36*, 105–140.

Shriberg, L. D., & Kent, R. D. (1995). *Clinical phonetics* (2nd ed.). Allyn & Bacon.

Shriberg, L. D., & Kwiatkowski, J. (1994). Developmental phonological disorders. I: A clinical profile. *Journal of Speech and Hearing Research, 37*, 1100–1126.

Shriberg, L. D., Austin, D., Lewis, B. A., McSweeney, J. L., & Wilson, D. L. (1997). The percentage of consonants correct (PCC) metric: Extensions and reliability data. *Journal of Speech, Language, and Hearing Research, 40*(4), 708–722.

Shriberg, L., & Kwiatkowski, J. (1982). Phonological disorders III: A procedure for assessing severity of involvement. *Journal of Speech and Hearing Disorders, 47*, 256–270.

Shriberg, L., & Widder, C. (1990). Speech and prosody characteristics of adults with mental retardation. *Journal of Speech and Hearing Research, 33*, 627–653.

Shriberg, L., Fourakis, M., Hall, S., Karlsson, H., Lohmeier, H., McSweeny, J., et al. (2010). Extensions to the speech disorders classification system (SDCS). *Clinical Linguistics and Phonetics, 24*, 795–824.

Shriberg, L., Potter, N., & Strand, E. (2011). Prevalence and phenotype of childhood apraxia of speech in youth with galactosemia. *Journal of Speech, Language, and Hearing Research, 54*, 487–519.

Shriberg, L., Tomblin, J., & McSweeny, J. (1999). Prevalence of speech delay in 6-year old children and comorbidity with language impairment. *Journal of Speech, Language, and Hearing Research, 42*, 1461–1481.

Shuster, L. I. (2009). The effect of sublexical and lexical frequency on speech production: An fMRI investigation. *Brain and Language, 111*(1), 66–72. https://doi.org/10.1016/j.bandl.2009.06.003

Shuster, L. I., & Lemieux, S. K. (2005). An fMRI investigation of covertly and overtly produced mono- and multisyllabic words. *Brain and Language, 93*, 20–31.

Sigafoos, J. (2000). Creating opportunities for augmentative and alternative communication: Strategies for involving people with developmental disabilities. *Augmentative and Alternative Communication, 16*, 183–190.

Sigafoos, J., O'Reilly, M., Seely-York, S., & Edrisinha, C. (2004). Teaching students with developmental disabilities to locate their AAC device. *Research in Developmental Disabilities, 25*(4), 371–383.

Silliman, E. R., & Wilkinson, L. C. (2004). Collaboration for language and literacy learning. In E. R. Silliman & L. C. Wilkinson (Eds.), *Language and literacy learning in schools* (pp. 3–38). Guilford Press.

Silver, C., Beitler, J., Shaha, A., Rinaldo, A., & Ferlito, A. (2009). Current trends in initial management of laryngeal cancer: The declining use of open surgery.

European Archives of Oto-Rhino-Laryngology, 266, 1333–1352.

Silverman, R., & Doyle, B. (2013). Vocabulary and comprehension instruction for ELLs in the era of Common Core State Standards. In S. B. Neuman & L. B. Gambrell (Eds.), *Quality reading instruction in the age of common core standards* (pp. 121–135). Newark, DE: International Reading Association.

Simmons-Mackie, N. (2018). *Aphasia in North America.* Aphasia Access.

Simon-Cereijido, G., & Méndez, L.I. (2018). Using language-specific and bilingual measures to explore lexical–grammatical links in young Latino dual-language learners. *Language, Speech, and Hearing Services in Schools, 49,* 537–550.

Singer, B., & Bashir, A. (2004). EmPOWER, A strategy of teaching students with language learning disabilities how to write expository text. In E. R. Silliman & L. C. Wilkinson (Eds.), *Language and literacy learning in schools* (pp. 239–272). Guilford Press.

Singer, C., Hessling, A., Kelly, E., Singer, L., & Jones, R. (2020). Clinical characteristics associated with stuttering persistence: A meta-analysis. *Journal of Speech, Language, and Hearing Research, 63,* 2995–3018.

Singleton, N. C., & Shulman, B. B. (2014). Language development: Foundations, processes, and clinical applications (2nd ed.). Jones & Bartlett Learning.

Sitren, A., & Vallila-Rohter, S. (2019). How well do we use our technology?: Examining iPad navigation skills in individuals with aphasia and older adults. *American Journal of Speech-Language Pathology, 28,* 1523–1536.

Sitzer, D. I., Twamley, E. W., & Jeste, D. V. (2006). Cognitive training in Alzheimer's disease: A meta-analysis of the literature. *Acta Psychiatrica Scandinavica, 114*(2), 75–90.

Skarakis-Doyle, E., Dempsey, L., & Lee, C. (2008). Identifying language comprehension impairment in preschool children. *Language, Speech, and Hearing Services in Schools, 39,* 54–65.

Skebo, C. M., Lewis, B. A., Freebairn, L. A., Tag, J., Avrich Ciesla, A., & Stein, C. M. (2013). Reading skills of students with speech sound disorders at three stages of literacy development. *Language, Speech, and Hearing Services in Schools, 44,* 360–373.

Skibbe, L. E., Grimm, K. J., Stanton-Chapman, T. L., Justice, L. M., Pence, K. L., & Bowles, R. P. (2008). Reading trajectories of children with language difficulties from preschool through fifth grade. *Language, Speech, and Hearing Services in Schools, 39,* 475–486.

Small, J. A., & Perry, J. (2005). Do you remember?: How caregivers question their spouses who have Alzheimer's disease and the impact on communication. *Journal of Speech, Language, and Hearing Research, 48*(1), 125–136.

Smit, A., Hand, B., Freilinger, J., Bernthal, J., & Bird, A. (1990). The Iowa Articulation Norms Project and its Nebraska replication. *Journal of Speech and Hearing Disorders, 55,* 779–798.

Smith, A. L., & Hustad, K. (2015). AAC and early intervention for children with cerebral palsy: Parent persepctives and child risk factors. *Augmentative and Alternative Communication, 31*(4), 336–350.

Smith, A. L., Barton-Hulsey, A., & Nwosu, N. (2016). AAC and families: Dispelling myths and empowering parents. *ASHA Perspectives Special Interest Group 12 Augmentative and Alternative Communication, 1*(12), 10–20. https://doi.org/10.1044/persp1.SIG12.10

Smith, A., & Weber, C. (2017). How stuttering develops: The multifactorial dynamic pathways theory. *Journal of Speech, Language, and Hearing Research, 60,* 2483–2505.

Smith, A., Sadagopan, N., Walsh, B., & Weber-Fox, C. (2010). Increasing phonological complexity reveals heightened instability in inter-articulatory coordination in adults who stutter. *Journal of Fluency Disorders, 35,* 1–18.

Smith, C. (2020). Culturally competent care for transgender voice and communication intervention. *Perspectives of the ASHA Special Interest Group, 5,* 457–462.

Smith, K. G., & Ryan, A. E. (2020). Relationship between single word reading, connected text reading, and reading comprehension in persons with aphasia. *American Journal of Speech-Language Pathology, 29,* 2039–2048.

Smith-Myles, B., Hilgenfeld, T., Barnhill, G., Griswold, D., Hagiwara, T., & Simpson, R. (2002). Analysis of reading skills in individuals with Asperger syndrome. *Focus on Autism and Other Developmental Disabilities, 17*(1), 44–47.

Smitheran, J., & Hixon, T. (1981). A clinical method for estimating laryngeal airway resistance during vowel production. *Journal of Speech and Hearing Disorders, 46,* 138–146.

Snell, M., Chen, L. Y., & Hoover, K. (2006). Teaching augmentative and alternative communication to students with severe disabilities: A review of intervention research 1997–2003. *Research and Practices for Persons with Severe Disabilities, 31,* 203–214.

Snow, C. E., Scarborough, H. S., & Burns, M. S. (1999). What speech-language pathologists need to know about early reading. *Topics in Language Disorders, 20*(1), 48–58.

Snow, J. (2010). Participation Through Circles of Support. In *The PATH & MAPS Handbook: Person Centered Ways to Build Community.* Inclusion Press.

Snowling, M. J., Duff, F. J., Nash, H. M., & Hulme, C. (2016). Language profiles and literacy outcomes of children with resolving, emerging, or persisting language impairments. *Journal of Child Psychology and Psychiatry, 57,* 1360–1369.

Snowling, M. J., Gallagher, A., & Frith, U. (2003). Family risk of dyslexia is continuous: Individual differences in the precursors of reading skill. *Child Development, 74*, 358–373.

Sohlberg, M. M., Ehlhardt, L., & Kennedy, M. (2005). Instructional techniques in cognitive rehabilitation: A preliminary report. *Seminars in Speech Language Pathology, 26*, 268– 279.

Sonies, B., Baum, B., & Shawker, T. (1984). Speech and swallowing in the elderly. *Gerontology, 3*, 279–283.

Soto, G. (2012). Training partners in AAC in culturally diverse families. *Perspectives on Augmentative and Alternative Communication, 21*(4), 144–149. https://doi.org/10.1044/aac21.4.144

Soto, G., & Yu, B. (2014, January). Considerations for the provision of services to bilingual children who use augmentative and alternative communication. *Augmentative and Alternative Communication, 30*(1), 83–92. https://doi.org/10.3109/07434618.2013.878751

Soto, G., Muller, E., Hunt, P., & Goetz, L. (2001). Critical issues in the inclusion of students who use augmentative and alternative communication: An educational team perspective. *Augmentative and Alternative Communication, 17*, 62–72.

Southwood, F., & Russell, A. F. (2004). Comparison of conversation, freeplay, and story generation as methods of language elicitation. *Journal of Speech, Language, and Hearing Research, 47*, 366–376.

Spanoudis, G. S., Papadopoulos, T. C., & Spyrou, S. (2019). Specific language impairment and reading disability: Categorical distinction or continuum? *Journal of Learning Disabilities, 52*, 3–14.

Spaulding, T. J, Plante, E., & Farinella, K. A. (2006). Eligibility criteria for language impairment: Is the low end of normal always appropriate? *Language, Speech, and Hearing Services in Schools, 37*, 61–72.

Spaulding, T. J., Plante, E., & Vance, R. (2008). Sustained selective attention skills of preschool children with specific language impairment: Evidence for separate attentional capacities. *Journal of Speech, Language, and Hearing Research, 51*, 16–34.

Spencer, E., Schuele, C. N., Guillot, K., & Lee, M. (2008). Phonological awareness skill of speech-language pathologists and other educators. *Language, Speech, and Hearing Services in Schools, 39*, 512–520.

Spencer, K., Paul, J., Brown, K. A., Ellerbrock, T., & Sohlberg, M. M. (2020). Cognitive rehabilitation for individuals with Parkinson's disease: Developing and piloting an external aids treatment program. *American Journal of Speech-Language Pathology, 29*, 1–19.

St Clair, M. C., Forrest, C. L., Kok Yew, S. G., & Gibson, J. L. (2019). Early risk factors and emotional difficulties in children at risk of developmental language disorder: A population cohort study. *Journal of Speech, Language, and Hearing Research, 62*, 2750–2771.

St Clair-Thompson, H. L., & Gathercole, S. E. (2006). Executive functions and achievements in school: Shifting, updating, inhibition and working memory. *Quarterly Journal of Experimental Psychology, 59*, 745–759.

Stadskleiv, K. (2017). Experiences from a support group for families of preschool children in the expressive AAC user group. *Augmentative and Alternative Communication, 33*(1), 3–13. https://doi.org/10.1080/07434618.2016.1276960

Stalpaert, J., Cocquyt, E., Criel, Y., Segers, L., Miatton, M., Van Langenhove, T., et al. (2020). Language and speech markers of primary progressive aphasia: A systematic review. *American Journal of Speech-Language Pathology, 29*, 2206–2225.

Stark, B. C. (2019). A comparison of three discourse elicitation methods in aphasia and age-matched adults: Implications for language assessment and outcome. *American Journal of Speech-Language Pathology, 28*, 1067–1083.

Starkweather, W. (1987). *Fluency and stuttering.* Prentice Hall.

Starkweather, W. (1997). Therapy for younger children. In R. F. Curlee & G. M. Siegel (Eds.), *Nature and treatment of stuttering: New directions* (2nd ed., pp. 143–166). Allyn & Bacon.

Starmer, H. (2017). Swallowing exercises in head and neck cancer. *Perspectives of the ASHA Special Interest Groups, 2*, 21–26.

Starmer, H., Gourin, C., Lua, L., & Burkhead, L. (2011). Pretreatment swallowing assessment in head and neck cancer patients. *Laryngoscope, 121*, 1208–1211.

Steele, C. (2012). Exercise-based approaches to dysphagia rehabilitation. *Nestle Nutrition Institute Workshop Series, 72*, 109–117.

Steele, C., & Van Lieshout, P. (2009). Tongue movements during water swallowing in healthy young and older adults. *Journal of Speech, Language, and Hearing Research, 52*, 1255–1267.

Steele, C., Alsanei, W., Ayanikalath, S., Barbon, C., Chen, J., Cichero, J., et al.. (2015). The influence of food texture and liquid consistency modification on swallowing physiology and function: A systematic review. *Dysphagia, 30*, 2–26.

Steele, C., Bayley, M., Peladeau-Pigeon, M., Nagy, Y., Namasivayam, A., Stokely, S., & Wolkin, T. (2016). A randomized trial comparing two tongue-pressure resistance training protocols for post-stroke dysphagia. *Dysphagia, 31*, 452–461.

Stella, M., Beckage, N. M., Brede, M., & De Domenico, M. (2018). Multiplex model of mental lexicon reveals explosive learning in humans. *Scientific Reports, 8*(1), 2259.

Stemple, J. (2007). *Principles of physiologic voice therapy.* Arizona State University.

Stemple, J., Roy, N., & Klaben, B. (2018). *Clinical voice pathology: Theory and management* (6th ed.). Plural Publishing.

Stepp, C. (2012). Surface electromyography for speech and swallowing systems: Measurement, analysis, and interpretation. *Journal of Speech, Language, and Hearing Research, 55,* 1232–1246.

Stillman, R., & Battle, C. (1984). Developing prelanguage communication in the severely handicapped: An interpretation of the Van Dijk method. *Seminars in Speech-Language Pathology, 5,* 159–170.

Stipancic, K., Borders, J. C., Brates, D., & Thibeault, S. L. (2019). Prospective investigation of incidence and co-occurrence of dysphagia, dysarthria, and aphasia following ischemic stroke. *American Journal of Speech-Language Pathology, 28,* 188–194.

Stoel-Gammon, C., & Herrington, P. (1990). Vowel systems of normally developing and phonologically disordered children. *Clinical Linguistics & Phonetics, 4,* 145–160.

Stoicheff, M. (1981). Speaking fundamental frequency characteristics of nonsmoking female adults. *Journal of Speech and Hearing Research, 24,* 437–441.

Story, B. (2002). An overview of the physiology, physics, and modeling of the sound source for vowels. *Acoustical Science and Technology, 23,* 195–206.

Strand, E. (2010). *An overview of dynamic temporal and tactile cueing for childhood apraxia of speech and other motor speech disorders* [Video]. (Available from Childhood Apraxia of Speech Association of North America, 416 Lincoln Avenue 2nd Fl., Pittsburgh, PA 15209)

Strand, E. (2019). Dynamic temporal and tactile cueing: A treatment strategy for childhood apraxia of speech. *American Journal of Speech-Language Pathology, 29,* 30–48. https://doi.org/10.1044/2019_AJSLP-19-0005

Strand, E. A., & McCauley, R. (1997, November). *Differential diagnosis of phonological impairment and developmental apraxia of speech.* Paper presented at the annual convention of the American Speech-Language-Hearing Association, Boston.

Strand, E., & McCauley, R. (2008). Differential diagnosis of severe speech impairment in young children. *The ASHA Leader, 13*(10). https://leader.pubs.asha.org/doi/10.1044/leader.FTR1.13102008.10

Strand, E., & Skinder, A. (1999). Treatment of developmental apraxia of speech: Integral stimulation methods. In A. Caruso & E. Strand (Eds.), *Clinical management of motor speech disorders in children* (pp. 109–148). Thieme.

Strand, E., McCauley, R., Weigand, S., Stoeckel, R., & Baas, B. (2013). A motor speech assessment for children with severe speech disorders: Reliability and validity evidence. *Journal of Speech, Language, and Hearing Research, 56,* 505–520.

Strand, E., Stoeckel, R., & Baas, B. (2006). Treatment of severe childhood apraxia of severe childhood apraxia of speech: A treatment efficacy study. *Journal of Medical Speech Pathology, 14,* 297–307.

Strange, W., & Broen, P. (1980). Perception and production of approximant consonants by 3-year-olds: A first study. In G. Yeni-Komshian, J. Kavanaugh, & C. A. Ferguson (Eds.), *Child phonology: Vol. 2. Perception.* Academic Press.

Streb, J., Hemighausen, E., & Rösler, F. (2004). Different anaphoric expressions are investigated by event-related brain potentials. *Journal of Psycholinguistic Research, 33,* 175–201.

Striano, T., Rochat, P., & Legerstee, M. (2003). The role of modeling and request type on symbolic comprehension of objects and gestures in young children. *Journal of Child Language, 30,* 27–45.

Strong, K. A., & Randolph, J. (2021). How do you do talk therapy with someone who can't talk?: Perspectives from mental health providers on delivering services to individuals with aphasia. *American Journal of Speech-Language Pathology, 30,* 2681–2692.

Suárez-González, A., Savage, S. A., Bier, N., Henry, M. L., Jokel, R., Nickels, L., & Taylor-Rubin, C. (2021). Semantic variant primary progressive aphasia: Practical recommendations for treatment from 20 years of behavioural research. *Brain Sciences, 11,* 1552–1570.

Suggate, S. P. (2014). A meta-analysis of the long-term effects of phonemic awareness, phonics, fluency, and reading comprehension interventions. *Journal of Learning Disabilities, 49*(1), 77–96.

Suiter, D. M., & Gosa, M. M. (2019). *Assessing and treating dysphagia: A lifespan perspective.* Thieme.

Suiter, D., & Leder, S. (2008). Clinical utility of the 3-ounce water swallow test. *Dysphagia, 23,* 244–250.

Suiter, D., Sloggy, J., & Leder, S. (2014). Validation of the Yale Swallow Protocol: A prospective double-blinded videofluoroscopic study. *Dysphagia, 29,* 199–203.

Sullivan, P. (2008). Gastrointestinal disorders in children with neurodevelopmental disabilities. *Developmental Disabilities Research Reviews, 14,* 128–136.

Sung, Y., Li, L., Blake, C., Betz, J. & Lin, F. R. (2015). Association of hearing loss and loneliness in older adults. *Journal of Aging and Health, 28*(6), 979–994. https://doi.org/10.1177/0898264315614570

Sung, J. E., Choi, S., Eom, B., Yoo, J. K., & Jeong, J. H. (2020). Syntactic complexity as a linguistic marker to differentiate mild cognitive impairment from normal aging. *Journal of Speech, Language, and Hearing Research, 63,* 1416–1429.

Sura, L., Madhavan, A., Carnaby, G., & Crary, M. (2012). Dysphagia in the elderly: management and nutritional considerations. *Clinical Interventions in Aging, 7,* 287–298.

Suttrup, I., & Warnecke, T. (2016). Dysphagia in Parkinson's disease. *Dysphagia, 31,* 24–32.

Swanson, H. L., & Beebe-Frankenberger, M. (2004). The relationship between working memory and mathematical problem solving in children at risk and not at risk for math disabilities. *Journal of Educational Psychology, 96,* 471–491.

Sweetow, R., & Sabes, J. (2006). The need for and development of an adaptive Listening and Communication Enhancement (LACE) program. *Journal of the American Academy of Audiology, 17*(8), 538–558.

Swineford, L. B., Thurm, A., Baird, G., Wetherby, A. M., & Swedo, S. (2014). Social (pragmatic) communication disorder: A research review of this new DSM-5 diagnostic category. *Journal of Neurodevelopmental Disorders, 6,* 41–49.

Szacka, K., Potulska-Chromik, A., Fronczewska-Wieniawska, K., Spychała, A., Kròlicki, L., & Kuźmza-Kozakiewicz, M. (2016). Scintigraphic evaluation of mild to moderate dysphagia in motor neuron disease. *Clinical Nuclear Medicine, 41,* e175–e180.

Tager-Flusberg, H., Paul, R., & Lord, C. E. (2005). Language and communication in autism. In F. Volkmar, R. Paul, A. Klin, & D. J. Cohen (Eds.), *Handbook of autism and pervasive developmental disorder: Vol. 1* (3rd ed., pp. 335–364). Wiley.

Tattersall, P., & Dawson, J., (2016). *Structured Photographic Articulation Test III—Featuring Dudsberry (SPAT-D3).* Janelle Publications.

Tattershall, S. (2004, November). *SLPs contributing to and learning within the writing process.* Paper presented at the annual convention of the American Speech-Language-Hearing Association, Philadelphia.

Templeton, S. (2003). The spelling/meaning connection. *Voices from the Middle, 10*(3), 56–57.

Templeton, S. (2004). Instructional approaches to spelling: The window on students' word knowledge in reading and writing. In E. R. Silliman & L. C. Wilkinson (Eds.), *Language and literacy learning in schools* (pp. 273–291). Guilford Press.

Terre, R, & Mearin, F. (2007). Prospective evaluation of oro-pharyngeal dysphagia after severe traumatic brain injury. *Brain Injury, 21*(13–14), 1411–1417.

Terrell, P., & Watson, M. (2018). Laying a firm foundation: Embedding evidence-based emergent literacy practices into early intervention and preschool environments. *Language, Speech, and Hearing Services in Schools, 49,* 148–164.

Terry, N. P. (2012). Examining relationships among dialect variation and emergent literacy skills. *Communication Disorders Quarterly, 33*(2), 67–77. https://doi.org/10.1177/1525740110368846

Thal, D., Jackson-Maldonado, D., & Acosta, D. (2000). Validity of a parent-report measure of vocabulary and grammar for Spanish-speaking toddlers. *Journal of Speech, Language, and Hearing Research, 43,* 1087–1100.

Themistocleous, C., Webster, K., Afthinos, A., & Tsapkini, K. (2021). Part of speech production in patients with primary progressive aphasia: An analysis based on natural language processing. *American Journal of Speech-Language Pathology, 30,* 466–480.

Therrien, M. C., Light, J., & Pope, L. (2016). Systematic review of the effects of interventions to promote peer interactions for children who use aided AAC. *Augmentative and Alternative Communication, 32*(2), 81–93.

Thibeault, S., Merrill, R., Roy, N., Gray, S., & Smith, E. (2004). Occupational risk factors associated with voice disorders among teachers. *Annals of Epidemiology, 14,* 786–792.

Thiemann, K. S., & Goldstein, H. (2004). Effects of peer training and written text cueing on social communication of school-age children with pervasive developmental disorder. *Journal of Speech, Language, and Hearing Research, 47,* 126–144.

Thiemann-Bourque, K., Brady, N., McGuff, S., Stump, K., & Naylor, A. (2016). Picture Exchange Communication System and pals: A peer-mediated augmentative and alternative communication intervention for minimally verbal preschoolers with autism. *Journal of Speech, Language, and Hearing Research, 59,* 1133–1145.

Thistle, J. J., Holmes, S. A., Horn, M. M., & Reum, A. M. (2018). Consistent symbol location affects motor learning in preschoolers without disabilities: Implications for designing augmentative and alternative communication displays. *American Journal of Speech Language Pathology, 27*(3), 1010–1017. https://doi.org/10.1044/2018_AJSLP-17-0129

Thistle, J. J., & Wilkinson, K. (2009). The effects of color cues on typically developing preschoolers' speed of locating a target line drawing: Implications for augmentative and alternative communication display design. *American Journal of Speech-Language Pathology, 18*(3), 231–240.

Thistle, J., & Wilkinson, K. (2017). Effects of background color and symbol arrangement cues on construction of multi-symbol messages by young children without disabilities: Implications for aided AAC design. *Augmentative and Alternative Communication, 33*(3), 160–169.

Thom, S., Hoit, J., Hixon, T., & Smith, A. (2006). Velopharyngeal function during vocalization in infants. *Cleft Palate Craniofacial Journal, 43,* 539–546.

Thomas, L. (1979). *The medusa and the snail: More notes of a biology watcher.* Viking.

Thomas, L., & Stemple, J. (2007). Voice therapy: Does science support the art? *Communicative Disorders Review, 1,* 49–77.

Thomason, K. M., Gorman, B. K., & Summers, C. (2007). English literacy development for English language learners: Does Spanish instruction promote or hinder? *EBP Briefs, 2*(2), 1–15.

Thompson Tetnowski, J., Tetnowski, J. A., & Damico, J. S. (2021). Patterns of conversation trouble source and repair as indices of improved conversation in aphasia: A multiple-case study using conversation analysis. *American Journal of Speech-Language Pathology, 30*, 326–343.

Thompson, C. K. (2004). Neuroimaging: Applications for studying aphasia. In L. L. LaPointe (Ed.), *Aphasia and related disorders* (pp. 19–38). Thieme.

Thompson, C. K., Shapiro, L. P., Kiran, S., & Sobecks, J. (2003). The role of syntactic complexity in treatment of sentence deficits in agrammatic aphasia: The Complexity Account of Treatment Efficacy (CATE). *Journal of Speech, Language, and Hearing Research, 46*, 591–607.

Thompson, P. A., Hulme, C., Nash, H. M., Gooch, D., Hayiou-Thomas, E., & Snowling, M. J. (2015). Developmental dyslexia: Predicting individual risk. *Journal of Child Psychology and Psychiatry, 56*, 976–987.

Thordardottir, E. T., & Ellis Weismer, S. (2002). Verb argument structure weakness in specific language impairment in relation to age and utterance length. *Clinical Linguistics & Phonetics, 16*, 233–250.

Thunstam, L. (2004). *Social networks and communication for children with deafness and additional impairments.* Unpublished master's thesis, Mälardalens University, Sweden.

Tichenor, S., & Yaruss, J. (2019). Stuttering as defined by adults who stutter. *Journal of Speech, Language, and Hearing Research, 62*, 4356–4369.

Tierney, L. M., Jr., McPhee, S. J., & Papadakis, M. A. (2000). *Current medical diagnosis and treatment* (39th ed.). Lange Medical Books/McGraw-Hill.

Tierney-Hendricks, C., Schliep, M. E., & Vallila-Rohter, S. (2022). Using an implementation framework to survey outcome measurement and treatment practices in aphasia. *American Journal of Speech-Language Pathology, 31*, 1133–1162.

Timler, G. R. (2018a, April 1). Similar . . . but very different: Determining when a child has social communication disorder versus autism spectrum disorder can be tricky. Here are some key considerations. *The ASHA Leader, 23*(4). 56–61

Timler, G. R. (2018b). Using language sample analysis to assess pragmatic skills in school-age children and adolescents. *Perspectives of the ASHA Special Interest Groups, 3*(1), 23–35.

Timler, G. R., Vogler-Elias, D., & McGill, K. F. (2007). Strategies for promoting generalization of social communication skills in preschoolers and school-aged children. *Topics in Language Disorders, 27*, 167–181.

Titze, I. R. (1994). *Principles of voice production.* Prentice Hall.

Titze, I., Lemke, J., & Montequin, D. (1997). Populations in the U.S. workforce who rely on voice as a primary tool of trade: A preliminary report. *Journal of Voice, 11*, 254–259.

Tjaden, K., & Liss, J. (1995). The influence of familiarity on judgments of treated speech. *American Journal of Speech-Language Pathology, 4*, 38–39.

Tobii Dynavox. (2018). *The Story of Core.* http://tdvox.web-downloads.s3.amazonaws.com/Core%20First/TD-TheStory_of_Core.pdf

Tolins, J., Namiranian, N., Akhtar, N., & Fox Tree, J. E. (2017). The role of addressee backchannels and conversational grounding in vicarious word learning in four-year-olds. *First Language, 37*, 648–671.

Tomas, E., Demuth, K, & Petocz, P. (2017). The role of frequency in learning morphophonological alternations: implications for children with specific language impairment. *Journal of Speech, Language, and Hearing Research, 60*, 1316–1329. https://doi.org/10.1044/2016_JSLHR-L-16-0138

Tomblin, J. B., Zhang, X., Buckwalter, P., & O'Brien, M. (2003). The stability of primary language disorder: Four years after kindergarten diagnosis. *Journal of Speech, Language, and Hearing Research, 46*, 1283–1296.

Tomblin, J., Harrison. M., Ambrose, S., Walker, E., Oleson, J., & Moeller, M. (2015). Language outcomes in young children with mild to severe hearing loss. *Ear and Hearing, 36*(10), 76S–91S.

Tomes, L. A., Kuehn, D. P., & Peterson-Falzone, S. J. (1997). Behavioral treatment of velopharyngeal impairment. In K. R. Bzoch (Ed.), *Communicative disorders related to cleft lip and palate* (4th ed., pp. 529–562). PRO-ED.

Tompkins, C. A., Baumgaertner, A., Lehman, M. T., & Fassbinder, W. (2000). Mechanisms of discourse comprehension impairment after right hemisphere brain damage: Suppression of lexical ambiguity resolution. *Journal of Speech, Language, and Hearing Research, 43*, 62–78.

Tompkins, C., Blake, M. T., Wambaugh, J., & Meigh, K. (2011). A novel, implicit treatment for language comprehension processes in right hemisphere brain damage: Phase I data. *Aphasiology, 25*, 789–799.

Tompkins, C., Fassbinder, W., Blake, M., Baumgaertner, A., & Jayaram, N. (2004). Inference generation during text comprehension by adults with right hemisphere brain damage: Activation failure vs. multiple activation? *Journal of Speech, Language, and Hearing Research, 47*, 1380–1395.

Tompkins, C., Klepousniotou, E., & Scott, G. (2013). Treatment of right hemisphere disorders. In I. Papathanasiou, P. Coppens, & C. Potagas (Eds.), *Aphasia and related neurogenic communication disorders* (pp. 345–364). Jones & Bartlett.

Tompkins, C., Lehman-Blake, M., Baumgaertner, A., & Fassbinder, W. (2001). Mechanisms of discourse comprehension impairment after right hemisphere brain damage: Suppression in inferential ambiguity resolution. *Journal of Speech, Language, and Hearing Research, 44*, 400–415.

Tompkins, C., Scharp, V., Meigh, K., & Fassbinder, W. (2008). Coarse coding and discourse comprehension in adults with right hemisphere brain damage. *Aphasiology, 22*, 204–223.

Torgesen, J. K. (2000). Individual difference in response to early interventions in reading: The lingering problem of treatment resisters. *Learning Disabilities Research and Practice, 15*, 55–64.

Torgesen, J. K. (2005). Recent discoveries from research on remedial interventions for children with dyslexia. In M. Snowling & C. Hulme (Eds.), *The science of reading: A handbook* (pp. 521–537). Blackwell.

Tostanoski, A., Lang, R., Raulston, T., Carnett, A., & Davis, T. (2014). Voices from the past: Comparing the rapid prompting method and facilitated communication. *Developmental Neurorehabilitation, 17*(4), 219–223. https://doi.org/10.3109/17518423.2012.749952

Tosto, M. G., Hayiou-Thomas, M. E., Harlaar, N., Prom-Wormley, E., Dale, P. S., & Plomin, R. (2017). The genetic architecture of oral language, reading fluency, and reading comprehension: A twin study from 7 to 16 years. *Developmental Psychology, 53*, 1115–1129.

Tourne, L. (1991). Growth of the pharynx and its physiologic implications. *American Journal of Orthodontics and Dentofacial Orthopedics, 99*, 129–139.

Towey, M., Whitcomb, J., & Bray, C. (2004, November). *Print-sound-story-talk, a successful early reading first program.* Paper presented at the annual convention of the American Speech-Language-Hearing Association, Philadelphia.

Trabasso, T., & Wiley, J. (2005). Goal plans of action and inferences during comprehension of narratives. *Discourse Processes, 39*(2–3), 129–164. https://doi.org/10.1207/s15326950dp3902&3_3

Travers, J. C., Tincani, M. J., & Lang, R. (2014). Facilitated communication denies people with disabilities their voice. *Research & Practice for Persons with Severe Disabilities, 39*(3), 195–202. https://doi.org/10.1177/1540796914556778

Treffert, D. A. (2009). *Hyperlexia: Reading precociousness or savant skill?* Wisconsin Medical Society. www.wisconsinmedicalsociety.org/savant_syndrome/savant_articles/hyperlexia.

Trembath, D., Paynter, J., Keen, D., & Ecker, U. K. (2015). "Attention: Myth Follows!" Facilitated communication, parent and professional attitudes towards evidence-based practice, and the power of misinformation. *Evidence Based Communication Assessment and Intervention, 9*(3), 113–126. https://doi.org/10.1080/17489539.2015.1103433

Troche, M., & Mishra, A. (2017). Swallowing exercises in patients with neurodegenerative disease: What is the current evidence? *Perspectives of the ASHA Special Interest Groups, 2*, 13–20.

Truong, K., & Cunningham, L. (2011, July/August). Is a temporary threshold shift harmless? *Audiology Today.* 64–65

Tsao, F., Liu, H., & Kuhl, P. K. (2004). Speech perception in infancy predicts language development in the second year of life: A longitudinal study. *Child Development, 75*, 1067–1084.

Tucker, J., & Tucker, G. (1979). A clinical perspective on the development and anatomical aspects of the infant larynx and trachea. In G. Healy & T. McGill (Eds.), *Laryngo-tracheal problems in the pediatric patient* (pp. 3–8). Charles C. Thomas.

Tumanova, V., Conture, E., Lambert, E., & Walden, T. (2014). Speech disfluencies of preschool-age children who do and do not stutter. *Journal of Communication Disorders, 49*, 25–41.

Tunmer, W. E., & Chapman, J. W. (2012). Does set for variability mediate the influence of vocabulary knowledge on the development of word recognition skills? *Scientific Studies of Reading, 16*, 122–140.

Tye-Murray, N. (2009). *Foundations of aural rehabilitation: Children, adults, and their family members* (3rd ed.). Delmar Cengage Learning.

Tymms, P., Merrell, C., & Bailey, K. (2018) The long-term impact of effective teaching. *School Effectiveness and School Improvement, 29*, 242–261.

U.S. Census Bureau. (2013). *Language use in the United States.* Author.

U.S. Census Bureau. (2020, December). *Los Angeles, California population.* https://worldpopulationreview.com/us-cities/los-angeles-ca-population

U.S. Department of Health and Human Services. (2007). *Child maltreatment, 2007.* www.acf.hhs.gov/programs/cb/pubs/cm07/summary.htm

U.S. Department of Housing and Urban Development. (2021) *U.S. Housing and Urban Development 2020 annual homeless assessment report part 1* (HUD No. 21-041). https://www.hud.gov/press/press_releases_media_advisories/hud_no_21_041

U.S. Food and Drug Administration (FDA). (2022) *Cochlear implants.* https://www.fda.gov/medical-devices/implants-and-prosthetics/cochlear-implants

Ukrainetz, T. A., Harpell, S., Walsh, C., & Coyle, C. (2000). A preliminary investigation of dynamic assessment with Native American kindergarteners. *Language, Speech, and Hearing Services in Schools, 31*, 142–154.

Utianski, R., & Duffy, J. (2022). Understanding, recognizing, and management functional speech disorders:

Current thinking illustrated with a case series. *American Journal of Speech-Language-Pathology, 31,* 1205–1220.

Valian, V., & Aubry, S. (2005). When opportunity knocks twice: two-year-olds' repetition of sentence subjects. *Journal of Child Language, 32,* 617–641.

Valian, V., & Casey, L. (2003). Young children's acquisition of *wh-* questions: The role of structured input. *Journal of Child Language, 30,* 117–143.

Vallotton, C. D. (2012). Infant signs as intervention? Promoting symbolic gestures for preverbal children in low-income families supports responsive parent-child relationships. *Early Childhood Research Quarterly, 27*(3), 401–415. https://doi.org/10.1016/j.ecresq.2012.01.003

Van Borsel, J., De Cuypere, G., Rubens, R., & Destaerke, B. (2000). Voice problems in female-to-male transsexuals. *International Journal of Language and Communication Disorders, 35,* 427–442.

Van den Berg, J. (1958). Myoelastic-aerodynamic theory of voice production. *Journal of Speech and Hearing Research, 1,* 227–244.

Van der Merwe, A. (2004). The voice use reduction program. *American Journal of Speech-Language Pathology, 13,* 208–218.

Van Kleeck, A. (2008). Providing preschool foundations for later reading comprehension: The importance of and ideas for targeting inferencing in storybook-sharing interventions. *Psychology in the Schools, 45,* 627–643. https://doi.org/10.1002/pits.20314

Van Kleeck, A., & Schuele, C. M. (2010). Historical perspectives on literacy in early childhood. *American Journal of Speech-Language Pathology, 19,* 341–355.

Van Kleeck, A., Vander Woude, J., & Hammett, L. (2006). Fostering literal and inferential language skills in Head Start preschoolers with language impairment using scripted book-sharing discussions. *American Journal of Speech-Language Pathology, 15,* 85–95.

Van Lancker Sidtis, D., Choi, J., Alken, A., & Sidtis, J. J. (2015). Formulaic language in Parkinson's disease and Alzheimer's disease: Complementary effects of subcortical and cortical dysfunction. *Journal of Speech, Language, and Hearing Research, 58,* 1493–1507.

Van Meter, A. M., Nelson, N. W., & Ansell, P. (2004, November). *Developing spelling and vocabulary skills in curriculum writing activities.* Paper presented at the annual convention of the American Speech-Language-Hearing Association, Philadelphia.

Van Riper, C. (1982). *The nature of stuttering.* Prentice Hall.

Van Riper, C. (1992). *The nature of stuttering* (2nd ed.). Waveland Press.

Van Riper, C., & Emerick, L. (1984). *Speech correction: An introduction to speech pathology and audiology* (7th ed.). Englewood Cliffs, NJ: Prentice Hall.

Van Stan, J., Roy, N., Awan, S., Stemple, J., & Hillman, R. (2015). A taxonomy of voice therapy. *American Journal of Speech-Language Pathology, 24,* 101–125.

Van Tatenhove, G. (2014). Issues in language sample collection and analysis with children using AAC. *Perspectives on Augmentative and Alternative Communication, 23*(2), 65–74. https://doi.org/10.1044/aac23.2.65

Vanderheiden, G., & Yoder, D. E. (1986). *Overview.* American Speech-Language-Hearing Association.

Vanryckeghem, M., & Brutten, G. (2006). *KiddyCAT Communication Attitude Test for Preschool and Kindergarten Children Who Stutter.* Plural Publishing.

Vanryckeghem, M., Brutten, G., & Hernandez, L. (2005). A comparative investigation of the speech-associated attitude of preschool and kindergarten children who do and do not stutter. *Journal of Fluency Disorders, 30,* 307–318.

Vaughn, S., & Klingner, J. (2004). Teaching reading comprehension to students with learning disabilities. In C. A. Stone, E. R. Silliman, B. J. Ehren, & K. Apel (Eds.), *Handbook of language and literacy: Development and disorders* (pp. 541–555). Guilford Press.

Venkatagiri, H. S. (1999). Efficient keyboard layouts for sequential access in augmentative and alternative communication. *Augmentative and Alternative Communication, 15*(2), 126–134.

Verdolini, K. (1998). *Resonant voice therapy.* National Center for Voice and Speech.

Verdolini, K., Rosen, C., & Branski, R. (2006). *Classification manual for voice disorders–I.* Erlbaum.

Vermiglio, A. (2014). On the clinical entity in audiology: Central auditory processing and speech recognition in noise disorder. *Journal of the American Academy of Audiology, 25,* 904–917.

Victorino, K. R., & Schwartz, R. G. (2015). Control of auditory attention in children with specific language impairment. *Journal of Speech, Language, and Hearing Research, 58,* 1245–1257.

Vihman, M. M. (2017). Learning words and learning sounds: Advances in language development. *British Journal of Psychology, 108,* 1–27. https://doi.org/10.1111/bjop.12207

Virtue, S., & van den Broek, P. (2004). Hemispheric processing of anaphoric inferences: The activation of multiple antecedents. *Brain and Language, 93,* 327–337.

Virtue, S., Haberman, J., Clancy, Z., Parrish, T., & Beeman, M. (2006). Neural activity of inferences during story comprehension. *Brain Research, 1084,* 104–114.

Vogel, I., Verschuure, H., Van der Ploeg, C., Brug, J., & Raat, H.(2010). Estimating adolescent risk for hearing loss based on data from a large school-based survey. *American Journal of Public Health, 100*(6), 1095–1100.

Vugs, B., Hendriks, M., Cuperus, J., & Verhoeven, L. (2014). Working memory performance and executive function behaviors in young children with SLI. *Research in Developmental Disabilities, 35,* 62–74. Wadman. R., Durkin, K., & Conti-Ramsden, G. (2008). Self-esteem, shyness, and sociability in adolescents with specific language impairment (SLI). *Journal of Speech, Language, and Hearing Research, 51,* 938–52. https://doi.org/10.1044/1092-4388(2008/069)

Wadman, R., Durkin, K., & Conti-Ramsden, G. (2008). Self-esteem, shyness, and sociability in adolescents with specific language impairment (SLI). *Journal of Speech, Language, and Hearing Research, 51,* 938–952.

Wagner, D. K. (2018). Building augmentative communication skills in homes where English and Spanish are spoken: Perspectives of an evaluator/interventionist. *Perspectives on Augmentative and Alternative Communication, 3*(12), 173–184. https://doi.org/10.1044/persp3.SIG12.172

Wahlberg, T., & Magliano, J. P. (2004). The ability of high-functioning individuals with autism to comprehend written discourse. *Discourse Processes, 38*(1), 119–144.

Waite, M. C., Theodoros, D. G., Russell, T. G., & Cahill, L. M. (2010). Internet-based telehealth assessment of language using the CELF-4. *Language, Speech, and Hearing Services in Schools, 41,* 445–458.

Walker, E., Sapp, C., Dallapiazza, M., Spratford, M., & McCreery, R. (2020). Language and reading outcomes in fourth-grade children with mild hearing loss compared to age-matched peers. *Language, Speech and Hearing Services in Schools, 51*(1), 17–28.

Wallace, S. E., Knollman-Porter, K., Brown, J. A., & Hux, K. (2019). Narrative comprehension by people with aphasia given single versus combined modality presentation. *Aphasiology, 33,* 731–754.

Waltzman, S. B., & Roland, J. T. (2005). Cochlear implantation in children younger than 12 months. *Pediatrics, 116,* e487–e493.

Wambaugh, J., & Bain, B. (2002). Make research methods an integral part of your clinical practice. *The ASHA Leader, 7*(21), 1, 10–13.

Wambaugh, J., Mauszycki, S., & Ballard, K. (2013). Advances in the treatment of acquired apraxia of speech. *Perspectives on Neurophysiology and Neurogenic Speech and Language Disorders, 23,* 112–119.

Wang, P., & Spillane, A. (2009). Evidence-based social skills interventions for children with autism: A meta-analysis. *Education and Training in Developmental Disabilities, 44*(3), 318–342.

Washington, J.A., Branum-Martin, L., Sun, C., & Lee-James, R. (2018). The impact of dialect density on the growth of language and reading in African American children. *Language, Speech, and Hearing Services in Schools, 49,* 232–247.

Webster, W. (1993). Evidence in bimanual finger tapping of an attentional component to stuttering. *Behavioural Brain Research, 37,* 93–100.

Weinstein, B., Sirow, L., & Moser, S. (2016). Relating hearing aid use to social and emotional loneliness in older adults. *American Journal of Audiology, 25,* 54–61.

Weismer, S., Tomblin, J. B., Zhang, X., Buckwalter, P., Gaura Chynoweth, J., & Jones, M. (2000). Non-word repetition performance in school-age children with and without language impairment. *Journal of Speech, Language, and Hearing Research, 43,* 865–878.

Wendt, O., & Miller, B. (2013). Systematic review documents emerging empirical support for certain applications of iPods® and iPads® in intervention programs for individuals with developmental disabilities, but these are not a "one-size-fits-all" solution. *Evidence-Based Communication Assessment & Intervention, 7*(3), 91–96.

Werfel, K. L., Eisel Hendricks, A., & Schuele, C. M. (2017). The potential of past tense marking in oral reading as a clinical marker of specific language impairment in school-age children. *Journal of Speech, Language and Hearing Disorders, 60,* 3561–3572.

Westby, C. E. (2004). A language perspective on executive functioning, metacognition, and self-regulation in reading. In C. A. Stone, E. R. Silliman, B. J. Ehren, & K. Apel (Eds.), *Handbook of language and literacy: Development and disorders* (pp. 398–427). Guilford Press.

Westby, C. E. (2005). Assessing and remediating text comprehension problems. In H. W. Catts & A. G. Kamhi (Eds.), *Language and reading disabilities* (2nd ed., pp. 157–232). Allyn & Bacon.

Westerveld, M. F., Paynter, J., & Wicks, R. (2020). Shared book reading behaviors of parents and their verbal preschoolers on the autism spectrum. *Journal of Autism and Developmental Disorders, 50,* 3005–3017.

Wheeler-Hegland, K., Frymark, T., Schooling, T., McCabe, D., Ashford, J., Mullen, R., et al. (2009). Evidence-based systematic review: Oropharyngeal dysphagia behavioral treatments. Part V—Applications for clinicians and researchers. *Journal of Rehabilitation & Development, 46,* 215–222.

Whitehurst, G. J., & Lonigan, C. J. (2001). Emergent readers: Development from prereaders to readers. In S. B. Neuman & D. K. Dickinson (Eds.), *Handbook of early literacy research* (pp. 11–29). Guilford Press.

Whitmire, K. A. (2000). Adolescence as a developmental phase: A tutorial. *Topics in Language Disorders, 20*(2), 1–14.

Wiig, E. H., Zureich, P. Z., & Chan, H. H. (2000). A clinical rationale for assessing rapid automatized naming with language disorders. *Journal of Learning Disabilities, 33*, 359–374.

Wilcox, K., & Morris, S. (1999). *Children's speech intelligibility measure.* Psychological Corporation.

Wilder, J., & Granlund, M. (2006, August). *Presymbolic children in Sweden: Interaction, family accommodation and social networks.* Proceedings from the 12th ISAAC Research Conference, Düsseldorf.

Wilkinson, K., Carlin, M., & Thistle, J. (2008). The role of color cues in facilitating accurate and rapid location of aided symbols by children with and without Down syndrome. *American Journal of Speech-Language Pathology, 17*, 179–193.

Williams, A. (2000a). Multiple oppositions: Case studies of variables in phonological intervention. *American Journal of Speech-Language Pathology, 9*, 282–288.

Williams, A. (2000b). Multiple oppositions: Theoretical foundations for an alternative contrastive intervention approach. *American Journal of Speech-Language Pathology, 9*, 282–288.

Williams, G. J., Larkin, R. F., Rose, N. V., Whitaker, E., Roeser, J., & Wood, C. (2021). Orthographic knowledge and clue word facilitated spelling in children with developmental language disorder. *Journal of Speech, Language, and Hearing Research, 64*, 3909–3927. https://doi.org/10.1044/2021_JSLHR-20-00710

Williams, K. J., Walker, M. A., Vaughn, S., & Wanzek, J. (2017). A synthesis of reading and spelling interventions and their effects on spelling outcomes for students with learning disabilities. *Journal of Learning Disabilities, 50*(3), 286–297.

Williams, R. (2015). *The ethics of gatekeeping in trans healthcare.* https://www.philpercs.com/2015/11/the-ethics-of-gatekeeping-in-trans-healthcare.html

Williams-Sanchez, V., McArdle, R., Wilson, R., Kidd, G., Wilson, C., & Bourne, A. (2014). Validation of screening tests of auditory function using the telephone. *Journal of the American Academy of Audiology, 25*(10), 937–951.

Wilson, S. M., Eriksson, D. K., Brandt, T. H., Schneck, S. M., Lucanie, J. M., Burchfield, A. S., et al. (2019). Patterns of recovery from aphasia in the first 2 weeks after stroke. *Journal of Speech, Language, and Hearing Research, 62*, 723–732.

Wilson, S., Thach, B., Brouillette, R., & Abu-Osba, Y. (1981). Coordination of breathing and swallowing in human infants. *Journal of Applied Physiology, 50*, 851–858.

Wilson, T., & Hyde, M. (1997). The use of Signed English pictures to facilitate reading comprehension by deaf students. *American Annals of the Deaf, 142*(4), 333–341.

Windsor, J., Scott, C. M., & Street, C. K. (2000). Verb and noun morphology in the spoken and written language of children with language learning disabilities. *Journal of Speech, Language, and Hearing Research, 43*, 1322–1336.

Wise, R. J. S., Scott, S. K., Blank, S. C., Mummery, C. J., Murphy, K., & Warburton, E. A. (2001). Separate neural subsystems within "Wernicke's area." *Brain, 124*, 83–95.

Wisenburn, B., & Mahoney, K. (2009). A meta-analysis of word-finding treatments for aphasia. *Aphasiology, 23*(11), 1338–1352.

Wittke, K., & Spaulding, T. J. (2018). Which preschool children with specific language impairment receive language intervention? *Language, Speech, and Hearing Services in Schools, 49*, 59–71.

Wolf, M., & Katzir-Cohen, T. (2001). Reading fluency and its intervention. *Scientific Studies in Reading, 5*, 211–239.

Wolfe, J., Morais, M., & Schaefer, E. (2015). Improving hearing performance for cochlear implant recipients with use of a digital, wireless, remote-microphone, audio-streaming accessory. *Journal of the American Academy of Audiology, 26*(6), 532–539.

Woll, B., & Morgan, G. (2012). Language impairments in the development of sign: Do they reside in a specific modality or are they modality-independent deficits? *Bilingualism: Language and Cognition, 15*(1), 75–87.

Wolter, J. A., & Pike, K. (2015). Dynamic assessment of morphological awareness and third-grade literacy success. *Language, Speech, and Hearing Services in Schools, 46*, 112–126.

Wolter, J. A., Wood, A., & D'zatko, K. W. (2009). The influence of morphological awareness on the literacy development of first-grade children. *Language, Speech, and Hearing Services in Schools, 40*, 286–298.

Wombles, K. (2014). Some fads never die—they only hide behind other names: Facilitated communication is not and never will be augmentative and alternative communication. *Evidence Based Communication Assessment and Intervention, 8*(4), 181–186. https://doi.org/10.1080/17489539.2015.1012780

Won, J., & Rubinstein, J. (2012). CI performance in prelingually deaf children and postlingually deaf adults. *The Hearing Journal, 65*(9), 32–34.

Wong, B. Y. (2000). Writing strategies instruction for expository essays for adolescents with and without learning disabilities. *Topics in Language Disorders, 20*(4), 244.

Wong, B. Y., Butler, D. L., Ficzere, S. A., & Kuperis, S. (1996). Teaching low achievers and students with learning disabilities to plan, write, and revise opinion essays. *Journal of Learning Disabilities, 29*(2), 197–212.

Wong, W. (2020). Economic burder of Alzheimer disease and managed care considerations. *American Journal of Managed Care, 26*(8), S177–S183.

Woods, J. J., & Wetherby, A. M. (2003). Early identification of and intervention for infants and toddlers who are at risk for autism spectrum disorder. *Language, Speech, and Hearing Services in Schools, 34,* 180–193.

World Health Organization (WHO). (2001a). *International classification of functioning, disability and health* (ICF). https://www.who.int/standards/classifications/international-classification-of-functioning-disability-and-health

World Health Organization (WHO). (2001b). *The world health report 2001—Mental illness: New understanding, new hope.* www.whoint/whr/en/

World Health Organization (WHO). (2006). *Addressing the global challenges of craniofacial anomalies. Report of a WHO meeting on International Collaborative Research on Craniofacial Anomalies.* Author.

World Health Organization (WHO). (2016). *Preterm birth.* http://www.who.int/mediacentre/factsheets/fs363/en/

World Health Organization. (2017). *World Report on Hearing.* https://www.who.int/teams/noncommunicable-diseases/sensory-functions-disability-and-rehabilitation/highlighting-priorities-for-ear-and-hearing-care

World Health Organization. (WHO). (n.d.). *Deafness and hearing loss.* http://www.who.int/mediacentre/factsheets/fs300/en/

Worldometers Info. (2022, March). *Worldometers Real Time World Population.* https://www.worldometers.info/

Worldometers. (2022, March). *Worldometers real time world population.* https://www.worldometers.info/

Wright Karem, R., Washington, K. N., Crowe, K., Jenkins, A., Leon, M., Kokotek, L., et al. (2019). Current methods of evaluating the language abilities of multilingual preschoolers: A scoping review using the International Classification of Functioning, Disability and Health–Children and Youth Version. *Language, Speech and Hearing Services in Schools, 50,* 434–451.

Wright, C. A., Kaiser, A. P., Reikowsky, D. I., & Roberts, M. Y. (2013). Effects of a naturalistic sign intervention on expressive language of toddlers with Down syndrome. *Journal of Speech, Language, and Hearing Research, 56,* 994–1008.

Xia, W., Zheng, C., Lei, Q., Tang, Z., Hun, Q., Zhang, Y., & Zhu, S. (2011). Treatment of post-stroke dysphagia by Vital-Stim therapy coupled with conventional swallowing training. *Journal of Huazhong University of Science and Technology [Medical Sciences], 31,* 73–76.

Xue, S. A., & Hao, G. J. (2003). Changes in the human vocal tract due to aging and the acoustic correlates of speech production: A pilot study. *Journal of Speech, Language, and Hearing Research, 46,* 689–701.

Yairi, E. (1981). Disfluencies of normally speaking 2-year-old children. *Journal of Speech Language, and Hearing Research, 24,* 301–307.

Yairi, E. (1982). Longitudinal studies of disfluencies in 2-year-old children. *Journal of Speech and Hearing Research, 25,* 402–404.

Yairi, E. (1983). The onset of stuttering in 2- and 3-year-old children: A preliminary report. *Journal of Speech and Hearing Disorders, 48,* 171–177.

Yairi, E. (2004). The formative years of stuttering: A changing portrait. *Contemporary Issues in Communication Science and Disorders, 31,* 92–104.

Yairi, E., & Ambrose, N. (1992a). A longitudinal study of children: A preliminary report. *Journal of Speech and Hearing Research, 35,* 755–760.

Yairi, E., & Ambrose, N. (1992b). Onset of stuttering in preschool children: Selected factors. *Journal of Speech and Hearing Research, 35,* 782–788.

Yairi, E., & Ambrose, N. (1999). Early childhood stuttering I: Persistency and recovery rates. *Journal of Speech, Language, and Hearing Research, 42*(5), 1097–1112.

Yairi, E., & Ambrose, N. (2004). Stuttering: Recent developments and future directions. *The ASHA Leader, 18,* 4–5, 14–15.

Yairi, E., & Ambrose, N. (2013). Epidemiology of stuttering: 21st century advances. *Journal of Fluency Disorders, 38*(2), 66–87.

Yairi, E., & Lewis, B. (1984). Disfluencies at the onset of stuttering. *Journal of Speech and Hearing Research, 27,* 154–159.

Yairi, E., Ambrose, N., & Cox, N. (1996). Genetics of stuttering: A critical review. *Journal of Speech and Hearing Research, 39,* 771–784.

Yairi, E., Ambrose, N., Paden, E., & Throneburg, R. (1996). Predictive factors of persistence and recovery: Pathways of childhood stuttering. *Journal of Communication Disorders, 29,* 51–77.

Yairi, E., Watkins, R., Ambrose, N., & Paden, E. (2001). What is stuttering? [Letter to the editor]. *Journal of Speech, Language, and Hearing Research, 44,* 585–592.

Yang, H., & Gray, S. (2017). Executive function in preschoolers with primary language impairment. *Journal of Speech, Language, and Hearing Research, 60,* 379–392.

Yao, L., Zhao, H., Shen, C., Liu, F., Qiu, Li, & Fu, L. (2020). Low-frequency repetitive transcranial magnetic stimulation in patients with poststroke aphasia: Systematic review and meta-analysis of its effect upon communication. *Journal of Speech, Language, and Hearing Research, 63,* 3801–3815.

Yaruss, J. (1997). Clinical measurement of stuttering behaviors. *Contemporary Issues in Communication Science and Disorders, 24,* 33–44.

Yaruss, J., & Pelczarski, K. M. (2007). Evidence-based practice for school-age stuttering: Balancing existing research with clinical practice. *EBP Briefs, 2*(4), 1–8.

Yaruss, J., & Quesal, R. (2006). Overall assessment of speaker's experience of stuttering (OASES): Documenting multiple outcomes in stuttering treatment. *Journal of Fluency Disorders, 31,* 90–115. https://doi.org/10.1016/j.jfludis.2006.02.002

Yaruss, J., Coleman, C., & Quesal, R. (2012). Stuttering in school-age children: A comprehensive approach to treatment. *Language, Speech, and Hearing Services in Schools, 43,* 536–548.

Yavas, M. (1998). *Phonology: Development and disorders.* Singular.

Yavas, M., & Goldstein, B. (1998). Phonological assessment and treatment of bilingual speakers. *American Journal of Speech-Language Pathology, 7*(2), 49–60.

Yilmaz, T., Kuscu, O., Sozen, T., & Suslu, A. (2017). Anterior glottic web formation for voice feminization: Experience of 27 patients. *Journal of Voice, 31,* 757–762.

Ylvisaker, M., & DeBonis, D. (2000). Executive function impairment in adolescence: TBI and ADHD. *Topics in Language Disorders, 20*(2), 29–57.

Ylvisaker, M., & Feeney, T. J. (1998). *Collaborative brain injury intervention: positive everyday routines.* Singular.

Yoder, P. J., Molfese, D., & Gardner, E. (2011). Initial mean length of utterance predicts the relative efficacy of two grammatical treatments in preschoolers with specific language impairment. *Journal of Speech, Language, and Hearing Research, 54,* 1170–1181.

Yonick, T., Reich, A., Minifie, F., & Fink, B. (1990). Acoustical effects of endotracheal intubation. *Journal of Speech and Hearing Disorders, 55,* 427–433.

Yont, K. M., Hewitt, L. E., & Miccio, A. W. (2000). A coding system for describing conversational breakdowns in preschool children. *American Journal of Speech Language Pathology, 9,* 300–309.

Yorkston, K. M., Smith, E., & Beukelman, D. R. (1990). Extended communication samples of augmentative communicators: I. A comparison of individualized versus standard single-word vocabularies. *Journal of Speech and Hearing Disorders, 55,* 217–224.

Yorkston, K., & Beukelman, D. (2013). Evidence supporting dysarthria intervention: An update of systematic reviews. *Perspectives on Neurophysiology and Neurogenic Speech and Language Disorders, 23,* 105–111. https://doi.org/10.1044/nnsld23.3.105

Yorkston, K., Beukelman, D., Strand, E., & Hakel, M. (2010). *Management of motor speech disorders in children and adults* (3rd ed.). PRO-ED.

Yorkston, K., Miller, R., & Strand, E. (2004). *Management of Speech and Swallowing in Degenerative Diseases* (2nd ed.). PRO-ED.

Yoshinaga-Itano, C., Sedey, A. L., Coulter, D. K., & Mehl, A. L. (1998). Language of early- and later-identified children with hearing loss. *Pediatrics, 102*(5), 1161–1171. https://doi.org/10.1542/peds.102.5.1161

Zajac, D. (1997). Velopharyngeal function in young and older adult speakers: Evidence from aerodynamic studies. *Journal of the Acoustical Society of America, 102,* 1846–1852.

Zambrana, I. M., Pons, F., Eadie, P., & Ystrom, E. (2014). Trajectories of language delay from age 3 to 5: Persistence, recovery and late onset. *International Journal of Language & Communication Disorders, 49,* 304–316. https://doi.org/10.1111/1460-6984.12073

Zebrowski, P. (1991). Duration of the speech disfluencies of beginning stutterers. *Journal of Speech and Hearing Research, 343,* 483–491.

Zebrowski, P., & Wolf, A. (2011). Working with teenagers who stutter: Simple suggestions for a complex challenge. *Perspectives on Fluency and Fluency Disorders, 21,* 37–42.

Zemlin, W. R. (1998). *Speech and hearing sciences: Anatomy and physiology* (4th ed.). Allyn & Bacon.

Zerbeto, A. B., Soto, G., C. R., Chun, R. Y. S., de Lurdes Zanolli, M., Rezende, A. C. F. A., & Clarke, M. (2020). Use and implementation of the International Classification of Functioning, Disability and Health with children and youth within the context of augmentative and alternative communication: An integrative literature review. *CEFAC, 22*(6).

Zerbeto, A. B., Soto, G., C. R., Zanolli, M. d., Rezende, A. C., & Clarke, M. (2020). Use and implementation of the international classification of functioning, disability and health with children and youth within the context of augmentative and alternative Communicaiton: An Integrative literature review. *CEFAC, 22*(6). https://doi.org/10.1590/1982-0216/20202268020

Zhao X., Leotta, A., Kustanovich, V., Lajonchere, C., Geschwind, D. H., Law, K., et al. (2007). A unified genetic theory for sporadic and inherited autism. *Proceedings of the National Academy of Science, 31,* 12831–12836.

Zraick, R., Kempster, G., Conner, N., Thibeault, S., Klaben, B., Bursac, Z., et al. (2011). Establishing validity of the consensus auditory-perceptual evaluation of voice (CAPE-V). *American Journal of Speech-Language Pathology, 20,* 14–22.

Zumach, A., Gerrits, E., Chenault, M., & Antenuis, L. (2010). Long-term effects of early-life otitis media on language development. *Journal of Speech, Language, and Hearing Research, 53*(1), 34–43.

NAME INDEX

A

Abitbol, J., 297
Abraham, C., 87–88, 357, 366, 370, 371, 372, 373
Abrams, H. B., 389–390, 425, 426
Abrams, M., 299, 325, 326
Acar, B., 426
Acoustical Society of America, 8
Adams, C., 106
Adesope, O., 150
Affoo, R. H., 263
Aikens, N. L., 183
Allen, A., 478
Alloway, R. G., 185
Alloway, T. P., 185
Al Otaiba, S., 176
Altman, K. W., 41
Altmann, L., 202
Alzheimer's Association, 257, 258
Ambrose, N., 269–270, 271, 272, 273, 275, 276, 278, 281, 282
Amendah, D., 109
American Academy of Audiology (AAA), 8, 393, 414, 420, 427
American Academy of Pediatrics, 120
American Cancer Society, 304
American Psychiatric Association (APA), 112, 115, 183, 257
American Speech-Language-Hearing Association (ASHA), 4, 7, 8, 9, 12, 17, 23, 33, 38, 43, 47, 51, 108, 131, 156, 175, 236, 244, 246, 258, 358, 374, 399, 420, 442–443, 445, 446, 450, 462
ANCDS TBI Writing Committee, 254
Anderson, J., 326
Anderson, N., 375
Andrews, C., 288
Andrews, G., 269
Andrus, J., 322
Anthony, J. L., 99
Apel, K., 48, 195, 199, 205
Archer, B., 241
Archibald, L. M., 105
Aristotle, 277
Aronson, A. E., 74
Arvedson, J., 41, 363–364, 377–378
Ash, B., 364
Ashford, J. R., 377–378
Aubry, S., 96

B

Baade, A., 450
Babb, M., 237
Bacon, E. C., 128
Bailey, R., 369

Bain, B., 48
Bainbridge, K., 390
Baker, E., 167
Baker, S., 207
Ball, L. J., 472
Balsamo, L., 220
Bangert, K. J., 136
Barbarin, O., 183
Barczi, 41
Barker, R. M., 478
Barkley, 101–102
Barkmeier-Kraemer, J., 309, 322
Barnes, G., 369
Barth, A. E., 197
Bashir, A., 211
Baum, S., 247
Baylor, C., 240, 349
Bear, D. R., 199, 205, 208
Bedore, L. M., 133–134, 192
Beebe-Frankenberger, M., 105
Behrman, A., 297
Bell, A. G., 18
Bell, A. M., 18
Belmonte. M. K., 109
Beltyukova, S., 288
Benelli, B., 100
Bent, T., 74
Bergman, R. L., 120
Berlin, C., 431
Bernard-Bonnin, A. C., 41
Berni, M., 148
Berninger, V. W., 181, 199, 201, 205, 207
Bernstein Ratner, N., 14
Bernthal, J., 152, 153, 161, 163, 167, 168
Beukelman, D. R., 351, 445, 447, 459, 460, 463, 467, 468, 471, 478
Bhasin et al., 2006, 113
Bhatnagar, S., 333, 337
Bhattacharyya, N., 12, 41, 299
Biggs, E. E., 478
bilingualnamingtherapy.psu.edu, 243
Binos, P., 431, 437
Bishop, D. V. M., 104, 106
Bitetti, D., 180
Blachman, B., 194–195
Black, L. I., 12, 40, 299
Blackstone, S. W., 464, 468
Blake, M. L., 244, 246–247
Bleile, K. M., 146, 161, 220
Bliss, L. S., 129
Bloodstein, O., 269, 273, 274, 275
Blumenthal, M., 165
Boberg, E., 277, 284, 285
Boersma, P., 12
Boey, R., 289
Boggs, T., 363–364, 377–378
Boi, R., 426

Boisclair, A., 181
Boisvert, I., 432
Bolderson, 136
Boliek, C., 67, 167, 322
Bondy, A. S., 452
Boone, D. R., 293, 298, 299, 303, 304, 312
Bornstein, H., 392
Bornstein, M. H., 99
Boswell, S., 9
Bothe, A., 288
Boudreau, D. M., 114, 188, 194, 196, 1325
Bourgeois, M. S., 258, 263
Bourgeron, T., 109
Boutsen, F., 322, 353–354
Boyle, M., 113, 290
Brackenbury, T., 14, 16
Brackett, K., 41
Brady, N. C., 114, 477
Branson, D., 460
Brault, M. W., 12
Breadmore, H. L., 185
Brea-Spahn, M. R., 207
Brignell, A., 102
Brinton, B., 105, 186
Broadfoot, C., 353–354, 363–364
Brock, K., 455
Brooks, G., 207
Brosnahan, S., 59, 62
Brown, J., 256
Brown, J. A., 242
Brownlie, E. B., 104
Brumberg, J. S., 448, 458
Brundage, S., 279
Brunner, M., 256
Brutten, G., 281
Bulow, M., 380
Burgess, S., 133–134
Burridge, A., 98
Bus, A. G., 175
Butler, L., 277
Byeon, H., 299
Byrd, C., 287

C

Cabré, M., 41
Caccamise, D., 178
Cafiero, J., 452
Cain, K., 101, 179
Calculator, S. N., 447
Calder, S. D., 136
Calvert, D., 154
Calvert, P., 290
Campbell, T., 152, 153
Capps, L., 185

563

SUBJECT INDEX

A

AAA. *See* American Academy of Audiology (AAA)

AAA Scope of Practice, 393

AAC. *See* Alternative communication system (AAC); Augmentative and alternative communication (AAC) devices

"AAC and Families: Dispelling Myths and Empowering Parents" (Smith), 461

AAC input, 451, 459

AAC output, 451, 458–459

ABCD mnemonic, 49

Abdominal aponeurosis, 61

Abdominal binder, 350

Abdominal content, 58, 60, 61

Abdominal wall, 58, 60–61, 65

Abduction, 70

ABR. *See* Auditory brainstem response (ABR)

Academy of Dispensing Audiologists, 487

Academy of Rehabilitative Audiology, 487

Access barriers, 463

Accessory characteristics, 273

Accessory nerve (XI), 339

Acoustical Society of America, 8

Acoustic neuroma, 406

Acquired conditions, 444

Acquired problems, 34–35

Acquired sensorineural hearing losses, 405

Activity limitation, 387

Acute laryngitis, 303, 306

AD. *See* Alzheimer disease (AD)

ADA. *See* Americans with Disabilities Act of 1990 (ADA)

Adam's apple, 69

Adapted toys and books, play and access to, 474

Additions, 162–164

Adduction, 70, 72

ADHD. *See* Attention-deficit/hyperactivity disorder (ADHD)

Adolescence. *See* School-age children and adolescents

Adult communicators, 461–462

Adult dysphagia, etiologies of, 361–364

Adulthood

  language development in, 217–218

  language form in, 218

  use of various communication techniques in, 217–218

  vocabulary content in, 218

Adult language disorders, 215–266

  aphasia, 222–244

  cognitive impairment, 256–263

  language development beyond childhood, 217–218

  nervous system and, 219–222

  right-hemisphere damage, 244–249

  traumatic brain injury, 249–256

Adults

  augmentative and alternative communication and, 478

  cochlear implants in, 432

  hearing aids in, 425–426

  hearing loss in, 389–390

Advanced age

  communication disorders in, manifestation of, 42

  communication features of, 32

AEPs. *See* Auditory evoked potentials (AEPs)

Affricates, 144

Age of onset, 404

Agnosia, 225

Agrammatism, 225

Aided AAC communication systems, 452–456

  symbolic representation of aided symbols, 452–454

Aided language stimulation, 459, 472

Aided symbols

  orthography and orthographic print symbols, 455–456

  pictorial symbols, 455

  symbolic representation of, 452–454

  tangible symbols, 454

Air conduction testing, 417–419

ALDs. *See* Assistive listening devices (ALDs)

Alport's syndrome, 405

ALS. *See* Amyotrophic lateral sclerosis (ALS)

Alternative communication system (AAC), 138

Alternative-language users, 443

Alveolar processes, 76

Alveolar sounds, 143

Alveoli, 59–60, 67

Alzheimer disease (AD), 258–260

Alzheimer's Association, 259

American Academy of Audiology (AAA), 8, 390, 393, 420, 427, 434, 487

American Academy of Otolaryngology—Head and Neck Surgery, 487

American Academy of Speech Correction, 18

American Auditory Society, 487

American Coalition of Citizens with Disabilities, 18

American Psychiatric Association (APA), 106

American Sign Language (ASL), 29, 391–393, 433, 450–451

American Speech-Language-Hearing Association (ASHA), 4, 8, 485–486

  AAC defined by, 443

  advocacy for individuals with communicative disabilities, 486

  audiology defined by, 393

  career information, 8, 9

  Certificate of Clinical Competence in Audiology, 7

  Certificate of Clinical Competence in Speech-Language Pathology, 9

  clinical service in speech-language pathology and audiology, 485–486

  Code of Ethics, 48

  credentials needed in audiology and speech-language pathology, 9

  evidence-based practice, information on, 17

  Health Care Survey in Speech-Language Pathology, 2021, 357–358

  history of, 18

  maintenance of ethical standards, 486

  National Outcomes Measurement System, 246

  professional articles on reading disorders, 183

  scientific study of the processes and disorders of human communication, 485

  Working with Culturally and Linguistically Diverse Students in Schools, 47

Americans with Disabilities Act of 1990 (ADA), 3

Amplitude, 395

Amyotrophic lateral sclerosis (ALS), 306, 308, 343

Anatomy, 57. *See also* Organ systems involved in swallowing and speech production

ANCDS TBI Writing Committee, 254

Aneurysm, 230

Angular gyrus, 222

Anomia, 225

Anomic aphasia, 227, 228

ANSD. *See* Auditory neuropathy spectrum disorder (ANSD)

APA. *See* American Psychiatric Association (APA)

APD. *See* Auditory processing disorder (APD)

Aphasia, 222–244, 346, 347

  assessment for, 234–237

  causes of, 229–230

  conclusion, 244

  deficits caused by, 223–225

  defined, 13, 222

  differential diagnosis of, 229

  evidence-based practice for, 242–243

  fluent aphasias, 226–228

  intervention for, 237–243

  lifespan issues, 231–233

  nonfluent aphasias, 226, 227, 228–229

  other neurogenic disorders with, 224

  patterns of behavior in, 224

  patterns of recovery in, 224

  primary progressive aphasia, 243–244

  severity of, 223, 224

  stroke as cause of, 222, 229–230

  terms used in, 225

  types of, 223, 226–229

Aphonia, 304, 307

Aplasia, 404, 405

Apraxia Kids, 157

Apraxia of speech, 36, 314, 339, 345–347

  aphasia and, 346, 347

  defined, 345

  evidence-based practice with, 354

  lifespan issues, 346, 347

  management of, 352–354

  motor speech production process in, 345

  speech of individuals with, 345–346

Arteriovenous malformation, 230

Articulation, 150–151

  disorders of, 36

  lifespan view of, 31–32

  in speech, 27–28